PERSPECTIVES IN HYPERTENSION
Volume 3

New Therapeutic Strategies in Hypertension

PERSPECTIVES IN HYPERTENSION SERIES

Series Editors
Barry M. Brenner, Norman M. Kaplan,
and John H. Laragh

Vol. 3 New Therapeutic Strategies in Hypertension, *edited by Norman M. Kaplan,*
Barry M. Brenner, and John H. Laragh, 336 pp., 1989.

Vol. 2 Endocrine Mechanisms in Hypertension, *edited by John H. Laragh,*
Barry M. Brenner, and Norman M. Kaplan, 384 pp., 1989.

Vol. 1 The Kidney in Hypertension, *edited by Norman M. Kaplan, Barry M. Brenner,*
and John H. Laragh, 288 pp., 1987.

PERSPECTIVES IN HYPERTENSION
Volume 3

New Therapeutic Strategies in Hypertension

Editors

Norman M. Kaplan, M.D.

University of Texas
Health Science Center at Dallas
Dallas, Texas

Barry M. Brenner, M.D.

Department of Medicine
Harvard Medical School
Boston, Massachusetts

John H. Laragh, M.D.

Cardiovascular Center
The New York Hospital
Cornell Medical Center
New York, New York

Raven Press 🐦 New York

Raven Press, 1185 Avenue of the Americas, New York, New York 10036

Made in the United States of America

The material contained in this volume was submitted as previously unpublished material, except in the instances in which credit has been given to the source from which some of the illustrative material was derived.

Great care has been taken to maintain the accuracy of the information contained in the volume. However, neither Raven Press nor the editors can be held responsible for errors or for any consequences arising from the use of the information contained herein.

Materials appearing in this book prepared by individuals as part of their official duties as U.S. Government employees are not covered by the above-mentioned copyright.

9 8 7 6 5 4 3 2 1

Library of Congress Cataloging-in-Publication Data

New therapeutic strategies in hypertension / editors, Norman M.
 Kaplan, Barry M. Brenner, John H. Laragh.
       p.   cm. — (Perspectives in hypertension ; vol. 3)
    Includes bibliographies and index.
    ISBN 0-88167-528-8
    1. Hypertension—Chemotherapy. 2. Hypotensive agents.
I. Kaplan, Norman M., 1931-M. II. Brenner, Barry M., 1937–
III. Laragh, John H., 1924–   IV. Series: Perspectives in
hypertension series ; v. 3.
    [DNLM: 1. Antihypertensive Agents—therapeutic use.
2. Hypertension—therapy.   W1 PE871APH v. 3 / WG 340 N5326]
RC685.H8N49   1989
616.1'3206—dc20
DNLM/DLC
for Library of Congress   86-43104
                                                                    CIP

Preface

This third volume in the series *Perspectives in Hypertension* provides a thorough, up-to-date review of the treatment of hypertension. The coverage is complete, including every currently available class of drug and a number that are still under investigation (described in the chapter by Taylor and Kaplan). New insights into the use of agents that are "old," have also been provided.

This multiauthored text provides ample documentation of the major issues involved in the treatment of hypertension today. The reader will find excellent coverage both by type of therapy and by type of patient. Each chapter is written by recognized experts in the field.

Most of these experts were chosen because of their long and deep interest in the area of their chapter. With those covering specific drugs, a certain degree of extra enthusiasm about their usefulness may come through, but the advice is well documented.

Beyond the coverage of individual drugs, the management of multiple problem patients is described including those with concomitant diabetes, cardiovascular disease, or renal dysfunction as well as those who are elderly, pregnant, or severely hypertensive. Lastly, both the use of various non-drug therapies and the value of withdrawal of drug therapy are given appropriate coverage.

This book will be useful to cardiologists, pharmacologists, nephrologists, and to all practitioners who are involved in the management of hypertensive patients.

The Editors

Contents

1 Aim and Goals of Therapy
Göran Berglund

5 Nonpharmacologic Therapy of Hypertension:
An Update
Norman M. Kaplan

17 Diuretics
John M. Flack and Richard H. Grimm

33 Centrally Acting Antihypertensive Agents
*Michael A. Weber, William F. Graettinger,
and Deanna G. Cheung*

51 Alpha Blockers
Rafael F. Schäfers and John L. Reid

71 Beta-Adrenergic Blockers in Hypertension:
An Updated Review
William H. Frishman and Howard B. Mayer

97 Angiotensin Converting Enzyme Inhibitors
Bernard Waeber, Jürg Nussberger, and Hans R. Brunner

115 Calcium Blockers
Fritz R. Bühler

125 New Antihypertensive Drugs
D. G. Taylor and H. R. Kaplan

141 Strategies in Choosing Therapy for Hypertension
John H. Laragh

171 Withdrawal of Drug Therapy in the Treatment of
Hypertension
Michael H. Alderman and Bernard Lamport

183 Treatment of Severe Hypertension
Lionel H. Opie

199   Treatment of Hypertension in Patients with Cardiovascular
         Disorders
         Robert J. Cody

211   Treatment of Hypertension in the Elderly
         Charles P. Tifft and Aram V. Chobanian

231   Hypertension in Pregnancy
         Jay M. Sullivan

253   The Effects of Antihypertensive Therapy on Renal Function
         John H. Bauer and Garry P. Reams

289   Hypertension with Diabetes
         Sharon Anderson and Barry M. Brenner

307   Subject Index

Contributors

Michael H. Alderman
*Department of Epidemiology and
    Social Medicine
Albert Einstein College of Medicine
Bronx, New York 10461*

Sharon Anderson
*Department of Medicine
Harvard Medical School
Boston, Massachusetts 02115*

John H. Bauer
*Hypertension Section, Division of
    Nephrology
Department of Medicine
University of Missouri
Columbia, Missouri 65212*

Göran Berglund
*Department of Medicine
University of Lund
Malmo General Hospital
S-214 01 Malmo, Sweden*

Barry M. Brenner
*Department of Medicine
Harvard Medical School
Boston, Massachusetts 02115*

Hans R. Brunner
*Division of Hypertension
Centre Hospitalier Universitaire
    Vaudois
1011 Lausanne, Switzerland*

Fritz R. Bühler
*Department of Research
University Hospital Basel
4031 Basel, Switzerland*

Aram V. Chobanian
*Evans Memorial Department of
    Clinical Research
Boston University
School of Medicine
Boston, Massachusetts 02118*

Deanne G. Chung
*Veterans Administration Medical
    Center
Long Beach, California 90822*

Robert J. Cody
*Division of Cardiology
Department of Medicine
The Ohio State University Hospital
Columbus, Ohio 43210*

John M. Flack
*Division of Epidemiology
School of Public Health
University of Minnesota
Minneapolis, Minnesota 55455*

William H. Frishman
*Department of Medicine,
    Epidemiology and Social Medicine
Albert Einstein College of Medicine
Bronx, New York 10461*

Richard H. Grimm
*Department of Prevention Cardiology
Division of Epidemiology
University of Minnesota
Minneapolis, Minnesota 55455*

H. R. Kaplan
*Department of Pharmacology
Parke-Davis Research Division
Warner-Lambert Company
Ann Arbor, Michigan 48105*

Norman M. Kaplan
*Department of Internal Medicine
University of Texas Southwestern
    Medical Center
Dallas, Texas 75235*

Bernard Lamport
*Department of Epidemiology and
    Social Medicine
Albert Einstein College of Medicine
Bronx, New York 10461*

John H. Laragh
Cardiovascular Center
The New York Hospital
Cornell Medical Center
New York, New York 10021

Howard B. Mayer
Department of Medicine
Mount Sinai Hospital and Medical
Center
New York, New York 10032

Jurg Nussberger
Division of Hypertension
Centre Hospitalier Universitaire
Vaudois
1011 Lausanne, Switzerland

Lionel H. Opie
Department of Medicine and
Hypertension Clinic
University of Cape Town Medical
School and Groote Schuur
Hospital
Observatory 7925, South Africa

Garry P. Reams
Hypertension Section
Division of Nephrology
Department of Medicine
University of Missouri 65212

John L. Reid
Department of Materia Medica and
Therapeutics
Stobhill General Hospital
University of Glasgow
Glasgow G21 3UW, Scotland

Rafael F. Schäfers
Department of Materia Medica and
Therapeutics
Stobhill General Hospital
University of Glasgow
Glasgow G21 3UW, Scotland

Jay M. Sullivan
Department of Medicine
Division of Cardiovascular Diseases
The University of Tennessee
Memphis, Tennessee 37501

D. G. Taylor
Department of Pharmacology
Parke-Davis Research Division
Warner-Lambert Company
Ann Arbor, Michigan 48105

Bernard Waeber
Division of Hypertension
Centre Hospitalier Universitaire
Vaudois
1011 Lausanne, Switzerland

Michael A. Weber
Veterans Administration Medical
Center
Long Beach, California 90822

PERSPECTIVES IN HYPERTENSION
Volume 3

New Therapeutic Strategies in Hypertension

New Therapeutic Strategies in Hypertension,
edited by Norman M. Kaplan,
Barry M. Brenner, and John H. Laragh.
Raven Press, Ltd., New York © 1989.

Aim and Goals of Therapy

Göran Berglund

Department of Medicine, University of Lund, Malmö General Hospital, S-214 01 Malmö, Sweden

Hypertension is an entity associated with an increased risk of atherosclerotic cardiovascular complications, most commonly coronary heart disease and stroke (5,6). Although often asymptomatic, it is associated with several metabolic aberations such as obesity, glucose intolerance or overt diabetes, hyperinsulinemia and hyperlipidemia, all known to increase the risk of atherosclerosis (7).

From the above facts it is obvious that any treatment for hypertension must meet several requirements. This chapter aims to describe the objectives of antihypertensive therapy.

The goals of treatment of hypertension are in most recommendations (4,8) "the lower, the better", i.e., the lowest possible blood pressure (BP) should be attained. This recommendation is based on the assumption that the risk of cardiovascular complications will follow the same downward slope when BP is abruptly lowered as the well-known upward slope relationship shown to be present in epidemiological studies between BP and later (often decades) occurrence of cardiovascular complications. Recently, however, certain doubts as to the truth of this assumption have been raised in several trials whose results indicate a J-shaped, instead of a straight positive, relationship between achieved BP level and occurrence of cardiovascular events (1,2,3,9). A second aim of this chapter is, therefore, to discuss the strategies and goals of antihypertensive treatment.

DIAGNOSIS OF HYPERTENSION

Before discussing the objective of the treatment, a few words on how to set the diagnosis of hypertension properly are needed. Most cases of hypertension have mild hypertension, i.e., diastolic BP 90 to 105 mmHg according to the WHO criteria (4). This means that the risk of developing a cardiovascular complication within the next 6 to 12 months is low. Ample time should, therefore, be allotted for the establishment of a safe diagnosis of hypertension. It should be set first when several BP measurements have been taken; the milder the BP elevation the more BP measurements should be taken. Several of these BP measurements can be made by a nurse. As a guide, I usually recommend at least six BPs to be taken at six different visits during 4 to 6 months. In cases of moderate to severe hypertension, i.e., diastolic BP above 105 mmHg, the diagnosis can be made after fewer BP measurements. Hypertension is said to be at hand when the mean of the BPs is ≥ 90 mmHg diastolic. This limit applies irrespective of the age of the patient.

Women have a distinctly lower risk of cardiovascular complications than men at corresponding BP levels. Although it has been seriously discussed whether white women with mild hypertension and no other cardiovascular risk factors should be at all treated with antihypertensive drugs, such a discussion falls outside the scope of this chapter. Unitl further data are gathered, men and women should be treated according to the same criteria.

THE AIM OF ANTIHYPERTENSIVE THERAPY

The ultimate aim of antihypertensive treatment is to eliminate the increased risk of cardiovascular complications in a particular hypertensive patient. It is, thus, a primary preventive treatment in most cases. As most patients are asymptomatic, the given therapy should be largely without side effects. As the following chapters will show, antihypertensive therapy consists of both nondrug therapies and a large arsenal of drugs. Specific combinations of nonpharmacological and pharmacological strategies must be chosen in certain subgroups of hypertensive patients as discussed in separate chapters (See Chapters 12 to 17).

To decrease the risk of cardiovascular complications, the treatment must aim to:

1. decrease BP towards normal
2. decrease the burden of other cardiovascular risk factors, such as:

smoking
hypercholesterolemia
hypertriglyceridemia
hyperinsulinemia
impaired glucose tolerance and clinically overt diabetes
central obesity and/or alcohol problems.

As can be seen from this list of aims, antihypertensive treatment is *not* a simple therapeutic task that any physician can solve properly without prolonged and intensive training. It calls for a physician carefully trained in changing patient behavior to a healthier way of eating, drinking, and exercising. The physician must also be knowledgeable in history taking and physical examinations, and in using the correct drug or drug combination in a particular hypertensive patient. He/she must also be aware of the importance of an administrative system that invites the patients to check-up visits, and sees that those not applying for a scheduled visit will be called again. This will help to decrease the otherwise high drop-out frequency. To improve patient interaction, the physician in charge of a hypertensive patient must see to it that the patient gets proper information regarding the disease and *detailed* instructions of how to change smoking, eating, drinking, and exercise habits in order to decrease BP and associated cardiovascular risk factors. To optimize patient cooperation the physician should use, or develop, a system of feedback to the patient of changes in BP and risk factors during the course of treatment.

Thus, there is no doubt that antihypertensive treatment, if it shall fulfill all its aims, is a complex task to undertake. It takes a physician knowledgeable in behavioral changes as well as in sophisticated drug treatment. In the future more attention must be paid to teaching physicians a practical method of how to attain behavioral changes. This is not only true for hypertension; most of the common severe diseases (cardiovascular diseases, diabetes, alcoholism, and cancer) are to a large extent caused by faults in the way we smoke, eat, drink, or exercise, i.e., the way we behave.

TREATMENT STRATEGIES AND GOALS

As previously stated antihypertensive treatment aims at preventing cardiovascular complications prone to occur in hypertensive patients. To reach this goal each hypertensive patient should be given individual treatment goals adjusted to the patient's risk-factor profile (e.g., smoking, alcohol and dietary habits, overweight, blood lipids, physical exercise, etc.); and one *partial* goal is to reduce diastolic BP < 90 mmHg.

The antihypertensive therapy should always include nonpharmacological methods as described in the following chapter. If drugs become necessary, treatment should be instituted with one of the first-line drugs discussed in the subsequent chapters, preferably a nonselective beta blocker or a thiazide diuretic. If no effect on BP is achieved by the first drug, the second drug should be tried, or alternatively, the two types of drugs could be combined. If normotension is not achieved, other third-line drugs could be added when patient compliance to the treatment has been assured.

Treatment of high BP might, in the initial phase, need rather intensive contacts with the patient. However, when normotension has been achieved, one or two visits with the physician would be enough contact in most uncomplicated cases. Home BP measurement should be encouraged to give a better picture of the usual BP level. If BP has been normal for several years, dose reduction and eventually withdrawal of all drugs could be tried under careful BP supervision. Previously the BP goal often has been set "as low as possible without side effects." This doctrine might very well be true, but recently more and more data suggesting a U-shaped or a J-shaped relationship between achieved BP control and cardiovascular morbidity (1,2,3,9) have been presented. Thus, Cruickshank et al., (3) showed a J-shaped relationship with higher congenital heart disease (CHD) death rates for hypertensives with mean in-study DBP < 85 mmHg. A similar pattern was found by Coope and Warrender (2), both for treated and untreated hypertensives, which points to the possibility that other factors than the antihypertensive treatment per se might explain the J-shaped curve. The J-shaped relationship between attained BP and cardiovascular events has been confirmed in two separate large studies (1,9). Dividing hypertensives into discrete subgroups according to their attained BP,

and then calculating mortality or morbidity rates in these subgroups has some inherited problems that must be taken into account when interpreting the data. Thus, adjustment for varying CHD risk at entry must be made. A hypertensive with a high risk of a coronary event will carry this high risk with him into the trial. This must be statistically adjusted if the true influence of the attained BP should be determined. Influences of differences in follow-up time, intensity of antihypertensive treatment, and changes in other risk factors must be taken into account. However, keeping these inherited shortcomings in mind, properly analysed trials indicate that low-achieved DBPs (< 85 mmHg) are associated with increased risk of cardiovascular complications, especially CHD. This might explain why, in most studies, antihypertensive drug treatment has been unsuccessful in reducing CHD. Further analyses of trials including both an actively-treated group and a placebo-treated group are urgently needed. Until results from these analyses are at hand BP should not be forced below 85 mmHg.

REFERENCES

1. Berglund, G. (1989): Is there a point beyond which pressure reduction is dangerous? *Am. J. Hypertens.* In press.
2. Coope, J. and Warrender, T. S. (1987): Lowering blood pressure. *Lancet,* ii:518.
3. Cruickshank, J. M., Thorp, J. M., and Zacharias, F. J. (1987): Benefits and potential harm of lowering high blood pressure. *Lancet,* i:581–584.
4. Guidelines for the treatment of mild hypertension: Memorandum from a WHO/ISH meeting (1983): *Lancet,* i:457–458.
5. Kannel, W. B. (1974): Role of blood pressure in cardiovascular morbidity and mortality. Progr. Cardiovasc. Dis., 17:5–24.
6. Kannel, W. B., Schwartz, M. J., and McNamara, P. M. (1969): Blood pressure and risk of coronary heart disease. The Framingham Study. *Dis. Chest,* 56:43–52.
7. Larsson, B. (1985): Obesity and prospective risk of associated diseases. In: *Metabolic Complications of Human Obesity. Excerpta Medica, Amsterdam.*
8. Report. (1984): The 1984 report of the Joint Na-

tional Committee on Detection, Evaluation, and Treatment of High Blood Pressure. U.S. Department of Health and Human Services, Public Health Service, National Institutes of Health. NIH Publication No. 84–1088.

9. Samuelsson, O., Wilhelmsen, L., Anderson, O. K., Pennert, K., and Berglund, G. (1987): Cardiovascular morbidity in relation to change in blood pressure and serum cholesterol levels in treated hypertension. Results from the Primary Prevention Trial in Göteborg, Sweden. *JAMA*, 258:1768–1776.

New Therapeutic Strategies in Hypertension,
edited by Norman M. Kaplan,
Barry M. Brenner, and John H. Laragh.
Raven Press, Ltd., New York © 1989.

Nonpharmacologic Therapy of Hypertension: An Update

Norman M. Kaplan

University of Texas Southwestern Medical Center, Dallas, Texas 75235

More and more, the use of various non-pharmacologic therapies is being advocated as the first treatment for the majority of patients with hypertension (61). The reasons are multiple, including:

1. The inclusion into active therapy of a larger portion of the 75% of all hypertensives who have mild hypertension, i.e., diastolic blood pressure (DBP) from 90 to 104 mm Hg. This group, almost 40 million in the United States alone, is inherently at less risk for the rapid development of the various cardiovascular complications than are those with more severe hypertension. Practitioners, therefore, are more willing to try nonpharmacologic therapies, even if they are less effective than drugs.

2. The realization that drugs, as they have been used, have not provided protection against coronary disease (43). This is accompanied by the recognition that many of the risk factors for coronary disease—hypercholesterolemia, low (levels of) high density lipoprotein (HDL)-cholesterol, obesity, physical inactivity, stress—are approachable through the same nonpharmacological strategies that are useful in treating hypertension. In particular, the recent emphasis directed toward dietary control of hypercholesterolemia will likely reflect favorably on hypertension as well.

3. The continued publication of properly controlled trials of various nonpharmacologic therapies which show clear evidence that they will lower the blood pressure in many users. As will be detailed subsequently, this has been particularly true for potassium and calcium supplements, physical exercise, and moderation of ethanol so that these now join previously accepted techniques—sodium restriction and weight reduction—in the generally accepted lists of effective nonpharmacologic therapies.

4. A public less enamored of drugs and more interested in changing their lifestyle as a way to prevent and cure disease, along with the replacement of older generations of authoritarian, drug-oriented physicians with younger graduates who espouse a holistic view toward medicine and more active participation of their patients in a partnership arrangement.

5. As these nonpharmacologic therapies are being used increasingly, it is likely that practitioners are becoming more certain of both their ability to gain patient's acceptance of them and the patient's successful responsiveness to their application.

As I have written elsewhere (31):

Two caveats must be recognized about the acceptance of non-drug approaches: first, their efficacy need not be great in degree or uniform in occurrence; second, their ability to protect against cardiovascular disease need not have been demonstrated. As to the first of these caveats, a 5 mm Hg fall in blood pressure in many patients may be all that can be expected from the use of one or another non-drug approaches. However, if that can be accomplished with relative ease, little or no cost, and no adverse effects, it may bring many patients' pressure down to a level needing no or less drug therapy and thereby well worth having. The effect should be obtainable by a significant portion, though certainly not all, of the hypertensive population.

"As to the second caveat, non-drug therapies may never be shown to provide protection against cardiovascular disease. Consider the difficulty in showing such protection with antihypertensive drugs, which have many fold greater potency than most non-drug approaches. Consider further the difficulty in monitoring adherence to their use in the thousands of patients who would need to be followed for 5 to 10 years or longer to establish their protective capacity. Here we find that scientific principle is gotten the better of by practice. Therefore, non-drug approaches must be accepted on their promise to lower the blood pressure and the premise, therefrom, that they will thereby reduce cardiovascular disease."

With these preliminaries out of the way, each of the nonpharmacologic treatments will be briefly reviewed, with emphasis upon the more recent evidence of their efficacy, updating my 1985 review (28) and 1986 chapter (29).

WEIGHT REDUCTION

A major breakthrough has occurred in our understanding of the association between obesity and hypertension, revolving around hyperinsulinemia (60). As shown in Fig 1, this association is largely limited to upper body obesity, which is now recognized to be the major distinguishing characteristic that leads to the high prevalence of hypertension, diabetes, and hypertriglyceridemia in obese people.

The failure to recognize the special pathogenicity of upper body obesity likely is responsible for the continued debate about the degree of risk for coronary and other cardiovascular diseases associated with obesity; some find that the risks are higher for lean hypertensives (21), others that obese hypertensives are at more risk (5).

Only if the proportion of obesity that is in the upper body is taken into account, will the association between the risks and the degree of obesity become clear (13). From such data, it is obvious that the risks are related not to the total degree of obesity but to its distribution.

The recognition that hyperinsulinemia is the common pathway for most of the complications of upper body obesity has been accompanied by the realization that hyperinsulinemia is also present in nonobese hypertensives, secondary to insulin resistance (18). Therefore, increasing attention will be directed toward the effect of various antihypertensive therapies upon this hormone.

We have some evidence that weight loss will reduce insulin levels. Rocchini, et al., (63) have shown that the fall in blood pressure that accompanied weight loss achieved by caloric restriction was correlated with a fall in plasma insulin levels measured during an oral glucose tolerance test. Moreover, they found that both the blood pressure and plasma insulin levels fell more if the subjects performed regular physical exercise.

Cautions About Weight Loss

In hopes of reducing plasma insulin as a way of enhancing the antihypertensive effect of weight loss, caution has been advised about the use of the type of lower-calorie diet—low in fat and higher in carbohydrate—that is often used to achieve gradual weight loss (55). When a group of nonobese hypertensives were given a diet with only 25% of the calories from fat and 56% from carbohydrate, their plasma-insulin response to a glucose load was greater than after a diet with 41% fat and 40% carbohydrate. Therefore, a lower carbohydrate diet may be particularly effective in reducing the blood pressure in obese hypertensives.

Meanwhile, increasing attention has been directed to very low-calorie diets, in the range of 400 per day, as being both safe and

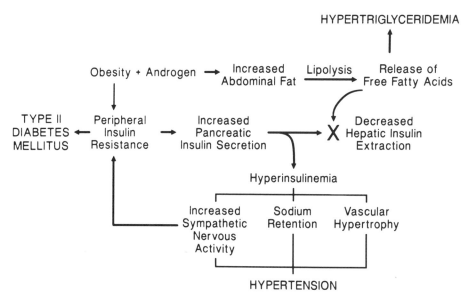

FIG. 1. A possible schema for the development of hypertension, type 2 diabetes mellitus, and hypertriglyceridemia with upper body obesity.

efficacious in achieving all of the desired effects of weight loss more rapidly than usual diets (2). Despite evidence that much of the initial weight loss is water loss (37), large numbers of massively obese people have successfully and safely used these protein, vitamin, and mineral enriched supplements (35). For those who are 100 pounds or more overweight, a very low-calorie diet in concert with a structured counseling and exercise program is more likely to be successful and considerably safer than surgery or other alternatives.

There are concerns about the long-term consequences of current weight-loss practices. For example, people who repeatedly lose a good deal of weight on such crash diets might end up with more resistant obesity. The postobese appear to have about 15% lower metabolic rates than control subjects of the same weight who have always been lean (20). This lower BMR may be countered by regular exercise, another reason to encourage those who are obese and hypertensive to remain physically active.

Another concern has risen from studies on rats who develop hypertension when refed after periods of starvation (15). Their hypertension persisted after 4 periods of supplemented fasting.

Finally, there is concern over the pressor effects of commonly-used sympathomimetic agents to reduce appetite. This concern may be lessened if one of a group of serotonin re-uptake inhibitors, fluoxetine, now available for treatment of depression, also is able to suppress carbohydrate craving and cause weight loss as preliminary trials indicate (17).

The Potential for Prevention

Weight loss may be the only proven and practical way to prevent the development of hypertension. In an 11-year longitudinal survey of 2,925 schoolchildren in Muscatine, Iowa, those who lost weight tended to have a fall in blood pressure, those who gained weight, a rise (10). The magnitude of the change in blood pressure was related directly to the change in body weight and not dependent on the initial blood pressure.

Weight loss should be encouraged for all hypertensives who are overweight. Thereby, the blood pressure will likely fall and, as an extra benefit, the plasma lipid profile may also improve. The regimen for weight loss should be whatever the patient will accept and follow. For some, a structured, carefully monitored, very low-calorie program may be best. For others, a more gradual reprogramming of daily dietary practices based on behavioral modification may be more effective. With caution against the use of diet pills which contain sympathomimetics which may raise the blood pressure, any weight loss regimen that works should be tried, remembering that with persistence, success is more likely than many assume.

MODERATE SODIUM RESTRICTION

About half of patients with hypertension will lower their blood pressure by 5 mm Hg or more when they reduce their daily dietary sodium intake from the usual 150 to 200 mmol to 80, the amount in 2 g of sodium or 5 g of NaCl. More rigid restriction will usually lower blood pressure more. In a controlled trial of 50, 110, and 190 mmol of sodium/day, each for 4 weeks, supine blood pressures fell 17/10, 9/6, and 1/1 mm Hg on the 3 levels (44).

It may be helpful to identify sodium sensitivity, although the easier course might be to simply try moderate sodium restriction with all patients and, if this does not help, allow the patient to return to the prior intake. The more sodium-sensitive patients include those with higher levels of pressure, older age, less responsive sympathetic nervous system, black race (16), and a haptoglobin 1-1 phenotype (80).

Moderate sodium restriction seems useful for all patients since it not only often lowers the blood pressure but also enhances the antihypertensive efficacy of all drugs save calcium entry blockers (40) and re-

duces the degree of potassium wastage with diuretic therapy (32).

POTASSIUM SUPPLEMENTATION

The combination of a lower sodium and a higher potassium intake may be more effective than either alone in reducing the blood pressure according to the findings of some (53) but not others (78). Potassium supplements by themselves may lower the blood pressure: in a 15-week double blind placebo-controlled trial, 48 mmol/day of K+ given to 37 patients effected a 14/10 mm Hg fall in supine blood pressure, whereas the placebo-treated had a slight rise in blood pressure (70). Others found a lesser fall with potassium supplements: blood pressure fell only 3.4/1.8 mm Hg compared to placebo in a trial using 120 mmol/day of K+ for 8 weeks (76).

It may be possible to achieve whatever antihypertensive effect is obtainable from increased potassium intake by altering the diet, substituting low-sodium, high-potassium natural foods for high-sodium, low-potassium processed foods. Thereby, with relatively little increase in dietary potassium intake it also may be possible to protect against stroke, as was found in a 12-year prospective study of 859 men and women aged 50 to 79 years (34).

CALCIUM SUPPLEMENTATION

The issues as to whether calcium deficiency is associated with more hypertension and whether calcium supplements will lower the blood pressure remain unsettled. The data on lesser calcium intake are very soft (30), and more and more of the controlled studies fail to find a fall in blood pressure with 1 to 2 g/day of extra calcium (7,52,69,82). However, some do find an effect (41), whereas others find that only a portion of the hypertensive population respond to supplemental calcium (22,75). The responders seem to be hypertensives who have hypercalcuria (possibly secondary to high dietary sodium intake) leading to lower ionized calcium and mild elevations in blood parathyroid hormone (PTH). PTH is a pressor hormone and when it is reduced, as by supplemental calcium or vitamin D (39), the blood pressure may fall (Fig. 2).

It is not worth the trouble to search out the patients, probably a minority, who are "calcium-sensitive." This is because the remaining patients may experience a rise in blood pressure with extra calcium, and there is a potential for increasing kidney stone formation. The best advice is to encourage an adequate dietary calcium intake and not to give supplemental calcium.

MAGNESIUM SUPPLEMENTATION

Even in the absence of significant falls in serum magnesium, magnesium deficiency may develop, particularly with the use of diuretics. Although magnesium supplements do not lower the blood pressure when given to unselected hypertensives, they may do so when given to those on long-term thiazide diuretic therapy who are magnesium deficient (66).

Adoption of a vegetarian diet may lead to a reduction in blood pressure (3); the increased fiber in the vegetarian diet may be responsible. In a controlled study on a weight reducing diet for 12 weeks, 30 over-weight women given 6 g/day of extra fiber in tablets lost 8.5 kg and had a fall in blood pressure of 9/9 mm Hg, whereas the 30 women given placebo tablets lost 6.7 kg and had a 0/4 mm Hg fall in blood pressure (72).

Regardless of how it works, a high-fiber intake has been found to reduce mortality from ischemic heart disease in a 12-year prospective study (33).

Fat and Fish Oil

Men in both California (81) and southern Italy (65) who ingest more mono- and poly-unsaturated fat as part of their usual diet have been found to have lower blood pressures than those who do not. The addition of polyunsaturated fats with concomitant reduction in saturated fat has been shown to cause a 5/4 mm Hg fall in blood pressure in a 6-week controlled study on 179 people in North Karelia, Finland (51). The previously noted findings of Parillo, et al., (55) should be recalled: when they placed a group of hypertensives on a low-saturated-fat, high-carbohydrate diet, plasma insulin levels rose higher during a glucose tolerance test.

On the one hand, despite a great deal of enthusiasm about the use of omega-3 fatty acids from fish oils, recent papers have failed to document an antihypertensive effect (26). On the other hand, they have been

Sodium-sensitive, Low-renin Hypertension

$$\text{Volume expansion} \longrightarrow \uparrow U_{Ca} \longrightarrow \downarrow plasma_{Ca} \longrightarrow \uparrow PTH \longrightarrow \uparrow BP$$

$$\begin{array}{c}\uparrow Ca \\ \text{intake} \end{array} \longrightarrow \left[\begin{array}{c} \text{further} \\ \uparrow U_{Ca} \end{array} \right] \longrightarrow \uparrow plasma_{Ca} \longrightarrow \downarrow PTH \longrightarrow \downarrow BP$$

FIG. 2. A potential explanation for a hypotensive action of increased dietary calcium intake.

shown to raise serum cholesterol (79) and worsen diabetic control in noninsulin dependent diabetic patients (19).

CAFFEINE

Acutely, caffeine may raise the blood pressure and have an additive effect to the pressor response to mental stress (57). However, even the acute response is not uniform and tolerance quickly develops with repeated consumption, so there appear to be no long-term pressor effects from caffeine ingestion (49).

ALCOHOL

Heavy alcohol abuse is unquestionably a major health problem but moderate alcohol intake, less than 2 ounces per day as would be present in 4 usual portions of beer, wine, or whiskey, may be associated with less coronary mortality than seen in those who abstain (48). This apparent protection against coronary disease has been claimed to reflect not a protective effect of ethanol but an association with other good health practices among those who are light to moderate drinkers (67). At the same time, concerns about a higher incidence of stroke with increasing ethanol consumption appear to have been settled: ischemic or occlusive strokes do not seem to be increased but hemorrhagic strokes are increased (36).

This in turn may reflect what has become increasingly obvious: alcohol consumption beyond 1.5 to 2 ounces/day will raise the blood pressure, and reduction of alcohol intake from heavier levels will often lower the blood pressure (42). Some find that, whereas, it takes more than an average of 3 ounces of ethanol a day for an association with more hypertension to be evident, nonetheless, alcohol may be the cause of the hypertension in 4 to 9% of men with hypertension (6).

The manner by which ethanol raises the blood pressure remains unsettled, with many possibilities supported by both human and animal experimentation. These include: alterations in prostaglandin metabolism (9); reduction in baroreceptor reflex sensitivity (1); insulin resistance with hyperinsulinemia (68); alterations in sodium and calcium fluxes across cells (73); and suppression of endothelium-dependent relaxation (12).

EXERCISE

Regular physical exercise may provide multiple benefits including a fall in blood pressure in patients with mild hypertension (Fig. 3) (44,50). The tendency for blood pressure to come down appears to result from a fall in peripheral resistance which is, in turn, secondary to a fall in sympathetic nervous system activation as reflected by lower levels of plasma catecholamines (44,50). In addition, a reduction of blood volume may contribute to the antihypertensive effect of repetitive chronic isotonic exercise (77).

In view of the previously noted hyperinsulinemia seen in both obese and nonobese hypertensives which may be at least in part responsible for the elevated blood pressure, another effect of long-term physical training—an increased sensitivity to insulin manifested by an enhancement of insulin-stimulated glucose uptake and a lesser rise in plasma-insulin levels after a glucose load (38,64)—could also contribute to the fall in blood pressure.

Acutely, during strenuous *isotonic* exercise, systolic blood pressure rises by 30 to 60 mm Hg, whereas diastolic pressure rises much less (62), and in some who are conditioned and who thereby have a greater vasodilatory capacity (45), diastolic pressures may fall. Those with hypertension often display abnormal left ventricular systolic function that is not related either to left ventricular hypertrophy (LVH) or ischemic heart disease (46). An exaggerated rise in systolic pressure during isotonic exercise in normotensive people may be an early man-

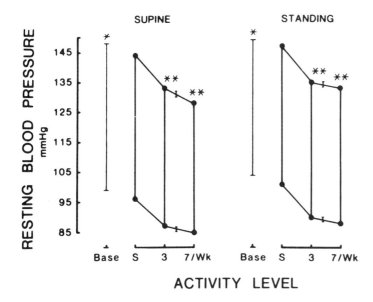

FIG. 3. Resting supine and standing blood-pressure at 3 levels of physical activity. Baseline measurement (Base), sedentary activity (S), 3 times/week exercise (3), and 7 times/week exercise (7). *$p < 0.05$, difference from sedentary value for both systolic and diastolic blood pressure; **$p < 0.01$. (Reprinted with permission from Nelson, L., Esler, M. D., Jennings, G. L., and Korner, P. I. (1986): Effect of changing levels of physical activity on blood-pressure and haemodynamics in essential hypertension. *Lancet,* 2:473–6.)

ifestation of developing hypertension but is more likely a super-normal response (27), and should not be taken as an indication for the future development of hypertension.

Acutely, during *isometric* exercise both systolic and diastolic pressures rise markedly, to extremely high levels in those such as weightlifters who do intense isometric exercise and a Valsalva maneuver (54). The response to isometric exercise, which is exaggerated further in patients with hypertension, is not reduced by treatment with beta-blockers but is suppressed somewhat by treatment with alpha$_1$-blockers (23).

The additional benefits of regular isotonic exercise may also include a greater amount of weight loss among obese subjects than can be achieved by caloric restriction alone (25). The extra weight loss provided by exercise may be minimal but it includes more fat and less lean body mass than would be achieved by caloric restriction alone (25).

Perhaps the most impressive benefit of regular exercise for hypertensive patients is an overall reduction in the incidence of coronary heart disease (CHD); this assumes that hypertensives would benefit equally, if not more, than would the general population. The evidence for the favorable effect of physical activity on CHD incidence is very impressive (58) and may reflect physical fitness, rather than the actual level of physical activity (71). In turn, the protection against CHD provided by physical activity may reflect a lower incidence of hypertension (4) than can be detected even in children (74), as well as favorable effects on plasma lipids (24).

RELAXATION

The manner by which exercise helps reduce cardiovascular risk in general, and blood pressure in particular, may also involve a sense of relaxation and relief of tension. Whereas the blood pressure falls immediately after both exercise and relaxation (59), there is considerably stronger evidence, as reviewed in the preceding section, that the blood pressure falls are sustained and persistent with exercise, whereas the evidence concerning relaxation is weaker. To be sure, some find a significant and long-lasting antihypertensive effect from relaxation therapy, even as provided by general practitioners (56). Others find no effects (47) whereas the majority finding is a small effect little beyond that noted by repeated blood pressure monitoring (8).

CESSATION OF SMOKING

This, the last of the nonpharmacologic therapies for hypertension, will do little for the blood pressure but a great deal for the overall cardiovascular health of the patient. Patients who stop smoking may actually experience a slight rise in blood pressure, largely from the 5- to 10-pound (or more) weight gain that so frequently follows smoking cessation. Nonetheless, the cardiovascular risks of smoking, including a 2- to 10-fold increased likelihood of stroke (11), are so great that the most important step a smoker can take to reduce these risks is to stop smoking.

CONCLUSION

Not all hypertensive patients need to use all of these nonpharmacologic therapies and not all who use them will achieve a fall in blood pressure. Nonetheless, they will cause no harm, and little if any interference, with the quality of life. Since most will also reduce other cardiovascular risks beyond the blood pressure, their use should be encouraged for all who are hypertensive.

REFERENCES

1. Abdel-Rahman, A-RA., Merrill, R. H., and Wooles, W. R. (1987): Effect of acute ethanol administration on the baroreceptor reflex control of heart rate in normotensive human volunteers. *Clin. Sci.*, 72:113–22.
2. Amatruda, J. M., Richeson, J. F., Welle, S. L., Brodows, R. G., and Lockwood, D. H. (1988): The safety and efficacy of a controlled low-energy ('very-low-calorie') diet in the treatment of non-insulin-dependent diabetes and obesity. *Arch. Intern. Med.*, 148:873–77.
3. Beilin, L. J., Armstrong, B. K., Margetts, B. M., Rouse, I. L., and Vandongen, R. (1987): Vegetarian diet and blood pressure. *Nephrology*, 4(Suppl. 1):37–41.
4. Blair, S. N., Goodyear, N. N., Gibbons, L. W., and Cooper, K. H. (1984): Physical fitness and

incidence of hypertension in healthy normotensive men and women. *JAMA*, 252:487–90.
5. Bloom, E., Reed, D., Yano, K., and MacLean, C. (1986): Does obesity protect hypertensives against cardiovascular disease? *JAMA*, 256:2972–75.
6. Bulpitt, C. J., Shipley, M. J., and Semmence A. (1987): The contribution of a moderate intake of alcohol to the presence of hypertension. *J. Hypertension*, 5:85–91.
7. Cappuccio, F. P., Markandu, N. D., Singer, D. R. J., Smith, S. J., Shore, A. C., and MacGregor, G. A. (1987): Does oral calcium supplementation lower high blood pressure? A double blind study. *J. Hypertension*, 5:67–71.
8. Chesney, M. A., Black, G. W., Swan, G. E., and Ward, M. M. (1987): Relaxation training for essential hypertension at the worksite: 1. The untreated mild hypertensive. *Psychosomatic Med.*, 49:250–63.
9. Clark, L. T., Hoover, E. L., Crandall, D. L., Cervoni, P., Haynes, S., and El Sherif, N. (1987): Atrial natriuretic peptide and prostaglandin responses to alcohol induced hypertension (abstract). *Clin. Res.*, 35:440A.
10. Clarke, W. R., Woolson, R. F., and Lauer, R. M. (1986): Changes in ponderosity and blood pressure in childhood: The Muscatine study. *Am. J. Epidemiol.*, 124:195–206.
11. Colditz, G. A., Bonita, R., Stampfer, M. J., et al. (1988): Cigarette smoking and risk of stroke in middle-aged women. *N. Engl. J. Med.*, 318:937–41.
12. Criscione, L., Powell, J. R., Burdet, R., Engesser, S., Schlager, F., and Schopfer, A. (1988): Ethanol suppresses endothelium-dependent relaxation in isolated, perfused mesenteric arterial beds of the rat (abstract). 12th International Society of Hypertension, p. 1314. Kyoto, Japan.
13. Dohanue, R. P., Abbott, R. D., Bloom, E., Reed, D. M., and Yano, K. (1987): Central obesity and coronary heart disease in men. *Lancet*, 1:821–23.
14. Duncan, J. J., Farr, J. E., Upton, S. J., Hagan, R. D., Oglesby, M. E., and Blair, S. N. (1985): The effects of aerobic exercise on plasma catecholamines and blood pressure in patients with mild essential hypertension. *JAMA*, 254:2609–13.
15. Ernsberger, P., and Nelson, D. O. (1988): Refeeding hypertension in dietary obesity. *Am. J. Physiol.*, 254:R47–55.
16. Falkner, B. (1988): Sodium sensitivity: A determinant of essential hypertension. *J. Am. Coll. Nutr.*, 7:35–41.
17. Ferguson, J. M., and Feighner, J. P. (1987): Fluoxetine-induced weight loss in overweight non-depressed humans. *Intl. J. Obesity*, 11(Suppl. 3):163–70.
18. Ferrannini, E., Buzzigoli, G., Bonadonna, R., Giorico, M.A., Oleggini, M., Graziadei, L., Pedrinelli, R., Brandi, L., and Bevilacqua, S. (1987): Insulin resistance in essential hypertension. *N. Engl. J. Med.*, 317:350–57.
19. Glauber, H., Wallace, P., Griver, K., and Brechtel, G. (1988): Adverse metabolic effect of omega-

3 fatty acids in non-insulin-dependent diabetes mellitus. *Ann. Intern. Med.,* 108:663–68.

20. Geissler, C. A., Miller, D. S., and Shah, M. (1987): The daily metabolic rate of the post-obese and the lean. *Am. J. Clin. Nutr.,* 45:914–20.

21. Goldbourt, U., Holtzman, E., Cohen-Mandelzweig, L., and Neufeld, H. N. (1987): Enhanced risk of coronary heart disease mortality in lean hypertensive men. *Hypertension,* 10:22–28.

22. Grobbee, D. E., and Hofman, A. (1986): Effect of calcium supplementation on diastolic blood pressure in young people with mild hypertension. *Lancet,* 2:703–7.

23. Hamada, M., Kazatani, Y., Shigematsu, Y., Ito, T., Kokubu, T., and Ishise, S. (1987): Enhanced blood pressure response to isometric handgrip exercise in patients with essential hypertension: Effects of propranolol and prazosin. *J. Hypertension,* 5:305–9.

24. Hespel, P., Lijnen, P., Fagard, R., Van Hoof, R., Rosseneu, M., and Amery, A. (1988): Changes in plasma lipids and apoproteins associated with physical training in middle-aged sedentary men. *Am. Heart J.,* 115:786–92.

25. Hill, J. O., Sparling, P. B., Shields, T. W., and Heller, P. A. (1987): Effects of exercise and food restriction on body composition and metabolic rate in obese women. *Am. J. Clin. Nutr.,* 46:622–30.

26. Houwelingen, R. V., Nordoy, A., van der Beek, E., Houtsmuller, U., de Metz, M., and Hornstra, G. (1987): Effect of a moderate fish intake on blood pressure, bleeding time, hematology, and clinical chemistry in healthy males. *Am. J. Clin. Nutr.,* 46:424–36.

27. Iskandrian, A. S., and Heo, J. (1988): Exaggerated systolic blood pressure response to exercise: A normal variant or a hyperdynamic phase of essential hypertension? *Intl. J. Cardiol.,* 18:207–17.

28. Kaplan, N. M. (1985): Non-drug treatment of hypertension. *Ann. Intern. Med.,* 102:359–73.

29. Kaplan, N. M. (1986): Treatment of hypertension: Nondrug therapy and the rationale for drug therapy. In: *Clinical Hypertension,* 4th edition, edited by Kaplan, N. M., pp. 147–179. Williams and Wilkins, Baltimore.

30. Kaplan, N. M. (1988): Calcium and potassium in the treatment of essential hypertension. *Semm. Nephrol.,* 8:176–84.

31. Kaplan, N. M. (1988): Nonpharmacologic approaches to hypertension management. In: *Evolving Concepts in the Management of Hypertension.* Scientific Therapeutics Information, Fort Lee, N.J.

32. Kaplan, N. M., Carnegie, A., Raskin, P., et al. (1985): Potassium supplementation in hypertensive patients with diuretic-induced hypokalemia. *N. Engl. J. Med.,* 312:746–49.

33. Khaw, K.-T., and Barrett-Connor, E. (1987): Dietary fiber and reduced ischemic heart disease mortality rates in men and women: A 12-year prospective study. *Am. J. Epidemiol.,* 126:1093–1102.

34. Khaw, K.-T., and Barrett-Connor, E. (1987): Di-etary potassium and stroke-associated mortality: A 12-year prospective population study. *N. Engl. J. Med.,* 316:235–40.

35. Kirschner, M. A., Schneider, G., Ertel, N. H., and Gorman, J. (1988): An eight-year experience with a very-low-calorie formula diet for control of major obesity. *Intl. J. Obesity,* 12:69–80.

36. Klatsky, A. L. (1987): Alcohol and stroke (abstract). *JACC,* 9:78A.

37. Kreitzman, S. N. (1988): Total body water and very-low-calorie diets. *Lancet,* 1:111.

38. Krotkiewski, M., Mandroukas, K., Sjostrom, L., Sullivan, L., Wetterqvist, H., and Bjorntorp, P. (1979): Effects of long-term physical training on body fat, metabolism, and blood pressure in obesity. *Metabolism,* 28:650–58.

39. Lind, L., Wengle, B., and Ljunghall, S. (1987): Blood pressure is lowered by vitamin D (alpha-calcidol) during long-term treatment of patients with intermittent hypercalcaemia. *Acta Med. Scand.,* 222:423–27.

40. Luft, F. C., and Weinberger, M. H. (1988): Review of salt restriction and the response to antihypertensive drugs: Satellite symposium on calcium antagonists. *Hypertension,* 11(Suppl. I):I–229–32.

41. Lyle, R. M., Melby, C. L., Hyner, G. C., Edmondson, J. W., Miller, J. Z., and Weinberger, M. H. (1987): Blood pressure and metabolic effects of calcium supplementation in normotensive white and black men. *JAMA,* 257:1772–76.

42. MacMahon, S. (1987): Alcohol consumption and hypertension. *Hypertension,* 9:111–21.

43. MacMahon, S. W., Cutler, J. A., Furberg, C. D., Payne, G. H. (1986): The effects of drug treatment for hypertension on morbidity and mortality from cardiovascular disease: A review of randomized controlled trials. *Prog. Cardiovasc. Dis.,* 29(Suppl. 1):99–118.

44. Markandu, N. D., Singer, D. R. J., Sagnella, G. A., Cappuccio, F. P., Sugden, A. L., and MacGregor, G. A. (1988): A double blind study of three sodium intakes, and the long term effects of sodium restriction in essential hypertension (abstract). 12th International Society of Hypertension Meeting, p. 202. Kyoto, Japan.

45. Martin, W. H. III, Montgomery, J., Snell, P. G., Corbett, J. R., Sokolov, J. J., Buckey, J. C., Maloney, D. A., and Blomquist, C. G. (1987): Cardiovascular adaptations to intense swim training in sedentary middle-aged men and women. *Circulation,* 75:323–30.

46. Miller, D. D., Ruddy, T. D., and Zusman, R. M., et al. (1987): Left ventricular ejection fraction response during exercise in asymptomatic systemic hypertension. *Am. J. Cardiol.,* 59:409–13.

47. van Montfrans, G., Karemaker, J., Wieling, W., and Dunning, A. J. (1988): Effect of relaxation therapy on 24-hours continuous ambulatory blood pressure: One-year follow up (abstract). 12th International Society of Hypertension Meeting, p. 786. Kyoto, Japan

48. Moore, R. D., and Pearson, T. A. (1986): Mod-

erate alcohol consumption and coronary artery disease: A review. *Medicine*, 65:242–67.

49. Myers, M. G. (1988): Effects of caffeine on blood pressure. *Arch. Intern. Med.*, 148:1189–93.

50. Nelson, L., Esler, M. D., Jennings, G. L., and Korner, P. I. (1986): Effect of changing levels of physical activity on blood-pressure and haemodynamics in essential hypertension. *Lancet*, 2:473–76.

51. Nissinen, A., Pietinen, P., Tuomilehto, J., Vartiainen, E., Iacono, J. M., and Puska, P. (1987): Predictors of blood pressure change in a series of controlled dietary intervention studies. *J. Human Hypertens.*, 1:167–73.

52. Nowson, C., and Morgan, T. (1986): Effect of calcium carbonate on blood pressure. *J. Hypertension*, 4(Suppl. 6):S673–75.

53. Nowson, C. A., and Morgan, T. O. (1988): Change in blood pressure in relation to change in nutrients effected by manipulation of dietary sodium and potassium. *Clin. Exp. Pharmacol. Physiol.*, 15:225–42.

54. Palatini, P., Mos, L., Di Marco, A., Mormino, P., Munari, L., Del Torre, M., Valle, F., Pessina, A. C., and Dal Palu, C. (1987): Intra-arterial blood pressure recording during sports activities. *J. Hypertension*, 5(Suppl. 5):S479–81.

55. Parillo, M., Coulston, A., Hollenbeck, C., and Reaven, G. (1988): Effect of a low fat diet on carbohydrate metabolism in patients with hypertension. *Hypertension*, 11:244–48.

56. Patel, C., and Marmot, M. (1988): Can general practitioners use training in relaxation and management of stress to reduce mild hypertension? *Br. Med. J.*, 296:21–24.

57. Pincomb, G. A., Lovallo, W. R., Passey, R. B., and Wilson, M. F. (1988): Effect of behavior state on caffeine's ability to alter blood pressure. *Am. J. Cardiol.*, 61:798–802.

58. Powell, K. E., Thompson, P. D., Caspersen, C. J., and Kendrick, J. S. (1987): Physical activity and the incidence of coronary heart disease. *Ann. Rev. Public Health*, 8:253–87.

59. Raglin, J. S., and Morgan, W. P. (1987): Influence of exercise and quiet rest on state anxiety and blood pressure. *Med. Sci. Sports Exerc.*, 19:456–63.

60. Reaven, G. M., and Hoffman, B. B. (1987): A role for insulin in the aetiology and course of hypertension? *Lancet*, 2:435–37.

61. Report. (1988): 1988 Joint National Committee. The 1988 Report of the Joint National Committee on Detection, Evaluation, and Treatment of High Blood Pressure. *Arch. Intern. Med.*, 148:1023–38.

62. Robinson, T. E., Sue, D. Y., Huszczuk, A., Weiler-Ravell, D., and Hansen, J. E. (1988): Intra-arterial and cuff blood pressure responses during incremental cycle ergometry. *Med. Sci. Sports Exerc.*, 20:142–49.

63. Rocchini, A. P., Katch, V., Schork, A., and Kelch, R. P. (1987): Insulin and blood pressure during weight loss in obese adolescents. *Hypertension*, 10:267–73.

64. Rodnick, K. J., Haskell, W. L., Swislocki, A. L. M., Foley, J. E., and Reaven, G. M. (1987): Improved insulin action in muscle, liver, and adipose tissue in physically trained human subjects. *Am. J. Physiol.*, 253:E489–95.

65. Rubba, P., Mancini, M., and Fidanza, F., et al. (1987): Adipose tissue fatty acids and blood pressure in middle-aged men from southern Italy. *Intl. J. Epidemiol.*, 16:528–31.

66. Saito, K., Hattori, K., Omatsu, T., Hirouchi, H., Sano, H., and Fukuzaki, H. (1988): Effects of oral magnesium on blood pressure and red cell sodium transport in patients receiving long-term thiazide diuretics for hypertension. *Am. J. Hypertens.*, 1:71S–74S.

67. Shaper, A. G., Phillips, A. N., Pocock, S. J., and Walker, M. (1987): Alcohol and ischaemic heart disease in middle aged British men. *Br. Med. J.*, 294:733–37.

68. Shelmet, J. J., Reichard, G. A., Skutches, C. L., Hoeldtke, R. D., Owen, O. E., and Boden, G. (1988): Ethanol causes acute inhibition of carbohydrate, fat, and protein oxidation and insulin resistance. *J. Clin. Invest.*, 81:1137–45.

69. Siani, A., Strazzullo, P., and Guglielmi, S., et al. (1988): Controlled trial of low calcium versus high calcium intake in mild hypertension. *J. Hypertension*, 6:253–56.

70. Siani, A., Strazzullo, P., Russo, L., et al. (1987): Controlled trial of long term oral potassium supplements in patients with mild hypertension. *Br. Med. J.*, 294:1453–56.

71. Sobolski, J., Kornitzer, M., De Backer, G., et al. (1987): Protection against ischemic heart disease in the Belgian physical fitness study: Physical fitness rather than physical activity? *Am. J. Epidemiol.*, 125:601–10.

72. Solum, T. T., Ryttig, K. R., Solum, E., and Larsen, S. (1987): The influence of a high-fibre diet on body weight, serum lipids and blood pressure in slightly overweight persons: A randomized, double-blind, placebo-controlled investigation with diet and fibre tablets (Dumo Vital^R). *Intl. J. Obesity*, 11(Suppl. 1):67–71.

73. Stokes, G. S., Monaghan, J. C., Willcocks, D., Jones, M. P., and Marwood, J. F. (1987): Erythrocyte cation fluxes in the normotensive and hypertensive clients of a health screening clinic. *J. Hypertension*, 5:285–91.

74. Strazzullo, P., Cappuccio, F. P., Trevisan, M., et al. (1988): Leisure time physical activity and blood pressure in schoolchildren. *Am. J. Epidemiol.*, 127:726–33.

75. Strazzullo, P., Siani, A., Guglielmi, S., et al. (1986): Controlled trial of long-term oral calcium supplementation in essential hypertension. *Hypertension*, 8:1084–88.

76. Svetkey, L. P., Yarger, W. E., Feussner, J. R., DeLong, E., and Klotman, P. E. (1987): Double-blind, placebo-controlled trial of potassium chloride in the treatment of mild hypertension. *Hypertension*, 9:444–50.

77. Urata, H., Tanabe, Y., and Kiyonaga, A., et al. (1987): Antihypertensive and volume-depleting

effects of mild exercise on essential hypertension. *Hypertension*, 9:245–52.

78. Valori, C., Bentivoglio, M., and Corea, L., et al. (1987): Dietary sodium restriction versus low-sodium/high-potassium salt as ancillary treatment in hypertension. *J. Hypertension*, 5(Suppl. 5):S315–17.

79. Vandongen, R., Mori, T. A., Codde, J. P., Stanton, K. G., and Masarei, J. R. L. (1988): Hypercholesterolaemic effect of fish oil in insulin-dependent diabetic patients. *Med. J. Aust.*, 148:141–43.

80. Weinberger, M. H., Miller, J. Z., Fineberg, N. S., Luft, F. C., Grim, C. E., and Christian, J. C. (1987): Association of haptoglobin with sodium sensitivity and resistance of blood pressure. *Hypertension*, 10:443–46.

81. Williams, P. T., Fortmann, S. P., and Terry, R. B., et al. (1987): Associations of dietary fat, regional adiposity, and blood pressure in men. *JAMA*, 257:3251–56.

82. Zoccali, C., Mallamaci, F., and Delfino, D. (1986): Long-term oral calcium supplementation in essential hypertension: A double-blind, randomized, crossover study. *J. Hypertension*, 4(Suppl. 6):S676–78.

New Therapeutic Strategies in Hypertension,
edited by Norman M. Kaplan,
Barry M. Brenner, and John H. Laragh.
Raven Press, Ltd., New York © 1989.

Diuretics

John M. Flack and Richard H. Grimm

*Division of Epidemiology, School of Public Health, University of Minnesota,
Minneapolis, Minnesota 55455*

A new era of antihypertensive therapy was launched when chlorothiazide was introduced in 1958. Since then thiazides have been the foundation of the stepped-care approach for antihypertensive therapy. Thiazides continue to be the most commonly-prescribed class of antihypertensive agents (89). There are four major classes of diuretics: thiazides, thiazide-like, loop or "high ceiling", and potassium-sparing diuretics (Table 1).

Diuretics have contributed significantly to the effective management of elevated blood pressure which has resulted in significant declines in the incidence of stroke, congestive heart failure, progressive hypertension, and renal failure. However, the ability of diuretics to reduce the incidence of coronary heart disease (CHD) incidence remains questionable.

Thiazides were initially recommended in the 1977 Joint National Committee (JNC) report (45) as the preferred initial choice for drug therapy of hypertension. The 1988 Fourth Joint National Committee report (46) recommends thiazides as one of several choices for initial therapy which includes beta-blockers, calcium blockers, and angiotensin converting enzyme (ACE) inhibitors. The majority of clinical trials involving drug treatment of mild hypertension have used thiazide diuretics alone or as the base for a multidrug regimen (Table 2). Diuretic use has been recently questioned because of increased concerns about diuretic-induced metabolic disturbances which include hy-pokalemia, hypercholesterolemia, hypertriglyceridemia, hyperuricemia, hyperglycemia, and hypomagnesemia.

Questions have also been raised about the efficacy of thiazides from the results of several large scale trials which have suggested the possibility of differential subgroup effects on cardiac morbidity and mortality (41). Specific hypertensive subgroups, such as those with left ventricular hypertrophy (LVH) or occult CHD, probably represented a significant portion of the study participants with resting ECG abnormalities who experienced adverse effects possibly related to high-dose diuretic treatment. The Multiple Risk Factor Intervention Trial (MRFIT) Study used thiazide doses that are quite high by today's standards (up to 100 mg/day of hydrochlorothiazide or chlorthalidone); curiously, this dose level was considered moderate when the study was planned. As a result of these studies, "low-dose" diuretic therapy is now much more common. 12.5 mg/day of chlorthalidone or hydrochlorothiazide is recommended as a reasonable starting dose by the most recent JNC Report (46).

Thiazide and thiazide-like diuretics owe their longevity as first-line blood pressure therapy to their low cost, efficacy in blood pressure control, and reasonable patient acceptance. Moreover, diuretics are easy to titrate and are relatively safe, especially at the lower doses. Therefore, thiazides continue to play an important role in the treatment of many patients with uncomplicated

Table 1. *Diuretics*

Type	Dosing range (mg/day)	Pill size (mg)
Thiazide		
Bendroflumethiazide	2.5–5	2.5, 5, 10
Benzthiazide	12.5–50	50
Chlorothiazide	125.0–500	250, 500
Cyclothiazide	1.0–2	2
Hydrochlorothiazide	12.5–50	25, 50, 100
Hydroflumethiazide	12.5–50	50
Methyclothiazide	2.5–5	2.5, 5
Polythiazide	1.0–4	1, 2, 4
Trichlormethiazide	1.0–4	2, 4
Thiazide-like		
Chlorthalidone	12.5–25	25, 50, 100
Indapamide	2.5–5	2.5
Metolazone	1.25–5	2.5, 5, 10
Quinethazone	25.0–100	50
Loop#		
Bumetanide	0.5–5	0.5, 1.0
Ethacrynic acid	25.0–100	20, 50
Furosemide	20.0–320	20, 40, 80
Potassium-sparing		
Amiloride	5.0–10	5
Spironolactone	25.0–100	25, 100
Triamterene	50.0–100	50

Adapted from ref. 106.

essential hypertension. It should be noted, however, that thiazides are of little value in treating hypertensive emergencies since it may take several days for their blood pressure lowering effect to be manifest.

MECHANISM OF ACTION

Thiazide diuretics initially lower blood pressure by causing a prompt diuresis and natriuresis which results in contraction of the extracellular fluid volume (ECFV). The ECFV is reduced by approximately two liters within the first 48 h of therapy (22). Leth (53) and Tarazi et al. (88) have shown that the thiazide-induced contraction of the plasma volume is maintained long term; although probably not to the degree of the short-term plasma volume changes.

Thiazides inhibit active sodium and chloride reabsorption in the cortical thick ascending limb of Henle where 15 to 30% of the filtered sodium load is reabsorbed

(17,48). Freis et al. (22) showed that the initial fall in blood pressure is associated with a reduction in cardiac output and unchanged peripheral resistance. Later, cardiac output increases back to baseline and peripheral resistance falls below pretreatment levels (12).

Nonrenal mechanisms of blood pressure lowering may possibly contribute to the thiazides ability to lower blood pressure by reducing peripheral resistance. Possible mechanisms for this phenomenon include a reduced vasoconstrictor response to pressor substances (24,75), and secondary hyperreninism (26), which may stimulate production of vasodilatory prostaglandins. Also, Resnick has suggested that sodium may stimulate the cellular uptake of calcium (76). Theoretically, this could occur in response to high dietary sodium intake and/ or reduced renal sodium excretion; thereby, leading to increased vascular resistance and elevated blood pressure.

Sodium overload of the arterial wall has been considered to be a potential cause of elevated vascular resistance and vascular hyperreactivity. Increased vessel wall sodium has been demonstrated in the large arteries of hypertensives (74) but not in the smaller arterioles which are the primary resistance vessels. Conceivably, thiazides could reduce vascular resistance directly or indirectly by reducing vessel wall sodium content. However, a direct action on the arteriolar wall by thiazides has not been proven to explain the fall in peripheral resistance that occurs with chronic therapy. Although the initial fall in blood pressure with thiazides appears due to the loss of plasma volume, the long-term decline in blood pressure is most likely due to the combined effect of a contracted plasma volume as well as a decrease in vascular resistance (14). Several mechanisms have been proposed for the lower resistance; however, at this time, it is unclear as to the primary mechanism(s) involved. Tobian (90) has proposed "reverse autoregulation"

Table 2. *Major drug trials of treatment of mild to moderate hypertension*

Trial	Entry DBP Range (mm Hg)	No. of Patients	Drug	Years F/U
Active Tx vs placebo				
VA, 1970	90–114	380	HCTZ/RS HDRZ	3.8
USPHS, 1977	90–114	389	CTZ/RS	7–10
Australian, 1980	95–109	3,247	CTZ	4.0
Oslo, 1980	90–109	785	HCTZ	5–6.5
MRC, 1985	95–109	17,354	BDRZ/PRO	4.9
EWPHE, 1985	90–119	840	HCTZ/TMTR	4.6
Non-placebo control				
HDFP, 1979	90–104	10,940	CTD and/or SPL/TMTR	5.0
MRFIT, 1982	90+	12,866	CTD/HCTZ SPL/TMTR	7.0
IPPPSH, 1985	100–125	6,357	OXPR/NBB	3.9
HAPPHY, 1987	100–130	3,297	ATEN/MTP BDRZ/HCTZ	3.8

HCTZ = hydrochlorothiazide; CTZ = chlorothiazide; RS = rauwolfia serpentina; BDRZ = bendroflumethiazide; PRO = propranolol; TMTR = triamterene; CTD = chlorthalidone; SPL = spironolactone; OXPR = oxyprenolol; NBB = non-beta-blocker; ATEN = atenolol; MTP = metoprolol.
VA = Veterans Administration Cooperative Study; USPHS = United States Public Health Service Study; Australian = Australian Therapeutic Trial; Oslo = Oslo Hypertension Study; MRC = Medical Research Council Trial; EWPHE = European Working Party on Hypertension in the Elderly; MRFIT = Multiple Risk Factor Intervention Trial; IPPPSH = International Prospective Primary Prevention Study in Hypertension; HAPPHY = Heart Attack Primary Prevention in Hypertension Trial.
Adapted from ref. 107.

as a possible explanation for the reduction in vascular resistance. The initial diuretic-induced contraction of the ECFV results in reduced venous return, central venous pressure and cardiac output. According to theory, this may result in mechanical activation of reflexes that reduce peripheral resistance, thereby allowing the cardiac output to increase back to pretreatment values. Also, as Lund-Johansen points out, thiazides may actually differ in their individual mechanisms of blood pressure reduction (55). Regardless of findings suggesting non-renal mechanism(s) of action for the thiazide diuretics, it should be noted that thiazides are ineffective in lowering blood pressure when the glomerular filtration rate is less than 25 ml/min.

Efficacy

Thiazides are effective blood pressure lowering agents in most forms of hypertension when used alone or as part of multidrug regimens. Diuretics enhance the blood pressure lowering effects of other major classes of antihypertensives. Tolerance to the blood pressure lowering effect of the thiazides rarely occurs. The pretreatment renin profile does not predict the blood pressure lowering obtained with thiazide diuretics; however, an exaggerated activation of the renin-aldosterone axis may limit further blood pressure reduction during upward dose titration of the thiazides (96).

Thiazides and beta-blockers reduce blood pressure by similar magnitude (Table 3). Moreover, diuretics are also similar in blood pressure lowering compared to other nondiuretic antihypertensives (3,67,83,95, 99). Approximately 50 to 60% of hypertensives should have acceptable blood pressure control with thiazide doses ranging between 12.5 to 50 mg of hydrochlorothiazide per day. When combined with ACE-inhibitors (37,94,99) or beta-blockers (95), thia-

Table 3. *Blood pressure reduction: thiazides versus beta-blockers*

Study	Fall in blood pressure (mm Hg)
VA Coop Study, 1982 (93)	
Hydrochlorothiazide	18/12
Propranolol	10/12
MRC Trial (57)	
Bendroflumethiazide	13/5
Propranolol	10/4
MRFIT (30)	
Chlorthalidone/	15/10
Hydrochlorothiazide	
HAPPHY (102)	
Bendroflumethiazide/	25/16
Hydrochlorothiazide	
Atenolol/Metoprolol	25/17

See Table 2 abbreviations.

zide diuretics considerably enhance blood pressure lowering.

Use of Thiazides in Black Patients

Black hypertensives appear more likely to have "salt-sensitive," low-renin hypertension with normal to mildly increased plasma volume (104); however, peripheral resistance tends to be elevated and cardiac output is frequently reduced compared to white hypertensives (100). Thiazide diuretics are very effective agents in reducing blood pressure in black hypertensives. Blacks may respond better in blood pressure lowering to thiazide diuretics compared to monotherapy with beta-blockers (93,95) and ACE-inhibitors (94). Although the majority of both blacks and whites respond well to all these agents, other classes of antihypertensive drugs usually result in an even greater blood pressure reduction (94,95). Though questions have been raised concerning differential blood pressure effects overall by race, diuretics appear to reduce blood pressure to a similar degree in black and white hypertensives (93).

Diuretic Use in the Elderly

Elderly hypertensives tend to have "salt sensitive," low-renin hypertension with contracted plasma volumes (105). Peripheral resistance tends to be increased and cardiac output is often reduced in elderly hypertensives. Ironically, diuretics are very effective agents for lowering blood pressure in the elderly, despite the fact that plasma volume is usually contracted.

Analysis of data from the pilot Systolic Hypertension in the Elderly Program (SHEP) (42) showed that 88% of elderly persons with isolated systolic hypertension treated with chlorthalidone alone achieved their goal blood pressure. In this group, 56% required just 25 mg/day of chlorthalidone to achieve goal blood pressures. At the end of one year, systolic and diastolic pressures were reduced 17/6 mmHg from baseline in the chlorthalidone group compared to placebo. Diuretic therapy was well tolerated by this elderly group and adherence was maintained at a high level with minimal adverse metabolic disturbances.

DIURETIC SIDE EFFECTS

Many of the thiazide-related metabolic disturbances, and to a lesser degree side effects, are dose related. The goal of diuretic therapy should be to use the lowest possible diuretic dose to achieve adequate blood pressure control. This approach, along with nonpharmacologic adjunctive therapy including weight loss, dietary sodium and alcohol reduction, and increased physical activity will help to minimize the adverse metabolic effects of thiazide therapy while maximizing blood pressure control.

Metabolic Effects of Thiazides

Hypokalemia is defined conventionally as a serum potassium of less than 3.5 mEq/L. Hypokalemia is the most common thiazide-induced metabolic disturbance; it occurs in 10 to 36% of thiazide-treated hypertensives and is clearly dose-related (30,39). In one study only 10% of thiazide-treated hypertensives had serum potassium levels less than 3.0 mEq/L (30). Most often, the fall in serum potassium ranges between 0.3 to 1.2 mEq/L depending on the dose and type of thiazide prescribed. Dose for dose, the prevalence of hypokalemia is greater with chlorthalidone than hydrochlorothiazide (30). The fall in serum potassium may occur during the first week of thiazide treatment (59). Hypertensives who are hypokalemic in the absence of diuretic therapy should be evaluated for other conditions such as primary hyperaldosteronism.

Thiazides produce hypokalemia by several mechanisms. First, they contract the ECFV which may result in hyperreninemic hyperaldosteronism thereby enhancing Na^+-K^+ exchange in the distal tubule. Also, diuretics increase the delivery of sodium ions to the distal tubule which provides more substrate for Na^+-K^+ exchange. In addition, thiazide-induced chloride depletion, which, independent of ECFV contraction, increases renal potassium secretion. Finally, metabolic alkalosis and increased serum catecholamines, both consequences of diuretic therapy (17,35), result in a shift of potassium ions to an intracellular location where they are more efficiently secreted by the kidneys.

Potassium Homeostasis

The relevance of serum potassium and total body potassium to the genesis of arrhythmias is still a major question. Approximately 95% of the total body potassium is located in the intracellular space. The total body/serum potassium ratio may be important; however, total body potassium is difficult to measure. Studies have suggested that diuretic use only minimally effects total body potassium (16,87). In addition, other cations such as magnesium and calcium may also play an important role.

Although there is much more to be learned concerning the clinical relevance of hypokalemia, prudent medical practice involves monitoring serum potassium and in-

itiating treatment should hypokalemia develop. Diet has been advocated as a means to increase potassium intake, although it is very difficult by means of diet alone to sufficiently increase dietary potassium and improve serum potassium levels. Although a potassium-rich diet can be advised, most patients with hypokalemia will require discontinuation of the diuretic, potassium supplementation, or the addition of a potassium-sparing diuretic to normalize their serum potassium.

Hypokalemia and Ventricular Arrhythmias

Historically, hypokalemia no doubt has generated the most concern of all of the adverse metabolic effects associated with thiazide therapy. This is primarily due to the deeply-held conventional view that hypokalemia promotes cardiac ventricular irritability. The strongest evidence associating diuretic use to ventricular arrhythmias comes from recent analysis of data from the MRFIT, which found a positive relationship between diuretic use, hypokalemia, and the incidence of ventricular premature beats (VPBs) (11).

Hypokalemia has long been suspected to cause ventricular arrhythmias. Although the causal relationship between diuretic-induced hypokalemia and ventricular arrhythmias recently has been questioned (71,72), other studies have found a positive correlation (11,39).

Ventricular premature beats are associated with an increased risk of sudden death in persons with CHD (47). Moreover, contrary to previous reports (71,72), apparently healthy men with VPBs may be at increased risk for sudden death (1). Obese hypertensives and hypertensives with left ventricular hypertrophy (LVH) are at increased risk for VPBs, complex ventricular arrhythmias, and sudden death (61,62). Furthermore, it has been shown that diuretic-treated hypertensives with LVH may have more ventricular arrhythmias when di-uretic-induced hypokalemia develops (36). Savage (79) has pointed out that the major-ity of hypertensives with LVH are not ap-propriately diagnosed by a standard surface ECG. Moreover, the majority of patients with CHD (who are at increased risk for arrhythmias and sudden death) also go un-diagnosed.

It remains controversial whether potas-sium supplementation is effective in de-creasing or abolishing ventricular ectopy. Some investigators have demonstrated re-duced VPBs in diuretic-treated hyperten-sives with hypokalemia after potassium supplementation (10,38) although, this is not an invariable observation (72). Other potassium-conserving measures such as the addition of potassium-sparing diuretics or an ACE-inhibitor to a thiazide diuretic may also reduce VPBs (21,40).

Additional analyses of data from the MRFIT suggests that diuretic treatment may be harmful in men with resting ECG abnormalities (including tall R waves and negative T waves) (69). These ECG abnor-malities may represent men with occult CHD and/or LVH. Moreover, these ECG abnormalities have been positively corre-lated with an increased baseline prevalence of VPBs (11). Men randomized to the spe-cial intervention (SI) group with resting base-line ECG abnormalities who were treated intensively with either hydrochlo-rothiazide or chlorthalidone experienced a 65% excess of CHD deaths compared to usual care (UC) men. UC men, in general, were treated less intensively, usually with lower thiazide dose levels. Within-group analysis in the SI group suggested an ad-verse interaction between the presence of resting baseline ECG abnormalities and di-uretic treatment. Data from the Oslo hy-pertension trial and the Hypertension De-tection and Follow-Up Program (HDFP) is consistent with the MRFIT findings, at least in white men with base-line resting ECG ab-normalities (41,50).

Hypokalemic hypertensives with VPBs may be at increased risk for more complex ventricular arrhythmias which may possibly lead to an increased risk for sudden death. Clearly, hypokalemia increases the risk for ventricular arrhythmias in patients taking digitalis (70,85) and in the setting of an acute myocardial infarction (77), therefore, thia-zide diuretics should be used very cau-tiously or avoided in these situations. How-ever, the management of mild hypokalemia in diuretic-treated hypertensives with no clinical evidence of underlying heart dis-ease (by far the most common clinical sce-nario) continues to be a topic of intense de-bate (28).

Treatment of Hypokalemia

Few would argue that severe hypokale-mia (<3.0 mEq/L) should be avoided in all diuretic-treated patients. However, the management of mild hypokalemia (3.0–3.5 mEq/L) continues to be a major question. Diuretic therapy should be avoided, if pos-sible, in hypertensives prone to arrhyth-mias. However, this is not always practical; therefore, diuretic-induced hypokalemia should be prevented or promptly treated should it occur. Moreover, serum potas-sium levels are not static, and may fall pre-cipitously in response to catecholamine surges or acute alkalosis associated with ex-ercise, anxiety, or acute myocardial infarc-tion. Thus, there seems to be ample ration-ale to maintain the serum potassium levels above 3.5 mEq/L in diuretic-treated pa-tients.

Several methods are available to mini-mize thiazide-induced problems with potas-sium, including use of low-dose thiazide therapy, potassium-sparing diuretics, ACE-inhibitors, or possibly beta-blockers as ad-juncts to the thiazides, and a diet moder-ately restricted in sodium and high in po-tassium.

Even with intensive hygienic measures many patients will require potassium supplements or discontinuation of thiazides to restore potassium levels to normal. Usual clinical doses range from 15 to 100 mEq daily for potassium chloride. Individuals who are refractory to potassium supplementation should be screened for hypomagnesemia and/or metabolic alkalosis; both of these conditions may promote increased renal potassium loss.

Hypomagnesemia

Magnesium deficiency is associated with vague clinical symptomatology such as weakness, tremors, and anorexia (44). As with other thiazide-induced metabolic disturbances, hypomagnesemia is probably dose-related. Persons with a local soft water supply, the elderly, those who abuse alcohol, and the malnourished are at increased risk for the development of hypomagnesemia when treated with diuretics. Hypomagnesemia increases the likelihood of digitalis toxicity (81). Experimentally, it has been shown that hypomagnesemia leads to a decreased intracellular potassium concentration (81) and to increased myocardial uptake of digitalis (44). Hollifield (39) reported increased VPBs in thiazide-treated patients who developed hypomagnesemia. Moreover, Whang et al. (101) pointed out the difficulty in raising serum potassium levels in hypomagnesemic patients.

Serum magnesium levels should be periodically checked in diuretic-treated hypertensives, although lymphocyte or red cell magnesium may be more informative than serum magnesium levels. Low-dose thiazide therapy and adjunctive therapy with a potassium-sparing diuretic (39,56) have been helpful in preventing hypomagnesemia.

Hyperuricemia

Thiazides cause hyperuricemia by decreasing the glomerular filtration rate and renal blood flow. In addition, thiazides act as competitive inhibitors of renal tubular uric acid secretion (23). Hyperuricemia is a common complication of thiazide diuretic therapy and is also likely dose-related. Hyperuricemia occurs in 26 to 33% of untreated mild hypertensives (60). On average, the rise in serum uric acid observed with thiazides is less than 1 mg/dl. For most patients this change in uric acid is clinically insignificant. Clinical gout occurs predominantly in men and the incidence of this complication has been less than 5% over years of thiazide treatment in major hypertension trials (13,102).

Messerli et al. (60) correlated elevated serum acid levels with elevated renal vascular resistance and reduced renal blood flow in hypertensive patients. Furthermore, Korbin et al. (49) found that hypertensives with hyperuricemia had a significantly greater LV mass than those without hyperuricemia. Possibly, uric acid elevations are a marker for hypertensive renal and cardiac end-organ damage. Hyperuricemia is also a concern because it has been found to be an independent risk factor for subsequent myocardial infarction; although, a causal relationship for hyperuricemia and CHD has not been established.

Most hypertensives who develop hyperuricemia can remain on thiazides without treatment. Those with uric acid levels of greater than 10 mg/dl should be considered for thiazide withdrawal or long-term treatment of the hyperuricemia with allopurinol or probenecid. Attacks of acute gout can be managed with typical antigout therapy using nonsteroidal antiinflammatory agents.

Glucose Intolerance

Thiazide diuretic use is infrequently associated with clinical problems in glucose tolerance if pretreatment glucose values are normal. Only 2.9% of diuretic-treated men in the Heart Attack Primary Prevention in Hypertension (HAPPHY) trial developed glucose intolerance over 45 months of treatment (102). Results from the thiazide-treated group in MRC and the MRFIT trials also suggest that glucose intolerance is not a major problem and is reversible once the diuretic is discontinued (30,58).

The mechanism(s) of thiazide-induced impaired glucose tolerance most likely relates to impaired insulin release from the pancreatic beta cells (18) and/or peripheral insulin resistance (27). Hypertensives may be predisposed to developing glucose intolerance with thiazide treatment. Untreated hypertensives have been found to possess a defect in nonoxidative glucose metabolism indicative of peripheral insulin resistance (20), and also demonstrate an exaggerated rise in glucose and insulin levels after a standard glucose load (27). Hypokalemia may decrease pancreatic insulin secretion or decrease the conversion of proinsulin to insulin, either of which could impair glucose tolerance. In addition, preservation of potassium balance and avoiding hypokalemia may prevent thiazide-induced hyperglycemia (33). Moreover, adjunctive use of the ACE-inhibitor captopril may blunt thiazide-induced hyperglycemia, possibly by preserving potassium balance (99).

Advancing age and increasing duration of therapy may increase the risk for hyperglycemia. Diabetics may occasionally experience a deterioration in glucose levels within a few weeks of initiating thiazide therapy (82). This may necessitate a dose reduction, correction of hypokalemia, stopping of thiazide treatment, or switching to a loop diuretic.

Although the clinical significance of glucose changes associated with thiazide therapy is unknown, it seems prudent to avoid hyperglycemia if at all possible. Preventing hypokalemia, maintenance of ideal body weight, and use of low-dose thiazide therapy may lower the incidence of thiazide-induced hyperglycemia.

Lipids

Thiazide diuretics were first reported possibly to cause hypercholesterolemia in 1964 (80). However, little attention was paid to this observation until the late 1970s (4). Subsequently, thiazides have been documented to increase total cholesterol, LDL-cholesterol, and triglycerides while producing only minor reductions in HDL-cholesterol (29,32,51,64).

The adverse lipid effects observed in thiazide-treated men with the MRFIT were further examined in an ancillary study which utilized a modified Latin square design (32). Grimm et al. reports in this study that thiazides produce elevations of total cholesterol, LDL-cholesterol, and triglycerides, and that a cholesterol-lowering diet prescribed simultaneously blunts the thiazide lipid changes. These results were highly consistent with the thiazide-related lipid changes observed over 72 months of treatment in the larger MRFIT study. A substantial literature on thiazides and lipids has developed since the original MRFIT observations and several reviews have summarized these studies (52,78,98).

It has been speculated that thiazide-induced lipid changes are short-term, however this hypothesis rests on a fragile, highly-select database without any plausible metabolic explanation put forward to explain the proposed long-term adaptation. Lipid results from the Hypertension Detection and Follow-Up Program have been the foundation for most of the speculation on the duration of thiazide-induced lipid changes (13). In the HDFP stepped-care cohort, largely treated with chlorthalidone, total cholesterol was elevated compared to baseline but returned back to baseline by the second year of the study, and was actually below baseline by the end of the study. Unfortunately, this data adds little to our understanding of the duration thiazide lipid effects because this HDFP study lacked an appropriate control group for changes in lipids. A multitude of factors, apart from diuretic-induced changes, could have confounded the observed lipid changes. Such factors include a large proportion of the cohort ceasing to use diuretics over the course of the study, weight loss, and changes in diet, etc.; these all seem as likely to account for the observed secular changes in lipids as a short-term diuretic effect. The evidence in support of long-term thiazide-induced lipid effects comes from several major prospective trials with control groups demonstrating persistence of lipid changes long term, including the MRFIT where the adverse lipid effects were observed over 72 months (29,51). Results of studies which involve the systematic withdrawal of diuretics after long-term treatment using well controlled experimental designs also support the long-term lipid effect (31,84). In these situations serum cholesterol goes down significantly when diuretics are withdrawn, compared to controls. At least one study did not find a long-term diuretic lipid effect compared to appropriate controls (42). This study may be different because it utilized smaller doses of diuretics and, in general, studied older patients (higher pretreatment cholesterol) which may have influenced the results.

There is no direct evidence that thiazide lipid changes increase an individual's risk for CHD; however, there is little reason to believe that these changes are inconsequential. Data from the recently completed PROCAM Trial (7) found that hypercholesterolemia and hypertension clustered in their study population. Moreover, a marked increase in the four-year risk for CHD was observed in hyperlipidemic hypertensives compared to hypertensives with normal lipids (unpublished observations by Flack and Wiist found that the prevalence of hypertension increases with increasing cholesterol levels; thus confirming observations made in the PROCAM Trial). The recently reported Helsinki Heart Study (25) lends credence to the concept that favorable concurrent changes in non-LDL lipoproteins may act as amplifiers of CHD risk reduction when LDL-cholesterol is reduced.

The mechanism(s) of diuretic lipid changes is unknown. Most likely, increased production and/or impaired catabolism of lipoproteins are involved. Possibly, hypertensives are predisposed to lipid derangements because of pretreatment insulin resistance, diuretic-induced insulinopenia, and/or thiazide-induced increases in catecholamine levels. These metabolic derangements may alter lipoprotein metabolism in such a way as to favor increased lipid levels.

Thiazide lipid changes are potentially important for several reasons: (1) other CHD risk factors tend to "cluster" in hypertensives adding to their baseline CHD risk; (2) a major cardiovascular event in hypertensives is coronary heart disease; (3) the majority of hypertensives are treated with diuretics; and (4) thiazide lipid changes are largely preventable. Moreover, these lipid changes could potentially negate some or all of the expected CHD reduction after the blood pressure has been lowered.

The 1988 report from the JNC (3) endorses the concept of treating hypertension without adversely affecting other CHD risk factors. A lipid profile should be obtained prior to initiating antihypertensive therapy. Diuretics should be avoided, if possible, in persons with "high-risk" LDL-cholesterol levels (≥ 160 mg/dl). When thiazides are prescribed in persons with LDL-cholesterol levels equal to, or greater than, 130 mg/dl, a cholesterol lowering diet should be implemented and reinforced at each subsequent patient visit. Approximately 6 to 8 weeks after initiation of diuretic therapy, the lipid profile should be repeated. Increased dietary intake of soluble dietary fiber (blackeyed peas, lentils, oat bran, etc.) may aid in reducing cholesterol levels (6). The lowest possible diuretic dose should be used, and consideration to discontinuing diuretic therapy should be given in patients with continued "high-risk" LDL-cholesterol levels. It is recommended in hypertensive patients where lipids are a concern, that thiazides be avoided as initial therapy. Moreover, if thiazides are used, they may substantially reduce the cholesterol lowering effect of a low-fat/low-cholesterol diet (51). In these patients, first line therapy should be agents which are beneficial to lipids, the selective alpha$_1$-inhibitors, or agents which are likely lipid neutral such as ACE-inhibitors, calcium channel blockers, ISA beta-blockers, central adrenergic inhibitors, vasodilators, and indapamide.

Other Metabolic Effects

Thiazide diuretics may cause hyponatremia. They inhibit generation of "free water" in the thick ascending limb of Henle, thereby impairing renal diluting mechanisms. Hyponatremia occurs infrequently during thiazide treatment. Occasionally, excessive water intake overwhelms renal-diluting mechanisms and hyponatremia may occur. Those at increased risk for thiazide-induced hyponatremia include the elderly, persons consuming diets severely restricted in sodium, and edematous patients.

Thiazides decrease the renal clearance of calcium. Mild hypercalcemia may be rarely observed during thiazide treatment, and is usually of no clinical consequence. Other uncommon thiazide-related complications include azotemia, alkaline phosphatase elevations, and renal zinc wastage.

Thiazide-related Side Effects

Thiazide diuretics, although usually well tolerated, do sometimes cause side effects severe enough to result in drug discontinuation. Bendrofluazide was discontinued in 17.1% of men and 12.8% of women during the five year MRC Trial (58). In the HDFP trial, where active drug therapy was chlorthalidone based, approximately 33% of the drug-treated active participants were withdrawn from medication by the end of the five-year study (13).

Thiazides, like other blood pressure lowering drugs, can be associated with impotence. 16.2% of diuretic treated MRC participants reported impotence after 12 weeks of therapy. For the entire trial, there were 19.6 cases of impotence/1,000 patient-years of follow-up in diuretic treated men compared to 0.9/1,000 patient-years in the placebo group (58). Moreover, it may be presumptious to assume that sexual dysfunction occurs only in diuretic-treated men.

Less common diuretic-related side effects include dizziness, lethargy, dry mouth, palpitations, orthostatic hypotension, headaches, nausea, and muscle cramps. Rarely reported clinical conditions associated with thiazide therapy include acute pancreatitis, skin rash, interstitial nephritis, vasculitis, thrombocytopenia, leukopenia, and hemolytic anemia.

INDAPAMIDE

Indapamide is a two-methyindoline thiazide-like diuretic which has been used in Europe since 1974. This agent became available for clinical use in the United States in 1983. With indapamide, blood pressure is normalized in one-half to two-thirds of persons with mild to moderate hypertension who are treated with doses of between 2.5 to 5 mg/day (66).

Indapamide lowers blood pressure via renal as well as nonrenal mechanisms. Sodium, chloride, and water reabsorption are inhibited in the cortical-diluting segment of the distal convoluted tubule. Renal blood flow, glomerular filtration rate (GFR) and cardiac output are usually unaffected; however, peripheral resistance falls during indapamide therapy (103). Indapamide is highly lipophilic compared to the more commonly-used thiazide diuretics. This may explain, at least in part, how indapamide accumulates in vascular smooth muscle where it may exert a calcium channel blocking effect (65,73).

Metabolic side effects tend to be less severe and occur less frequently with indapamide. In particular, indapamide does not have an adverse impact on blood lipids (9,97). Although usually neutral with respect to lipids, HDL-cholesterol levels may increase during indapamide therapy (63). Elevations of uric acid, similar to those seen with the thiazides, may occur. Glucose intolerance occurs infrequently. Hypokalemia develops in approximately 10% of indapamide-treated patients.

The main advantage of indapamide over the cheaper and more commonly prescribed thiazides is that similar blood pressure lowering is obtained without adversely impacting on blood lipids. Moreover, other adverse metabolic disturbances are less frequently encountered. However, unlike the thiazides, indapamide may lower blood pressure in azotemic hypertensives (2). The potential advantages of indapamide therapy over more commonly-used thiazides must be counter-balanced against a significantly higher cost of drug therapy.

LOOP DIURETICS

Loop diuretics (furosemide, ethacrynic acid, bumetanide) are the most potent class of diuretics currently available. They may be administered via oral or intravenous routes. Loop diuretics are less frequently indicated for uncomplicated essential hypertension than are the thiazides, largely due to the smaller reduction in blood pressure obtained with these agents compared to the thiazides (5,8).

Loop diuretics are most often indicated and may be preferable to the thiazides in refractory hypertension, diabetic hypertension, and hypertension associated with CHF. Moreover, loop diuretics lower blood pressure more effectively than do thiazides when renal function is compromised (GFR < 25 cc/min).

Loop diuretics inhibit sodium and chloride cotransport in the medullary thick ascending limb of Henle (8). They cause a rapid diuresis and natriuresis that is shorter in duration but similar in magnitude to that observed with thiazide diuretics (8); therefore, the loop diuretics are usually prescribed at least twice daily. Metabolic side effects such as hypocholesterolemia, hypokalemia, hypomagnesemia, etc., occur during loop diuretic therapy although less frequently than during therapy with thiazide diuretics. Moreover, when these adverse metabolic side effects do occur they tend to be less severe.

POTASSIUM-SPARING DIURETICS

The potassium-sparing diuretics (amiloride, spironolactone, triamterene) are most often prescribed combined with a thiazide or loop diuretic. By themselves they are relatively weak diuretics (8). Accordingly, their major clinical use is as adjunctive therapy to the thiazide diuretics, due to their potassium- and magnesium-sparing properties. The hydrochlorothiazide/potassium-sparing diuretic combination is associated with smaller reductions in serum magnesium than observed with thiazide-diuretic monotherapy and may be superior to potassium supplements in maintaining serum potassium levels (54,56,68). Indications for using potassium-sparing diuretics include persistence of diuretic-induced hypomagnesemia or hypokalemia after hygienic measures have failed to maintain electrolyte homeostasis. In addition, diuretic-treated individuals who are predisposed to developing ventricular arrhythmias are candidates for potassium-sparing diuretics. Adjunctive prophylactic use of these agents in uncomplicated essential hypertension is not recommended due to the expense as well as the observation that most patients treated with diuretics, particularly with low doses of thiazides, do not develop hypokalemia.

Potassium-sparing diuretics exert their main antikaliuretic and natriuretic effect in the cortical collecting duct. Intraluminal negativity and distal tubular sodium-potassium exchange are primary determinants of renal potassium secretion (8). Spironolactone is a competitive inhibitor of aldosterone and therefore inhibits potassium secretion. Amiloride and triamterene decrease renal potassium secretion by lowering luminal membrane permeability to sodium ions which, independent of aldosterone, reduces potassium ion excretion. Hydrogen ion secretion is also reduced. As a consequence of increased luminal sodium, electronegativity is reduced. Diuretics which exert their natriuretic effect more proximally and increase the delivery of sodium to the distal nephron enhance the effectiveness of the potassium-sparing agents.

In some instances, potassium-sparing diuretics may be preferrable to oral potassium supplements due to their dual ability to preserve both potassium and magnesium. In addition, they may help to prevent ventricular arrhythmias (86). In some instances, a cost differential may exist between potassium-sparing diuretics and oral potassium supplements favoring the former, particularly when high doses of the potassium supplements are used.

Hyperkalemia is the most serious side effect which may rarely occur with potassium-sparing diuretics. Hyperkalemia usually occurs in patients with reduced renal function but may also occur in patients taking ACE-inhibitors, nonsteroidal antiinflammatory drugs and oral potassium supplements; thus, concomitant therapy with potassium-sparing diuretics, ACE-inhibitors, or potassium supplements should be avoided. Over-the-counter potassium-containing salt substitutes pose a similar threat. Diabetics, because of their propensity for hyporeninemic hypoaldosteronism and reduced renal function, are also at increased risk for hyperkalemia. These agents usually do not adversely affect carbohydrate metabolism. Triameterene may increase uric acid levels. Other side effects include GI distress, diarrhea, and hyperchloremic metabolic acidosis. Antiandrogenic effects such as tender breasts, gynecomastia, and impotence may occur during spironolactone therapy, though suprisingly, the incidence of impotence appears to be quite low. In this

same report, spironolactone was found to adversely affect plasma lipids by significantly increasing LDL-cholesterol (19). Potassium-sparing diuretics are contraindicated in persons with renal disease. Moreover, triamterene undergoes extensive hepatic metabolism and should be avoided in patients with liver disease.

INDICATIONS

Thiazide diuretics are reasonable therapeutic choices for most forms of nonazotemic hypertension. They effectively lower blood pressure until the creatinine clearance is less than 25 cc/min (creatinine 2.5 mg/dl). Alternative drug therapy to the thiazides should be prescribed, if possible, for hypertensives with elevated blood lipids, abnormal resting ECGs, and/or ventricular arrhythmias. When thiazides are prescribed in such patients they should be given in the lowest dose possible combined with a cholesterol-lowering diet. In patients predisposed to ventricular arrhythmias, cation electrolyte homeostasis should be diligently maintained. Thiazides should also be avoided or used cautiously in diabetic patients because of the hyperglycemia associated with thiazide treatment. Moreover, diabetic patients often have lipid profiles which are adversely influenced by thiazide diuretics.

Thiazides should be prescribed at the lowest dose that is effective in obtaining the desired level of blood pressure control. Ideally, the dose range for the initiation of thiazide therapy should be 12.5 to 25 mg/day. The maximum daily dose should never exceed 50 mg/day of HCTZ or chlorothalidone or an equivalent amount of another thiazide diuretic (3).

CONCLUSIONS

Thiazide diuretics are inexpensive and provide a relatively safe way to lower blood pressure. They have been proven effective in reducing most pressure-related complications of hypertension such as stroke, congestive heart failure, renal failure, etc. (34,43,57,91,92).

A strong rationale for including thiazides in multi-drug regimens is that they have a dose-sparing effect on all other nondiuretic hypertensives. This should reduce the overall cost of therapy when compared to single drug therapy using a more expensive agent to achieve the same level of blood pressure control. Moreover, thiazides help prevent the development of pseudotolerance which may occur with some other nondiuretic agents.

Although initial cost of thiazides is less than most other antihypertensives, the cost differential narrows considerably when the expense of monitoring for thiazide-induced metabolic disturbances is considered. For example, periodic ascertainment of serum magnesium, potassium, lipid, and glucose levels add significantly to the cost of diuretics-based antihypertensive regimens. Therefore, when the cost of diuretic therapy is compared to other classes of antihypertensive agents, the expense of increased subsequent follow-up should be factored in as well as the possibility that thiazide lipid changes may be associated with more major atherosclerotic events over subsequent years of therapy; however, thiazides should continue to play a major role in the drug treatment of hypertension for the foreseeable future.

ACKNOWLEDGMENT

This work was supported in part by U.S. Public Health Service grant #09014139.

REFERENCES

1. Abdalla, I. S. H., Prineas, R. J., Neaton, J. D., Jacobs, D. J., and Crow, R. S. (1987): Relation between ventricular premature complexes and sudden cardiac death in apparently healthy men. *Am. J. Cardiol.,* 60:1036–1042.
2. Acchiardo, S. R., and Skoutakis, V. (1983): Clinical efficacy, safety, and pharmacokinetics of indapamide in renal impairment. *Am. Heart J.,* 106:237–244.
3. Alderman, M. H., Davis, T. K., and Carroll, L. (1986): Initial antihypertensive therapy: Comparison of prazosin and hypochlorothiazide. *Am. J. Med.,* 80(Suppl. 2A):120–125.
4. Ames, R. P., and Hill, P. (1976): Elevation of serum lipid levels during diuretic therapy of hypertension. *Am. J. Med.,* 61:748–757.
5. Anderson, J., Godfrey, B. E., Hill, D. M., Munro-Faure, A. D., and Sheldon, J. (1971): A comparison of the effects of hydrochlorothiazide and of furosemide in the treatment of hypertensive patients. *Quarterly Journal of Med.,* XL:541–560.
6. Anderson, J. W. (1987): Dietary fiber, lipids and atherosclerosis. *Am. J. Cardiol.,* 60:17G–22G.
7. Assman, G., And Schulte, H. (1987): The Prospective Cardiovascular Munster Study: Prevalence and prognostic significance of hyperlipidemia in men with systemic hypertension. *Am. J. Cardiol.,* 59:9G–17G.
8. Bariso, C. R., Hanenson, I. B., and Gaffney, T. E. (1970): A comparison of the antihypertensive effects of furosemide and chlorothiazide. *Curr. Ther. Res.,* 12:333–340.
9. Beling, S., Vukovich, R. A., Neiss, E. S., Zisblatt, M., Webb, E., and Losi, M. (1983): Longterm experience with indapamide. *Am. Heart J.,* 106:258–262.
10. Carlais, P. V., Materson, B. J., and Perez-Stable, E. (1984): Potassium and diuretic-induced ventricular arrhythmias in ambulatory hypertensive patients. *Miner Electrolyte Metab.,* 10:148–154.
11. Cohen, J. D., Neaton, J. D., Prineas, R. J., and Daniels, K. A. (1987): Diuretics, serum potassium and ventricular arrhythmias in the Multiple Risk Factor Intervention Trial. *Am. J. Cardiol.,* 60:548–554.
12. Conway, J., and Lauwers, P. (1960): Hemodynamic and hypertensive effects on long-term therapy with chlorothiazide. *Circulation,* 21:21–27.
13. Curb, J. D., Maxwell, M. H., Schneider, K. A., Taylor, J. O., and Shulman, N. B. (1986): Adverse effects of antihypertensive medications in the Hypertension Detection and Follow-up Program. *Prog. Cardiovasc. Dis.,* 29(Suppl. 1):73–78.
14. DeCarvalho, J. G. R., Dunn, F. G., Lohmoller, G., and Frohlich, E. D. (1977): Hemodynamic correlates of prolonged thiazide therapy: Comparison of responders and nonresponders. *Clin. Pharm. Ther.,* 22:875–880.
15. Duke, M. (1978): Thiazide-induced hypokalemia associated with acute myocardial infarction and ventricular fibrillation. *JAMA,* 239:43–45.
16. Edmonds, C. J., and Jasoni, B. (1972): Total body potassium in hypertensive patients during prolonged diuretic therapy. *Lancet,* 2:8–12.
17. Eknoyan, G. (1981): Understanding diuretic therapy. *Drug Therapy,* 11:47–58.
18. Fajans, S. S., Floyd, J. C., Knopf, R. F., Rull, J., Guntsche, E. M., and Conn, J. W. (1966): Benzothiadiazine suppression of insulin release from normal and abnormal islet tissue in man. *J. Clin. Invest.,* 45:481–502.
19. Falch, D., and Schreiner, A. (1983): The effect of spironolactone on lipid, glucose and uric acid

levels in blood during long-term administration to hypertensives. *Acta Med. Scand.*, 213:27–30.

20. Ferrannini, E., Giuseppe, B., Bonadonna, R., Giorico, M. A., Oleggini, M., Graziadei, L., Pedrinelli, R., Brandi, L., and Bevilacqua, S. (1987): Insulin resistance in essential hypertension. *N. Engl. J. Med.*, 317:350–357.

21. Ferroni, C., Raffaeli, S., Botta, G., and Paciaroni, E. (1986): Diuretic-induced hypokalemia in uncomplicated systemic hypertension: Effect of captopril on blood pressure, plasma potassium and ventricular ectopic activity (abstract). *Postgrad. Med.*, 62(Suppl. 1):131.

22. Freis, E. D. (1986): How diuretics lower blood pressure. *Am. Heart J.*, 106:185–187.

23. Freis, E. D., and Sappington, R. F. (1966): Long-term effect of probenecid on diuretic-induced hyperuricemia. *JAMA*, 198:147–149.

24. Freis, E. D., Wanko, A., Schnaper, H. W., and Frohlich, E. D. (1960): Mechanism of the altered blood pressure responsiveness produced by chlorothiazide. *J. Clin. Invest.*, 39:1277–1281.

25. Frick, M. H., Ello, O., Happa, K., Heinonen, O. P., Heinsalmi, P., Helo, P., Huttunen, J. K., Kaitaniemi, P., Koskinen, P., Manninen, V., Mäenpää, H., Mälokönen, M., Mänttäri, M., Norola, S., Pasternack, S., Pikkarainen, J., Romo, M., Sjöblom, T., and Nikkilä, E. A. (1987): Helsinki Heart Study: Primary prevention trial in middle-aged men with dyslipidemia. *N. Engl. J. Med.*, 317:1237–1245.

26. Frohlich, E. D. (1987): Diuretics in hypertension. *J. Hypertension*, 5(Suppl. 3):S43–S49.

27. Fuh, M., Shieh, S-M., Wu, D-A., Chen, Y-D., and Reaven, G. M. (1987): Abnormalities of carbohydrate and lipid metabolism in patients with hypertension. *Arch. Intern. Med.*, 147:1035–1038.

28. Goldenberg, K., Setara, J. F., Black, H. R., Moser, M., and Barnes, H. V. (1988): Potassium maintenance in hypertensive patients receiving diuretics is indicated in all cases. In: *Debates in Medicine*, edited by G. Gitnick, pp. 138–165.

29. Goldman, A. I., Steele, B. W., Schnaper, H. W., Fitz, A. E., Frohlich, E. D., and Perry, H. M. (1980): Serum lipoprotein levels during chlorthalidone therapy. *JAMA*, 244:1691–1695.

30. Grimm, R. H., Cohen, J. D., Smith, W. M., Falvo-Gefard, L., and Neaton, J. D. (1985): Hypertension management in the Multiple Risk Factor Intervention Trial (MRFIT). Six-year intervention results for men in special intervention and usual care groups. *Arch. Intern. Med.*, 145:1191–1199.

31. Grimm, R., Kofron, P., Neaton, J., Elmer, P., and Svendsen, K. (1987): Evidence for long-term adverse effects of antihypertensive drugs on lipids (abstract). *CVD Epidemiology Newsletter*, 41:15

32. Grimm, R. H., Leon, A. S., Hunninghake, D. B., Lenz, K., Hannan, P., and Blackburn, H. (1981): Effects of thiazide diuretics on plasma lipids and lipoproteins in mildly hypertensive patients. *Ann. Intern. Med.*, 94:7–11.

33. Helderman, J. H., Elahi, D., Andersen, D. K., Raizes, G. S., Tobin, J. D., Shocken, D., and Andres, R. (1983): Prevention of glucose intolerance of thiazide diuretics by maintenance of body potassium. *Diabetes*, 32:106–111.

34. Helgeland, A. (1980): Treatment of mild hypertension: A five-year controlled drug trial: The Oslo Study. *Am. J. Med.*, 69:725–732.

35. Henry, D. P., Luft, F. C., Weinberger, M. H., Fineberg, N. S., and Grim, C. E. (1980): Norepinephrine in urine and plasma following provocative maneuvers in normal and hypertensive subjects. *Hypertension*, 2:20–28.

36. Holland, O. B. (1986): Ventricular ectopic activity with diuretic-induced hypokalemia [abstract]. *Clin. Res.*, 34:480A.

37. Holland, O. B., Kuhnert, L. V., Campbell, W. B., and Anderson, R. . (1983): Synergistic effect of captopril with hydrochlorothiazide for treatment of low-renin hypertensive black patients. *Hypertension*, 5:235–239.

38. Holland, O. B., Nixon, J. V., and Kuhnert, L. (1981): Diuretic-induced ventricular ectopic activity. *Am. J. Med.*, 70:762–768.

39. Hollifield, J. W. (1986): Thiazide treatment of hypertension. Effects of thiazide diuretics on serum potassium, magnesium and ventricular ectopy. *Am. J. Med.*, 80(Suppl. 4A):8–12.

40. Hollifield, J. W., and Slaton, P. E. (1981): Thiazide diuretics, hypokalemia and cardiac arrhythmias. *Acta Med. Scand.*, 647(Suppl. 1): 67–73.

41. Holme, I., Helgeland, A., Hjermann, I., Leren, P., and Lund-Larsen, P. G., (1984): Treatment of mild hypertension with diuretics: The importance of ECG abnormalities in the Oslo Study and in MRFIT. *JAMA.*, 251:1298–1299.

42. Hulley, S. B., Furberg, C. D., Gurland, B., McDonald, R., Perry, H. M., Schnaper, H. W., Schoenberger, J. A., Smith, W. M., and Vogt, T. M. (1980): Systolic Hypertension in the Elderly Program (SHEP): Antihypertensive efficacy of chlorthalidone. *Am. J. Cardiol.*, 56:913–920.

43. Hypertension Detection and Follow-up Cooperative Group (1979): Five-year findings of the Hypertension Detection and Follow-up Program. I. Reduction in mortality of persons with high blood pressure, including mild hypertension. *JAMA.*, 242:2562–2571.

44. Iseri, L. T., Freed, J., and Bures, A. R. (1975): Magnesium deficiency and cardiac disorders. *Am. J. Med.*, 58:837–846.

45. Joint National Committee (1977): The Report of the Joint National Committee on Detection, Evaluation and Treatment of High Blood Pressure: A cooperative study. *JAMA.*, 237:255–261.

46. Joint National Committee (1988): The 1988 report of the Joint National Committee on Detection, Evaluation, and Treatment of High Blood Pressure. *Arch. Intern. Med.*, 148:1023–1038.

47. Kannel, W. B., McGee, D. L., and Schatzkin,

A. (1984): An epidemiological perspective of sudden death. 26-year follow-up in the Framingham Study. *Drugs,* 28 (Suppl. 1):1–16.

48. Kokko, J. P. (1984): Site and mechanism of action of diuretics. *Am. J. Med.,* 77 (Suppl. 5A):11–17.

49. Korbin, I., Frohlich, E. D., Ventura, H. O., and Messerli, F. H. (1986): Renal involvement follows cardiac enlargement in essential hypertension. *Arch. Intern. Med.,* 146:272–276.

50. Kuller, L. H., Hulley, S. B., Cohen, J. D., and Neaton, J. (1986): Unexpected effects of treating hypertension in men with electrocardiographic abnormalities: A critical analysis. *Circ.,* 73:114–123.

51. Lasser, N. L., Grandits, G. W., Caggiula, A. W., Cutler, J. A., Grimm, R. H., Kuller, L. H., Sherwin, R. W., and Stamler, J. (1984): Effects of anti-hypertensive therapy on plasma lipids and lipoproteins in the Multiple Risk Factor Intervention Trial. *Am. J. Med.,* 76(Suppl. 2A):51–65.

52. Leren, P. (1987): Effects of antihypertensive drugs on lipid metabolism. *Clin. Ther.,* 9:326–332.

53. Leth, A. (1970): Changes in plasma and extracellular fluid volumes in patients with essential hypertension during long-term treatment with hydrochlorothiazide. *Circulation,* 42:479–485.

54. Licht, J. H., Haley, R. J., Pugh, B., and Lewis, S. B. (1983): Diuretic regimens in essential hypertension. A comparison of hypokalemic effects, blood pressure control and cost. *Arch. Intern. Med.,* 143:1694–1699.

55. Lund-Johansen, P. (1970): Hemodynamic changes in long-term diuretic therapy of essential hypertension. *Acta. Med. Scand.,* 187:509–518.

56. Maronde, R. F., Chan, L., and Vlachakis, N. (1986): Hypokalemia in thiazide-treated systemic hypertension. *Am. J. Cardiol.,* 58:18A–21A.

57. Medical Research Council Working Party (1985): MRC trial of treatment of mild hypertension: Principal results. *Br. Med. J.,* 291:97–104.

58. Medical Research Council Working Party on Mild to Moderate Hypertension (1981): Adverse reactions to bendrofluazide and propranolol for the treatment of mild hypertension. *Lancet,* 2:539–543.

59. Melby, J. C. (1986): Selected mechanisms of diuretic-induced electrolyte changes. *Am. J. Cardiol.,* 58:1A–4A.

60. Messerli, F. H., Frohlich, E. D., Dreslinski, G. R., Suarez, D. H., and Aristimuno, G. E. (1980): Serum Uric Acid in essential hypertension: An indicator of renal vascular involvement. *Ann. Int. Med.,* 93:817–821.

61. Messerli, F. H., Nunez, B. D., Ventura, H. O., and Snyder, D. W. (1987): Overweight and sudden death. Increased ventricular ectopy in cardiopathy of obesity. *Arch. Intern. Med.,* 147:1725–1728.

62. Messerli, F. H., Ventura, H. O., and Elizardi, D. J. (1984): Hypertension and sudden death: Increased ventricular ectopic activity in left ventricular hypertrophy. *Am. J. Med.,* 77:18–22.

63. Meyer-Sabellek, W., Heitz, J., Arntz, J. R. et al. (1984): The influence of indapamide on serum lipoproteins in essential hypertension. *Methods Find. Exp. Clin. Pharmacol.,* 6:471–474.

64. Middeke, M., Weisweiler, P., Schwandt, P., and Holzgreve, H. (1987): Serum lipoproteins during antihypertensive therapy with beta blockers and diuretics: A controlled long-term comparative trial. *Clin. Cardiol.,* 10:94–98.

65. Mironneau, J. (1988): Indapamide-induced inhibition of calcium movement in smooth muscles. *Am. J. Med.,* 84(Suppl. 1B):10–14.62.

66. Moreledge, J. H. (1983): Clinical efficacy and safety of indapamide in essential hypertension. *Am. Heart J.,* 106:229–232.

67. Moser, M., Lunn, J., and Materson, B. J. (1985): Comparative effects of diltiazem and hydrochlorothiazide in blacks with hypertension. *Am. J. Cardiol.,* 56:101H–104H.

68. Multicenter Diuretic Cooperative Study Group (1981): Multiclinic comparison of amiloride, hydrochlorothiazide and hydrochlorothiazide plus amiloride in essential hypertension. *Arch. Intern. Med.,* 141:482–486.

69. Multiple Risk Factor Intervention Trial Research Group (1985): Baseline rest electrocardiographic abnormalities, antihypertensive treatment, and mortality in the multiple Risk Factor Intervention Trial. *Am. J. Cardiol.,* 55:1–15.

70. Page, E. (1955): Precipitation of ventricular arrhythmias due to digitalis by carbohydrate administration. *Am. J. Med.,* 19:169–176.

71. Papademetriou, V., Burris, J. F., Notargiacoma, A., Fletcher, R. D., and Freis, E. D. (1988): Thiazide therapy is not a cause of arrhythmia in patients with systemic hypertension. *Arch. Intern. Med.,* 148:1272–1276.

72. Papademetriou, V., Fletcher, R., Khatri, I. M., and Freis, E. D. (1983): Diuretic-induced hypokalemia in uncomplicated systemic hypertension: Effect of plasma potassium on cardiac arrhythmias. *Am. J. Cardiol.,* 52:1017–1022.

73. Pruss, T., and Wolf, P. S. (1983): Preclinical studies of indapamide, a new two-methylindoline antihypertensive diuretic. *Am. Heart J.,* 106:208–211.

74. Redleaf, P. O., and Tobian, L. (1958): The question of vascular hyperresponsiveness in hypertension. *Circ. Res.,* 6:185–193.

75. Reid, W. D., and Laragh, J. H. (1965): Sodium and potassium intake, blood pressure and pressor response to angiotensin. *Proc. Soc. Exp. Biol. Med.,* 120:26–29.

76. Resnick, L. (1986): Calcium metabolism, renin activity and the antihypertensive effects of calcium channel blockade. *Am. J. Med.,* 81(Suppl. 6A):6–14.

77. Reuben, S. R., and Thomas, R. D. (1982): The relationship between serum potassium and car-

diac arrhythmias following cardiac infarction in patients aged over 65 years. *Curr. Med. Res. Opin.,* 7(Suppl. 1):79–82.

78. Rohlfing, J. J. and Brunzell, J. D. (1986): The effects of diuretics and adrenergic-blocking agents on plasma lipids. *West. J. Med.,* 145:210–218.

79. Savage, D. D. (1987): Overall risk of left ventricular hypertrophy secondary to systemic hypertension. *Am. J. Cardiol.,* 60:8I–12I.

80. Schoenfeld, M. R. and Goldberger, E. (1964): Hypercholesterolemia induced by thiazides: A pilot study. *Curr. Ther. Res.,* 6:180–184.

81. Seller, R. H., Cangiano, J., Kim, K. E., Mendelssohn, S., Brest, A. B., and Swartz, C. (1970): Digitalis toxicity and hypomagnesemia. *Am. Heart J.,* 79:57–68.

82. Shapiro, A. P., Benedek, T. G., and Small, J. C. (1961): Effect of thiazides on carbohydrate metabolism in patients with hypertension. *N. Engl. J. Med.,* 265:1028–1033.

83. Stamler, R., Stamler, J., Gosch, F. C., Berkson, D. M., Dyer, A., and Hershinow, P. (1986): Initial antihypertensive drug therapy: Alpha blocker or diuretic. *Am. J. Med.,* 80(Suppl. 2A):90–93.

84. Stamler, R., Stamler, J., Grimm, R., Gosch, F. C., Elmer, P., Dyer, A., Berman, R., Fishman, J., Van Heel, N., Civinelli, J., and McDonald, A. (1987): Nutritional therapy for high blood pressure. Final report of a four-year randomized controlled trial—The Hypertension Control Program. *JAMA,* 257:1484–1491.

85. Steiness, E., and Olesen, K. H. (1976): Cardiac arrhythmias induced by hypokalemia and potassium loss during maintenance digoxin therapy. *Br. Heart J.,* 38:167–172.

86. Stewart, D. E., Ikram, H., Espiner, E. A., and Nicholls, M. G. (1985): Arrhythmogenic potential of diuretic-induced hypokalemia in patients with mild hypertension effects of furosemide and chlorothiazide. *Curr. Ther. Res.,* 12:333–340.

87. Talso, P. J., and Carballo, A. J. (1960): Effects of benzothiadiazines on serum and total body electrolytes. *Ann. NY Acad. Sci.,* 88:975–989.

88. Tarazi, R. C., Dustan, H. P., and Frohlich, E. D. (1970): Long-term thiazide therapy in essential hypertension evidence for persistent alteration in plasma volume and renin activity. *Circulation,* 41:709–717.

89. Gallup, G., and Cotugno, H. E. (1986): Preferences and practices of Americans and their physicians in antihypertensive therapy. *Am. J. Med.,* 81(Suppl. 6C):20–24.

90. Tobian, L. (1974): How sodium and the kidney relate to the hypertensive arteriole. *Fed. Proc.,* 33:138–142.

91. U.S. Public Health Service Hospitals Cooperative Study Group (1977): Treatment of mild hypertension. Results of a ten-year intervention trial. *Cir. Res.,* 40:I98–I105.

92. Veterans Administration Cooperative Study on Antihypertensive Agents (1970): Effects of treatment on morbidity in hypertension: II. Results of patients with diastolic pressures averaging 90 through 114 mm Hg. *JAMA,* 213:1143–1151.

93. Veterans Administration Cooperative Study Group in Antihypertensive Agents (1982): Comparison of propranolol and hydrochlorothiazide for the initial treatment of hypertension. Results of short-term titration with emphasis on racial differences in response. *JAMA,* 248:1996–2003.

94. Veterans Administration Cooperative Study Group on Antihypertensive Agents (1982): Racial differences in response to low-dose captopril are abolished by the addition of hydrochlorothiazide. *Br. J. Clin. Pharmac.* 14:97S–101S.

95. Veterans Administration Cooperative Study Group on Antihypertensive Agents (1983): Efficacy of Nadolol alone and combined with bendroflumethiazide and hydralazine for systemic hypertension. *Am. J. Cardiol.,* 52:1230–1237.

96. Weber, M. A., Lopez-Ovejero, J. A., Drayer, J. I., Case, D. B., and Laragh, J. H. (1977): Renin reactivity as a determinant of responsiveness to antihypertensive treatment. *Arch. Intern. Med.,* 137:284–289.

97. Weidmann, P., Meir, A., and Mordasini, R., et al. (1981): Diuretic treatment and serum lipoproteins: Effects of tienilic acid and indapamide. *Klin. Wocheschr.,* 59:343–346.

98. Weidmann, P., Uehlinger, D. E., and Gerber, A. (1985): Antihypertensive treatment and serum lipoproteins. *J. Hypertension,* 3:297–306.

99. Weinberger, M. H. (1982): Comparison of captopril and hyprochlorothiazide alone and in combination in mild to moderate essential hypertension. *Br. J. Clin. Pharmacol.,* 14:127S–131S.

100. Weir, M. R., and Saunders, E. (1988): Pharmacologic management of systemic hypertension in blacks. *Am. J. Cardiol.,* 61:46H–52H.

101. Whang, R., and Aikawa, J. K. (1977): Magnesium deficiency and refractoriness to potassium repletion. *J. Chron. Dis.,* 30:65–68.

102. Wilhelmsen, L., Berglund, G., Elmfeldt, D., Fitzsimons, T., Holzgreve, H., Hosie, J., Hörnkvist, P., Pennert, K., Tuomiehto, J., and Wedel, H. (1987): Beta-blockers versus diuretics in hypertensive men: Main results from the HAPPHY Trial. *J. Hypertension,* 5:561–572.

103. Wilson, P., and Kem, D. C. (1988): Indapamide. *In: Drugs for the Heart and Circulation,* edited by F. H. Messerli, W. B. Saunders, Philadelphia.

104. Wright, J. T. (1988): Profile of systemic hypertension in black patients. *Am. J. Cardiol.,* 61:41H–45H.

105. Zemel, M. B., and Sowers, J. R. (1988): Salt sensitivity and systemic hypertension in the elderly. *Am. J. Cardiol.,* 61:7H–12H.

106. Materson, B. J. (1983): Insights into intrarenal sites and mechanisms of action of diuretic agents. *Am. Heart J.,* 106:188–208.

107. Grimm, R. H., Neaton, J. D., and Prineas, R. J. (1987): Primary prevention trials and the rationale for treating mild hypertension. *Clin. Therapeutics,* 9:20–30.

New Therapeutic Strategies in Hypertension,
edited by Norman M. Kaplan,
Barry M. Brenner, and John H. Laragh.
Raven Press, Ltd., New York © 1989.

Centrally Acting Antihypertensive Agents

Michael A. Weber, William F. Graettinger, and Deanna G. Cheung

Veterans Administration Medical Center, Long Beach, California 90822 and University of California, Irvine, California

Centrally acting sympathetic nervous system inhibitors have been available since the early 1950s, and were among the first drugs used in treating hypertension. Despite the recent development of new classes of antihypertensive agents, centrally acting agents continue to have an important role in the management of hypertension. These agents effectively reduce blood pressure in a broad group of hypertensive patients, and can be administered to patients with renal insufficiency, diabetes mellitus, obstructive airway disease, and coronary artery disease. This class of drugs is widely used and well tolerated in treating mild to severe hypertension in both young and elderly patients.

While the importance of blood pressure reduction is central in the management of hypertension, there is increasing recognition that competent management should minimize symptomatic side effects and adverse metabolic changes. Additionally, optimal treatment should reduce or eliminate left ventricular hypertrophy and improve myocardial function. Centrally active antihypertensive agents have been associated with regression of left ventricular hypertrophy, and have minimal effects on glucose metabolism and the plasma lipid profile.

Side effects such as dry mouth and drowsiness appear to occur far less frequently than previously thought, as experience with lower doses of these agents has accumulated. The characteristics and use of the centrally acting agents and their use in monotherapy and in combination with other drugs will be described in this chapter.

PHARMACOLOGY OF INDIVIDUAL AGENTS

Currently available centrally acting agents include clonidine, guanabenz, guanfacine, and reserpine. These drugs work primarily by decreasing sympathetic outflow from the central nervous system, but differ in their mechanisms of action.

The growing evidence for a role of the sympathetic nervous system in mediating hypertension has been recently reviewed in detail (83). It has been claimed, for example, that plasma norepinephrine concentrations are higher in hypertensive than in normal patients, and that in hypertensive patients there is a correlation between the plasma catecholamine concentration and the blood pressure (28,84). Hypertensive patients, and individuals prone to hypertension, may have exaggerated sympathetic responses to stressful stimuli (16,29). Beyond its direct effects, the sympathetic nervous system may also influence blood pressure through its interactions with other mechanisms, such as the renin-angiotensin system, and through its effects on sodium and water balance (7,101). The centrally acting agents themselves have helped to provide further evidence supporting a role for sympathetic activity in hypertension; thus, it has been shown that there is a close correlation between the decreases in blood pressure produced by agents such as clonidine and their inhibitory effects on central and peripheral nerve tone (79).

Although these agents all influence central sympathetic outflow, there are differences between them in their actions on the peripheral components of the sympathetic nervous system and in their effects on the heart and on endocrine function. For this reason, these agents will be considered separately.

Clonidine

Although it was introduced more recently than reserpine or methyldopa, clonidine has been studied in greater detail than the other agents and has become the model upon which central nervous system mechanisms of action have been best defined (85). As with the other drugs in this group, as well as with some of the beta-blocking agents, clonidine can produce side effects such as drowsiness or dry mouth that tend to indicate an action in the central nervous system. But more specifically, when clonidine is injected directly into the intracerebral ventricles (74) or the cisterns (47) it produces decreases in blood pressure and in heart rate.

A major concept in the regulation of blood pressure by the central nervous system is that alpha-adrenergic receptors within specific neurons mediate cardiovascular events when stimulated by naturally occurring sympathomimetic substances or by exogenously administered drugs. Specifically, when these alpha receptors, which are situated in the lower brain stem in the nucleus tractus solitarii of the medulla oblongata, are activated, there is a decrease in sympathetic outflow to the cardiovascular system (88). Thus, it has been concluded that the antihypertensive action of clonidine is probably dependent upon its alpha receptor agonist properties within central nervous system which produce in-

hibitory effects on peripheral sympathetic activity. In confirmation of this idea, it has been shown that pretreatment with the alpha receptor blocking agents phentolamine will antagonize clonidine's blood pressure lowering action (8).

The alpha adrenergic stimulating properties of clonidine might produce an interesting, but opposing, effect in the peripheral circulation to that accomplished by its actions in the central nervous system. Within minutes of administering clonidine to hypertensive persons there is a small but definite increase in blood pressure. This phenomenon usually is short lived; it is soon overwhelmed by the antihypertensive effect of clonidine's action in the central nervous system. But it has been suggested that the pressor dose-response relationship in the periphery sometimes may exist for clonidine concentrations over a wider range than for clonidine's effect in the central nervous system; that is, the centrally mediated hypotensive action of clonidine might reach plateau stage while the peripheral blood pressure-raising action may continue to parallel with the increasing doses. If this concept is true, it suggests that high doses of clonidine could be counterproductive and may even have a lesser overall antihypertensive effect than lower doses.

In addition to its action at the post-synaptic alpha receptor, clonidine also has an agonist effect at the presynaptic receptor, which, by activating mechanisms that inhibit neurotransmittor release, thereby might contribute to the decrease in plasma norepinephrine concentrations found during treatment. The importance of this effect in the overall antihypertensive action of clonidine is not yet clear. However, a recent report (79) showing close correlations between both cerebrospinal and plasma norepinephrine concentrations and clonidine-induced decrements in blood pressure indicate that the primary effect of clonidine on plasma norepinephrine levels originates from its actions in the central nervous system.

As previously mentioned, sympathetic mechanisms may raise blood pressure by impairing the sensitivity of baroreflex function. Thus, the action of clonidine in the nucleus tractus solitarius of the vasomotor center may restore sensitivity to baroreflex mechanisms. Indeed, such an action of clonidine in reversing baroreceptor impairment has been shown both in hypertensive animals (50) as well as in patients with essential hypertension (32). The modest decrease in heart rate often observed with clonidine is at least partly due to direct stimulatory effects on vagal mechanisms (48,49).

The actions of clonidine on the renin-angiotensin-aldosterone system potentially could contribute to its antihypertensive properties. It is likely that the inhibition of renin release produced by clonidine is secondary to its inhibition of sympathetic activity, although it is also possible that a direct drug action within the kidney might contribute to the renin-lowering effect (66). It has been shown that there may be separate renin-dependent and renin-independent components to the antihypertensive action of clonidine. In one study using repeated measurement (8), on the first day of treatment with a low dose of clonidine in hypertensive patients, a close correlation was observed between decreases in plasma-renin activity and decreases in blood pressure. Thereafter, blood pressure continued to fall during a period of several days by a mechanism that clearly was unrelated to the effect of clonidine on renin release. Even in low-renin patients, in whom clonidine did not cause any change in plasma-renin activity, there was an appreciable fall in blood pressure. Interestingly, clonidine can cause a suppressive effect on aldosterone production that also might contribute to its antihypertensive action. This effect might be independent of changes in the renin-angiotensin system and might result directly from clonidine's central action, perhaps mediated by changes in adrenocorticotrophic hormone (ACTH) release (98).

The hemodynamic properties of clonidine are summarized and compared with the other centrally-acting agents in Table 1. During chronic administration, blood pressure and heart rate remain decreased in both the supine and erect postures (10). Despite the inhibition of sympathetic mechanisms, there is an appropriate cardiac output response during exercise in patients receiving clonidine (9). It has been speculated that the preservation of cardiovascular reflexes during clonidine treatment is due to the predominance of the central nervous system action, which allows peripheral effector mechanisms to remain virtually intact. This characteristic may help explain the particularly low incidence of orthostatic symptoms with clonidine (8,68). Renal blood flow and glomerular filtration rate are well preserved during treatment with clonidine; the decrease in renovascular resistance produced by the drug appears to compensate for any fall in renal perfusion pressure (76). Clonidine may be particularly valuable to patients with renal insufficiency; it is effective in lowering blood pressure in both severe and milder forms of hypertension associated with renal failure and does not appear to cause deterioration in the level of renal function (37,53). Because renal clearance is important in the elimination of clonidine, its dosage should be modified in accordance with glomerular filtration rate.

Clinical experience has shown clonidine to be a highly effective antihypertensive agent (71,106). The addition of a diuretic potentiates its antihypertensive effect in many patients; it has been estimated that the clonidine-diuretic combination will adequately control blood pressure in more than 70% of patients with mild to moderate hypertension (39,82). In many instances, the antihypertensive effects of clonidine can be achieved with dosages of 0.4 mg daily or less; adherence to lower dosage regimens not only minimizes side effects, but virtually eliminates the possibility of re-

Table 1. *Hemodynamic effects of centrally acting sympathetic inhibitors*

Antihypertensive agent	Cardiac output	Plasma volume	Glomerular filtration rate	Orthostasis	Total peripheral vascular resistance	Plasma renin activity
Clonidine	↓	↔	↔	−	↓	↓ or ↔
Guanabenz	↓	↔	↔	−	↓	↓ or ↔
Guanfacine	↓	↔	↔	−	↓	↓ or ↔
Methyldopa	↓	↑	↔	+	↓	↓
Reserpine	↓	↑	↓	+	↓	↓

bound problems if the treatment is precipitously discontinued. Comparative studies have shown that clonidine is at least as effective as agents such as methyldopa (61,68). It has been suggested that clonidine may be less likely than methyldopa to produce orthostatic symptoms. In other studies, clonidine has been shown to be at least as effective in lowering blood pressure as propranolol (97) or prazosin (45). The use of clonidine in combination with other antihypertensive agents is discussed below.

Table 2 lists adverse effects that may occur during treatment with clonidine. The most common side effects are drowsiness or sedation and dry mouth. These effects are seen soon after the institution of therapy but tend to decrease in severity during the first few weeks of treatment (62). Approximately 7% of patients will discontinue treatment because they consider the side effects to be intolerable (54). As discussed later, the use of clonidine in its transdermal preparation may markedly reduce the frequency and severity of unwanted symptomatic side effects.

Guanabenz

Guanabenz penetrates the central nervous system, decreases sympathetic discharge and thereby decreases blood pressure by a central mechanism (6). Studies have indicated that the action of guanabenz is mediated by stimulation of alpha receptors, by demonstrating inhibition of its effects by concurrent alpha-adrenergic blockade. Competitive binding studies using brain homogenates have indicated that guanabenz has a strong affinity for the alpha-2-subtype; this selectivity may be even greater than that observed for clonidine (24). The same studies have indicated that the affinity of guanabenz for the alpha-2 receptor is approximately 1,300-fold greater than that for the alpha-1 receptor. In hy-

Table 2. *Clinical adverse effects of centrally acting antihypertensive agents*

Effect	Reserpine	Methyldopa	Clonidine	Guanabenz	Guanfacine
Depression	+ +	r	−	−	−
Drowsiness	r	+	+ +	+ +	+
Dry mouth	−	+	+ +	+ +	+ +
Sexual dysfunction	+	+ +	+	+	+
Fluid retention	+ +	+ +	−	−	−
Weight gain	+	+	−	−	−
Headache	+	+	+	+	+
Nightmares	+ +	+	r	−	−
Nasal congestion	+ +	r	−	−	−

r = rare; + = infrequent; + + = common.

pertensive patients, the decrease in blood pressure produced by guanabenz predictably is associated by decreases in peripheral resistance. At the same time, there are only minimal changes in heart rate, myocardial contractility, or cardiac output (77). Moreover, the response of the heart to exercise does not appear to be affected by this agent.

The effects of guanabenz on renal function have been studied closely in the dog (78). In this species, guanabenz has been found to increase glomerular filtration rate and sodium excretion. There is no change in renal blood flow, but urine osmolality is decreased. The apparent increase in water excretion seems to be related to an alpha-2 specific inhibitor effect of guanabenz on the release of antidiuretic hormone. The mechanism of the increase of sodium excretion is not as well understood, but may be partly dependent on an increase in glomerular filtration rate. It also is possible that guanabenz has a direct effect on renal tubular alpha receptors that mediate sodium excretion. Experience with other centrally acting agents indicates that an inhibitory action on aldosterone production could contribute to this effect (98), although this mechanism has not yet been studied directly with guanabenz. Experience with guanabenz in human subjects has indicated that it has relatively little effect on renal function. Importantly, long-term treatment with this agent does not cause retention of sodium or water, and does not appear to produce changes in plasma or blood volume (4,30). Clinically, weight gain and edema do not occur. This characteristic of guanabenz enables it to be considered for single-agent therapy of mild to moderate hypertension.

As would be predicted with an agent that inhibits sympathetic outflow, it has been established that guanabenz decreases plasma concentrations of catecholamines and dopamine β-hydroxylase activity (5,105). It has also been shown that the greatest decreases in catecholamines occur in those patients whose resting catecholamines levels are highest, suggesting that hypertension characterized by increased sympathetic activity is particularly susceptible to this form of treatment (20). This study has also shown that guanabenz attenuates the increases in plasma concentrations of both norepinephrine and epinephrine during exercise, whereas clonidine seems to diminish only the concentrations of norepinephrine. Thus, it is possible that these two agents might have differing effects on adrenomedullary responsiveness to sympathetic stimuli. Guanabenz also has a modest inhibitory effect on plasma renin activity. Although there is little change in renin values in low-renin hypertensive patients during guanabenz treatment, most patients with normal or high-renin values tend to have decreases in plasma-renin activity during treatment.

The metabolic effects of guanabenz may be of clinical relevance. It has been shown to reduce serum concentrations of total cholesterol (90,91), sometimes by as much as 10 percent. The decrease appears to be due primarily to a reduction in the low density lipoprotein fraction (44), and it has also been reported that triglyceride concentrations may be reduced. These effects may be related, at least in part, to direct actions of the drug on hepatic synthesis and on fatty acid oxidation (13). Guanabenz does not appear to influence glucose metabolism (21,91). Measurements of insulin, glucogen, and growth hormone remain unchanged during chronic treatment with this agent (21). Moreover, in a multicenter study in diabetic hypertensive patients, we found that no changes in diabetic therapy were necessitated by concurrent antihypertensive therapy with guanabenz (96).

Guanfacine

Guanfacine is a centrally acting agent with characteristics essentially resembling those of clonidine and guanabenz. Recently available for clinical use in the United States, its once-daily efficacy may add to its acceptance in the clinical setting. Preliminary studies in animal models have documented that guanfacine, like clonidine, is an alpha-adrenergic agonist in both the central nervous system and the peripheral arterial circulation. Low-dose infusions in the dog have shown that whereas intravenous guanfacine produced no consistent hemodynamic effect, administration directly into the vertebral artery produced marked blood pressure-lowering responses. Moreover, these effects were prevented by pretreatment with phentolamine (75). Guanfacine also has been shown to decrease sympathetic outflow from the central nervous system as measured directly in studies of sympathetic nerve flow (89). This agent slightly slows the heart rate, presumably through its facilitation of reflex bradycardia (57). It produces the expected transitory pressor responses when given to the pithed rat (75); these effects can be blocked by phentolamine, yohimbine, and prazosin (46,63). However, guanfacine has a far greater selectivity for the alpha II adrenergic receptor than the alpha-1 receptor (52).

Guanfacine produces strong antihypertensive effects (72) in hypertensive patients. There are concomitant decreases in plasma concentrations of catecholamines and renin activity, but the relationship between these changes and those in blood pressure have not been directly established (72). Other metabolic changes include decreases in serum prolactin, but not in growth hormone (34). The plasma lipid concentrations, including total cholesterol and triglycerides, also are slightly decreased; there appears to be no change in glucose metabolism as judged by glucose tolerance tests (34). Hemodynamically, guanfacine works primarily by decreasing peripheral resistance. Interestingly, it also appears to reduce right atrial pressure, suggesting that it may be a useful agent in patients with ventricular dysfunction in whom a reduction in preload may be of value (72).

Studies with guanfacine as antihypertensive monotherapy have established its efficacy used once-daily, most typically in doses of 1 mg (23,80,103). It has been found to be significantly more effective than placebo in decreasing blood pressure, and to have efficacy similar to that of guanabenz. In these studies it did not alter measurements of plasma volume, emphasizing its potential suitability as a single agent for the treatment of hypertension. However, guanfacine also has been shown to be highly effective when used as a second-line agent, in addition to pretreatment with a diuretic. When added to chlorthalidone (56), it has been shown to produce significant further decrements in blood pressure. Interestingly, this effect of guanfacine occurs in a very narrow dosage range: 0.5 mg daily was found not to be more effective than placebo, whereas doses of 2 to 3 mg daily were no more effective than just 1 mg daily. This study, as well as a further wide-scale multicenter experience (104), emphasized that the incidence of significant symptomatic adverse effects was low, and that only a very small percentage of patients voluntarily discontinued treatment. As with all drugs of this type, sudden discontinuation of treatment with guanfacine results in an increase in blood pressure, but the rate of rise is less than that observed with clonidine (104). A large multinational study, conducted primarily in Europe, has confirmed the efficacy and good side-effect profile of guanfacine when administered in low doses. This experience has documented the use of this agent, either alone or in combination with a variety of other drugs, for up to 7 years, and has reported that antihypertensive efficacy and patient acceptance of guanfacine appears to be sustained during chronic administration (40).

Methyldopa

As with clonidine, methyldopa, which has been available for general use since 1963, appears to produce its antihypertensive action through its effects in the central nervous system. Injections of small doses of methyldopa directly into the vertebral artery or into the cerebral ventricle produce reductions in arterial blood pressure. It is likely that the antihypertensive action of methyldopa is dependent on stimulation of alpha-adrenergic receptors that are probably located in the nucleus tractus solitarii of the medulla. In confirmation of this idea that an alpha agonist mechanism is involved, the antihypertensive action of methyldopa can be blocked by pretreatment with the alpha-blocking agents phentolamine (86). The activation of these receptors is not directly by methyldopa itself, but by its metabolite alpha-methylnorepinephrine, which is formed within the brain. Indeed, inhibition of dopamine-β-hydroxylase, which is an essential factor in the formation of alpha-methylnorepinephrine, decreases the antihypertensive efficacy of methyldopa (15). Injection of the metabolite directly into the cerebral ventricle produces decreases in blood pressure that actually are greater than those produced by methyldopa itself (35).

Actions of methyldopa in the periphery also may contribute to its antihypertensive effect. The false neurotransmitter theory was long considered the best explanation for methyldopa's antihypertensive action. It has been shown that methyldopa and its metabolite, alpha-methylnorepinephrine, like norepinephrine, are taken up by the adrenergic nerve endings. At neuronal discharge, alpha-methylnorepinephrine is released together with the native norepinephrine and competes with it at the postsynaptic alpha-adrenergic receptor. It is likely that alpha methylnorepinephrine is less potent than norepinephrine in producing vasoconstrictor effects when interacting with the alpha receptor, and therefore causes an overall reduction in vascular tone and blood pressure. In animal studies, however, this mechanism has not been consistently verified (33), and it has not been com-

pletely possible to be certain that the antihypertensive action of methyldopa is due directly to the generation of alpha-methylnorepinephrine (87).

It has been postulated that methyldopa may also interfere with the biosynthesis of norepinephrine. Methyldopa may inhibit the enzyme dopa decarboxylase that is responsible for the formation of dopamine from dopa and is a necessary part of the production of the final neurotransmittor, norepinephrine. Although inhibition of norepinephrine appears to be an effective way to reduce blood pressure, it now seems less likely that methyldopa works through this mechanism, for while the racemic (DL) preparation of methyldopa is required for the full antihypertensive action (26), only the L isomer poses decarboxylation properties (67). As with clonidine, methyldopa also has an inhibitory effect on renin release. Although this mechanism has not been highly studied, it has been shown that the antirenin action of methyldopa can potentially play a part during its use as single-agent therapy (102) or in combination with a diuretic (43).

The hemodynamic effects of methyldopa are summarized in Table 1. During chronic treatment there is a decrease in total peripheral resistance with a maintenance of cardiac output at base-line levels (65). Although there is a tendency for blood pressure to be decreased to a greater extent in the standing than in the supine posture, this orthostatic effect is less than that seen with peripheral adrenergic blockers such as guanethidine (64). Like clonidine, the antihypertensive action of methyldopa is not associated with decreases in glomerular filtration rate or renal blood flow, factors that enhance the usefulness of this agent in patients with renal insufficiency (11).

The maximum antihypertensive effect of methyldopa occurs approximately 6 hours after an oral dose, and some antihypertensive effectiveness may persist for up to 48 hours. As single-agent therapy, methyldopa controls blood pressure in up to 70% of patients with mild hypertension and is also effective in patients with more severe forms of hypertension (41). The addition of a diuretic to methyldopa adds considerable antihypertensive effect: approximately two-thirds of patients with mild, moderate, or severe hypertension can have their blood pressure normalized with this combination. Since methyldopa given alone frequently causes compensatory retention of salt and water (which then decreases its long-term antihypertensive effectiveness), it has become customary for this agent to be given in combination with a diuretic. Moreover, the addition of the diuretic often enables blood pressure control to be obtained with relatively modest doses of each drug.

The most common adverse effect with methyldopa, as shown in Table 2, is drowsiness or excessive sedation; this is troublesome in approximately one-quarter of all patients. The drowsiness will usually diminish with continued use of the drug. Less well defined problems with mentation, including difficulty in concentrating and amnesia-like episodes, and difficulties in calculation or the retention of newly obtained information, also may occur (1). Postural dizziness is seen in about 15% of patients taking methyldopa. Dry mouth, sexual disfunction, and gastrointestinal upsets also are seen occasionally. Approximately 5 to 10% of patients will be forced to discontinue treatment with methyldopa because of adverse effect.

Methyldopa has been associated with the development of a positive direct Coomb's test, hemolytic anemia, hepatitis, or drug fever. The positive direct Coomb's reaction occurs in approximately 25% of patients taking methyldopa; the antibody is directed against Rh locus, not against the drug (51). However, only about 5% of patients with a Coomb's reaction (that is, less than 1% of all patients given methyldopa) will actually develop hemolytic anemia. A form of hepatitis indistinguishable from viral hepatitis occurs in approximately 2% of patients receiving methyldopa. This phenomenon is manifested by elevated liver enzymes and requires termination of the methyldopa treatment. Usually the liver function chemistries will return to normal after the drug has been stopped (22). Drug fever, either with or without associated liver findings, occurs in approximately 1% of patients receiving this drug (27). It is advised that methyldopa not be given to patients with a history of liver disease or hypersensitivity to the drug.

Despite these rate adverse effects, methyldopa has for a long time represented a palatable and effective form of antihypertensive therapy. Its future role will become clearer as it is compared with newer types of antihypertensive agents. Recently, this agent was a principal form of treatment in a major clinical trial of the benefits of antihypertensive therapy in the elderly (2); the positive findings of this study, as discussed elsewhere in this volume, have again emphasized that this long-available agent may still have an important role to play in the management of clinical hypertension.

Reserpine

Despite the effects it exerts at other sites, reserpine clearly has important central mechanisms of action. It depletes norepinephrine and serotonin stores in the brain and in peripheral adrenergic nerve endings. In animal studies, tissue catecholamine concentrations begin to fall 1 hour after administration of reserpine and reach their nadir by 24 hours. There are two mechanisms postulated by which this effect could be achieved. First, it has been suggested that reserpine enhances the degradation of norepinephrine by blocking its incorporation into protective chromaffin granules. Second, it is possible that reserpine blocks the uptake of dopamine into the storage granules in which it would be converted to norepinephrine (73). Within the central nervous system, these actions of reserpine presumably occur in the vasomotor center in the medulla oblongata and also in the hypothalamus (59).

Despite the importance of its action in the central nervous system, reserpine works in a fashion different from that postulated for clonidine, guanabenz, or methyldopa; it appears to have an inhibitory effect on adrenergic mechanisms rather than the agonist action suggested for the other agents. However, centrally determined side effects such as drowsiness and sedation occur as frequently with reserpine as with the other agents. There also appears to be an increase in vagal tone similar to that produced by clonidine, a factor which may explain the decrease in heart rate seen with reserpine (14). There is an increase in gastric acid secretion during reserpine treatment that also may be mediated through an increase in vagal tone. The cardiovascular effects of reserpine are summarized in Table 1, and its adverse effects in Table 2. Reserpine remains an effective antihypertensive drug, is inexpensive, and has the convenience of once-daily dosage. Concern about some of its adverse effects has resulted, however, in a gradual decrease in its use during the last few years.

CLINICAL EFFECTS OF CENTRALLY ACTING ANTIHYPERTENSIVE AGENTS

Among the wide range of antihypertensive agents currently available, the selection of a particular drug may be a matter of personal preference or experience of the prescribing physician. Table 3 summarizes the dose regimens of the currently available centrally acting agents. The centrally acting agents continue to play an important role in antihypertensive therapy because of their generally safe profile and effectiveness. These agents are effective in a wide range of patients (Table 4). While they tend to have slightly more symptomatic side effects than are found with newer types of agents, such as the converting enzyme inhibitors or the calcium channel blockers, a growing experience with the centrally acting drugs has indicated that their use in low dosages will minimize unwanted side effects without causing substantial decreases in efficacy. Moreover, these agents are effective and safe in treating hypertension when it occurs together with a number of other disorders (Table 5). This comparison suggests that there are circumstances where the centrally acting drugs might be preferable. Moreover, a major clinical trial, recently completed in the United Kingdom by the Medical Research Council, with a diuretic and a beta blocker suggested that the incidence of adverse effects with these types of drugs was comparatively high (58).

The centrally acting agents can be used at virtually any stage of a stepped-care approach to the treatment of hypertension. As previously discussed, these agents work well in combination with diuretics. Such a combination can allow good results to be

Table 3. *Dosages of centrally acting antihypertensive agents*

	Starting dose (mg)	Recommended range (mg)	Maximum dose (mg)	Usual regimen
Clonidine	0.1	0.1–0.4	1.2	b.i.d.
Guanabenz	4	4–16	32	b.i.d.
Guanfacine	1.0	1.0–3.0	3.0	q.d.
Methyldopa	250	250–1,000	1,500	b.i.d.
Reserpine	0.1	0.1–0.25	0.25	q.d.

The dose should be divided as indicated by the usual regimen employed. Lower starting doses can be employed, especially in elderly patients or when used in combination therapy.

Table 4. *Clinical range of three types of antihypertensive agents*

Demographic group	Centrally-acting agents	β-blockers	Diuretics
Black patients	Effective	Less effective	Less effective
White patients	Effective	Effective	Less effective
Young patients	Effective	Effective	Less effective
Elderly patients	Effective	Less effective	Less effective

achieved with comparatively low doses of the agents employed. These agents also work well in combination with vasodilators such as hydralazine or minoxidil. For example, it has been shown that clonidine is at least as effective as propranolol when given together with hydralazine and a diuretic in patients with more severe forms of hypertension (60). In patients with treatment-resistant hypertension it also has been found that the superimposition of clonidine on complex multidrug antihypertensive regimens can be highly effective in inducing blood pressure control (53).

The combination of clonidine or other centrally acting agents with the beta-blocking agent propranolol (Table 6) is synergistic, and results in decreases in blood pressure fall greater than with either agent given alone (97). This suggests that these two types of agents have differing antihypertensive mechanisms; whereas the antirenin action of propranolol (together with its other as-yet-poorly-understood mechanisms of action) contributes importantly to its blood pressure-lowering activity (12), clonidine, while also exhibiting part of its antihypertensive action through its renin-lowering effect, works largely through inhibition of sympathetic activity. Interestingly, the heart rate-lowering effects of these two agents also are additive. Propranolol presumably works through its direct inhibitory action on the heart, whereas clonidine lowers heart rate through its enhancement of vagal tone.

It is also of interest to consider the interaction of clonidine with the alpha-adrenergic blocking agent prazosin (Table 5). The sites of the principal antihypertensive actions of these 2 agents are different; clonidine works chiefly within the central nervous system, whereas prazosin works at the peripheral postsynaptic alpha-adrenergic receptor. Despite this difference, both agents ultimately have the same effect, which is blocking the vasoconstriction produced when the sympathetic nervous system, through its neurotransmitter norepinephrine, stimulates the postsynaptic alpha-adrenergic receptor. Thus, it is not surprising that it has been found that the addition of prazosin in patients already being treated with clonidine fails to bring

Table 5. *Clinical effects of three types of antihypertensive therapy*

Condition	Centrally acting agents	β-blockers	Diuretics
Concurrent diabetes mellitus	Safe and effective	Caution with insulin-taking patients	May influence concurrent diabetes therapy
Hypercholesterolemia	Improved	Possibly worsened	Possibly worsened
Adverse metbolic changes	None or rare	None or rare	Potassium and several other factors influenced
Exercise tolerance	No change	Decrease	Decrease
Left ventricular abnormalities	Potential improvement	Inconsistent or no change	No change

Table 6. *Blood pressure values (mean ± SEM) in crossover studies*[a]

Treatment	Systolic blood pressure (mm Hg)	Diastolic blood pressure (mm Hg)
Control	158 ± 7	100 ± 3
Clonidine alone	142 ± 5[b]	92 ± 3[b]
Prazosin alone	144 ± 5	94 ± 1[b]
Clonidine + prazosin	143 ± 8[b]	93 ± 6[b]
Control	166 ± 5	109 ± 2
Clonidine alone	149 ± 3[b]	96 ± 3[b]
Propranolol alone	149 ± 5[b]	100 ± 3[b]
Clonidine + propranolol	146 ± 7[b]	93 ± 3[b]

[a] Comparison of clonidine (0.3 mg a day) with prazosin (15 mg a day) (n = 13); clonidine (0.3 mg a day) with propranolol (120 mg a day) (n = 8), or a combination of these agents.

[b] $p < 0.05$ or better when compared with control value.

All measurements were in the seated position.

about further antihypertensive effects (38). It is likely that the central action of clonidine (and presumably of guanabenz or methyldopa) in suppressing sympathetic outflow is so effective that there is virtually no peripheral sympathetic vascular drive remaining to be blocked by the prazosin action. A further unproductive combination is that between reserpine and guanethidine; however, because each of these agents is now used infrequently, the likelihood of this combination is small.

Occasionally, the sudden cessation of treatment with the centrally acting agents can provoke a rapid rise in blood pressure to its pretreatment values, or to even higher levels. This effect, sometimes described as a discontinuation syndrome, has been described in detail elsewhere in this volume (93). When given in combination with beta-blocking agents, it is wise to gradually withdraw the beta blocker before discontinuing the centrally-acting agent.

ALTERNATIVE DELIVERY SYSTEMS

Clonidine may be administered transdermally using a small skin-colored patch that contains sufficient drug to provide treatment for seven days at a time. Three differing sizes of this device are available, providing, respectively, 0.1 mg, 0.2 mg, or 0.3 mg clonidine per day. The skin patches are water resistant, adhere well to the skin, and allow patients to undertake a full range of physical activities while wearing them.

Transdermal clonidine has pharmacokinetic characteristics which underlie its main potential advantages as an antihypertensive therapy. After the skin patch is first applied it takes from 2 to 3 days for the clonidine to reach its stable plasma concentration owing to an initial period of skin sequestration of the drug. Once the clonidine has reached its plateau level, it remains constant on a relatively permanent basis. When one patch is removed (after approximately 1 week), the clonidine disappears only slowly from the plasma owing to the accumulated drug in the skin reservoir. Thus, when a new patch is administered, typically at another site, it starts providing sufficient clonidine so that, together with the residual drug from the previous patch, the plasma-drug concentration remains constant. The actual amount of clonidine able to pass through the skin varies slightly according to the location used; the most practical and effective areas appear to be the chest or the upper outer arm.

The evenness of the plasma-clonidine concentrations during transdermal therapy result in a significant decrease in patient perceptions of side effects. When conventional oral medications are used their plasma concentrations tend to reach high-peak concentrations soon after the tablets are ingested; thereafter, there is a steady decline in plasma concentration to the trough level that immediately precedes administration of the next tablet. It is likely that symptomatic side effects associated with drug administration are associated with the peak plasma concentrations. Thus, it is not surprising that when transdermal clonidine has been substituted for the oral form of the agent, there has been a marked reduction in the incidence of symptomatic side effects (94).

Skin reactions constitute the most common complaint with the transdermal clonidine preparation. They usually occur between 3 weeks and 9 months of the start of treatment. Up to 20% of patients treated with this device complain of a localized reaction that typically occurs under the patch itself. This reaction can vary from a mild nonspecific superficial irritation to a localized allergic response. Occasionally, this latter reaction can be associated with formation of small vesicles or superficial ulcerations. Regardless of the type of reaction, cessation of treatment is associated with disappearance of the skin lesion. If the skin reaction is not severe, patients may elect to continue treatment; there have been no reports of systemic or generalized reactions to this form of treatment that are of clinical concern. Moreover, subsequent challenging of patients who have experienced allergic reactions to the skin patch with large oral doses of clonidine have reactivated the skin responses in only one or two instances; again, cessation of the treatment resulted in rapid disappearance of these manifestations. Patients most likely to incur a skin reaction are those with very fair skin; it is also possible that women are slightly more susceptible than men.

Multiple clinical trials with transdermal clonidine have shown its efficacy across the full demographic spectrum of hypertensive patients (99). It has been found to work well in elderly patients as well as in the young, and to be equally effective in black and white patients. Moreover, it works well in patients with renal insufficiency and in those with diabetes mellitus. As with other forms of antihypertensive therapy, it is effective as monotherapy in approximately 60% of patients with mild to moderate essential hypertension.

The most significant advantage of transdermally administered clonidine is its con-

Table 7. *Transdermal clonidine therapy in patients switched from treatment with oral antihypertensive agents*

Response	Patients (%)	Physicians (%)
Highly satisfied	46	43
Satisfied	32	36
Indifferent or dissatisfied	20	20
Highly dissatisfied	2	1

Results were obtained in 3,059 patients and 451 physicians responding to questionnaires concerning transdermal clonidine therapy.
From ref. 36, with permission.

venience and avoidance of generalized side effects. Table 6 summarizes physician and patient evaluations of this form of treatment as compared with previous forms of antihypertensive therapy. In this surveillance of more than 3,000 patients (36) there is clearly a strong acceptance of this newer form of treatment (Table 7). The attraction of taking medication on a once-weekly basis appears to be strong, allowing patients to go for long periods of time without being reminded of their requirements for medical support. It is also of practical value in some older or infirm patients who are unable for physical or emotional reasons to be responsible for taking their medications. The administration of this treatment can be easily undertaken in such individuals by relatives or other personnel. Overall, the interesting characteristics of this innovative form of therapy should make it attractive in a substantial proportion of hypertensive patients. Where unwanted side effects, poor compliance, or inadequate results have occurred with conventional forms of treatment, the transdermal clonidine preparation might offer a good alternative for achieving satisfactory and well tolerated control of blood pressure.

CENTRAL ADRENERGIC AGENTS IN TREATING ELDERLY PATIENTS

Because the centrally acting antihypertensive agents inhibit sympathetic mechanisms, they are appropriate forms of therapy for older hypertensive patients. There has been an extensive experience with clonidine in treating elderly patients. Both the oral and the transdermal form of this agent effectively decrease the predominantly systolic hypertension found in this age group. This antihypertensive effect has been shown to occur without producing unwanted changes in cerebral blood flow (69). In an earlier study in patients with predominantly systolic hypertension, it was found that effective antihypertensive effects could be produced by low doses of clonidine administered in combination with the diuretic chlorthalidone (31). Moreover, these results were achieved in a majority of patients with a single nighttime dosage, thereby adding to the convenience of the treatment and minimizing its potential symptomatic side effects.

A large-scale analysis of treatment with guanabenz in the elderly also has been carried out (95). Approximately 50% of these patients, aged 61 to 76 years, had decreases in systolic blood pressure of at least 20 mm Hg when treated with guanabenz alone; similar results were found in patients receiving a combination of guanabenz and hydrochlorothiazide. As with clonidine, this agent was found to be generally well tolerated by the patients. Recently, methyldopa was used in a large-scale European study of the long-term benefits of treating hypertension in the elderly. In these subjects, whose age averaged 72 years, and who were followed for up to 7 years, the combination of a diuretic with methyldopa produced sustained antihypertensive effects (2). Of even greater importance, major cardiovascular events and cardiovascular mortality were decreased by approximately 40% in patients receiving these active medications, as compared with those receiving only placebo. Thus, a significant number of studies indicate that the centrally-acting antihypertensive agents might be particularly appropriate as antihypertensive therapy in elderly subjects.

THE EFFECT OF CENTRALLY ACTING AGENTS ON LEFT VENTRICULAR STRUCTURE

Left ventricular hypertrophy is a common complication of hypertension. It may constitute a risk factor independent of the increased blood pressure (42). The level of blood pressure itself, the associated increase in cardiac work, the effects of the renin angiotensin system, and increased age may all contribute to the establishment of left ventricular hypertrophy. However, there is strong evidence that the sympathetic nervous system is a predominant cause of left ventricular muscular hypertrophy. Norepinephrine has been shown to produce hypertrophy independently of other humoral or hemodynamic factors. Moreover, studies in spontaneously hypertensive rats have shown that left ventricular mass correlates with plasma norepinephrine concentrations, and that sympathetic blockade can produce regression of hypertrophy (81). These changes produced by sympatholytic agents were found to be independent of their effects on blood pressure, whereas vasodilators were found to be ineffective in reversing left ventricular hypertrophy despite their ability to decrease blood pressure (81). For this reason, there has been a growing interest in the use of the centrally acting antihypertensive agents in patients whose hypertension may be associated with hypertrophic changes of the muscle of the left ventricle.

Methyldopa has been found to be particularly effective in producing regression of echocardiographically measured hypertrophy. In studies in which diuretics failed to cause changes in left ventricular muscle mass despite clear falls in blood pressure, addition of methyldopa produced clear regression of the hypertrophy (25,70). Moreover, methyldopa has been found to produce significant reductions in left ventricular muscle mass as well as in the thickness of the interventricular septum and the

Table 8. *Atrial emptying index in hypertensive subjects before and after 16 weeks of therapy*

	Baseline	Treatment	Significance
Clonidine (n = 6)	0.40	0.48	p < 0.05
Propranolol (n = 5)	0.47	0.46	NS

From ref. 100, with permission.

left ventricular posterior wall even in patients in whom it has not been effective in decreasing blood pressure (17). When used as monotherapy, it is likely that the centrally acting agents are even more effective in producing regression of left ventricular hypertrophy than when added to a diuretic (18). This property has also been demonstrated for guanabenz in patients with left ventricular hypertrophy (92). Clonidine has been shown to produce decreases in muscle mass both when used in combination with a low-dose diuretic (55) or when given as a single agent (3). Moreover, functional changes may occur. Table 8 shows average values for left atrial emptying index (AEI) in patients treated with either propranolol or clonidine (100). AEI is quantified echocardiographically as the proportion of posterior motion of the posterior aortic echogram that occurs during the first third of diastole. It measures early diastolic emptying of the atrium and thus is related to the early filling characteristics of the left ventricle (19). The data in Table 8 thus suggest that clonidine treatment may actually enhance cardiac diastolic function in hypertensive patients.

SUMMARY

Centrally acting antihypertensive agents constitute an important class of clinically useful drugs in the contemporary treatment of hypertension. Their broad range of efficacy and safety in hypertensive patients allows their use in treating patients with concurrent conditions such as renal insufficiency, ischemic heart disease, chronic obstructive lung disease, and diabetes mellitus. The apparent absence of adverse metabolic effects along with possible improvements in plasma-lipid profiles during therapy with these drugs are particularly advantageous in treating patients at high risk for progression of atherosclerosis. In addition, this class of agents appears to induce regression of left ventricular hypertrophy and may improve left ventricular diastolic function. Symptomatic side effects, primarily dry mouth and drowsiness, constitute the major limitations associated with the use of these drugs. However, the side effects can be minimized by using lower total daily doses, or by administrating the drug nocturnally, or via a transdermal system which releases the drug at a slow rate. Used alone or in combination with other agents, centrally acting antihypertensive agents represent a form of therapy with significant advantages in the treatment of hypertension in a broad range of clinical situations.

REFERENCES

1. Adler, S. (1974): Methyldopa-induced decrease in mental activity. *JAMA*, 230:1428.
2. Amery, A., Birkenhager, W., Brixko, P., Bulpitt, C., Clement, D., Deruyttere, M., De Schaepdryver, A., Dollery, C., Fagard, R., Forette, F., Forte, J., Hamdy, R., Henry, J. F., Joossens, J. V., Leonetti, G., Lund-Johansen, P., O'Malley, K., Petrie, J., Strasser, T., Tuomilehto, J., and Williams, B. (1985): Mortality and morbidity results from the European Working Party on high blood pressure in the elderly trial. *Lancet*, 1(8442):1349.
3. Arevalo, J. V. (1983): Clonidine and left ventricular function in patients with arterial hypertension. *Tribuna Medica*, 68:29.
4. Bauer, J. H. (1983): Effects of guanabenz therapy on renal function and body fluid composition. *Arch. Intern. Med.*, 143:1163.
5. Bauer, J. H., and Burch, R. N. (1983): Comparative studies: Guanabenz versus propranolol as first-step therapy for the treatment of primary hypertension. *Cardiovasc. Rev. Rep.*, 4:9.
6. Baum, T., Shropshire, A. T. (1976): Studies on the centrally mediated hypotensive activity of guanabenz. *Eur. J. Pharmacol.*, 37:31.
7. Bickerton, R. K., and Buckley, J. P. (1961): Evi-

dence for a central mechanism in angiotensin induced hypertension. *Proceed. Soc. Exper. Biol. Med.*, 106:834.

8. Bolme, P., and Fuxe, K. (1971): Pharmacologic studies on the hypotensive effects of clonidine. *Eur. J. Pharmacol.*, 13:168.

9. Brest, A. N. (1980): Hemodynamic and cardiac effects of clonidine. *J. Cardiovasc. Pharmacol.*, 2(Suppl. 1):39.

10. Brod, J., Horbach, L., and Just, H. (1972): Acute effects of clonidine on central and peripheral hemodynamics and plasma renin activity. *Eur. J. Clin. Pharmacol.*, 4:107.

11. Brodwall, E. K., Myrhe, E., Stenbaek, O., and Hansen, T. (1966): The effect of methyldopa on renal function in patients with renal insufficiency. *Acta Med. Scand.*, 191:339.

12. Buhler, F. R., Laragh, J. H., Baer, L., and Sealey, J. (1972): Propranolol inhibition or renin secretion. *New. Engl. J. Med.*, 287:1209.

13. Capuzzi, D. M., and Cevallos, W. H. (1984): Inhibition of hepatic cholesterol and triglyceride synthesis by guanabenz acetate. *J. Cardiovasc. Pharmacol.*, 6:s847–s852.

14. Cohen, S. I., Young, M. W., and Lau, S. H. (1968): Effects of reserpine therapy on cardiac output and atrioventricular conduction during rest and controlled heart rates in patients with essential hypertension. *Circulation*, 37:738.

15. Day, M. D., Roach, A. G., and Whiting, R. L. (1973): The mechanisms of the antihypertensive action of alpha-methyldopa in hypertensive rats. *Eur. J. Pharmacol.*, 21:271.

16. Doyle, A. E., and Fraser, J. R. E. (1961): Essential hypertension and inheritance of vascular reactivity. *Lancet*, 11:509.

17. Drayer, J. I. M., Gardin, J. M., and Weber, M. A. (1982): Changes in cardiac anatomy and function during therapy with alpha-methyldopa: An echocardiographic study. *Curr. Ther. Res.*, 32:856.

18. Drayer, J. I. M., Weber, M. A., and Gardin, J. M. (1984): Mediators of changes in left ventricular mass during antihypertensive therapy. In: *Cardiac LVH*, edited by H. E. D. J. Keurs and J. J. Schipperheyn, p. 224. Martinus Nijhoff, Boston.

19. Dreslinski, G. R., Frolich, E. D., Dunn, F. G., Messerli, F. H., Suarez, D. H., and Reisin, E. (1981): Echocardiographic diastolic ventricular abnormality in hypertensive heart disease: Atrial emptying index. *Am. J. Cardiol.*, 47:1087.

20. Dziedzic, S. W., Elijovich, F., Felton, K., Yeager, K., and Krakoff, L. R. (1983): Effect of guanabenz on blood pressure response to posture and exercise. *Clin. Pharmacol. Ther.*, 33:151.

21. Eldridge, J. C., Strandhoy, J., and Buckalew, V. M., Jr. (1984): Endocrinologic effects of antihypertensive therapy with guanabenz or hydrochlorothiazide. *J. Cardiovasc. Pharmacol.*, 6:s776–s780.

22. Elkington, S. G., Schreiber, W. M., and Conn, H. O. (1969): Hepatic injury caused by L-alphamethyldopa. *Circulation*, 40:589.

23. Fillingim, J. M., Blackshear, J. L., Strauss, A., and Strauss, M. (1986): Guanfacine as monotherapy for systemic hypertension. *Am. J. Cardiol.*, 57:50E–54E.

24. Fluck, E. R., Homan, C. A., Knowles, J. A., and Ruelius, H. W. (1983): Differential binding of guanabenz and its metabolites to cerebral alpha-2 receptors. *Drug Develop. Res.*, 3:91.

25. Fouad, F. M., Nahashima, Y., and Tarazi, R. C., et al. (1983): Differential binding of guanabenz and its metabolites to cerebral alpha-2 receptors. *Drug. Dev. Res.*, 3:91.

26. Gillespie, L. Jr., Oates, J. A., Crout, J. R., and Sjoersdma, A. (1962): Clinical and chemical studies with alpha-methyldopa in patients with hypertension. *Circulation*, 25:281.

27. Glontz, G. E., and Saslow, S. (1968): Methyldopa fever. *Arch. Int. Med.*, 122:445.

28. Goldstein, D. S. (1980): Plasma catecholamines in essential hypertension: An analytical review. *Hypertension*, 5:86.

29. Goldstein, D. S., Lake, C. R., Chernow, B., Ziegler, M. G., Coleman, M. D., Taylor, A. A., Mitchell, J. R., Kopin, I. J., and Keiser, H. R. (1983): Age-dependence of hypertensive-normotensive differences in plasma norepinephrine. *Hypertension*, 5:100.

30. Golub, M. S., Eggena, P., Barrett, J. D., Thananopavarn, C., and Sambhi, M. P. (1982): Fluid volumes during antihypertensive therapy with guanabenz in mild hypertension. *Clin. Pharmacol. Ther.*, 2:230.

31. Gray, D. R., Weber, M. A., and Drayer, J. I. M. (1983): Effects of low-dose antihypertensive therapy in elderly patients with predominant systolic hypertension. *J. Gerontol.*, 38:302.

32. Guthrie, A., Jr., and Kotchen, T. A. (1983): Effects of oral clonidine on baroreflex function in patients with essential hypertension. *Chest*, 83(Suppl.):327.

33. Haefely, W., Hurlimann, A., and Thoeneu, H. (1966): The effect of stimulation of sympathetic nerves in the cat treated with reserpine, alphamethyldopa, and alpha-methylmetatyrosine. *Br. J. Pharmacol.*, 26:172.

34. Hauger-Klevene, J. H., Balossi, E. C., and Scornavacchi, J. C. (1986): Effects of guanfacine on growth hormone, prolactin, renin, lipoproteins and glucose in essential hypertension. *Am. J. Cardiol.*, 57:27E–31E.

35. Heise, A., and Kroneberg, G. (1972): Alphasympathetic receptor stimulation in the brain and hypotensive activity of alpha-methyldopa. *Eur. J. Pharmacol.*, 17:315.

36. Hollifield, J. (1986): Clinical acceptability of transdermal clonidine: A large-scale evaluation by practitioners. *Am. Heart. J.*, 112:900.

37. Hoobler, S. W., and Sagastume, E. (1971): Clonidine hydrochloride in the treatment of hypertension. *Am. J. Cardiol.*, 28:67.

38. Hubbell, F. A., Weber, M. A., and Drayer, J. I. M. (1981): Neutralization of prazosin's anti-

hypertensive effect in the presence of clonidine (abstract). *Clin. Res., 29:*272A.

39. Igloe, M. C. (1973): Antihypertensive efficacy and safety of a clonidine-chlorthalidone combination. *Curr. Ther. Res.,* 15:559.

40. Jerie, P. (1986): Long-term evaluations of therapeutic efficacy and safety of guanfacine. *Am. J. Cardiol.,* 57:55E–59E.

41. Johnson, P., Kitching, A. A., and Lowther, C. P. (1972): Treatment of hypertension with methyldopa. *Br. Med. J.,* 1:133.

42. Kannel, W. B. (1983): The Framingham study. *Am. J. Med.,* 75:4.

43. Kaplan, N. M. (1975): Antihypertensive drugs in combination. *Arch. Int. Med.,* 135:660.

44. Kaplan, N. M. (1984): Effects of guanabenz on plasma lipid levels in hypertensive patients. *J. Cardiovasc. Pharmacol.,* 6:s841–s846.

45. Kirkendall, W. M., Hammond, J. J., Thomas, J. C., Overturf, M. L., and Zama, A. (1978): Prazosin and clonidine for moderately severe hypertension. *JAMA,* 240:2553.

46. Kleinlogel, H., Scholtysik, G., and Sayers, A. C. (1975): Effects of clonidine and BS 100–141 on the EEG sleep pattern in rats. *Eur. J. Pharmacol.,* 33:159.

47. Kobinger, W., and Walland, A. (1967): Investigations into the mechanism of the hypotensive effect of 2-(2,6-dichlorophenylamino)-2-imidazoline HCL. *Eur. J. Pharmacol.,* 2:155.

48. Kobinger, W., and Walland, A. (1972): Evidence for a central activation of vagal cardiodepressor reflex by clonidine. *Eur. J. Pharmacol.,* 19:203.

49. Kobinger, W., and Walland, A. (1972): Facilitation of vagal reflex bradycardia by an action of clonidine on central alpha receptors. *Eur. J. Pharmacol.,* 19:210.

50. Korner, P. I., Oliver, J. R., Sleight, P., Robinson, J. S., and Chalmers, J. P. (1975): Assessment of cardiac autonomic excitability in renal hypertensive rabbits using clonidine-induced resetting of the baroreceptor-heart rate reflex. *Eur. J. Pharmacol.,* 33:353.

51. Lo Buglio, A. F., and Jandl, J. H. (1967): The nature of the alpha-methyldopa red-cell antibody. *N. Engl. J. Med.,* 176:658.

52. Louis, W. J., Summers, R. J., Dynmon, M., and Jarrott, B. (1982): New developments in alpha-adrenoceptor drugs for the treatment of hypertension. *J. Cardiovasc. Pharmacol.* 76:299P.

53. Lubbe, W. F. (1974): Clonidine in the management of uncontrolled hypertension. *S. Afr. Med. J.,* 48:391.

54. McMahon, F. G. (1978): *Management of Essential Hypertension,* Futura, Mt. Kisco, New York.

55. McMahon, F. G., Michael, R., Ryan, J. R., LaCorte, W. S., and Jain, A. (1985): Regression of left ventricular hypertrophy in nineteen hypertensive patients treated with clonidine for eighteen months: A prospective study. In: *Low Dose Oral and Transdermal Therapy of Hypertension,* edited by M. A. Weber, J. I. M. Drayer,

and R. Kolloch, p. 81. Steinkopff-Verlag, Darmstadt.

56. Materson, B. J., Kessler, W. B., Alderman, M. H., Canosa, F. L., and Finnerty, F. A., et al. (1986): A multicenter, randomized, double-blind dose response evaluation of step-2 guanfacine versus placebo in mild to moderate hypertension. *Am. J. Cardiol.,* 57:32E–37E.

57. Medgett, I. C., and McCulloch, M. W. (1979): Effects of clonidine, guanfacine and three imidazoline derivatives related to clonidine on blood pressure, heart rate and gastric acid secretion in the anesthetized rat. *Arch. Int. Pharmacodyn.,* 240:158.

58. Medical Research Council Working Party (1985): MRC trial of treatment of mild hypertension: Principal results. *Br. Med. J.,* 219(6488):97.

59. Molzbauer, M., and Vogt, M. (1956): Depression by reserpine of the noradrenaline concentration in the hypothalamus of the cat. *J. Neurochemistry,* 1:8.

60. Mroczek, W. J., and Davidov, M. E. (1978): A randomized clinical trial of clonidine and propranolol in hypertensive patients receiving a diuretic and a vasodilator. *Curr. Ther. Res.,* 23:294.

61. Mroczek, W. J., Leibel, B. A., and Finnerty, F. A. (1972): Comparison of clonidine and methyldopa in a hypertensive patient receiving a diuretic. *Am. J. Cardiol.,* 29:712.

62. Multer, H. N., Licht, J. H., Ilnicki, L. P., and Singh, S. (1979): Clinical efficacy and pharmacokinetics of clonidine in hemodialysis and renal insufficiency. *J. Lab. Clin. Med.,* 94:223.

63. Nagakawa, Y., Chin, W., and Imai, S. (1982): Effects of guanfacine on pre- and postsynaptic α-adrenoceptors studied in comparison with those of clonidine. *Folia Pharmacol. Jpn.,* 79:431.

64. Oates, J. A., Seligmann, A. W., and Clark, M. A. (1965): The relative efficacy of guanethidine, methyldopa and paragyline as antihypertensive agents. *N. Engl. J. Med.,* 273:729.

65. Onesti, G., Brest, A. N., Novack, P., and Moyer, J. H. (1962): Pharmacodynamic effects and clinical use of alpha-methyldopa at rest and during exercise in patients with arterial hypertension. *Acta Med. Scand.,* 171:75.

66. Pettinger, W. A., Keeton, T. K., Campbell, W. B., Harper, D. C. (1976): Evidence for a renal adrenergic receptor inhibiting renin release. *Circ. Res.,* 38:338.

67. Porter, C. C., Totaro, J. A., and Leiby, C. M. (1961): Some biochemical effects of alpha-methyl- 3,4-dihydroxyphenylalanine and related compounds in mice. *J. Pharmacol. Exp. Ther.,* 134:139.

68. Putzeys, M. R., and Hoobler, S. W. (1972): Comparison of clonidine and methyldopa on blood pressure and side effects in hypertensive patients. *Am. Heart. J.,* 83:467.

69. Reed, W. G., Devous, M., Kirk, L. M., et al. (1985): Effects of catapres-TTS on cerebral

blood flow in elderly hypertensive patients In: *Low Dose Oral and Transdermal Therapy of Hypertension*, edited by Weber, M. A., Drayer, J. M., and Kolloch, R., p. 22. Springer-Verlag, New York.

70. Reichek, N., Franklin, B. B., Chandler, T., Muhammad, A., Plapper, G. T., St. John Sutton, M. (1982): Reversal of left ventricular hypertrophy by antihypertensive therapy. *Eur. Heart. J.*, 3(Suppl. A):165.

71. Rosenman, R. H. (1975): Combined clonidine-chlorthalidone therapy in hypertension: Two years' experience in 30 patients. *Arch. Int. Med.*, 135:1236.

72. Rosenthal, J. H. (1986): Hemodynamic and endocrine responses to guanfacine in normotensive volunteers and hypertensive patients. *Am. J. Cardiol.*, 57:22E–26E.

73. Rutledge, C. O., and Weiner, N. (1967): The effect of reserpine upon the synthesis of norepinephrine in the isolated rabbit heart. *J. Pharmacol. Exp. Ther.*, 157:290.

74. Schmitt, H., and Schmitt, H. (1969): Localization of the hypotensive effect of 2-(2,6-dichlorophenylamino)-2-imidazoline hydrochloride. *Eur. J. Pharmacol.*, 6:8.

75. Scholtysik, G., Lauener, H., Eichenberger, E., Burki, H., Salzmann, R., Muller-Schweinitzer, E., and Waite, R. (1975): Pharmacological actions of the antihypertensive agent N-amidino-2-(2,6-dichlorophenyl)acetamide hydrochloride (BS 100–141). *Arzneimittelforsch*, 25:1483.

76. Schwartz, A. B., Kim, K. E., Swartz, C., and Onesti, G. (1973): Cardiac and renal hemodynamic effects of clonidine. In: *Hypertension*, edited by G. Onesti, p. 381. Grune & Stratton, New York.

77. Shah, R. S., Walker, B. R., Vanov, S. K., and Helfant, R. H. (1976): Guanabenz effects on blood pressure and noninvasive parameters of cardiac performance in patients with hypertension. *Clin. Pharmacol. Ther.*, 19:732.

78. Standhoy, J. W., Morris, M., and Buckalew, V. M. (1982): Renal effects of the antihypertensive guanabenz in the dog. *J. Pharmacol. Exper. Ther.*, 221:347.

79. Sullivan, P. A., DeQuattro, V., Foti, A., and Curzon, G. (1986): Effects of clonidine on central and peripheral nerve tone in primary hypertension. *Hypertension*, 8:611.

80. Szam, I., and Hollo, J. (1982): Long-term antihypertensive therapy with guanfacine. *Int. J. Clin. Pharmacol. Ther. Toxicol.*, 20:388.

81. Tarazi, R. C., Sen, S., Saracoga, M., and Fouad, F. (1982): The multifactorial role of catecholamines in hypertensive cardiac hypertrophy. *Eur. Heart. J.*, 3(Suppl. A):103.

82. Toubes, D. B., McIntosh, T. J., Kirkendal, W. M., and Wilson, W. R. (1971): Hypotensive effects of clonidine and chlorthalidone. *Am. Heart. J.*, 81:312.

83. Tuck, M. L. (1987): The sympathetic nervous system in essential hypertension. *Am. Heart. J.*, 112:877, 1986.

84. Tuck, M. L., Stern, N., and Sowers, J. R. (1985): Enhanced 24-hour norepinephrine and renin secretion in young patients with essential hypertension: Relation with circadian pattern of arterial blood pressure. *Am. J. Cardiol.*, 55:112.

85. Van Zwieten, P. A. (1973): The central action of antihypertensive drugs, mediated via central alpha-receptors. *J. Pharmac. Pharmacol.*, 25:89.

86. Van Zwieten, P. A. (1973): Antihypertensive drugs with a central action. *Prog. Pharmacol.*, 1:1.

87. Van Zwieten, P. A. (1976): Centrally mediated action of alpha-methyldopa. In: *Regulation of Blood Pressure by the Central Nervous System*, edited by G. Onesti, M. Fernandes, and K. E. Kim, p. 293. Grune & Stratton, New York.

88. Van Zwieten, P. A. (1980): Pharmacology of centrally acting hypotensive drugs. *Br. J. Clin. Pharmacol.*, 10:13.

89. Waite, R. (1975): Inhibition of sympathetic nerve activity, resulting from central alpha-adrenoceptor stimulation. In: *Recent Advances in Hypertension*. Vol. II, edited by P. Miliez and M. Safar, pp. 27–31. Boehringer Ingelheim Reims.

90. Walker, B. R., Deitch, M. W., Gold, J. A., and Levey, B. A. (1982): Evaluation of guanabenz added to hydrochlorothiazide therapy in hypertension. *J. Int. Med. Res.*, 10:131.

91. Walker, B. R., Schneider, B. E., and Gold, J. A. (1980): A two-year evaluation of guanabenz in the treatment of hypertension. *Curr. Ther. Res.*, 27:786.

92. Walson, P. D., Graver, P., Rath, A., Kilbourne, K., and Deitch, M. W. (1984): Effects of guanabenz in adolescent hypertension. *J. Cardiovasc. Pharmacol.*, 6:S814.

93. Weber, M. A. (1980): Discontinuation syndrome following cessation of treatment with clonidine and other antihypertensive agents. *J. Cardiovasc. Pharmacol.*, 2(Suppl. 1):S73.

94. Weber, M. A., and Drayer, J. I. M. (1984): Clinical experience with rate-controlled delivery of antihypertensive therapy by a transdermal system. *Am. Heart. J.*, 108:231.

95. Weber, M. A., and Drayer, J. I. M. (1986): Treatment of hypertension in the elderly. *South. Med. J.*, 79:323.

96. Weber, M. A., Drayer, J. I. M., and Deitch, M. W. (1984): Hypertension in patients with diabetes mellitus: Treatment with a centrally acting agent. *J. Cardiovasc. Pharmacol.*, 6:s823–s829.

97. Weber, M. A., Drayer, J. I. M., and Laragh, J. H. (1978): The effects of clonidine and propranolol separately and in combination on blood pressure and plasma renin activity in essential hypertension. *J. Clin. Pharmacol.*, 18(516):233.

98. Weber, M. A., Drayer, J. I. M., Hubbell, F. A., and Laragh, J. H. (1983): Effects on the renin-angiotensin system of agents acting at central

and peripheral adrenergic receptors. *Chest*, 83(Suppl.):374.

99. Weber, M. A., Drayer, J. I. M., McMahon, F. G., Hamburger, R., Shah, A., and Kirk, L. (1984): Transdermal administration of clonidine for treatment of high BP. *Arch. Int. Med.*, 144:1211.

100. Weber, M. A., Graettinger, W. F., and Drayer, J. I. M. (1987): The adrenergic inhibitors. *Med. Clin. N. Am.*, 71(5):959.

101. Weber, M. A., Tonkon, M. J., and Klein, R. C. (1987): Blood pressure monitoring for assessing the duration of action of antihypertensive treatment. *J. Clin. Pharmacol.*, 27:751–755.

102. Weidmann, P., Hirsch, D., and Maxwell, M. H., et al. (1974): Plasma renin and blood pressure during treatment with methyldopa. *Am. J. Cardiol.*, 34:671.

103. Westelink, K., and Michotte, Y. (1982): Low dose guanfacine once-a-day for the treatment of hypertension in general practice: A multicentre pilot study. *Curr. Med. Res. Opin.*, 7:631.

104. Wilson, M. F., Haring, O., Lewin, A., Bedsole, G., Stepansky, W., Fillingim, J., Hall, D., Roginsky, M., McMahon, F. G., Jagger, P., and Strauss, M. (1986): Comparison of guanfacine versus clonidine for efficacy, safety and occurrence of withdrawal syndrome in step-2 treatment of mild to moderate essential hypertension. *Am. J. Cardiol.*, 57:43E–49E.

105. Winer, N., and Carter, C. H. (1982): Effects of abrupt discontinuation of guanabenz and clonidine in hypertensive patients. *Clin. Pharmacol. Ther.*, 32:282.

106. Yeh, B. K., Nantel, A., and Goldberg, L. I. (1971): Antihypertensive effect of clonidine: its use alone and in combination with hydrochlorothiazide and guanethidine in the treatment of hypertension. *Arch. Int. Med.*, 127:233.

New Therapeutic Strategies in Hypertension,
edited by Norman M. Kaplan,
Barry M. Brenner, and John H. Laragh.
Raven Press, Ltd., New York © 1989.

Alpha Blockers

Rafael F. Schäfers and John L. Reid

Department of Materia Medica and Therapeutics, University of Glasgow, Glasgow G21 3UW Scotland

Antagonists of alpha adrenergic receptors were among the earlier drugs to be evaluated in the treatment of hypertension. Early alpha blockers included phenoxybenzamine (noncompetitive) and phentolamine (competitive antagonist). Both still are used in the control of hypertensive crises in pheochromocytoma. However, neither agent proved useful in long-term clinical control of hypertension. Phenoxybenzamine was associated with profound and long-lasting postural hypotension, while phentolamine was short-acting and of limited use as long-term therapy.

The identification of subtypes of alpha receptors (the recognition that phentolamine and phenoxybenzamine were relatively nonselective) was followed by the recognition that prazosin was a selective alpha$_1$ antagonist. Up until then, prazosin had been characterized as a nonspecific vasodilator, phosphodiesterase inhibitor, or "atypical" alpha-blocker. It is now apparent that most, if not all, actions of prazosin at therapeutic doses are a consequence of competitive antagonism of alpha$_1$ receptors. Although prazosin is the prototype there are now several related quinazolines, terazosin, doxazosin, and trimazosin, as well as other drugs in which alpha$_1$ blockade may contribute to their actions (labetalol, ketanserin, urapidil).

HEMODYNAMICS

Central Hemodynamics

The primary pathophysiological and hemodynamic abnormality of established essential hypertension is an increased total peripheral resistance (TPR) associated with a normal or decreased cardiac output (83,84).

Chronic treatment with prazosin or doxazosin (i.e., 2 weeks to 1 year) lowers resting and exercise blood pressure by decreasing the TPR at rest (72,83,85,88,107), during dynamic (83,85,88,107) as well as isometric (88) exercise, and during a variety of other cardiovascular stress tests including cold pressor test (88) and lower body negative pressure (107) (Table 1). Cardiac output at rest and during dynamic exercise remains unaltered or may slightly increase (72,83, 85,88,107,135), even after treatment periods of up to one year (83,85). In contrast beta blockers may reduce cardiac output (83,84). There is some evidence that prazosin hemodynamically compensates for the cardiodepressant effect of a beta-blocker (atenolol) in combination therapy (78).

Cardiovascular reflex-control mechanisms are preserved during long-term prazosin treatment as demonstrated by unaltered responses to various cardiovascular stimuli and unchanged baroreceptor sensitivity (53,70,88,107). The physiological circadian pattern of blood pressure control is maintained during prazosin treatment (166).

In summary, prazosin and related compounds control blood pressure by directly interfering with the primary hemodynamic abnormality of the "disease," maintaining or even improving cardiac output.

Table 1. *Summary of reported hemodynamic effects (% change) of prazosin and doxazosin in essential hypertension*

Study	No. of evaluable patients	Duration of treatment (months)	Hemodynamic response at rest								
			Mean arterial pressure	Total peripheral resistance index	Cardiac index	Heart rate	Stroke index	Renal plasma flow	Renal blood flow	Renal vascular resistance	Glomerular filtration rate
Prazosin											
Koshy et al., 1977 (72)	14	2	−9[a]	−11[b]	+7[c]			−2			+0.5
O'Connor et al., 1979 (111)	12	1	−17[a]					+3	−0.3		−2
Falch et al., 1979 (43)	14	4	−10[a]	−11[a]	−1	−8[a]	+6	+15[a]			
Preston et al., 1979 (119)	10	1	−14[a]					+7	+5	−19[a]	−8
Bauer et al., 1984 (12)	12	5–6	−8[a]			−1		−4	−5	+6	+18
Lund-Johansen, 1975 (83)	10	12	−9[e]	−15[e]	+8[e]	−1[e]	+8[e]				
Mancia et al., 1980 (88)	7	0.5	−11[b]	−11[a,b]	+0.5[c]	−1					
Mulvihill-Wilson, et al., 1983 (107)	11	1	−6[a]	−13	No change	−8[e]	No change				
Scharf et al., 1984 (135)	10	2	−7[a]			−6	−0.5[d]				
Doxazosin											
Lund-Johansen et al., 1986 (85)	12	12	−13[a]	−19[a]	+8[a]	−0.3	+9				
Wilner, Ziegler, 1987 (169)	12	1.5	−8[a]		−3		+1	−1	−5	+8	

Results are expressed as mean % change from baseline or mean % change versus placebo (111,119).
After Lund-Johansen, ref. 84. Extended by results from refs. 12,85,135,169.
Reproduced with permission from ref. 84.
[a] Significance level p < 0.05 or less
[b] Total peripheral resistance
[c] Cardiac output
[d] Ejection fraction
[e] Level of significance not stated

Peripheral Hemodynamics

Effective antihypertensive treatment with prazosin, doxazosin, and related compounds in patients with normal kidney function does not result in any deterioration of renal function when studied after 1 to 6 months of therapy (12,43,72,95,111,119, 139,169). Renal plasma flow, renal blood flow, and glomerular filtration rate all show small, and in most cases statistically insignificant, changes (12,43,72,95,111,119,139, 169) (Table 1).

Whole blood volume and plasma volume have been reported to significantly increase due to sodium retention after 2 to 6 months. Prazosin administration and the effect may limit the long-term antihypertensive efficacy of prazosin in individual patients (12,72). Prazosin has no effect on the serum levels of potassium or on its renal handling (12). Doxazosin therapy for 5 to 8 days did not produce any significant change in the urinary excretion of sodium, potassium, and chloride (139).

Cerebral blood flow was unaffected by prazosin treatment in 8 elderly hypertensive patients (121). During long-term administration, prazosin does not modify forearm blood flow in essential hypertensives (35,107). Although the results of placebo-controlled trials of the therapeutic use of prazosin in patients with Raynaud's phenomenon or cold extremities are not consistent, they suggest that individual patients may derive benefit (110,145,170).

EFFECT ON PLASMA LIPIDS AND LIPOPROTEINS

A large body of epidemiological, pathological, and pharmacological evidence indicates that hypocholesterolemia is one of the major risk factors (or more accurately "risk predictors") of coronary heart disease mortality and morbidity (30,34,68, 146). A placebo-controlled study has provided strong evidence to suggest that "the magnitude of the risk associated with hypercholesterolemia is similar to the magnitude of risk associated with hypertension" (94). A high-cardiovascular risk is particularly associated with high levels of LDL-cholesterol, whereas high levels of HDL-cholesterol convey a relatively protective effect (30,68).

Lowering of plasma cholesterol by diet or drugs results in a reduction in the incidence of coronary heart disease (45,79,158) and may even delay the progression of established coronary atherosclerotic lesions (16,18). A drug-induced decline of approximately 10% in total cholesterol and a simultaneous, similar elevation in HDL-cholesterol in asymptomatic men with primary dyslipidemia was associated with 19% and 34% reductions in the incidence of fatal and nonfatal coronary heart disease in, respectively, the LRC-CPPT study (79) and the Helsinki Heart Study (45). The results of these 2 placebo-controlled trials studying samples of approximately 4,000 in each study highlight the potential impact which even relatively small changes in plasma lipoproteins may exert on cardiovascular risk. Similar, albeit more modest, changes in plasma lipoproteins are observed during treatment with alpha$_1$ antagonists.

In placebo-controlled trials as well as in comparative studies versus beta blockers and diuretics, treatment with prazosin, terazosin, or doxazosin is associated with reduction of total cholesterol and, in most studies increases in HDL-cholesterol (31, 33,44,46,61,77,108,125,144,156,160) (Tables 2–4). This results in an increase in the HDL-cholesterol/total-cholesterol ratio. Triglycerides tend to decline.

Both beta-blockers and diuretics may adversely affect this ratio by either decreasing the HDL-cholesterol fraction (beta blockers) or increasing total cholesterol (diuretics). Both classes of drugs consistently elevate triglycerides (Tables 3, 4) (3,74,76, 167). Prazosin tends to blunt these adverse lipid effects if it is added to an existing

Table 2. *Changes from baseline in serum lipids during alpha$_1$ blockade (placebo-controlled trials)*

	Doxazosin		Placebo			Terazosin		Placebo		
	n	Δ%	n	Δ%	p	n	Δ%	n	Δ%	p
Total cholesterol	142	−1.2	155	0.6	NS	128	−2.5	96	−0.1	<0.05
HDL cholesterol	142	7.6	155	4.8	NS	128	1.6	96	2.8	NS
HDL/total cholesterol	142	8.9	155	4.1	<0.05	128	4.2	96	2.9	NS
Triglycerides	142	−9.1	155	−3.0	NS	128	−6.8[a]	95	0.0[a]	NS

From Cox et al., 1986 (31), Deger, 1986 (33).
After Schäfers, Reid, from ref. 134.
Results from pooled data comprising 5 (doxazosin) and 3 (terazosin) placebo-controlled studies.
Dosage: Doxazosin, 1–16 mg once daily; Terazosin, 5, 10, and 20 mg once daily.
Duration: Doxazosin, 9–24 weeks; Terazosin, 4 weeks.
n, number of patients
Δ%, mean percentage change from baseline
p, significance level for *betweeen* group differences. NS, not significant.
[a] Median percentage change.

Table 3. *Changes from baseline in serum lipids during alpha₁ blockade. Comparative trials versus beta-blocker*

Author	No. of patients	Mean daily dosage (mg)	Duration (months)	Total-CH Δ%	HDL-CH Δ%	TG Δ%	DBP Δ%	BW Δ%
Leren et al. 1980 (77)	Pr = 23	4	2	−9[b]	−4 ns	−16[b]	−4 ns	+0.4 ns
	Pro = 23	160		−1 ns	−13[b]	+24[b]	−6 ns	+0.4 ns
Velasco et al.[a] 1986 (160)	Pr = 10	3.2	2	−11[b]	−16 ns	−14 ns	−15[b]	not reported
	Pro = 10	108.0		+4 ns	−8 ns	+16 ns	−17[b]	
Neusy, Lowenstein 1986 (108)	Pr = 11	5.4	6–12	−12[b]	ns	ns	−14[b]	ns
	Ate = 19	66		ns	ns	+17 ns	−14[b]	ns
Rouffy, Jaillard 1986 (125)	Pr = 29	8.9	6	−9[b]	+13[b]	−9[b]	−21[b]	+0.4 ns
	Ate = 30	150		+3[b]	−8[b]	+22[b]	−17[b]	+0.6 ns
Ferrara et al. 1986 (44)	Pr = 15	3.7	2.5	−7[b]	+13[b]	ns c	−10[b]	+0.7 ns
	Met = 15	193		ns c	−16[b] c	+16[b] c	−8[b]	+0.3 ns
Frick et al. 1986 (46)	Dox = 39	11.8	12	−2 NS	+4	−5 c	−6 (n = 60) c	ns
	Ate = 48	94.2		+3	−7	+43 c	−10 (n = 60) c	ns

After Schäfers, Reid, from ref. 134.

[a] This study was designed as a cross-over study. Since there were apparent carry over effects, the Δ% reported here relates to the comparison between baseline values at the end of the placebo run-in period with values at the end of the first treatment period.

Pr, prazosin; Dox, doxazosin; Pro, propranolol; Ate, atenolol; Met, metoprolol; CH, cholesterol; TG, triglycerides; DBP, diastolic blood pressure (supine); BW, body weight.

Δ%: mean percentage change from baseline (data as reported by author or calculated from the crude data given).

Significance level $p < 0.05$ or less.

[b] significant within group difference (baseline versus final value).

[c] significant between group difference (comparison of Δ%), compares the change from baseline in the alpha-blocker group with the change in baseline in the beta-blocker group.

ns, nonsignificant within group difference; NS, nonsignificant between group difference.

Table 4. *Changes from baseline in serum lipids during alpha₁ blockade. Comparative trials versus thiazide diuretic*

Author	No. of patients	Mean daily dosage (mg)	Duration (months)	Total-CH Δ%	HDL-CH Δ%	TG Δ%	DBP Δ%	BW Δ%
Stamler et al. 1986 (144)	Pr = 30	2–20		-2	not reported	-15	-11	ns
	HCT = 32	25–50	4.5	+4 [c]		+11 [c]	-9 [NS]	ns
Hjortdahl et al. 1987 (61)	Dox = 38–46	10.8	5.7	-4	-1	-7	-8	+0.2
	HCT = 39–41	89.1	5.4	+1 [c]	-13 [NS]	+8 [c]	-10 [NS]	-0.7 [NS]
Trost et al. 1987 (156)	Dox = 14–19	7.1	5.6	-6	+13	-17	-15	ns
	HCT = 12–16	81.3	5.7	+10 [c]	-8 [NS]	+26 [c]	-15 [NS]	ns

After Schäfers, Reid, from ref. 134.
Pr, prazosin; Dox, doxazosin; HCT, hydrochlorothiazide; CH, cholesterol; TG, triglycerides; DBP, diastolic blood pressure (supine); BW, body weight.
Δ%: mean percentage change from baseline (data as reported by author or calculated from the crude data given).
Significance level $p < 0.05$ or less.
[b] significant within group difference (baseline versus final value).
[c] significant between group difference (comparison of Δ%).
ns, nonsignificant within group difference; NS, nonsignificant between group difference.

diuretic or diuretic/beta-blocker regimen (49,65,97,105).

Most placebo-controlled primary prevention studies in hypertension have failed to demonstrate reductions in the incidence of myocardial infarction. Since most of these studies were based upon either diuretics or beta blockers, it has been proposed that the adverse metabolic effects, including the effects on lipids, may have compromised the potential beneficial effect of blood pressure reduction on cardiovascular mortality and morbidity (3,34,167). However, no large scale studies are yet available to provide evidence that the theoretical advantages of alpha$_1$ antagonists on plasma lipids do improve cardiovascular and cerebrovascular risks, whereas the beneficial effects of antihypertensive therapy with diuretics and beta blockers on cerebrovascular disease have been clearly identified (34).

ANTIHYPERTENSIVE EFFICACY

The antihypertensive efficacy and safety of prazosin is well established as previously reviewed (19,50,113,118,134,145,147). As initial monotherapy it is as effective as a beta-blocker, diuretic, or alpha-methyldopa (19,50,113,118,147) (Table 2) or "newer" antihypertensive agents such as captopril (114) or ketanserin (148). In patients whose blood pressure remains unsatisfactorily controlled on monotherapy, combination with a beta-blocker (149,152,159) or a diuretic (161) achieves a further reduction in blood pressure. Prazosin is as effective as other conventional vasodilator drugs (including hydralazine, labetalol, and nifedipine) when added to a standard diuretic/beta-blocker regimen (98,122). The combination of prazosin (2 mg b.i.d.) with the calcium antagonist verapamil (160 mg b.i.d.) is a safe and effective alternative for patients unresponsive to a combined diuretic/beta-blocker therapy (36).

The blood pressure lowering potential of doxazosin and terazosin is comparable to that of prazosin (31,132,154) and the newer agents can be given once daily. Terazosin has been safely and effectively combined with conventional beta-blocker and diuretic therapy (26,86,131). Up-to-date doxazosin has usually been given as a single agent. The antihypertensive efficacy of prazosin is well maintained during long-term treatment (to 7 years) in the large majority of patients as reviewed by Stanaszek et al. (145). Another study even reported a decrease in dose requirements (101), and tolerance was not observed in 61 patients completing more than 2 years of terazosin therapy (104). Prazosin in a single oral dose of 5 mg has been successfully used in the acute management of seriously elevated blood pressure (58).

Prazosin, doxazosin, and terazosin appear to have a safe side effect profile. The side effect most commonly associated with alpha$_1$ adrenoceptor blockers is a "first dose phenomenon" of orthostatic hypotension and, rarely, syncope (51,126,157). This largely can be avoided by careful dose titration and advice about postural change with the first small dose being given at bedtime (113,145).

Other side effects during long-term therapy include, in descending frequency: postural dizziness, headache, weakness and lack of energy, drowsiness, palpitations, peripheral edema, nausea, and blurred vision (13,118,143,154). Impotence is uncommon with alpha$_1$ antagonists (13,118,143). Although a very rare side effect, several cases of priapism associated with prazosin therapy have now been reported (1,20,89,137). Patients with renal failure may display a greater hypotensive response to prazosin (32,150) and the incidence of side effects is higher in this patient group (87).

The usual dose for antihypertensive therapy is 1 to 20 mg/day for prazosin, 1 to 16 mg/day for doxazosin, and 1 to 40 mg/day for terazosin (31,104,118,145). Due to its relatively short pharmacokinetic half-life of only 2 to 3 hours (145,163) prazosin has to be administered two or three times/day (145), although newer formulations may allow a single dose/day in the future (41). With their longer half-lives of 10 to 20 hours (39,142) doxazosin and terazosin effectively lower blood pressure on a single dose/day basis (26,31).

DOSE EFFECT RELATIONSHIP, PREDICTORS, AND DETERMINANTS OF RESPONSE

Early clinical observations described an apparent relationship between the initial oral dose of prazosin and severity and incidence of the "first dose" phenomenon (157). This finding is supported by the significant correlation between *plasma* prazosin concentrations and the fall in standing blood pressure after first time intravenous (11,138) and oral (37,151,164) administration in healthy (11,37,164) and hypertensive subjects (138,151).

Due to the lag between early peak blood levels after both intravenous and oral dosing and relatively delayed maximum hypotensive activity, such a direct linear relationship is not readily apparent for doxazosin (102,162). However, applying integrated pharmacokinetic-pharmacodynamic modeling (168), there is a significant correlation between the concentration of doxazosin in the "effect compartment" and its blood pressure lowering effect (102,162).

The degree of vascular alpha$_1$ adrenoceptor antagonism produced by prazosin (41) and doxazosin (162) in healthy volunteers also has been significantly related to plasma concentrations (41) or concentration in the "effect compartment" (162) respectively. This provides further evidence that vascular alpha$_1$ adrenoceptor antagonism is the underlying principle of the antihypertensive effect in humans (41,162), as suggested by classical pharmacological experiments (63,147).

Identification of factors that will predict the response to alpha antagonist drugs has proved difficult. One open clinical trial reported a better long-term therapeutic response in those patients who experienced an abrupt fall of blood pressure after the initial dose of prazosin (157). This has been found by other workers in a small controlled study applying pharmacokinetic-pharmacodynamic modeling (38), but not so by others who reported that the hypotensive activity of the first dose of prazosin was not significantly correlated with the blood pressure response to the final therapeutic steady state dosage (138). An alternative approach suggests that rather than the response to the initial dose the effect on systolic sitting and standing blood pressure during a short period of treatment (3 × 0.5 mg t.i.d.) may allow early identification of prazosin responders (138).

Although the relationship between baseline plasma-renin activity and therapeutic response to prazosin is not consistent (17,53,72), the renin-angiotensin system appears to be involved in the determination of response to alpha$_1$ blockade with prazosin. A significant inverse relationship between baseline plasma-renin activity and the orthostatic fall in blood pressure after the first dose has been reported (109). Essential hypertensives and hypertensive hemodialysis patients with high plasma-renin activity have been claimed to require higher doses than patients with normal renin activity (57,133). Blood pressure response was also claimed to be positively correlated to initial plasma noradrenaline levels (53). The responder rate to terazosin treatment was lower in black than in white patients (86). In summary, no reliable and clinically useful parameter of predictive value is yet available for optimization of the choice of alpha$_1$ adrenoceptor therapy. However, a good response to initial therapy does appear to make a favorable long-term response more likely.

ALPHA BLOCKERS IN THE ELDERLY

The EWPHE trial has provided evidence that antihypertensive therapy has beneficial effects on cardiovascular and cerebrovascular mortality in elderly hypertensives (2). Age-related changes in circulatory control mechanisms, such as attenuation of baroreceptor reflex function associated with adaptation in cerebrovascular autoregulation in longstanding hypertension, suggest that treatment of the elderly hypertensive should be undertaken with caution (54,155). Alpha$_1$ blockers theoretically may not appear the obvious first choice in older patients; however, actual clinical experience suggests that they are both effective and well tolerated in the elderly, (if patients with preexisting cardiovascular or cerebrovascular disease are excluded); prazosin, doxazosin, and terazosin have all been administered safely to groups of older patients (31,86,121,136,143). As changes in the pharmacokinetics (99,130) and pharmacodynamics (40) of prazosin and terazosin (99) have been described in the elderly, initiation and dose-titration of alpha$_1$-blocker therapy should be performed with particular care.

ALPHA BLOCKERS IN HYPERTENSION IN PREGNANCY

Prazosin has been used to control hypertension in pregnancy (82,128). It may prolong pregnancy (128) and, in combination with oxprenolol, has been reported to result in significantly higher birth weights than in pregnancies treated with bedrest alone (82).

ALPHA BLOCKERS IN HYPERTENSION AND CO-EXISTING DISEASES

Antihypertensive treatment poses particular problems in patients with other co-existing diseases, which often represent rela-

tive or absolute contraindications to many of the commonly-used antihypertensives. Efficacy in lowering blood pressure now is no longer sufficient, and antihypertensive therapy should also meet the following requirements:

1. It should not accelerate the natural history of any co-existing disease or compromise its therapeutic control (e.g., beta blockers in heart failure, peripheral vascular disease and asthma, diuretics in diabetes and gout).
2. It should not worsen cardiovascular risk profile. This is of particular importance for a co-existing disease such as diabetes which is a risk factor in its own right. Furthermore, most drugs depend on the liver or kidney for their elimination with the risk of accumulation and toxicity in co-existing liver or kidney failure. Individual dose adjustment may be necessary.
3. It should not compromise the quality of life of the patient on long-term antihypertensive therapy.

Alpha Blockers in the Patient With Chronic Heart Failure

Congestive cardiac failure is a major complication of untreated hypertension, which can be prevented by successful antihypertensive treatment (96). The concept of vasodilatation is now well established in the treatment of heart failure (62). Prazosin has been called a "balanced" or "mixed" vasodilator (i.e., it displays a vasodilating effect in both the venous and arterial vascular bed, thus "off-loading" the heart (4,62,63). This beneficial impact on central hemodynamics after *first* dose administration of prazosin in patients with heart failure has been confirmed by numerous trials as reviewed by Stanaszeck, et al. (145). Several placebo-controlled studies of up to 1 year duration have been conducted in small cohorts investigating the therapeutic use of prazosin in patients with congestive cardiac failure (60,91,123,145). The results of these trials are not consistent and the numbers of patients small. In general, they suggest some hemodynamic or clinical improvement only in individual patients.

A large scale (n = 642), double-blind, placebo-controlled trial with an average follow-up period of 2.3 years revealed no significant difference between placebo (n = 273) and prazosin (n = 183) on mortality and ejection fraction, whereas the addition of hydralazine/isosorbide dinitrate (n = 186) to the existing diuretic/digoxin regimen slightly, but significantly, improved both mortality and ejection fraction (28). Hypertension was an etiological factor in congestive heart failure in approximately 40% of patients in each group (27). However, even in the subgroup with a positive history of hypertension, prazosin failed to exert any apparent beneficial effect on mortality (27).

These results do not support the general use of prazosin in long-term therapy of congestive cardiac failure. The failure of prazosin to reduce mortality may be related to the development of tolerance to its hemodynamic effects (115,116). Rapid withdrawal of prazosin should be avoided in patients with congestive cardiac failure (55). Congestive cardiac failure modifies the pharmacokinetic handling of prazosin (127,145,163): the free fraction is increased in most patients (127), the area under the curve is enlarged, and the terminal elimination half-life (t1/2) prolonged (145,163). Nevertheless the average dose requirements of 2 to 30 mg/day in congestive cardiac failure exceed those for antihypertensive therapy (28,91,145). The disposition of terazosin was not significantly changed in patients with heart failure (142).

Alpha Blockers in the Patient With Chronic Renal Failure

Renal failure may be the cause as well as a complication of elevated blood pressure (52), and cardiovascular complications are a major cause of mortality in the hypertensive patient with impaired renal function (52,57). Prazosin as monotherapy and in most cases combination-therapy effectively lowers blood pressure in hypertensive patients with renal failure (even when requiring hemodialysis) without adverse influence on residual renal function (6,24,32,56,57, 59). Parameters of renal function such as plasma creatinine (6,32,59), blood urea (32), and estimations of glomerular filtration rate (GFR) (6,24,32) show no significant change during prazosin therapy lasting up to 6 months. Additionally terazosin for 14 days did not change creatinine clearance in 10 patients with renal impairment (67).

Unlike propranolol, prazosin had favorable effects on plasma lipids in hemodialysis patients (56). This "lipid aspect" may be of importance in dialysis patients who show an accelerated rate of atherosclerosis, which among other factors, is probably due to abnormalities in plasma lipids (52,56,57). Patients with renal failure demonstrate an exaggerated hypotensive response to prazosin (32,150). This possibly reflects changes in the disposition of prazosin in renal failure (145,163); higher peak plasma drug levels and a larger area under the curve (AUC) have been found by some investigators (145,150,163). A significantly increased free fraction of prazosin in chronic renal failure has also been observed (127). These pharmacokinetic changes may explain the increased blood pressure response in patients with renal failure, and may necessitate careful initiation of therapy and dose adjustments.

Only a few up-to-date studies have investigated the impact of impaired renal function on the pharmacokinetics and pharmacodynamics of terazosin (67) and doxazosin (23). No significant changes in the disposition of and the response to either drug have been found (23,67).

Alpha Blockers in Patients With Hepatic Failure

Although the main route of elimination of prazosin, doxazosin, and terazosin is by hepatic metabolism (39,142,163) information on the impact of impaired liver function on the pharmacokinetics of these drugs is limited. Since hepatocellular function is decreased in cirrhosis associated with various degrees of portal systemic shunting, higher plasma levels and a reduced clearance are likely to occur in cirrhotic patients (163). Furthermore, significantly elevated levels of free drug due to reduced protein binding with a close inverse linear correlation to plasma albumin have been found (127). Patients with impaired hepatic function therefore may respond to smaller than average doses of these drugs.

Alpha Blockers in Patients With Airways Disease

The sympathetic nervous system is intimately involved in the regulation of bronchial smooth muscle tone with beta receptor stimulation and alpha receptor blockade mediating bronchodilatation via an increase in intracellular cAMP levels (73). There is some evidence for an imbalance between alpha and beta receptors in asthma and atopic diseases with an augmented number of alpha and a reduction of beta receptors (106).

Placebo-controlled studies on the influence of an oral single dose of prazosin in patients with atopic airways disease provide evidence that prazosin has no adverse effect on bronchial function (15,92,93). Prazosin modestly increases the expiratory flow rate at 50% vital capacity (V_{50}) and the forced expiratory volume in one second (FEV_1) (92,93). The FEV_1 after a cold air hyperventilation challenge is unchanged by prazosin, but it does not protect against the cold-induced bronchoconstriction (15). *Inhaled* prazosin does not cause bronchodilatation, neither does it prevent histamine-induced bronchoconstriction in asthmatics (9,10). It does, however, partly inhibit exercise-induced bronchoconstriction (10). No information appears to be available on the impact of long-term prazosin therapy on bronchial function in asthmatic hypertensives. However, several case reports suggest that it does not aggravate respiratory function (73).

Thus, prazosin offers a safe alternative for the hypertensive asthmatic unlike beta-blockers which, irrespective of their ancillary pharmacological properties, should be avoided in these patients (29,73).

Alpha Blockers in Diabetic Patients

The prevalence of cardiovascular, renal vascular, peripheral arterial occlusive disease, and stroke is higher among diabetics than in nondiabetics (25,68). The risk of cardiovascular disease shows a substantial further increase, if the diabetes co-exists with other risk predictors like hypercholesterolemia, smoking, and hypertension (25,68). Hypertension occurs 2 to 3 times more frequently in a diabetic population (80).

The influence of prazosin on glucose homeostasis appears to differ after single and repeated dosing and also depends on the population studied. A *single* oral dose of prazosin increases fasting glucose levels in diabetic and nondiabetic hypertensives (7). Glucose disappearance and the early insulin response deteriorate after an intravenous glucose load in healthy volunteers (165). *Regular* treatment of 1 week (8), 5 weeks (22) and one year (81) in *nondiabetic* hypertensives did not change insulin and glucose levels in the fasting state (8,22,81) or after an *oral* glucose load (8,22). After an *intravenous* glucose load a decreased glucose tolerance has been observed (81).

There is no evidence to suggest that prazosin therapy worsens diabetic control in the *diabetic* hypertensive (8,71,75). After treatment for 1 week with 3 mg/day, an improved oral glucose tolerance has been claimed (8). The addition of an average of 2.4 mg prazosin/day to 100 mg hydrochlorothiazide did not alter glycosylated hemoglobin or fasting glucose levels after a 2 to 3 month observation (75).

Prazosin does not appear to adversely influence any diabetes-related complications. Sexual dysfunction improved when prazosin was substituted for methyldopa in hypertensive diabetic patients (80). As outlined earlier in this chapter in *Alpha blockers in the patient with chronic renal failure* section, residual renal function is preserved. Most of the studies referred to in *Alpha blockers in the patient with chronic renal failure* section, included patients with diabetic nephropathy (6,57,59). In placebo-controlled studies in nondiabetic hypertensives, prazosin did not affect the insulin-induced fall in plasma glucose. The concomitant tachycardia was not blunted and cardiac output was maintained while blood pressure fell (21,153).

Beta blockers, in particular propranolol, may lead to potentially dangerous hypoglycemic attacks (140). The physiological response to hypoglycemia is modified with blunting of tachycardia and marked rises in blood pressure (90,140). A hypertensive crisis caused by hypoglycemia and propranolol was successfully treated with prazosin (90). In addition, beta blockers may reduce peripheral (47,124) and, potentially, renal blood flow (111,112).

Thiazide diuretics worsen glucose tolerance in diabetic patients (48). A significant deterioration has also been demonstrated during long-term therapy in hypertensive nondiabetic patients (42,100). Although it has recently been claimed that long-term *low*-dose thiazide therapy is not diabetogenic (14), this study was not placebo controlled.

Both beta-blockers and thiazides may also interfere with sexual function (80,100).

Thus, prazosin can be regarded as a drug of choice for the hypertensive diabetic.

Alpha Blockers in Acute Inflammatory Disease

Prazosin is highly bound to alpha$_1$-acid glycoprotein which is elevated during severe acute inflammatory disease. A reduction in antihypertensive efficacy due to increased protein binding may therefore occur (127).

DRUG INTERACTIONS

Prazosin is often used in combination therapy to control blood pressure and many patients will also require drug therapy for co-existing diseases. Known and clinically important drug interactions are summarized below. Careful initial monitoring and individual dose adjustment is recommended if prazosin is to be administered in one of these combinations.

Interactions With Antihypertensive Drugs

Co-administration with a beta-blocker promotes the postural fall in blood pressure, blunts the reflex increase in heart rate and may increase the incidence of postural hypotension-related side effects (37,129). The pharmacokinetics of prazosin are not modified by this combination and thus cannot explain this change of hemodynamic effects (37,129).

Combination of prazosin with the calcium antagonists nifedipine (64,141) or verapamil (36,117) enhances the fall in supine and erect blood pressure in healthy volunteers (117) and hypertensive patients (36,64,141) and acute profound hypotensive responses have been observed in individual cases (64). This is in part due to an altered disposition of prazosin with higher peak plasma levels and an enlarged area under the curve (36,117); a pharmacodynamic interaction probably also contributes to this effect

(103). Although the combination of prazosin plus verapamil was found to be safe and effective during long-term therapy (36) caution is needed when initiating an alpha-blocker/calcium antagonist combination.

The combined use of clonidine and prazosin does not appear to achieve any clinically useful additive antihypertensive effect (66,69).

Interactions With Other Drugs

Nonsteroidal antiinflammatory drugs such as indomethacin reduce the antihypertensive effect of prazosin (129) and other antihypertensive drugs (5,120) probably by interference with renal prostaglandin synthesis (120). It has been suggested that sulindac is the nonsteroidal antiinflammatory drug (NSAID) of choice in these circumstances (120).

CONCLUSIONS

Prazosin and related selective alpha$_1$ antagonists are effective alone or in combination in a wide range of hypertensive patients.

They are relatively free of toxicity, especially severe tissue injury, and do not appear to impair intellectual or cognitive function or arousal. Where appropriate controlled comparisons have been undertaken, alpha$_1$ blockers appear to lower blood pressure by a similar magnitude in a similar proportion of patients to other widely-used drugs like beta blockers, diuretics, or ACE-inhibitors. Among the advantages of alpha blockers is the potential for safe use alone or in combination with most other drug groups. Alpha blockers are not relatively or absolutely contraindicated in patients with common or associated respiratory, cardiovascular, or metabolic diseases. They should be avoided or used with caution in patients with preexisting autonomic impairment and those who are volume depleted.

A potentially important and useful action of alpha$_1$ blockers on lipid metabolism results in a fall in total cholesterol and a rise in HDL cholesterol. Although these effects are modest, they appear to be an effect of this class of drugs and may result in potentially beneficial overall effects in more than one cardiovascular risk factor. Thus alpha$_1$ blockers deserve consideration for wider use in a broad-based approach directed not only to control of blood pressure but also to the more ambitious long-term goal of reversing or preventing atherosclerosis.

ACKNOWLEDGMENTS

We would like to thank Mrs. J. Hamilton for typing the manuscript.

REFERENCES

1. Adams, J. W., and Soucheray, J. A. (1984): Prazosin-induced priapism in a diabetic. *J. Urol.* 132:1208.
2. Amery, A., Birkenhäger, W., Brixko, P., et al. (1985): Mortality and morbidity results from the European Working Party on High Blood Pressure in the Elderly Trial. *Lancet*, 1:1349–1354.
3. Ames, R. P., and Hill, P. (1976): Elevation of serum lipid levels during diuretic therapy of hypertension. *Am. J. Med.*, 61:748–757.
4. Awan, N. A., Miller, R. R., Maxwell, K., and Mason, D. T. (1977): Effects of prazosin on forearm resistance and capacitance vessels. *Clin. Pharmacol. Ther.*, 22:79–84.
5. Baez, M. A., Alvarez, C. R., and Weidler, D. J. (1987): Effects of the non-steroidal anti-inflammatory drugs, piroxicam or sulindac on the antihypertensive actions of propranolol and verapamil. *J. Hypertens.*, 5(Suppl.5):S563–S566.
6. Bailey, R. R. (1977): Prazosin in the treatment of patients with hypertension and renal functional impairment. *Med. J. Aust.*, 2(Specl. Suppl.):42–45.
7. Barbieri, C., Caldara, R., Ferrari, C., et al. (1980): Metabolic effects of prazosin. *Clin. Pharmacol. Ther.*, 27:313–316.
8. Barbieri, C., Ferrari, C., Borzio, M., Piepoli, V., and Caldara, R. (1980): Metabolic effects of chronic prazosin treatment. *Horm. Metab. Res.*, 12:331–334.
9. Barnes, P. J., Ind, P., and Dollery, C. T. (1980): Inhaled prazosin in asthma. *Thorax*, 35:239.
10. Barnes, P. J., Wilson, N. M., and Vickers, H. (1981): Prazosin, an alpha-1-adrenoceptor antagonist, partially inhibits exercise-induced asthma. *J. Allergy. Clin. Immunol.*, 68:411–415.
11. Bateman, D. N., Hobbs, D. C., Twomey, T. M.,

Stevens, E. A., and Rawlins, M. D. (1979): Prazosin, pharmacokinetics and concentration effect. *Eur. J. Clin. Pharmacol.*, 16:177–181.

12. Bauer, J. H., Jones, L. B., and Gaddy, P. (1984): Effects of prazosin therapy on BP, renal function, and body fluid composition. *Arch. Intern. Med.*, 144:1196–1200.

13. Benson, D., Peterson, L. G., and Bartay, J. (1983): Neuropsychiatric manifestations of antihypertensive medications. *Psychiatr. Med.*, 1:205–214.

14. Berglund, G., Andersson, O. K., and Widgren, B. R. (1986): Low-dose antihypertensive treatment with a thiazide diuretic is not diabetogenic: A ten-year controlled trial with bendroflumethiazide. *J. Hypertens.*, 4(Suppl.5):S525–S527.

15. Bewtra, A., Nair, N., Alper, B., and Townley, R. (1982): The effect of prazosin on cold air hyperventilation challenges (CAHC). *J. Aller. Clin. Immunol.*, 69:152.

16. Blankenhorn, D. H., Nessim, S. A., Johnson, R. L., Sanmarco, M. E., Azen, S. P., and Cashin-Hemphill, L. (1987): Beneficial effects of combined colestipol-niacin therapy on coronary atherosclerosis and coronary venous bypass grafts. *JAMA*, 257:3233–3240.

17. Bolli, P., Amann, F. W., and Bühler, F. R. (1980): Antihypertensive response to postsynaptic alpha-blockade with prazosin in low- and normal-renin hypertension. *J. Cardiovasc. Pharmacol.*, (Suppl.3):S399–S406.

18. Brensike, J. F., Levy, R. I., Kelsey, S. F., et al. (1984): Effects of therapy with cholestyramine on progression of coronary arteriosclerosis: Results of the NHLBI Type II Coronary Intervention Study. *Circulation*, 69:313–324.

19. Brogden, R. N., Heel, R. C., Speight, T. M., and Avery, G. S. (1977): Prazosin: A review of its pharmacological properties and therapeutic efficacy in hypertension. *Drugs* 14:163–197.

20. Burke, J. R., and Hirst, G. (1980): Priapism and prazosin. *Med. J. Aust.*, 1:382–383.

21. Buzzeo, L. A., Steele, J. M., and Lowenstein, J. (1979): Unimpaired beta adrenergic responses during prazosin administration. *J. Pharmacol. Exp. Ther.*, 211:345–349.

22. Cambien, F., Plouin, P. F. (1985): Prazosin does not alter levels of plasma lipids, glucose and insulin. *J. Cardiovasc. Pharmacol.*, 7:516–519.

23. Carlson, R. V., Bailey, R. R., Begg, E. J., Cowlishaw, M. G., and Sharman, J. R. (1986): Pharmacokinetics and effect on blood pressure of doxazosin in normal subjects and patients with renal failure. *Clin. Pharmacol. Ther.*, 40:561–566.

24. Chopra, J. S., Parkash, C., Chabra, R., and Wadhwa, N. K. (1983): Prazosin in hypertension associated with chronic renal failure. *JAPI*, 31:159–161.

25. Christlieb, A. R. (1982): The hypertensions of diabetes. *Diabetes Care*, 5:50–58.

26. Chrysant, S. G., Black, H. R., Davidov, M., et al. (1986): Experience with terazosin administered in combination with other antihypertensive agents. *Am. J. Med.*, 80(Suppl.5B):55–61.

27. Cohn, J. N., Archibald, D. G., Francis, G. S., et al. (1987): Veterans Administration Co-operative Study on vasodilator therapy of heart failure: Influence of prerandomisation variables on the reduction of mortality by treatment with hydralazine and isosorbide dinitrate. *Circulation*, 75(Suppl.IV):49–54.

28. Cohn, J. N., Archibald, D. G., Ziesche, S., et al. (1986): Effect of vasodilator therapy on mortality in chronic congestive heart failure. *N. Engl. J. Med.*, 314:1547–1552.

29. Committee on Safety of Medicines. (1987): Fatal bronchospasm associated with beta-blockers. *Curr. Probl.*, 20.

30. Consensus Conference. (1985): Lowering Blood Cholesterol to Prevent Heart Disease. *JAMA*, 253:2080–2086.

31. Cox, D. A., Leader, J. P., Milson, J. A., and Singleton, W. (1986): The antihypertensive effects of doxazosin: A clinical overview. *Br. J. Clin. Pharmacol.*, 21:83S–90S.

32. Curtis, J. R., and Bateman, F. J. A. (1975): Use of prazosin in management of hypertension in patients with chronic renal failure and in renal transplant recipients. *Br. Med. J.*, 4:432–434.

33. Deger, G. (1986): Effect of terazosin on serum lipids. *Am. J. Med.*, 80(Suppl.5B):82–85.

34. Dollery, C. T. (1987): Risk predictors, risk indicators, and benefit factors in hypertension. *Am. J. Med.*, 82:(Suppl.1A):2–8.

35. Eklund, B., Hjemdahl, P., Seideman, P., and Atterhog, J-H. (1983): Effects of prazosin on hemodynamics and sympatho-adrenal activity in hypertensive patients. *J. Cardiovasc. Pharmacol.*, 5:384–391.

36. Elliott, H. L., Meredith, P. A., Campbell, L., and Reid, J. L. (1988): The combination of prazosin and verapamil in the treatment of essential hypertension. *Clin. Pharmacol. Ther.*, 43:554–560.

37. Elliott, H. L., McLean, K., Sumner, D. J., Meredith, P. A., and Reid, J. L. (1981): Immediate cardiovascular responses to oral prazosin: Effects of concurrent beta blockers. *Clin. Pharmacol. Ther.*, 29:303–309.

38. Elliott, H. L., Meredith, P. A., and Reid, J. L. (1986): Concentration-effect analysis of acute and long term prazosin in essential hypertension. *Eur. J. Clin. Invest.*, 16:A33.

39. Elliott, H. L., Meredith, P. A., and Reid, J. L. (1987): Pharmacokinetic overview of doxazosin. *Am. J. Cardiol.*, 59:78G–81G.

40. Elliott, H. L., Sumner, D. J., McLean, K., Rubin, P. C., and Reid, J. L. (1982): Effect of age on vascular alpha-adrenoceptor responsiveness in man. *Clin. Sci.*, 63:305s–308s.

41. Elliott, H. L., Vincent, J., Meredith, P. A., and Reid, J. L. (1988): Relationship between plasma prazosin concentrations and alpha antagonism in humans: Comparison of conventional and rate-controlled (Oros) formulations. *Clin. Pharmacol. Ther.*, 43:582–587.

42. European Working Party on Hypertension in the Elderly (EWPHE). (1978): Glucose intolerance during diuretic therapy. *Lancet*, 2:681–683.

43. Falch, D. K., Quist Paulsen, A., Odegaard, E., Norman, N. (1979): Central and renal circulation, renin and aldosterone in plasma during prazosin treatment in essential hypertension. *Acta Med. Scand.*, 206:489–494.

44. Ferrara, L. A., Marotta, T., Rubba, P., et al. (1986): Effects of alpha-adrenergic and beta-adrenergic receptor blockade on lipid metabolism. *Am. J. Med.*, 80(Suppl.2A):104–108.

45. Frick, M. H., Elo, O., Haapa, K., et al. (1987): Helsinki Heart Study: Primary-prevention trial with gemfibrozil in middle-aged men with dyslipidemia. *N. Engl. J. Med.*, 317:1237–1245.

46. Frick, M. H., Haltunen, P., Himanen, P., et al. (1986): A long-term double-blind comparison of doxazosin and atenolol in patients with mild to moderate essential hypertension. *Br. J. Clin. Pharmacol.*, 21:55S–62S.

47. Frohlich, E. D., Tarazi, R. C., and Dustan, H. P. (1969): Peripheral arterial insufficiency: A complication of beta-adrenergic blocking therapy. *JAMA*, 208:2471–2472.

48. Goldner, M. G., Zarowitz, H., and Akgun, S. (1960): Hyperglycemia and glycosuria due to thiazide derivatives in diabetes mellitus. *N. Engl. J. Med.*, 262:403–405.

49. Goto, Y. (1984): Effects of alpha- and beta-blocker antihypertensive therapy on blood lipids: A multicenter trial. *Am. J. Med.*, 76(Suppl.2A):72–78.

50. Graham, R. M., and Mulvihill-Wilson, J. (1980): Clinical Pharmacology of prazosin used alone or in combination in the therapy of hypertension. *J. Cardiovasc. Pharmacol.*, 2(Suppl.3):S387–S398.

51. Graham, R. M., Thornell, I. R., Gain, J. M., Bagnoli, C., Oates, H. F., and Stokes, G. S. (1976): Prazosin: The first-dose phenomenon. *Br. Med. J.*, 2:1293–1294.

52. Gunnells, J. C. (1983): Treating the patient with mild hypertension and renal insufficiency. *Am. J. Cardiol.*, 51:651–656.

53. Guthrie, G. P., Kotchen, T. A. (1983): Effects of prazosin and clonidine on sympathetic and baroreflex function in patients with essential hypertension. *J. Clin. Pharmacol.*, 23:348–354.

54. Hankey, G. J., and Gubbay, S. S. (1987): Focal cerebral ischaemia and infarction due to antihypertensive therapy. *Med. J. Aust.*, 146:412–414.

55. Hanley, S. P., Cowley, A., and Hampton, J. R. (1980): Danger of withdrawal of vasodilator therapy in patients with chronic heart failure. *Lancet*, 1:735–736.

56. Harter, H. R., Meltzer, V. N., Tindira, C. A., Naumovich, A. D., and Goldberg, A. P. (1986): Comparison of the effects of prazosin versus propranolol on plasma lipoprotein lipids in patients receiving hemodialysis. *Am. J. Med.*, 80((Suppl.2A):82–89.

57. Harter, H. R., Tindira, C. A., and Delmez, J.

A. (1981): Blood pressure control in hemodialysis patients: The long-term effects of prazosin. *J. Cardiovasc. Med.*, (Specl.Suppl.):49–59.

58. Hayes, J. M. (1980): Rapid control of serious high blood pressure with single large oral doses of prazosin. *Med. J. Aust.*, 1:31–32.

59. Heagerty, A. M., Russell, G. I, Bing, R. F., Thurston, H., and Swales, J. D. (1982): The addition of prazosin to standard triple therapy in the treatment of severe hypertension. *Br. J. Clin. Pharmacol.*, 13:539–541.

60. Higginbotham, M. B., Morris, K. G., Bramlet, D. A., Coleman, R. E., and Cobb, F. R. (1983): Long-term ambulatory therapy with prazosin versus placebo for chronic heart failure: Relation between clinical response and left ventricular function at rest and during exercise. *Am. J. Cardiol.*, 52:782–788.

61. Hjortdahl, P., Von Krogh, H., Daae, L., Holme, I., and Hjermann, I. (1987): A 24-week multicenter double-blind study of doxazosin and hydrochlorothiazide in patients with mild to moderate essential hypertension. *Acta Med. Scand.*, 221:427–434.

62. Hutton, I., and Hillis, W. S. (1986): Modern management of heart failure. *Br. J. Hosp. Med.*, 36:426–432.

63. Jauernig, R. A., Moulds, R. F. W., and Shaw, J. (1978): The action of prazosin in human vascular preparations. *Arch. Int. Pharmacodyn.*, 231:81–89.

64. Jee, L. D., and Opie, L. H. (1983): Acute hypotensive response to nifedipine added to prazosin in treatment of hypertension. *Br. Med. J.*, 287:1514.

65. Johnson, B. F., Romero, L., Johnson, J., and Marwaha, R. (1984): Comparative effects of propranolol and prazosin upon serum lipids in thiazide-treated hypertensive patients. *Am. J. Med.*, 76(Suppl.2A):109–112.

66. Jounela, A. J., Kanniainen, E., and Lilja, M. (1985): Interaction between clonidine and alpha blockers. *Clin. Cardiol.*, 8:641–642.

67. Jungers, P., Ganeval, D., Pertuiset, N., and Chauveau, P. (1986): Influence of renal insufficiency on the pharmacokinetics and pharmacodynamics of terazosin. *Am. J. Med.*, 80(Suppl.5B):94–99.

68. Kannel, W. B., and Sytkowski, P. A. (1987): Atherosclerosis risk factors. *Pharmacol. Ther.* 32:207–235.

69. Kapocsi, J., Farsang, C., and Vizi, E. S. (1987): Prazosin partly blocks clonidine-induced hypotension in patients with essential hypertension. *Eur. J. Clin. Pharmacol.*, 32:331–334.

70. Khatri, I. M., Levinson, P., Notargiacomo, A., and Freis, E. D. (1985): Initial and long-term effects of prazosin on sympathetic vasopressor responses in essential hypertension. *Am. J. Cardiol.*, 55:1015–1018.

71. Königstein, R. P. (1978): Die Behandlung der Hypertonie mit Prazosin bei "Altersdiabetikern". *Wien Med. Wochenschr.*, 128:27–30.

72. Koshy, M. C., Mickley, D., Bourgoignie, J., and

Blaufox, M. D. (1977): Physiologic evaluation of a new antihypertensive agent: Prazosin HCl. *Circulation*, 55:533–537.

73. Layton, C. R. (1981): Management of hypertension in patients with obstructive airways disease. *J. Cardiovasc. Med.*, (Specl.Suppl.):43–48.

74. Lehtonen, A. (1982): Betablockade und Plasmalipide, In: *Die Beta-Rezeptorenblockade aus Pathophysiologischer Sicht*, edited by H. Roskamm and H. Holzgreve, pp. 165–170. F. K. Schattauer Verlag, Stuttgart, New York.

75. Leichter, S. B., and Baumgardner, B. (1981): Effects of chronic prazosin therapy on intermediary metabolism in diabetic patients. *J. Cardiovasc. Med.*, (Specl.Suppl.):38–42.

76. Leren, P. (1987): Comparison of effects on lipid metabolism of antihypertensive drugs with alpha and beta-adrenergic antagonist properties. *Am. J. Med.*, 82(Suppl.1A):31–35.

77. Leren, P., Helgeland, A., Holme, I., Foss, P. O., Hjermann, I., and Lund-Larsen, P. G. (1980): Effect of propranolol and prazosin on blood lipids. *Lancet*, 2:4–6.

78. Lilja, M., Ikäheimo, M., Mattila, M. J., and Jounela, A. J. (1985): Haemodynamic effects of prazosin combinations during dynamic and isometric exercise. *Ann. Clin. Res.*, 17:316–322.

79. Lipid Research Clinics Program. (1984): The Lipid Research Clinics Coronary Primary Prevential Trial Results. I. Reduction in incidence of coronary heart disease. *JAMA*, 251:351–364.

80. Lipson, L. G. (1984): Treatment of hypertension in diabetic men: Problems with sexual dysfunction. *Am. J. Cardiol.*, 53:46A–50A.

81. Lithell, H., Berne, C., Waern, A. U., and Wibell, L. (1985): Glucose metabolism during long-term treatment with prazosin. *Diabetes Res.*, 2:297–299.

82. Lubbe, W. F., Hodge, J. V., and Kellaway, G. S. M. (1982): Antihypertensive treatment and fetal welfare in essential hypertension in pregnancy: A retrospective survey of experience with various regimes at National Women's Hospital, Auckland, 1970–1980. *N. Z. Med. J.*, 95:1–5.

83. Lund-Johansen, P. (1975): Hemodynamic changes at rest and during exercise in long-term prazosin therapy for essential hypertension. *Postgrad. Med.*, 58(Suppl.):45–54.

84. Lung-Johansen, P. (1986): Effects of antihypertensive therapy on the hemodynamics of hypertension: Clinical implications. *Clin. Ther.*, 8:382–397.

85. Lund-Johansen, P., Omvik, P., and Haugland, H. (1986): Acute and chronic haemodynamic effects of doxazosin in hypertension at rest and during exercise. *Br. J. Clin. Pharmacol.*, 21:45S–54S.

86. Luther, R. R., Glassman, H. N., Jordan, D. C., and Sperzel, W. D. (1986): Efficacy of terazosin as an antihypertensive agent. *Am. J. Med.*, 80(Suppl.5B):73–76.

87. MacCarthy, E. P., Thornell, I. R., and Stokes,

G. S. (1981): Prazosin: Long-term therapy of hypertension. *J. Cardiovasc. Med.*, (Specl. Suppl.):70–76.

88. Mancia, G., Ferrari, A., Gregorini, L., et al. (1980): Effects of prazosin on autonomic control of circulation in essential hypertension. *Hypertension*, 2:700–707.

89. Mandel, L. R. (1987): Priapism secondary to prazosin therapy. *Milit. Med.*, 152:523–524.

90. Mann, S. J., and Krakoff, L. R. (1984): Hypertensive crisis caused by hypoglycemia and propranolol. *Arch. Intern. Med.*, 144:2427–2428.

91. Markham, R. V., Corbett, J. R., Gilmore, A., Pettinger, W., Firth, B. G. (1983): Efficacy of prazosin in the management of chronic congestive heart failure: A 6-month randomized, double-blind, placebo-controlled study. *Am. J. Cardiol.*, 51:1346–1352.

92. Marlin, G. E., Thompson, P. J., Chow, C. M., Reddel, H. K., and Cheng, S. (1981): Bronchodilator action of prazosin. *Lancet*, 1:225.

93. Marlin, G. E., Thompson, P. J., Reddel, H. K., Chow, C. M., and Cheng S. (1982): Bronchodilator activity of prazosin in patients with allergic rhinitis and asthma. *Br. J. Clin. Pharmacol.*, 13:445–448.

94. Martin, M. J., Hulley, S. B., Browner, W. S., Kuller, L. H., and Wentworth, D. (1986): Serum cholesterol, blood pressure and mortality: Implications from a cohort of 361662 men. *Lancet*, 2:933–939.

95. Masoni, A., Tommasi, A. M., Baggioni, F., and Bagni, B. (1974): Hemodynamic study in men of medium-term treatment with a new amino-quinazoline antihypertensive agent (prazosin). In: *Prazosin-Evaluation of a New Antihypertensive Agent*, edited by D. W. K. Cotton, pp. 54–63. Excerpta Medica, Amsterdam; American Elsevier, New York.

96. Massie, B., and Chan, S. (1981): Management of hypertension in patients with congestive heart failure: Results of treatment with prazosin. *J. Cardiovasc. Med.*, (Specl.Suppl.):60–69.

97. Mauersberger, H. (1984): Effect of prazosin on blood pressure and plasma lipids in patients receiving a beta blocker and diuretic regimen. *Am. J. Med.*, 76(Suppl.2A):101–104.

98. McAreavey, D., Ramsay, L. E., Latham, L., et al. (1983): The "Third Drug" Trial: A comparative study of antihypertensive agents added to treatment when blood pressure is uncontrolled by a beta blocker plus thiazide diuretic. *J. Hypertens.*, 1(Suppl.2):116–119.

99. McNeil, J. J., Drummer, O. H., Conway, E. L., Workman, B. S., and Louis, W. J. (1987): Effect of age on pharmacokinetics of and blood pressure responses to prazosin and terazosin. *J. Cardiovasc. Pharmacol.*, 10:168–175.

100. Medical Research Council Working Party on Mild to Moderate Hypertension. (1981): Adverse reactions to bendrofluazide and propranolol for the treatment of mild hypertension. *Lancet*, 2:539–543.

101. Melkild, A. (1984): Prazosin ("Peripress"): A

long term study. *Curr. Med. Res. Opin.*, 9:214–228.

102. Meredith, P. A., Elliott, H. L., Kelman, A. W., and Reid, J. L. (1985): Application of pharmacokinetic-pharmacodynamic modelling for the comparison of quinazoline alpha-adrenoceptor agonists in normotensive volunteers. *J. Cardiovasc. Pharmacol.*, 7:532–537.

103. Meredith, P. A., Elliott, H. L., Pasanisi, F., and Reid, J. L. (1986): Prazosin and verapamil: A pharmacokinetic and pharmacodynamic interaction? *Br. J. Clin. Pharmacol.*, 21:85P.

104. Mersey, J. H., Abraham, P. A., Arnold, J. D., et al. (1986): Long-term experience with terazosin for treatment of mild to moderate hypertension. *Am. J. Med.*, 80(Suppl.5B):68–72.

105. Misson, R., Merkel, T., and Cutler, R. E. (1984): Comparison of blood pressure, plasma lipid and cardiac performance responses to prazosin versus propranolol in thiazide-treated hypertensive patients. *Am. J. Cardiol.*, 53:51A–54A.

106. Motulsky, H. J., and Insel, P. A. (1982): Adrenergic receptors in man: Direct identification, physiologic regulation and clinical alterations. *N. Engl. J. Med.*, 307:18–29.

107. Mulvihill-Wilson, J., Gaffney, F. A., Pettinger, W. A., Blomquist, C. G., Anderson, S., and Graham, R. M. (1983): Hemodynamic and neuroendocrine responses to acute and chronic alpha adrenergic blockade with prazosin and phenoxybenzamine. *Circulation*, 67:383–393.

108. Neusy, A. J., and Lowenstein, J. (1986): Effects of prazosin, atenolol and thiazide diuretic on plasma lipids in patients with essential hypertension. *Am. J. Med.*, 80(Suppl.2A):94–99.

109. Nicholson, J. P., Resnick, L. M., Pickering, T. G., Marion, R., Sullivan, P., and Laragh, J. H. (1985): Relationship of blood pressure response and the renin-angiotensin system to first dose prazosin. *Am. J. Med.*, 78:241–244.

110. Nielsen, S. L., Vitting, K., and Rasmussen, K. (1983): Prazosin treatment of primary Raynaud's phenomenon. *Eur. J. Clin. Pharmacol.* 24:421–423.

111. O'Connor, D. T., Preston, R. A., and Sasso, E. H. (1979): Renal perfusion changes during treatment of essential hypertension: Prazosin versus propranolol. *J. Cardiovasc. Pharmacol.*, 1(Suppl.):S38–S42.

112. O'Malley, K., O'Callaghan, W. G., Laher, M. S., McGarry, K., and O'Brien, E. (1983): Beta-adrenoceptor blocking drugs and renal blood flow with special reference to the elderly. *Drugs*, 25:(Suppl.2):103–107.

113. Okun, R. (1983): Effectiveness of prazosin as initial antihypertensive therapy. *Am. J. Cardiol.*, 51:644–650.

114. Okun, R., and Kraut, J. (1987): Prazosin versus captopril as initial therapy: Effect on hypertension and lipid levels. *Am. J. Med.*, 82(Suppl.1A):58–63.

115. Packer, M., Medina, N., and Yushak, M. (1986): Role of the renin-angiotensin system in the development of hemodynamic and clinical tolerance to long-term prazosin therapy in patients with severe chronic heart failure. *J. Am. Coll. Cardiol.*, 7:671–680.

116. Packer, M., Meller, J., Gorlin, R., and Herman, M. V. (1979): Hemodynamic and clinical tachyphylaxis to prazosin-mediated afterload reduction in severe chronic congestive heart failure. *Circulation*, 59:531–539.

117. Pasanisi, F., Elliott, H. L., Meredith, P. A., McSharry, D. R., and Reid, J. L. (1984): Combined alpha adrenoceptor antagonism and calcium channel blockade in normal subjects. *Clin. Pharmacol. Ther.*, 36:716–723.

118. Pitts, N. E. (1975): The clinical evaluation of prazosin, a new antihypertensive agent. *Postgrad. Med.*, (Suppl.):117–128.

119. Preston, R. A., O'Connor, D. T., and Stone, R. A. (1979): Prazosin and renal hemodynamics: Arteriolar vasodilatation during therapy of essential hypertension in man. *J. Cardiovasc. Pharmacol.*, 1:277–286.

120. Puddey, I. B., Beilin, L. J., Vandongen, R., Banks, R., and Rouse, I. (1985): Differential effects of sulindac and indomethacin on blood pressure in treated essential hypertensive subjects. *Clin. Sci.*, 69:327–336.

121. Ram, C. V. S., Meese, R., Kaplan, N. M., et al. (1987): Antihypertensive therapy in the elderly: Effects on blood pressure and cerebral blood flow. *Am. J. Med.*, 82:(Suppl.1A):53–57.

122. Ramsay, L. E., Parnell, L., and Waller, P. C. (1987): Comparison of nifedipine, prazosin and hydralazine added to treatment of hypertensive patients uncontrolled by thiazide diuretic plus beta-blocker. *Postgrad. Med. J.*, 63:99–103.

123. Reifart, N., Nadj, M., Kaltenbach, M., and Bussmann, W-D. (1985): Symptomatic and haemodynamic effects of prazosin in chronic congestive heart failure in a randomized double blind trial over one year. *J. Am. Coll. Cardiol.*, 5:461.

124. Roberts, D. H., Tsao, Y., Grimmer, S. F. M., Winstanley, P. A., Orme, M. L. E., and Breckenridge, A. M. (1987): Haemodynamic effects of atenolol, labetalol, pindolol and captopril: A comparison in hypertensive patients with special reference to changes in limb blood flow and left ventricular function. *Br. J. Clin. Pharmacol.*, 24:163–172.

125. Rouffy, J., and Jaillard, J. (1986): Effects of two antihypertensive agents on lipids, lipoproteins and apoproteins A and B. *Am. J. Med.*, 80(Suppl.2A):100–103.

126. Rubin, P. C., and Blaschke, T. F. (1980): Studies on the clinical pharmacology of prazosin I: Cardiovascular, catecholamine and endocrine changes following a single dose. *Br. J. Clin. Pharmacol.*, 10:23–32.

127. Rubin, P., and Blaschke, T. (1980): Prazosin protein binding in health and disease. *Br. J. Clin. Pharmacol.*, 9:177–182.

128. Rubin, P. C., Butters, L., Low, R. A., and Reid, J. L. (1983): Clinical pharmacological studies with prazosin during pregnancy complicated by

hypertension. *Br. J. Clin. Pharmacol.*, 16:543–547.

129. Rubin, P., Jackson, G., Blaschke, T. (1980): Studies on the clinical pharmacology of prazosin II: The influence of indomethacin and of propranolol on the action and disposition of prazosin. *Br. J. Clin. Pharmacol.*, 10:33–39.

130. Rubin, P. C., Scott, P. J. W., and Reid, J. L. (1981): Prazosin disposition in young and elderly subjects. *Br. J. Clin. Pharmacol.*, 12:401–404.

131. Rudd, P., Berenson, G., and Brown, M., et al. (1986): Cumulative experience with terazosin administered in combination with diuretics. *Am. J. Med.*, 80:(Suppl.5B):49–54.

132. Ruoff, G., Cohen, A., Hollifield, J. W., and McGarron, D. A. (1986): Comparative trials of terazosin with other antihypertensive agents. *Am. J. Med.*, 80(Suppl.5B):42–48.

133. Salvadeo, A., Segagni, S., Villa, G., Galli, F., Piazza, W., and Bovio, G. (1981): Prazosin in long term therapy of moderate/severe hypertension. *Curr. Ther. Res.*, 30:1055–1064.

134. Schäfers, R. F., and Reid, J. L. (1988): Alpha-1 adrenoceptor antagonists and sympatholytic drugs in the management of hypertension. In: *Handbook of Hypertension, Vol. 12. The Management of Hypertension*, edited by F. R. Bühler, pp. Elsevier, Amsterdam (in press).

135. Scharf, S. C., Lee, H-B., Wexler, J. P., and Blaufox, M. D. (1984): Cardiovascular consequences of primary antihypertensive therapy with prazosin hydrochloride. *Am J. Cardiol.*, 53:32A–36A.

136. Scott, P. J. W., Hosie, J., and Scott, M. G. B. (1988): A double-blind and cross-over comparison of once daily doxazosin and placebo with steady-state pharmacokinetics in elderly hypertensive patients. *Eur. J. Clin. Pharmacol.*, 34:119–123.

137. Segasothy, M. (1982): Prazosin and priapism. *Med. J. Malaysia.*, 37:384.

138. Seidemann, P., Grahnen, A., Haglund, K., Lindstrom, B., and Von Bahr, C. (1981): Prazosin dynamics in hypertension: Relationship to plasma concentration. *Clin. Pharmacol. Ther.*, 30:447–454.

139. Shionoiri, H., Yasuda, G., Yoshimura, H., et al. (1987): Antihypertensive effects and pharmacokinetics of single and consecutive administration of doxazosin in patients with mild to moderate hypertension. *J. Cardiovasc. Pharmacol.*, 10:90–95.

140. Skinner, D. J., and Misbin, R. I. (1975): Uses of propranolol, letter to the editor. *N. Engl. J. Med.*, 293:1205.

141. Sluiter, H. E, Huysmans, F. Th. M., Thien, Th. A., Koene, R. A. P. (1985): The influence of alpha-1-adrenergic blockade on the acute antihypertensive effect of nifedipine. *Eur. J. Clin. Pharmacol.*, 29:263–267.

142. Sonders, R. C. (1986): Pharmacokinetics of terazosin. *Am. J. Med.*, 80(Suppl.5B):20–24.

143. Sperzel, W. D., Glassman, H. N., Jordan, D. C., and Luther, R. R. (1986): Overall safety of

144. Stamler, R., Stamler, J., Gosch, F. C., Berkson, D. M., Dyer, A., and Hershinow, P. (1986): Initial antihypertensive drug therapy: Alpha blocker or diuretic. Interim report of a randomized controlled trial. *Am. J. Med.*, 80(Suppl.2A):90–93.

145. Stanaszek, W. F., Kellerman, D., Brogden, R. N., and Romankiewicz, J. A. (1983): Prazosin update: A review of its pharmacological properties and therapeutic use in hypertension and congestive heart failure. *Drugs*, 25:339–384.

146. Steinberg, D. (1987): Current theories of the pathogenesis of atherosclerosis. In: *Hypercholesterolemia and Atherosclerosis, Pathogenesis and Prevention*, edited by D. Steinberg, and J. M. Olefsky, pp. 5–24. Churchill Livingston, New York.

147. Stokes, G. S. (1984): Prazosin. In: *Handbook of Hypertension Vol. 5. Clinical Pharmacology of Antihypertensive Drugs*, edited by A. E. Doyle, pp. 350–375. Elsevier, Amsterdam.

148. Stokes, G. S., Mennie, B. A., and Marwood, J. F. (1986): Ketanserin and prazosin: A comparison of antihypertensive and biochemical effects. *Clin. Pharmacol. Ther.*, 40:56–63.

149. Stokes, G. S., Mennie, B. A., Gellatly, R., and Hill, A. (1983): On the combination of alpha- and beta-adrenoceptor blockade in hypertension. *Clin. Pharmacol. Ther.*, 34:576–582.

150. Stokes, G. S., Monaghan, J. C, Frost, G. W., and MacCarthy, E. P. (1979): Responsiveness to prazosin in renal failure. *Clin. Sci.*, 57:383s–385s.

151. Stokes, G. S., Monaghan, J. C., MacCarthy, E. P., and Oates, H. F. (1980): Responsiveness of hypertensive subjects to prazosin. *Clin. Exp. Pharmacol. Physiol.*, 7:215–217.

152. Stokes, G. S., Raftos, J., Lewis, R. G., et al. (1982): Combined use of prazosin and beta-blockers in hypertension. *J. Cardiovasc. Pharmacol.*, 4:S172–S175.

153. Takahashi, H., Watanabe, T., Iyoda, I., Ochiai, M., and Ijichi, H. (1985): Vasodepressor effects of prazosin during insulin-induced hypoglycemia in hypertensive patients. *Jpn. Heart. J.*, 26:965–973.

154. Torvik, D., and Madsbu, H-P. (1986): Multicentre 12-week double-blind comparison of doxazosin, prazosin and placebo in patients with mild to moderate essential hypertension. *Br. J. Clin. Pharmacol.*, 21:69S–75S.

155. Treatment of hypertension in the over-60s. (1985): *Lancet*, 1:1369–1370.

156. Trost, B. N., Weidmann, P., Riesen, W., Claessens, J., Streulens, Y., and Nelemans, F. (1987): Comparative effects of doxazosin and hydrochlorothiazide on serum lipids and blood pressure in essential hypertension. *Am. J. Cardiol.*, 59:99G–104G.

157. Turner, A. S., Watson, O. F., and Brocklehurst, J. E. (1977): Prazosin in hypertension: Clinical

studies with special reference to initiation of therapy. *Med. J. Aust.*, 2(Specl. Suppl.):33–37.

158. Tyroler, H. A. (1987): Lowering plasma cholesterol levels decreases risk of coronary heart disease: An overview of clinical trials. In: Steinberg, D., and Olefsky, J. M., eds. *Hypercholesterolemia and Atherosclerosis, Pathogenesis and Prevention*, edited by D. Steinberg and J. M. Olefsky, pp. 99–116. Churchill Livingstone, New York.

159. Vann Jones, J., and Steiner, J. M. (1980): Double-blind cross-over comparison of hydralazine and prazosin in hypertensive subjects on a beta-adrenoceptor blocking agent (atenolol) *Br. J. Clin. Pharmacol.*, 10:531–533.

160. Velasco, M., Hurt, E., Silva, H., Urbina-Quintana, A., et al. (1986): Effects of prazosin and propranolol on blood lipids and lipoproteins in hypertensive patients. *Am. J. Med.*, 80(Suppl.2A):109–113.

161. Veterans Administration Co-operative Study Group on Antihypertensive Agents. (1981): Comparison of prazosin and hydralazine in patients receiving hydrochlorothiazide: A randomized, double-blind clinical trial. *Circulation*, 64:772–779.

162. Vincent, J., Elliott, H. L., Meredith, P. A., and Reid, J. L. (1983): Doxazosin, an alpha-1-adrenoceptor antagonist: Pharmacokinetics and concentration-effect relationships in man. *Br. J. Clin. Pharmacol.*, 15:719–725.

163. Vincent, J., Meredith, P. A., Reid, J. L., Elliott, H. L., and Rubin, P. C. (1985): Clinical pharmacokinetics of prazosin, 1985. *Clin. Pharmacokinet.*, 10:144–154.

164. Von Bahr, C., Lindström, B., and Seideman, P. (1982): Alpha receptor function changes after the first dose of prazosin. *Clin. Pharmacol. Ther.*, 32:41–47.

165. Waern, A. U., Berne, C., Wibell, L., and Lithell, H. (1982): Short-term influence of a post-synaptic alpha-adrenoceptor blocking drug (prazosin) on carbohydrate metabolism. *Acta Med. Scand.*, (Suppl.)665:75–77.

166. Weber, M. A., Tonkon, M. J., and Klein, R. C. (1987): Effect of antihypertensive therapy on the circadian blood pressure pattern. *Am. J. Med.*, 82(Suppl.1A):50–52.

167. Weinberger, M. H. (1986): Antihypertensive therapy and lipids: Paradoxical influences on cardiovascular disease risk. *Am. J. Med.*, 80(Suppl.2A):64–70.

168. Whiting, B., and Kelman, A. W. (1980): The modelling of drug response. *Clin. Sci.*, 59:311–315.

169. Wilner, K. D., and Ziegler, M. G. (1987): Effects of alpha-1 inhibition on renal blood flow and sympathetic nervous activity in systemic hypertension. *Am. J. Cardiol.*, 59:82G–86G.

170. Wollersheim, H., Thien, T., Fennis, J., van Elteren, P. and, van't Laar, A. (1986): Double-blind, placebo-controlled study of prazosin in Raynaud's phenomenon. *Clin. Pharmacol. Ther.*, 40:219–225.

New Therapeutic Strategies in Hypertension,
edited by Norman M. Kaplan,
Barry M. Brenner, and John H. Laragh.
Raven Press, Ltd., New York © 1989.

Beta-Adrenergic Blockers in Hypertension: An Updated Review

William H. Frishman and Howard B. Mayer*

*Departments of Medicine Epidemiology and Social Medicine, The Albert Einstein College of Medicine; Bronx, New York 10461; and *Department of Medicine, Mt. Sinai Hospital and Medical Center, New York, New York 10003*

It is now recognized that beta-adrenergic blockers are effective in reducing the blood pressure of many patients with systemic hypertension (Table 1) (30). Although there is no consensus as to the mechanism(s) whereby the beta-blocking drugs lower blood pressure, it is probable that some, or all, of the mechanisms referenced in Table 1 are involved.

In whatever manner they work, beta blockers have been found to be useful in the treatment of systemic hypertension, although their definitive mechanism of action remains unclear. The various beta blockers differ in the presence or absence of intrinsic sympathomimetic activity (ISA), membrane-stabilizing activity (MSA), $beta_1$-selectivity, alpha-blocking properties, and relative potencies and duration of action. Whether these differences have any practical relevance in the clinical treatment of hypertension is uncertain. Nevertheless, all beta blockers to date appear to have blood pressure-lowering effects.

Three points can be made:

1. Beta-blocking drugs with intrinsic sympathomimetic activity (partial agonist activity) or alpha-blocking activity will cause less bradycardia.

2. The presence or absence of membrane-stabilizing effect seems to be irrelevant.

3. If a beta blocker has to be given to a potential asthmatic patient, it is best to use a $beta_1$-selective blocker, one with ISA, or one having alpha-blocking effects (33).

CLINICAL EXPERIENCES

The following is an updated review of the current literature on beta blockers, both old and new (Table 2), in the treatment of hypertension. It examines the adverse-effects of beta blockers, their effects in elderly patients, and on plasma lipids. The latter issue is still a highly controversial one. The true clinical significance in humans and the exact mechanism by which beta blockers alter plasma lipids and lipoproteins has yet to be definitively determined. Day et al. (16), suggested that the unopposed alpha stimulation occurring during beta-blockade inhibits lipoprotein lipase. This would then cause an increase in plasma triglyceride and a decrease in HDL cholesterol concentrations. Many investigators have further noted that beta blockers with relative $beta_1$-selectivity (16) and those with ISA (91), tend to produce fewer deleterious effects on plasma lipids.

There are several points to be noted when evaluating beta blocker trials in patients with hypertension:

1. Patients may vary in their individual dose requirements and rapidity of response. Hence, trials using small (or fixed) doses

Table 1. *Proposed mechanisms to explain the antihypertensive actions of beta blockers*

1. Reduction in cardiac output
2. Central nervous system effects
3. Inhibition of renin
4. Reduction in venous return and plasma volume
5. Reduction in peripheral vascular resistance
6. Resetting of baroreceptor levels
7. Effects on prejunctional beta receptors: reduction in norepinephrine release
8. Prevent the pressor response to catecholamines with exercise and stress

and short treatment periods may fail to show much effect.

2. In double-blind studies in which placebo follows active therapy, the duration of placebo therapy must be long enough to allow blood pressure to return to pretreatment levels. If this is not done, the thera-

peutic benefit of active drug will appear to be modest.

3. The best results of beta blockers in hypertension are achieved when the drugs are used in combination with other antihypertensive agents, especially diuretics.

Acebutolol (Sectral)

Acebutolol is a beta$_1$-selective beta blocker with weak ISA and MSA.

Trials Versus Placebo

Davidov (15) investigated the antihypertensive efficacy of acebutolol (200 to 600 mg twice-daily) versus placebo in a 27-week, multicenter, double-blind randomized study involving 237 patients. A greater re-

Table 2. *Pharmacodynamic properties of β-adrenoceptor blocking drugs*

Drug	β$_1$ = blockade potency ratio (propranolol = 1.0)	Relative β$_1$-selectivity	Intrinsic sympathomimetic activity	Membrane stabilizing activity
Acebutolol	0.3	+	+	+
Atenolol	1.0	+ +	0	0
Bevantolol	0.3	+ +	0	0
Bisoprolol	10.3	+ +	0	0
Bucindolol[d]		0	+	0
Carteolol	10.0	0	+	0
Carvedilol[a]	10.0	0	0	+ +
Celiprolol[b]	9.4	+	+ ?	0
Dilevalol[c]	1.0	0	+	0
Esmolol	0.02	+ +	0	0
Labetalol[d]	0.3	0	+ ?	0
Metoprolol	1.0	+ +	0	0
Nadolol	1.0	0	0	0
Oxprenolol	0.5–1.0	0	+	+
Penbutolol	1.0	0	+	0
Pindolol	6.0	0	+ +	+
Propranolol	1.0	0	0	+ +
Sotalol[e]	0.3	0	0	0
Tertatolol		0	0	0
Timolol	6.0	0	0	0
Isomer: *d*-propranolol				+ +

[a] Carvedilol has additional α$_1$-adrenergic blocking activity without peripheral β$_2$-agonism.
[b] Celiprolol may have additional peripheral α$_2$-adrenergic blocking activity at high doses.
[c] Dilevalol is an isomer of labetalol adrenergic with peripheral β$_2$-agonism but no α$_1$ blocking activity.
[d] Bucindolol and labetalol have additional α$_1$-adrenergic blocking activity and direct vasodilatory actions (β$_2$-agonism).
[e] Sotalol has additional type of antiarrhythmic activity.

duction in mean sitting diastolic blood pressure (from 99.2 ± 0.3 to 89.1 ± 0.9 mm Hg) was seen in acebutolol-treated patients than in those treated with placebo at the end of the 12-week dose titration phase. The antihypertensive effect of acebutolol was observed after 2 weeks of treatment, and was maintained throughout the remainder of the dose-titration period and the 12-week maintenance period which followed. During dose-titration, a significantly greater decrease in heart rate was seen in acebutolol-treated patients (from 78.4 ± 0.9 to 69.2 ± 0.9 b.p.m.) than in those treated with placebo.

Dose Interval Studies

Acebutolol 200 to 600 mg, given once-daily and twice-daily, was assessed by Weber and Drayer (98) in a multicenter, double-blind, placebo-controlled study of 192 patients. After three months of therapy, diastolic blood pressure was significantly lower in both treatment groups than in the placebo group. The percentage of patients whose blood pressure control was satisfactory was similar in the once daily and twice daily treatment groups.

Comparative Studies Versus Diuretics and Combination Therapy

A 27-week, multicenter, double-blind, randomized study of 360 patients was conducted by Wahl et al. (96), in order to compare the antihypertensive efficacies of acebutolol (200 to 600 mg twice-daily) and hydrochlorothiazide (25 to 50 mg twice-daily). Significant and comparable reductions in sitting and standing blood pressures were observed in the two treatment groups. A similar number of acebutolol-treated patients (72%) and hydrochlorothiazide-treated patients (63%) were classified as "responders" at the conclusion of the 15-week dose-titration phase. On subgroup

analysis, patients ≥ 65 years of age, responded equally well to acebutolol and to the diuretic, while black patients appeared to respond better to the diuretic.

One thousand four hundred two patients, (813 were newly diagnosed and 589 were known hypertensives), were treated with Secadrex (acebutolol 200 mg combined with hydrochlorothiazide 12.5 mg) once-daily for 12 weeks (63). A good response (MAP <113 or a decrease in MAP of $>15\%$) was observed in 86% of the newly-diagnosed hypertensives and in 77% of the known hypertensives. Heart rate decreased by 12.5% in the newly-diagnosed hypertensives and by 10% in the known hypertensives. Side effects that did not cause withdrawal from the study occurred at a rate of 53.1 per 100 known hypertensives on previous treatment, and decreased to 18.2 per 100 during treatment with Secadrex.

Studies Versus Other Beta Blockers

Wahl et al. (97) conducted a 29-week, multicenter, double-blind, randomized study of 376 patients in order to assess the comparative antihypertensive efficacies of acebutolol (200 to 800 mg twice-daily) and propranolol (60 to 240 mg twice-daily). The two agents produced significant and comparable reductions in sitting and standing blood pressure. At equivalent antihypertensive doses, acebutolol (13%) caused significantly less reduction in resting heart rate than propranolol (17%). Fewer acebutolol-treated (5.9%) than propranolol-treated patients (15.3%) were removed from the study because of side effects. Acebutolol was found to be more effective than propranolol in elderly patients.

In a double-blind, randomized, crossover study conducted by Turner, et al. (90) the antihypertensive efficacies of acebutolol (400 mg once-daily for 8 weeks) and atenolol (100 mg once-daily for 8 weeks) were assessed in 33 patients. The two agents produced significant and comparable reductions in mean arterial pressure after 4 weeks and 8 weeks of treatment. They also had similar effects on postexercise increases in systolic blood pressure and heart rate. Resting heart rate was reduced to a significantly greater extent by atenolol (18.3 b.p.m.) than by acebutolol (14.8 b.p.m.) after 4 weeks of treatment.

Comparative beta blocker studies with acebutolol are also included in other sections of this chapter.

Comparative Studies Versus Calcium-Entry Blockers and Combination Therapy

Sixty black hypertensive patients participated in a 40-week, double-blind, randomized trial which evaluated the comparative antihypertensive efficacies of acebutolol (mean dose 414 mg/day) and nitrendipine (mean dose 32 mg/day) (61). Both agents significantly reduced supine and standing blood pressure, although nitrendipine was significantly more effective than acebutolol. Supine diastolic blood pressure was reduced below 90 mm Hg in 67% of patients treated with nitrendipine and in 47% of patients treated with acebutolol. The addition of mefruside (12.5 to 25 mg daily) to either acebutolol or nitrendipine resulted in a further significant decrease in blood pressure in patients not controlled by monotherapy.

Trials In The Elderly

Salvetti et al. (81) conducted a multicenter, single blind, randomized, crossover trial to compare the antihypertensive effects of acebutolol (400 mg/day for 6 weeks) and hydrochlorothiazide (25 mg/day for 6 weeks) in 45 elderly (mean age 69.5 + 0.7 years) patients. Doses were increased to 600 mg/day and to 50 mg/day, respectively, after 4 weeks of treatment, for those patients whose diastolic blood pressure remained above 95 mm Hg. Both agents significantly reduced supine and standing blood pressures with no difference noted between the two regimens. Increasing the dose of either drug did not result in a further significant decrease in supine diastolic blood pressure.

Boyles (7) evaluated data from three multicenter, randomized, double-blind, parallel studies in order to assess the efficacy and safety of acebutolol in those patients 65 years of age or older. The three studies compared acebutolol to placebo, propranolol, and hydrochlorothiazide. Of the 54 elderly patients treated with acebutolol overall, 91% were "responders" (DBP <90 or ≥10% reduction in DBP from baseline). Acebutolol was more effective than any of the other regimens in terms of response rate. Acebutolol was well tolerated in all three studies, with only 3 patients (5.6%) being withdrawn from the study.

Effects On Plasma Lipids

Lehtonen (50) examined the effect on plasma lipids of acebutolol (400 to 800 mg once daily for 6 months) in 18 hypertensive patients. No significant changes were observed in very low density lipoprotein (VLDL) cholesterol, triglycerides, low-density lipoprotein (LDL) cholesterol, and plasma total cholesterol after 1, 3, and 6 months of treatment. There was a slight decrease in high density lipoprotein (HDL) cholesterol during treatment with acebutolol. Free fatty acid concentration was significantly reduced after 1 month of treatment with no further significant decrease thereafter. It was postulated that the neutral effect of acebutolol on plasma lipid levels may have been due to its ISA.

Atenolol (Tenormin)

Atenolol is a beta$_1$-selective beta blocker without ISA or MSA.

Studies Versus Other Beta Blockers

Comparative beta blocker studies with atenolol appear in other sections of this chapter.

Studies Versus Angiotensin-Converting Enzyme (ACE) Inhibitors

In a two-year, double-blind, randomized study, Andren et al. (3) compared the antihypertensive efficacies of captopril (25 to 100 mg 3 times daily) and atenolol (50 to 200 mg once-daily) in 50 patients. After the initial 12-week dose finding phase, comparable reductions in standing and recumbent blood pressures were observed in the atenolol group (30/20 and 24/18) and in the captopril group (33/19 and 31/20). This blood pressure lowering effect persisted during long-term treatment in both groups. Only atenolol reduced heart rate, and this effect was also maintained over two years. The addition of hydrochlorothiazide potentiated the antihypertensive effect of both agents to the same degree.

Bolzano et al. (6) compared the antihypertensive efficacies of atenolol (50 to 200 mg once-daily) and lisinopril (20 to 80 mg once-daily) in a 24-week, multicenter, double-blind, randomized, parallel-group study involving 490 patients. Patients whose blood pressures were still uncontrolled after 12 weeks of active treatment also received hydrochlorothiazide. Sitting diastolic blood pressures were significantly reduced by both regimens after 12 and 24 weeks. However, lisinopril was found to produce a greater reduction in sitting systolic blood pressure than atenolol during the entire study. Significantly more patients in the atenolol group (43.4%) than in the lisinopril group (32.5%) required the addition of a diuretic, although dual therapy with both agents resulted in similar significant further reduction in blood pressure.

Comparative Studies Versus Calcium-Entry Blockers and Combination Therapy

Escudero et al. (21) compared the antihypertensive efficacies of atenolol (50 mg twice-daily for 4 weeks) and verapamil (120 mg twice-daily for 4 weeks) in a double-blind, crossover study of 24 patients. Both agents reduced supine and upright blood pressures, with no difference noted. Hypertension was adequately stabilized in a similar number of patients during treatment with atenolol (71%) and verapamil (80%). Heart rate was significantly reduced only by atenolol, although a slight decrease was observed with verapamil.

Daniels et al. (14) conducted a double-blind, randomized, crossover trial in order to assess the comparative antihypertensive efficacies of atenolol (100 mg once daily for 4 weeks) and nifedipine (20 mg twice daily for 4 weeks) in 35 patients. Those who did not achieve both a supine and erect diastolic blood pressure of less than 90 mm Hg at the end of monotherapy received the two agents in combination for an additional 4 weeks. Atenolol had a significantly greater effect on supine and erect blood pressure than nifedipine. However, a significantly greater reduction in supine and erect blood pressure was observed with the combination (16 ± 2 and 21 ± 2 mm Hg, respectively) than with atenolol (9 ± 2 and 12 ± 2 mm Hg, respectively) or nifedipine (6 ± 2 and 5 ± 2 mm Hg, respectively) alone.

Studies Versus Alpha-Blocking Agents

Nash, et al. (69) compared the antihypertensive efficacies of atenolol (50 to 100 mg once-daily for 10 weeks) and doxazosin (1 to 16 mg once-daily for 10 weeks) in a double-blind, randomized, placebo-controlled study of 129 patients. Both atenolol ($-12/-12$ mm Hg) and doxazosin ($-13/-11$ mm Hg) produced significant reductions in standing blood pressure compared with placebo, without a significant difference noted. Parallel responses were observed for supine blood pressure. Unlike doxazosin, which had no effect on heart rate, atenolol significantly decreased both supine ($-9.9 ± 1.2$ beats/min) and standing $-11.2 ± 1.5$ beats/min) heart rate.

Frick et al. (28) further assessed the comparative antihypertensive efficacies of atenolol (50 to 100 mg once-daily) and doxazosin (1 to 16 mg once-daily) in a long-term, multicenter, double-blind, randomized study of 143 patients. Patients were followed for up to 52 weeks, with a minimum of 20 weeks of active therapy. It was found that although both agents significantly and comparably reduced standing blood pressure, atenolol was significantly more effective than doxazosin in reducing supine blood pressure.

Lange Andersen et al. (48) observed that atenolol (100 mg once-daily), but not prazosin (2 mg twice-daily), significantly lowered blood pressure and heart rate responses to exercise.

Trials In The Elderly

Andersen (2) conducted a 12-week, open, randomized study in order to compare the effects of atenolol (50 to 100 mg once-daily) and bendroflumethiazide (2.5 to 10 mg once-daily) in 162 middle-aged (50 to 64 years) and elderly (65 to 75 years) patients. Both agents significantly reduced blood pressure in the two age groups. There was no significant between-treatment difference noted in the elderly group, whereas atenolol was superior to bendroflumethiazide in reducing diastolic blood pressure in middle-aged patients.

Side-Effects Versus Other Beta Blockers

In a 24-week, single-blind study conducted by Fodor et al. (25) the comparative side-effect profiles of equally effective doses of atenolol and propranolol were assessed in 52 hypertensive patients with a prior history of adverse-effects related to lipophilic beta blocker therapy. Treatment began with propranolol (40 to 160 mg twice-daily for 8 weeks), was followed by atenolol (50 to 100 mg once-daily for 8 weeks), and ended with an additional 8 weeks of propranolol. The incidence and severity of adverse effects, particularly those related to

the central nervous system (CNS) (e.g., early awakenings, nightmares, depressed mood, insomnia, etc.), tended to improve significantly during the atenolol phase and worsen during readministration of propranolol. Severity scores followed this pattern, most notably in those patients who had experienced a particular side effect during the initial propranolol phase.

Foerster et al. (26) conducted a 24-week, randomized, crossover study of 107 patients in order to compare the side effects of atenolol (100 mg once-daily) and slow-release pindolol (20 mg once daily). A significant number of patients reported having experienced sleep disturbances, dreams, fatigue, and other such "side effects" prior to receiving beta blockers. The frequency of dreams and fatigue was significantly reduced with both agents. Sleep disturbances decreased significantly in atenolol-treated patients (38% to 18%) but increased significantly in pindolol-treated patients (33% to 44%). The investigators concluded that this latter finding was most likely due to the lower lipophilicity of atenolol.

Effects On Plasma Lipids

In a study mentioned elsewhere in this chapter, atenolol 100 mg daily was shown to significantly increase plasma triglycerides (although to a lesser extent than propranolol and oxprenolol) and to decrease HDL cholesterol (16).

In a 42-month, randomized, prospective study of 68 male hypertensives, Middeke et al. (66), compared the effects of atenolol (100 to 200 mg once-daily) and hydrochlorothiazide (50 to 100 mg once-daily) on serum lipoproteins. As in the previous study (16) these investigators noted a decrease in HDL cholesterol and an increase in triglycerides with atenolol. An additional observation, however, was that these changes were greater at increased beta blocker doses. Hydrochlorothiazide also increased serum triglycerides, but did not significantly affect HDL cholesterol. Only hydrochlorothiazide significantly raised LDL cholesterol. In contrast with atenolol, these diuretic-induced changes were not dose-dependent.

Rouffy and Jaillard (76) examined the effects of atenolol (100 to 200 mg once-daily) and prazosin (0.5 to 3 mg twice-daily) on plasma lipids in a 3-month, open, randomized, parallel-group study of 50 patients. Atenolol significantly reduced HDL cholesterol and A_1-lipoproteins, while raising LDL cholesterol, VLDL cholesterol, triglycerides and beta-lipoproteins. Prazosin therapy produced the opposite effects.

In a multicenter, double-blind study of 96 patients, Frick et al. (27) compared the serum lipid changes produced by atenolol (50 to 100 mg once-daily) versus doxazosin (1 to 16 mg once-daily) for up to 52 weeks. Again, atenolol caused unfavorable changes in plasma lipid concentrations (+triglycerides, −HDL cholesterol, −HDL/total cholesterol, +total cholesterol), whereas doxazosin had beneficial effects on these values.

Bevantolol (Ranestol)

Bevantolol is a new beta$_1$-selective beta blocker without ISA but with MSA.

A multicenter, double-blind, randomized, parallel-group study of 139 patients was conducted by Okawa (71) in order to assess the antihypertensive efficacy of bevantolol in dosages of 100, 200, 300, and 400 mg given twice-daily. Bevantolol, in doses of 200 to 400 mg, reduced diastolic blood pressure to a significantly greater extent than placebo. No difference was observed between the 200, 300, and 400 mg groups. Decreases in the 100 mg group however, were not significantly different than placebo. Similar reductions in systolic blood pressure were observed. Bevantolol also reduced resting heart rate in all 4 treatment groups.

One hundred twenty-five patients partic-ipated in 2 multicenter, double-blind studies conducted by Jain (43) in which the antihypertensive efficacy of bevantolol (100 to 400 mg daily) was assessed. The studies were similar in all aspects except for dosing intervals (once daily versus twice-daily administration). No significant difference in efficacy was observed between the once daily and twice daily treatment regimens.

Combination Therapy With Diuretics

Lucas et al. (56) carried out a multicenter, double-blind, randomized study of 244 patients in order to evaluate the antihypertensive effect produced by bevantolol (200 mg twice-daily for 4 weeks), when added after 4 weeks of therapy to hydrochlorothiazide 50 mg daily, hydrochlorothiazide 100 mg daily, or placebo. In all three groups, diastolic blood pressure was significantly lower after dual therapy with bevantolol than after monotherapy. Both hydrochlorothiazide groups produced significantly lower diastolic blood pressure values than did placebo during monotherapy and during combination therapy with bevantolol

Studies Versus Other Beta Blockers

Fairhurst (22) compared the antihypertensive efficacies of bevantolol (400 mg once daily for 12 weeks) and atenolol (100 mg once-daily for 12 weeks) in a randomized, double-blind trial in 229 patients. The two beta blockers produced significant and comparable reductions in systolic and diastolic blood pressure. However, the investigators found bevantolol's blood pressure lowering effect to be less rapid in onset. Although both agents significantly reduced heart rate, atenolol's effect was observed to be greater. In 104 patients, blood pressure and heart rate were measured every 24 hours after dosing. There was no significant between-treatment difference observed in this group after 12 weeks of active treatment.

Bisoprolol (Concor)

Bisoprolol is a new highly $beta_1$-selective beta blocker without ISA or MSA.

Pilot Studies

Ikeda et al. (41) evaluated the antihypertensive efficacy of bisoprolol in a study of 28 inpatients (5 to 20 mg once-daily for 4 weeks) and 68 outpatients (5 to 20 mg once-daily for 6 to 8 weeks). Bisoprolol significantly reduced systolic blood pressure, diastolic blood pressure, and heart rate in both patient groups. Responder rates were 73% and 62% in the two groups, respectively. Bisoprolol did not significantly alter diurnal variation of blood pressure. Bradycardia was the most common side effect of the drug, and was seen in 9 of 96 patients.

Dose-Finding Studies

In a double-blind, randomized study of 48 patients conducted by Weiner and Frithz (100) the antihypertensive efficacy of bisoprolol in dosages of 5, 10, and 20 mg once-daily for 8 weeks was assessed. Significant reductions in systolic blood pressure, diastolic blood pressure and heart rate (at rest and during bicycle exercise) were noted with all three doses of the drug. However, 20 mg once-daily caused the greatest decreases in supine blood pressure and heart rate. No differences were noted between the 5 mg and 10 mg groups. A further, significant reduction in blood pressure was not observed during a 10-month, open, dose-titration phase.

Studies Versus Other Beta Blockers

Bühler et al. (8) compared the antihypertensive efficacies of bisoprolol (10 to 20 mg once-daily for 8 weeks) and atenolol (50 to 100 mg once-daily for 8 weeks) in a randomized, double-blind, crossover, international multicenter study (BIMS) involving 104 patients. The investigators observed significantly greater reductions in blood pressure and heart rate with bisoprolol. The target blood pressure (DBP ≤ 95 mm Hg) was obtained in 68% of bisoprolol patients and in 56% of atenolol patients. In both treatment groups, patients under the age of 60 achieved the target blood pressure more often than those over 60. Regular cigarette smokers reached the target diastolic pressure more often with bisoprolol than with atenolol.

Effects On Plasma Lipids

Frithz and Weiner (34) studied the effects of bisoprolol (2.5 to 40 mg once-daily for 12 weeks) on serum lipid values in 43 patients, all of whom had achieved the target diastolic pressure of ≤ 90 mm Hg. Triglycerides, LDL, HDL, and total cholesterol values were unchanged compared with placebo, following 8 and 12 weeks of active treatment.

Forty-two patients participated in a double-blind, randomized study conducted by Lithell et al. (55), in which the effects of bisoprolol (10 and 20 mg once-daily for 6 months) and atenolol (50 and 100 mg once-daily for 6 months) on lipoprotein concentrations were assessed. Both doses of each beta-blocker were administered for a 3-month period. VLDL triglycerides increased significantly with both drugs. Whereas LDL cholesterol levels did not significantly change with either agent, HDL cholesterol significantly decreased with both bisoprolol and atenolol. Both agents also significantly lowered apolipoprotein A-1 levels in HDL. Overall, the 4 treatment regimens had similar effects on lipoprotein concentrations.

Bopindolol (Sandonorm)

Bopindolol is a new nonselective beta blocker with ISA and MSA.

Open Trials

In a study performed by Hulthen et al. (40), the antihypertensive efficacy of bopindolol (1 to 4 mg once-daily for 12 weeks) as related to age and plasma-renin activity was assessed. Bopindolol produced significant reductions in systolic and diastolic blood pressure. A diastolic blood pressure of less than 95 mm Hg was obtained in 19 of 23 (83%) patients. Diastolic blood pressure was decreased to a significantly greater extent in younger (19 to 35 years) than in older (36 to 59 years) patients. In addition, patients with normal or high-plasma-renin activity experienced a greater decrease in diastolic pressure than those with low-plasma-renin activity.

Dose-Finding Studies

In a multicenter, double-blind, randomized trial conducted by the Swiss Bopindolol Cooperative Study Group (104) the antihypertensive effects of bopindolol 1 and 2 mg once-daily, and atenolol 50 and 100 mg once-daily were assessed in 223 patients. If diastolic blood pressure was greater than 90 mm Hg after 4 weeks of treatment, the dosages were doubled. All 4 regimens produced a significant reduction in mean arterial blood pressure with no difference observed. Bopindolol 1 mg once-daily was equivalent in efficacy to the 2 mg dose, after 4 weeks and 8 weeks of active treatment. Bopindolol 1 mg once-daily maintained this antihypertensive effect in a 10-month, open phase which followed.

Schiess et al. (82) compared bopindolol (1 to 4 mg once-daily for 10 weeks), pindolol (7.5 to 30 mg once-daily for 10 weeks), and atenolol (50 to 200 mg once-daily for 10 weeks) in a multicenter, double-blind, randomized, parallel-group trial involving 369 patients. Hydrochlorothiazide was added if the target diastolic pressure of ≤90 mm Hg was not obtained after 6 weeks of active treatment. A significant reduction in sys-

tolic and diastolic blood pressure was observed in all three groups with no difference. Standing heart rate was reduced to a lesser degree by the two drugs with ISA (pindolol and bopindolol).

Effects On Plasma Lipids

The effect of bopindolol (1 to 4 mg once-daily) on plasma lipids and lipoprotein fractions was evaluated by Van Brummelen et al. (92) in a 12-week study of 24 hypertensive patients. No significant changes in total cholesterol, LDL cholesterol, and HDL cholesterol were observed. Plasma-triglyceride concentration was significantly increased after 4 and 8 weeks, but not after 12 weeks, of treatment.

Bucindolol

Bucindolol (MJ 13105) is a new nonselective beta blocker with ISA. It also has alpha-blocking and direct vasodilatory activity.

Chronic Effects

Rosendorff et al. (77) evaluated the antihypertensive efficacy of bucindolol (10 to 200 mg twice-daily for 12 weeks) in a long-term trial involving 30 patients. A significant reduction in both supine and standing blood pressure was noted after 12 weeks of therapy. In patients followed for one year, a significant reduction in mean blood pressure was observed in seven out of 12 months.

Comparative Studies Versus Diuretics and Combination Therapy

Rotmensch (79) evaluated the comparative antihypertensive effects of bucindolol (150 mg once-daily), hydrochlorothiazide (50 mg once-daily), and their combination. Each therapeutic regimen was for two weeks. Both bucindolol and hydrochlorothiazide significantly reduced standing diastolic blood pressure with no difference noted. The combination produced a further significant reduction in blood pressure compared with either agent alone.

Studies Versus Other Beta Blockers

In a double-blind, randomized, crossover, placebo-controlled study carried out by Webster et al. (99), the antihypertensive effects of single oral doses of bucindolol (50 to 200 mg) versus single oral doses of oxprenolol (40 to 160 mg) were compared. Bucindolol was found to be significantly more effective than oxprenolol or placebo in reducing blood pressure 1 to 2 hr post-dosing.

Carvedilol

Carvedilol (BM 14190) is a new combined nonselective beta blocker/precapillary vasodilator without ISA.

Open Studies

Heber et al. (38) studied the 24 hr blood pressure profile of carvedilol (25 to 50 mg twice-daily) after 4 weeks of therapy with this agent. Mean daytime reduction of blood pressure was 25 ± 3/19 ± 3 mm Hg. Mean decrease in heart rate was 22 ± 3 beats/min. Blood pressure during dynamic and isometric exercise was also reduced significantly. Carvedilol's antihypertensive effect began within 10 minutes of administration, and reached sustained maximal levels after 90 minutes.

Studies Versus Other Beta Blockers

In a double-blind, randomized study of 18 patients Meyer-Sabellek et al. (65) assessed the comparative antihypertensive effects of carvedilol (50 mg once-daily for 3 weeks) and metoprolol (200 mg once-daily for 3 weeks). Both agents significantly reduced supine and standing blood pressure. However, only carvedilol significantly lowered blood pressure during exercise.

Celiprolol (Selectol)

Celiprolol is a new beta$_1$-selective beta blocker with ISA but without MSA.

Open Trials

Hoffman and Hoffman (39) examined the effects of celiprolol in a six-week, multicenter study of 2,311 patients with mild to severe hypertension. All patients were treated initially with 200 mg once-daily celiprolol. In those patients whose blood pressure was not adequately lowered after three weeks, the dose was increased to 300 mg once-daily, or a diuretic was added, for the remaining three weeks. A majority of the patients (1,625) did not require the higher dose of celiprolol, or the addition of a diuretic in order to achieve blood pressure control. Overall, approximately 74% of the patients had a diastolic pressure less than 95 mm Hg after six weeks of therapy. Heart rate was lowered by a mean of 8 b.p.m., and mostly in those patients with tachycardia.

Trials Versus Placebo

Capone and Mayol (10) investigated the antihypertensive efficacy of once-daily celiprolol compared to placebo in an 18-week, multicenter, double-blind study involving 190 patients. Daily dosages of celiprolol ranged from 200 to 600 mg. Celiprolol produced a significant decrease in supine and standing blood pressure compared with placebo. A supine diastolic pressure of ≤90 mm Hg, or a decrease in this value by at least 10 mm Hg, was achieved in 66% of patients receiving celiprolol and in only 38% of those receiving placebo. Although the addition of chlorthalidone in "nonresponders" lowered blood pressure in both groups, the effect was greater in the celiprolol group than in the placebo group.

Studies Versus Other Beta Blockers

The antihypertensive efficacies of celiprolol (200 to 400 mg once-daily for 12 weeks) and propranolol (40 to 80 mg twice-daily for 12 weeks) were compared by Taylor et al. (87) in a double-blind, randomized study of 58 patients. The study consisted of a four-week dose-titration period followed by an eight-week maintenance phase. Celiprolol ($-14/-13$ mm Hg) and propranolol ($-11/-12$ mm Hg) produced comparable reductions in blood pressure at the end of the dose-titration period. However, at the end of the study, the antihypertensive effect of celiprolol ($-18/-14$ mm Hg) was found to be superior to propranolol ($-8/-9$ mm Hg). During the study, a greater reduction in heart rate was observed in the propranolol group than in the celiprolol group.

Dilevalol

Dilevalol, the R,R-isomer of labetalol, is a new nonselective beta blocker with alpha-blocker property and with ISA (? beta$_2$-selective).

Trials Versus Placebo

The antihypertensive efficacy of dilevalol was evaluated in a double-blind, parallel-group study conducted by Soberman et al. (85). Twenty-nine patients were randomized to either dilevalol (100 to 800 mg once-daily for 2 to 15 weeks) or placebo. This was followed by a maintenance phase lasting 4 weeks. Dilevalol reduced supine blood pressure to a significantly greater extent than placebo, both after the dose-titration period (difference of 17.3/10.5) and at the end of the maintenance phase (difference of 13.7/10.0). Similar reductions were noted with standing blood pressures. Dilevalol also produced a slight but significant reduction in heart rate as compared with placebo.

In a larger experience, Frishman et al. (32) demonstrated a greater blood pressure lowering effect with once daily dilevalol than with placebo. No effects on plasma lipids were seen.

Labetalol (Normodyne, Trandate)

Labetalol is a nonselective beta blocker with alpha-blocking, direct vasodilatory and intrinsic sympathomimetic activities. It has no membrane-stabilizing action.

Dose-Ranging Studies

The hypotensive efficacy of labetalol was investigated by Dux et al. (18) in a 14-week, single-blind study of 29 patients. Patients received, in succession, labetalol 0.6 g/day, labetalol 0.8 g/day and the latter plus hydrochlorothiazide 25 to 50 mg/day. Each treatment regimen was given for 4 weeks. Labetalol in either dose, or in conjunction with diuretic, significantly reduced supine and erect blood pressure as compared to placebo. A significant dose-dependent decrease in blood pressure was observed upon increasing the dose of labetalol from 0.6 g to 0.8 g/day. However, the addition of diuretic did not result in a significantly greater reduction in blood pressure than with labetalol 0.8 g/day alone.

Combination Therapy With Diuretics

In a multicenter, randomized, double-blind, parallel study carried out by the Labetalol/Hydrochlorothiazide Multicenter Study Group (47), the antihypertensive efficacy of labetalol (100 to 400 mg once-daily for 12 weeks) plus hydrochlorothiazide was assessed in 174 patients. The addition of labetalol to hydrochlorothiazide resulted in a further significant decrease in both supine and standing blood pressure as compared with placebo. There was no difference in response between black and white patients. Women tended to respond somewhat more than men, and subjects older than 55 years seemed to have a greater response than those younger than 55 years.

A multicenter, double-blind, randomized trial was conducted by Flamenbaum et al. (24), in order to compared the antihypertensive effects of labetalol (100 to 600 mg twice-daily) and propanolol (40 to 240 mg twice-daily) in 65 black and 75 white patients. They found that whereas labetalol was equally effective in black and white patients, propanolol was significantly less effective in blacks (-2.1 ± 1.6 mm Hg) than whites (-8.1 ± 3.3 mm Hg) in reducing standing diastolic blood pressure. Additionally, twice as many black patients receiving labetalol, compared to those receiving propranolol, achieved a standing diastolic blood pressure less than 90 mm Hg. Also, twice as many black patients treated with propranolol, compared to those treated with labetalol, required the addition of a diuretic in order to achieve blood pressure control.

Comparative Studies Versus Calcium-Channel Blockers and Combination Therapy

The antihypertensive efficacies of labetalol (200 to 400 mg twice-daily for six weeks), nifedipine (20 to 40 mg twice-daily for six weeks), and labetalol (200 mg twice-daily for four weeks) plus nifedipine (20 mg twice-daily for four weeks) were assessed in a randomized, double-blind, crossover trial involving 25 patients (70). All three treatment regimens significantly lowered supine and standing blood pressure compared to placebo. However, the investigators observed that labetalol was significantly more effective than nifedipine in lowering all blood pressure values except for supine diastolic blood pressure. Com-

bination therapy was significantly more effective in reducing blood pressure than either agent alone.

Combination Studies

Fifty-six patients whose blood pressure was not well controlled on a combination of atenolol (100 to 200 mg/day) and hydrochlorothiazide (50 mg/day) were randomly assigned to treatment with either labetalol (100 to 600 mg thrice-daily) plus hydrochlorothiazide (50 mg/day), or atenolol (200 mg/day) plus prazosin (0.5 to 7.0 mg thrice daily) and hydrochlorothiazide (50 mg/day) (93). Following six months of treatment on this schedule, systolic and diastolic blood pressures were reduced by 8.6 and 2.4 mm Hg in the labetalol group and by 7.7 and 5.0 mm Hg in the prazosin group. Fifty-two percent of the labetalol group and 58% of the prazosin group achieved a diastolic blood pressure less than 90 mm Hg.

Trials In The Elderly

Abernathy et al. (1) evaluated the efficacy of labetalol (100 to 400 mg twice-daily) in 20 patients older than 60 years, and in 19 patients younger than 60 years. The majority of the older patients had isolated systolic hypertension. A dose-titration period, lasting up to four weeks, was followed by a four-week maintenance period for those patients in whom blood pressure control was achieved. Standing systolic and diastolic blood pressure was significantly reduced in both age groups. However, 70% (14 of 20) of the older patients and only 32% (6 of 19) of the younger patients were controlled on 100 mg of labetalol twice daily. These investigators suggested that the efficacy of comparatively lower doses of labetalol in isolated systolic hypertension of the elderly may have been due to the drug's alpha$_1$-blocking property. They postulated that this led to improved peripheral vascular compliance in these patients.

Side-Effects Versus Other Beta Blockers

Burris et al. (9) assessed the side-effect profile of labetalol in 34 patients. All patients reported a recent history of beta blocker (i.e., propranolol, atenolol, pindolol, metoprolol, nadolol) related side effects, most notably fatigue (44%), impotence (21%), cold extremities (18%), and depression (15%). Only 3 of the 15 patients who reported fatigue on previous beta blocker therapy had a recurrence on labetalol. Similarly, only 1 of 7 and 1 of 5 patients, respectively, experienced recurrences of impotence and depression. None of the subjects reported cold extremities. Eighty-eight percent (30 of 34 patients) tolerated labetalol better than their previous beta blocker, and 24 of these patients (71%) preferred labetalol to their former beta-blocking drug.

Effects On Plasma Lipids

The effects of labetalol on plasma lipids have been studied by many investigators, with no adverse effects on lipids noted (31,62,73,86). Frishman et al. (31) conducted a double-blind, randomized, placebo-controlled study comparing the efficacies of labetalol and metoprolol in 70 hypertensive patients. Labetalol (300 to 1200 mg/daily) did not produce any changes in plasma cholesterol, triglycerides, LDL-cholesterol, HDL-cholesterol, or the HDL/total cholesterol ratio after 4 months of therapy.

Metoprolol (Betaloc, Lopressor)

Metoprolol is a beta$_1$-selective beta blocker without ISA or MSA.

The antihypertensive efficacy of once-daily conventional metoprolol (200 mg) was compared with two long-acting forms of metoprolol (film-coated metoprolol SR and metoprolol SA durules 200 mg once-daily) and with atenolol (100 mg once-daily), in a crossover study of 12 patients carried out by Silas et al. (84). Each treatment period lasted 4 weeks. At 3.5 hr after drug dosing, all 4 treatment regimens significantly reduced resting and exercise blood pressure and heart rate. However, at 24 hr post-dosing, only atenolol significantly reduced blood pressure and consistently produced a $\geq 10\%$ decrease in exercise heart rate. In contrast to the previous findings (105), slow-release metoprolol failed to cause a significant reduction in blood pressure after 24 hr. The efficacy and duration of action of the two slow-release formulations of metoprolol were, in fact, not found to be superior to once-daily conventional metoprolol.

Studies Versus Diuretics

In an open, multicenter, randomized study conducted by the Heart Attack Primary Prevention Hypertension Research Group (HAPPHY) (103), 6,569 males with mild to moderate hypertension received either a beta blocker (metoprolol 200 mg daily or atenolol 100 mg daily) or a thiazide diuretic (bendroflumethiazide 5 mg daily or hydrochlorothiazide 50 mg daily), and were followed for a total of 24,665 patient-years. Other antihypertensive drugs (e.g., hydralazine, spironolactone) were added if a diastolic blood pressure less than 95 mm Hg was not obtained with a single agent. These investigators observed no significant difference between the two groups in the frequency of coronary events (fatal and nonfatal) and in total mortality.

In contrast to the previous findings (103), Wikstrand et al. (101) (HAPPHY study) observed that in 3,234 male hypertensives (16,180 patient-years) metoprolol (mean dose 174 mg/day) reduced total coronary heart disease and stroke mortality to a significantly greater degree than thiazide diuretics. In addition, total mortality was significantly reduced in smokers who received metoprolol, as compared to those who received thiazide diuretics.

Studies Versus Other Beta Blockers

Comparative beta-blocker studies with metoprolol appear in other sections of this chapter.

Studies Versus Angiotensin Converting Enzyme (ACE) Inhibitors

The comparative antihypertensive efficacies of metoprolol (100 to 200 mg once-daily for 8 weeks) and lisinopril (40 to 80 mg once-daily for 8 weeks) were assessed in a multicenter, double-blind, randomized study of 179 patients (106). Both agents significantly reduced sitting diastolic blood pressure with no difference observed. It was noted, however, that patients treated with lisinopril had a significantly lower systolic blood pressure than those treated with metoprolol, after both 4 weeks and 8 weeks of therapy.

Comparative Studies Versus Calcium-Entry Blockers and Combination Therapy

Trimarco et al. (88) conducted a randomized, crossover, double-blind trial in 20 patients to compare the antihypertensive efficacies of metoprolol (100 mg twice-daily for 4 weeks) and diltiazem (600 mg four times daily for 4 weeks). Both agents significantly reduced supine and upright blood pressure with no significant difference noted. The percentage of patients who achieved a blood pressure below 150/90 mm Hg was similar with metoprolol and diltiazem. Only metoprolol significantly reduced the exercise-induced increase in systolic blood pressure.

Ekelund et al. (19) found that the addition of metoprolol (100 mg twice-daily) to nifedipine (10 mg thrice-daily) produced a further significant reduction in resting and exercise blood pressure.

Studies Versus Alpha-Blocking Agents

Leonetti et al. (52) conducted a randomized, crossover, double-blind trial in which the antihypertensive efficacy of metoprolol (100 mg twice-daily for 4 weeks) was compared to that of urapadil (30 mg twice-daily for 4 weeks) in 40 patients. Blood pressure, both in the upright and supine position, was significantly reduced by both agents with no significant difference noted. Heart rate was significantly reduced only after metoprolol with no values less than 50 beats/min observed. Exercise-induced increases in systolic blood pressure and heart rate were significantly reduced by metoprolol, but not by urapadil.

Trials In The Elderly

In a multicenter, randomized, double-blind study conducted by Wikstrand et al. (102), 562 elderly patients (60 to 75 years of age) received either metoprolol (100 mg once-daily) or hydrochlorothiazide (25 mg once-daily) for 4 weeks. If diastolic blood pressure remained greater than 95 mm Hg after this initial period, the dose was doubled in the hydrochlorothiazide group, while patients in the metoprolol group received, in addition, 12.5 mg hydrochlorothiazide. Systolic and diastolic blood pressure were significantly and similarly reduced by both drug regimens, after 4 and 8 weeks of treatment. The efficacy-tolerance index (a scoring system designed to measure antihypertensive efficacy, shifts in laboratory values, and in subjective symptoms) was significantly higher (more favorable) in patients treated with the metoprolol regimen than in those treated with hydrochlorothiazide.

Effects On Plasma Lipids

In a study mentioned elsewhere in this chapter, metoprolol 100 mg twice-daily was shown to significantly increase plasma tri-glycerides (though to a lesser extent than propranolol and oxprenolol) and decrease HDL cholesterol (16).

In a three-month, open, crossover study of 20 hypertensive patients, Rossner and Weiner (78) compared the effects of slow-release metoprolol (200 mg/day) and aten-olol (50 mg/day) on serum lipoproteins. Metoprolol significantly reduced HDL cho-lesterol and increased serum triglycerides and VLDL cholesterol. Atenolol, surpris-ingly, had no significant effect on these val-ues. The investigators postulated that aten-olol's neutral effect on lipids may have been a dose-related phenomenon.

In a 10-week, open, randomized trial in 30 hypertensive patients, Ferrara et al. (23) compared the lipid changes produced by metoprolol (100 to 200 mg daily) and pra-zosin (0.5 to 4 mg daily). Again metoprolol significantly lowered HDL cholesterol and increased triglycerides. In contrast, prazo-sin increased HDL cholesterol and had a neutral effect on plasma triglycerides. Pra-zosin also reduced total serum cholesterol.

Nadolol (Corgard)

Nadolol is a nonselective beta blocker with no ISA or MSA.

Trials Versus Placebo

Dupont et al. (17) examined the antihy-pertensive and renal effects of nadolol (80 mg once-daily for 4 weeks) in a randomized, double-blind, crossover study of 10 pa-tients. Nadolol significantly lowered mean ambulatory blood pressure and heart rate. Renal blood flow and glomerular filtration rate were unchanged, in spite of the fact that nadolol had a negative effect on cardiac out-put. These findings are in agreement with others that, unlike propranolol, nadolol lowers blood pressure without altering renal hemodynamics.

Comparative Studies Versus Diuretics and Combination Therapy

In a randomized, double-blind study con-ducted by the Veterans Administration Cooperative Study Group (95), 365 male pa-tients received nadolol (80 to 240 mg once-daily for 12 weeks), bendroflumethiazide (5 to 10 mg once-daily for 12 weeks), or a com-bination of these two agents for 12 weeks. The diuretic reduced systolic (but not dias-tolic) blood pressure to a significantly greater degree than nadolol. The combina-tion produced significantly greater reduc-tions in systolic and diastolic blood pressure than either agent alone. The antihyperten-sive efficacy of nadolol was significantly greater in whites than in blacks. Con-versely, bendroflumethiazide was more ef-fective in blacks than in whites. Adding hy-dralazine (25 to 100 mg twice-daily) to those patients whose blood pressure was uncon-trolled produced further and comparable re-ductions in diastolic blood pressure in all three treatment groups.

Twenty-seven patients, 24 of whom had decreased renal function, participated in a crossover study comparing nadolol (120 mg/day) with atenolol (100 mg/day) (68). Sitting and lying blood pressures were lowered to a significantly greater degree with atenolol. Heart rate was reduced similarly by both agents. Glomerular filtration rate and effec-tive plasma flow were not significantly al-tered by either beta blocker.

Studies Versus Prazosin

In an open, crossover study of 20 male patients uncontrolled on diuretic mono-therapy, Okun and Kraut (72) compared the antihypertensive effects of nadolol (mean dose 63.15 mg/day) plus polythiazide versus prazosin (mean dose 3.3 mg/day) plus po-lythiazide. Sitting, standing, and supine blood pressures were similarly reduced by both treatment regimens. Neither agent in combination with a thiazide diuretic had a negative effect on total body potassium.

Oxprenolol (Trasicor, Iset)

Oxprenolol is a nonselective beta blocker with ISA and MSA.

Trials Versus Diuretics

A multicenter, double-blind, randomized trial was conducted by the International Prospective Primary Prevention Study in Hypertension Group (IPPPSH) (42) in order to assess the degree to which treatment with slow-release oxprenolol (160 mg once-daily) affected the incidence of myocardial infarction, sudden cardiac death, and cerebrovascular accidents. A total of 6,357 patients (25,651 patient-years) participated in the trial and received, primarily, either oxprenolol or placebo. However, in the majority of patients in both groups, other antihypertensives (e.g., usually diuretics but also methyldopa, hydralazine, prazosin, clonidine, reserpine, etc.) were added in order to achieve better blood pressure control. There was no significant difference demonstrated between the two groups in the incidence of sudden death, myocardial infarction (fatal or nonfatal), or cerebrovascular accidents (fatal or nonfatal). However, on subgroup analysis, coronary event rate was significantly lower in nonsmoking males who received oxprenolol.

Comparative Studies Versus Diuretics and Combination Therapy

In a 12-week trial involving 143 patients, Friedman et al. (29) compared the antihypertensive efficacies of oxprenolol (160, 320, or 480 mg/day) versus hydrochlorothiazide (50, 100, or 150 mg/day). The study found that the blood pressure reduction achieved with oxprenolol was 6/2 mm Hg less than with hydrochlorothiazide.

Studies Versus Other Beta Blockers

Comparative beta blocker studies with oxprenolol appear in other sections of this chapter.

Studies Versus Calcium-Entry Blockers

Ruddel et al. (80) conducted a single-blind, randomized, long-term study in which 60 white males received either oxprenolol (160 to 320 mg once-daily) or nitrendipine (20 to 40 mg once-daily) for at least 4 months. Clinical casual blood pressure was significantly and similarly reduced by both agents. There was also no significant difference between the two groups in average blood pressure during ambulatory blood pressure monitoring; these values were not significantly different when compared with clinical casual blood pressure on the same day. Additionally, blood pressure during mental challenge (video game) increased to a similar degree in both groups.

The same group found that at similar levels of physical activity and at lower self-reported levels of arousal, patients treated with oxprenolol had lower ambulatory systolic blood pressure readings than those treated with nitrendipine. (83).

Effects On Plasma Lipids

In a study mentioned elsewhere in this chapter, oxprenolol 80 mg twice-daily was shown to significantly increase plasma triglycerides and decrease HDL cholesterol (16).

In a randomized, double-blind study of 20 patients, Ballantyne et al. (4) compared the effects of slow oxprenolol (160 to 320 mg once-daily) versus slow oxprenolol plus cyclopenthiazide (0.25 to 0.5 mg once-daily) on plasma lipids. Slow oxprenolol alone produced significant increases in LDL cholesterol and plasma cholesterol after 12 weeks of treatment. In contrast, slow oxprenolol combined with diuretic did not significantly alter LDL or plasma cholesterol. However, the combination did cause significant increases in plasma triglyceride and VLDL triglyceride.

Pindolol (Visken)

Pindolol is a nonselective beta blocker with ISA and no MSA.

Open Studies

A multicenter study of 7,324 patients was conducted by Marks et al. (58) in order to assess the antihypertensive efficacy of pindolol (5 to 10 mg twice-daily for 6 weeks) alone or in combination with a diuretic. The combination of pindolol plus a diuretic was not found to be superior to pindolol monotherapy in reducing blood pressure. Systolic and diastolic blood pressure was considerably reduced in blacks as well as whites. Pindolol was also found to be effective in reducing systolic and diastolic blood pressure in the elderly.

Comparative Studies Versus Diuretics and Combination Therapy

The antihypertensive efficacies of pindolol (15 mg once-daily for 8 weeks), hydrochlorothiazide (50 mg once-daily for 8 weeks), and pindolol (15 mg once-daily) plus hydrochlorothiazide (50 mg once-daily for 8 weeks) were assessed in a randomized, double-blind study involving 24 patients (44). Sitting, standing, and supine blood pressures were reduced to a greater extent with hydrochlorothiazide than with pindolol. However, the greatest reductions were achieved in those patients receiving the combination.

Studies Versus Other Beta Blockers

Comparative beta blocker studies with pindolol are presented in other sections of this chapter.

Comparative Studies Versus Calcium-Entry Blockers and Combination Therapy

A 12-week study involving 25 patients was carried out by Tsukiyama et al. (89) in order to assess the antihypertensive effects of pindolol (5 to 10 mg twice-daily) and nifedipine (10 to 30 mg twice-daily). Those patients who did not respond after 6 weeks of monotherapy received the 2 drugs in combination for the remaining 6 weeks. Nifedipine (6 of 12 patients) was more effective than pindolol (3 of 12 patients) in reducing blood pressure throughout the 12 weeks. However, the combination was found to be superior to either agent, producing a reduction in mean blood pressure from 128 ± 2 mm Hg to 103 ± 8 mm Hg.

Studies Versus Alpha-Blocking Agents

Sixty patients uncontrolled on diuretic therapy alone participated in a double-blind, randomized study comparing the antihypertensive effects of pindolol (5 to 10 mg twice-daily for 12 weeks) plus hydrochlorothiazide versus indoramin (25 to 50 mg twice-daily for 12 weeks) plus hydrochlorothiazide (57). Both regimens significantly reduced systolic and diastolic blood pressure after 2 weeks of therapy. This effect was maintained until the end of the study in both treatment groups. No significant difference in antihypertensive efficacy was noted between the two groups. Heart rate fell significantly with pindolol but was unchanged with indoramin.

Effects on Plasma Lipids

Lehtonen et al. (51) examined the effect on plasma lipids of pindolol (10 to 20 mg once-daily) in a 6-month study of 20 hypertensive patients. No significant change was observed in concentrations of triglyceride and free fatty acid. A significant rise in HDL cholesterol was observed after one month of therapy. Total cholesterol was reduced to a greater degree after six months than after one month of treatment. The absence of unfavorable changes on HDL cholesterol and triglycerides characteristic of other beta blockers (selective and nonselective) may be due to pindolol's ISA.

In a crossover study involving 16 hypertensive patients, Pasotti et al. (74) observed that pindolol, but not metoprolol, significantly increased HDL cholesterol.

In a long-term study of 11 hypertensive patients, Gretzer and Rossner (37) found that although pindolol (5 to 30 mg daily) significantly raised total triglycerides after two months of therapy, this increase was not observed at 16 months.

Propranolol (Inderal, Inderide, Inderal-LA)

Propranolol is a nonselective beta blocker without ISA but with MSA.

Comparative Studies Versus Diuretics (MRC Trial)

In a multicenter, single-blind, randomized, placebo-controlled study conducted by the Medical Research Council Working Party (64), 17,354 subjects were given either propranolol (up to 240 mg/day) or bendrofluazide (10 mg daily) and were observed for a total of 85,572 patient-years. The percentage of subjects with a diastolic blood pressure below 90 mm Hg was higher with bendrofluazide than with propranolol throughout the study. However, more patients receiving bendrofluazide required supplemental drug therapy (i.e., methyldopa, guanethidine) in order to achieve blood pressure control. Active treatment with either drug significantly decreased stroke rate compared with placebo (1.4 versus 2.6 per 1,000 patient-years, respectively). However, bendrofluazide caused a greater percentage reduction in stroke rate than propranolol. Whereas bendrofluazide decreased stroke rate in both nonsmokers and smokers, propranolol decreased stroke rate only in nonsmokers. Although the overall coronary event rate was not significantly altered by treatment, it was reduced

in nonsmokers treated with propranolol. Bendrofluazide did not reduce coronary event rate in either smokers or nonsmokers. Overall, the all cause mortality rate was also not significantly affected by treatment. However, treatment in men did result in a decrease in all cause mortality rate, while the opposite effect occurred in women.

Studies Versus Other Beta Blockers

Ravid et al. (75) conducted a prospective, double-blind, crossover, placebo-controlled study of 150 ambulatory patients in order to assess the comparative antihypertensive effects of slow-release propranolol (160 mg once-daily), atenolol (100 mg once-daily), slow-release oxprenolol (160 mg once-daily), and metoprolol (200 mg once-daily). Each beta blocker was administered for 4 weeks. Slow-release propranolol and atenolol significantly reduced supine, standing, and postexercise blood pressure. However, values obtained with metoprolol and slow-release oxprenolol were not significantly different from placebo.

Comparative beta blocker studies with propranolol are also shown in other parts of this chapter.

Trials Versus Angiotensin-Converting Enzyme (ACE) Inhibitors

Two hundred seventy patients participated in a multicenter, double-blind, randomized study carried out by the Captopril Research Group Of Japan (11) in which the antihypertensive efficacies of propranolol (20 to 40 mg thrice-daily for 12 weeks) plus thiazide diuretic versus captopril (12.5 to 25 mg thrice-daily for 12 weeks) plus thiazide diuretic were compared. Prior to this study, all patients were uncontrolled on diuretic monotherapy. Diastolic blood pressure was significantly reduced by both agents, with no significant difference noted. However, systolic blood pressure was significantly lower in the captopril group, after 10 and 12 weeks of therapy. Pulse rate was significantly reduced by propranolol, but not by captopril. There were significantly fewer side effects in the captopril group (4.5%) than in the propranolol group (11.7%). However, a similar number of patients in each group were withdrawn from the study due to untoward side effects.

In a multicenter, randomized, double-blind study carried out by the Enalapril In Hypertension Study Group (UK) (20), the effects of propranolol (40 to 120 mg twice-daily for 12 weeks) and enalapril (5 to 20 mg twice-daily for 12 weeks) were assessed in 56 patients. Both agents significantly reduced systolic and diastolic blood pressure. However, as opposed to the previous investigators' findings (94), enalapril was significantly better than propranolol in reducing blood pressure. More patients treated with enalapril achieved a final diastolic blood pressure of 90 mm Hg or below.

Comparative Studies Versus Calcium-Entry Blockers and Combination Therapy

Massie et al. (60) compared propranolol (80 to 240 mg twice-daily) and sustained-release diltiazem (60 to 180 mg twice-daily) in a 6-month, multicenter, double-blind, parallel-group, randomized study of 196 patients. Both drugs produced a significant reduction in supine blood pressure, with no difference between them. The addition of hydrochlorothiazide, in patients uncontrolled on the highest drug doses, produced a greater fall in blood pressure when added to propranolol than when added to diltiazem. There was a greater decrease in heart rate with propranolol compared with diltiazem. Diltiazem was slightly more effective than propranolol in reducing systolic blood pressure in the elderly. However, this was not the case for diastolic blood pressure. Both agents were more effective in non-blacks than in blacks. However, within each race they were equally effective.

In contrast to other trials, Cubeddu et al.

(13) found that verapamil lowered sitting and standing blood pressure to a significantly greater extent than propranolol. They observed that the hypotensive effect of verapamil was superior to that of propranolol in both black and white patients.

Zusman et al. (107) compared sustained-release nifedipine (mean dose 80 mg/day for 12 weeks) and propranolol (mean dose 198 mg/day for 12 weeks) in a multicenter, double-blind, randomized study of 100 patients who were inadequately controlled on diuretic therapy alone. All patients continued to take diuretics during the trial. No significant difference in antihypertensive efficacy was noted between the two groups. A diastolic blood pressure under 90 mm Hg was obtained in 57% of the propranolol group, and in 63% of the nifedipine group. Only propranolol plus hydrochlorothiazide significantly reduced heart rate.

Studies Versus Prazosin

Twenty-seven patients with blood pressure uncontrolled on thiazide diuretics, participated in a randomized study comparing propranolol (40 to 240 mg twice-daily) and prazosin (1 to 10 mg twice-daily) when added to polythiazide (67). If blood pressure control was not achieved with the initial study drug, the other drug was added. The two agents, in combination with polythiazide, comparably reduced diastolic blood pressure to ≤85 mm Hg. However, of the six patients who required propranolol plus prazosin in order to achieve blood pressure control, five patients had originally received prazosin. Exercise-induced increases in systolic blood pressure were lowered only by propranolol.

Quality of Life

Croog et al. (12) conducted a multicenter, randomized, double-blind trial in 626 hypertensive men in order to compare the effects of propranolol (80 mg twice-daily), captopril (50 mg twice-daily), and methyl-dopa (500 mg twice-daily) on blood pressure and on the patients' quality of life. After 24 weeks of treatment all three agents significantly lowered sitting diastolic blood pressure with no difference noted between them. However, it was necessary to add a diuretic less often in patients taking propranolol. There were significantly fewer withdrawals due to side-effects in the captopril group (8%) than in the methyldopa group (20%). There was a slight but non-significant difference between the propranolol (13%) and captopril groups. No significant difference was observed between the groups in scores for social participation, visual memory, and sleep dysfunction. However, patients taking captopril had more favorable scores than those taking methyldopa on measures of general well-being, work performance, life satisfaction, cognitive function and physical symptoms. They also scored significantly higher than propranolol-treated patients on measures of general well-being, sexual dysfunction, and physical symptoms. Patients receiving propranolol scored higher on measures of work performance than those receiving methyldopa.

Trials in the Elderly

Nineteen elderly patients on diuretic therapy participated in a randomized, double-blind, crossover study comparing long-acting propranolol (160 mg once-daily for 4 weeks) versus conventional propranolol (40 mg thrice-daily for 4 weeks) (45). Both regimens significantly reduced supine, standing, and postexercise blood pressure. However, a slightly greater reduction in supine systolic blood pressure was noted with conventional propranolol than with the long-acting formulation.

Effects On Plasma Lipids

Leren et al. (53) studied the effects of propranolol (40 to 160 mg daily) and prazosin

(0.5 to 4 mg daily) on blood lipids in 23 men with mild hypertension. Propranolol significantly lowered HDL cholesterol, the fraction HDL cholesterol /LDL + VLDL cholesterol, and increased total serum triglycerides. Total cholesterol and LDL + VLDL cholesterol were unchanged. In contrast, prazosin did not significantly alter HDL cholesterol, but reduced total cholesterol, LDL + VLDL cholesterol, and total triglycerides. Combination therapy lowered HDL cholesterol, but to a lesser degree than with propranolol alone.

In a randomized, crossover trial involving 53 patients, Day et al. (16) observed that propranolol (80 mg twice-daily), oxprenolol (80 mg twice-daily), atenolol (100 mg daily), and metoprolol (100 mg twice-daily) all produced a significant rise in total and VLDL triglycerides. This increase, however, was significantly greater with the nonselective (propranolol and oxprenolol) than with the selective beta blockers (atenolol and metoprolol). HDL cholesterol was significantly lowered by all four beta blockers with the greatest reduction noted following treatment with propranolol. Plasma total and LDL cholesterol levels were unaltered.

Tertatolol

Tertatolol (S 2395) is a new, potent, non-selective beta blocker without ISA.

Open Studies

Komajda et al. (46) examined the anti-hypertensive effects of tertatolol (5 mg once-daily) in a 1-year open study involving 110 patients. After 12 months of therapy, 103 patients (93.6%) had achieved a supine diastolic blood pressure less than 95 mm Hg. The majority of these patients (80 of 103) did not require the addition of a diuretic or dihydralazine in order to achieve blood pressure control. Overall, tertatolol significantly reduced both systolic (-26.4 mm Hg) and diastolic (-19.9 mm Hg) blood pressure. Blood pressure control was similar in elderly (74.1%) and middle-aged patients (67.6%), and less in younger patients (100%).

Dose Finding Studies

Granier et al. (36) treated 40 patients with tertatolol 2.5, 5, and 10 mg once daily for two months in a double-blind, randomized, placebo-controlled study. Only the 5 and 10 mg doses significantly reduced blood pressure compared to placebo. No significant difference was observed between them.

Studies Versus Other Beta Blockers

Gallet et al. (35) conducted a single-blind, randomized study comparing the antihypertensive efficacies of tertatolol (5 mg once-daily) versus acebutolol (400 mg once-daily) in 32 patients. Supine, upright, and exercise blood pressures were significantly reduced by both agents after 3 months of treatment. No significant difference in efficacy was observed between them. However, these investigators noted that tertatolol achieved its maximal antihypertensive effect earlier than acebutolol.

Timolol (Blocadren, Timolide)

Timolol is a nonselective beta blocker with no ISA or MSA.

Open Studies

Bannon et al. (5) evaluated the antihypertensive efficacy of timolol maleate (10 mg twice-daily) in an open, multicenter study of 5,190 patients. Mean blood pressure was reduced by 20/13 mm Hg after one month of treatment. Greater reductions in mean diastolic blood pressure were observed in patients with moderate (17%) and severe (22%) hypertension than in those with mild hypertension (11%). Black and elderly patients responded less well than

other patient groups. Although approximately 20% of all patients experienced an adverse event, those most frequently reported were not related to beta-blockade.

Comparative Studies Versus Diuretics and Combination Therapy

In a randomized, crossover double-blind study of 20 patients, Chalmers et al. (54) compared the antihypertensive effects of timolol (10 mg 3 times daily for 8 weeks) versus hydrochlorothiazide (50 mg once-daily for 8 weeks). Both regimens significantly reduced lying and standing blood pressure. No significant difference in antihypertensive efficacy was noted between them.

Marsh et al. (59) performed a one-year, open study of 11,685 patients in order to assess the antihypertensive efficacy of timolol (10 to 40 mg once-daily) plus bendrofluazide (2.5 to 10 mg once-daily). Blood pressure was reduced by a mean of 31/19 mm Hg and heart rate was reduced by a mean of 11 beats/min. The combination effectively treated 69% (8,039) of the patients. The majority (61%) of these patients reached the target blood pressure on the lowest drug doses.

CONCLUSION

After almost 25 years of clinical use, the beta-adrenergic blockers have proven to be both safe and efficacious for the long-term treatment of systemic hypertension. Despite their common action in blocking beta-adrenergic receptor sites from being stimulated by catecholamines, clear differences between the drugs have been demonstrated. Some beta blockers are less effective in lowering blood pressure in black patients (e.g., propranolol, nadolol) than they are in white patients. Some drugs cause adverse effects on plasma lipids and lipoproteins while others do not (Table 3) (49). The side-effect profiles may vary from drug to drug, and some agents in this class need to be

Table 3. *Reported effects of various β-adrenergic blockers on lipids and lipoproteins*

	Pharmacologic properties			Lipids and lipoproteins				
	β-ISA	β$_1$-selectivity	α$_1$-blocking	Chol	HDL-chol	LDL-chol	VLDL-chol	Triglycerides
Acebutolol	+	+	0	↔	→	↓↔	↔	↔
Atenolol	0	+	0	↑ ↔	→ ↓	↔	←	←
Bisoprolol	0	+	0	↔	↔	↔	↔	↔
Bopindolol	+[a]	0	0	↔	↑	↔	↔	↑
Celiprolol	+[a]	+	+[b]	↔	↑	↔	↔	↑
Dilevalol	+[a]	0	0	↔	→	↔	↔	←
Labetalol	+[a]	0	+	↔	→ ↔	↔	← ↔	← ↔
Metoprolol	0	+	0	↔	→	↔	↑	↑ ←
Oxprenolol	+[c]	0	0	↔	→ ↔	↔	↔	↔
Pindolol	+	0	0	↔	→	↔	←	←
Propranolol	0	0	0	↔	→	↔		

[a] β-agonism is predominantly at peripheral β$_2$-receptor.
[b] Celiprolol may have selective α$_2$ adrenergic blocking activity.
[c] Oxprenolol has little measurable β-agonism.
Chol = cholesterol; ↑ increase; ↓ decrease; ↔ no change.

administered more frequently to patients than others.

One fact separates the beta-adrenergic blockers from all other antihypertensive drugs studied to date. They are the only drugs shown to reduce the risk of ischemic heart disease.

REFERENCES

1. Abernethy, D. R., Bartos, P., and Plachetka, J. R. (1987): Labetalol in the treatment of hypertension in elderly and younger patients. *J. Clin. Pharmacol.,* 27:902.
2. Andersen Gert Steen (1985): Atenolol versus bendroflumethiazide in middle-aged and elderly hypertensives. *Acta. Med. Scand.,* 218:165.
3. Andrew L., Karlberg, B. E., Svensson, A., Ohman, P., Nilsson, O. R., and Hansson, L. (1985): Long-term effects of captopril and atenolol in essential hypertension. *Acta. Med. Scand.,* 217:155.
4. Ballantyne, D., Ballantyne, F. C., and Mc-Murdo, A. (1981): Effect of slow oxprenolol and a combination of slow oxprenolol and cyclopenthiazide on plasma lipoproteins. *Atherosclerosis,* 39:301.
5. Bannon, J. A., Steward, K. A., DeLisser, O., and Schrogie, J. J. (1986): Clinical experience with timolol maleate monotherapy of hypertension. *Arch. Intern. Med.,* 146:654.
6. Bolzano, K., Arriaga, J., Bernal, R., et al. (1987): The antihypertensive effect of lisinopril compared to atenolol in patients with mild to moderate hypertension. *J. Cardiovasc. Pharmacol.,* 9 (Suppl 3):S43.
7. Boyles, P. W. (1985): Effects of age and race on clinical response to acebutolol in essential hypertension. *Am. Heart. J.,* 109:1184.
8. Buhler, F. R., Berglund, G., Anderson, O. K., et al. (1986): Double-blind comparison of the cardioselective β-blockers bisoprolol and atenolol in hypertension: The bisoprolol international multicenter study (BIMS). *J. Cardiovasc. Pharmacol.,* 8 (Suppl 11):S122.
9. Burris, J. F., Goldstein, J., Zager, P. G., Sutton, J. M., Sirgo, M. A., and Plachetka, J. R. (1986): Comparative tolerability of labetalol versus propranolol, atenolol, pindolol, metoprolol, and nadolol. *J. Clin. Hypertens.,* 3:285.
10. Capone, P., and Mayol, R. (1986): A placebo-controlled double-blind multicenter study of celiprolol in the treatment of mild and moderate hypertension. *J. Cardiovasc. Pharmacol.,* 8 (Suppl 4):S119.
11. Captopril Research Group of Japan. (1985): Clinical effects of low-dose captopril plus a thiazide diuretic on mild to moderate essential hypertension: A multicenter double-blind comparison with propranolol. *J. Cardiovasc. Pharmacol.,* 7:S77.
12. Croog, S. H., Levine, S., Testa, M. A., et al. (1986): The effects of anti-hypertensive therapy on the quality of life. *N. Engl. J. Med.,* 314:1657.
13. Cubeddu, L. X., Aranda, J., Singh, B., et al. (1986): A comparison of verapamil and propranolol for the initial treatment of hypertension: Racial differences in response. *JAMA,* 256:2214.
14. Daniels, A. R., and Opie, L. H. (1986): Atenolol plus nifedipine for mild to moderate systemic hypertension after fixed doses of either agent alone. *Am. J. Cardiol.,* 57:965.
15. Davidov, M. (1985): Acebutolol in essential hypertension: Results of two multicenter studies against placebo and propranolol. *Am. Heart. J.,* 109:1158.
16. Day, J. L., Metcalfe, J., and Simpson, C. N. (1982): Adrenergic mechanisms in control of plasma lipid concentrations. *Clin. Res.,* 284:1145.
17. Dupont, A. G., Vanderniepen, P., Bossuyt, A. M., Jonckheer, M. H., and Six, R. O. (1985): Nadolol in essential hypertension: Effect on ambulatory blood pressure, renal haemodynamics and cardiac function. *Br. J. Clin. Pharmacol.,* 20:93.
18. Dux, S., Grosskopf, I., Boner, G., and Rosenfeld, J. B. (1986): Labetalol in the treatment of essential hypertension: A single-blind dose ranging study. *J. Clin. Pharmacol.,* 26:346.
19. Ekelund, L-G., Ekelund, C., and Rossner, S. (1982): Antihypertensive effects at rest and during exercise of a calcium blocker, nifedipine, alone and in combination with metoprolol. *Acta Med. Scand.,* 212:71.
20. Enalapril in Hypertension Study Group (UK). (1984): Enalapril in essential hypertension: A comparative study with propranolol. *Br. J. Clin. Pharmacol.,* 18:51.
21. Escudero, J., Hernandez, H., and Martinez, F. (1986): Comparative study of the antihypertensive effect of verapamil and atenolol. *Am. J. Cardiol.,* 57:54D.
22. Fairhurst, G. J. (1986): Comparison of bevantolol and atenolol for systemic hypertension. *Am. J. Cardiol.,* 58:25E.
23. Ferrara, L. A., Marotta, T., Rubba, P., et al. (1986): Effects of alpha-adrenergic and beta-adrenergic receptor blockade on lipid metabolism. *Am. J. Med.,* 80 (2A):104.
24. Falmenbaum, W., Weber, M. A., McMahon, F. G., Materson, B. J., Carr, A. A., and Poland, M. (1985): Monotherapy with labetalol compared with propanolol: Differential effects by race. *J. Clin. Hypertens.,* 1:56.
25. Fodor, J. G., Chockalingam, A., Drover, A., Fifield, F., and Pauls, C. J. (1987): A comparison of the side effects of atenolol and propranolol in the treatment of patients with hypertension. *J. Clin. Pharmacol.,* 27:892.
26. Foerster, E.-Ch., Greminger, P., Siegenthaler, W., Vetter, H., and Vetter, W. (1985): Atenolol versus pindolol: Side effects in hypertension. *Eur. J. Clin. Pharmacol.,* 28 (Suppl):89.
27. Frick, M. H., Cox, D. A., Himanen, P., et al.

(1987): Serum lipid changes in a one-year multicenter, double-blind comparison of doxazosin and atenolol for mild to moderate essential hypertension. *Am. J. Cardiol.*, 59:61G.

28. Frick, M. H., Halttunen, P., Himanen, P., et al. (1986): A long-term double-blind comparison of doxazosin and atenolol in patients with mild to moderate essential hypertension. *Br. J. Clin. Pharmacol.*, 21:55S.

29. Friedman, B., Gray, J. M., Gross, S., and Levit, S. A. (1983): United States experience with oxprenolol in hypertension. *Am. J. Cardiol.*, 52:43D.

30. Frishman, W. H. (1988): β-Adrenergic Blockers. *Med. Clin. N. Amer.*, 72:37.

31. Frishman, W. E., Michelson, E., Johnson, B., et al. (1982): Effects of beta-adrenergic blockade on plasma lipids: A double-blind randomized placebo-controlled multicenter comparison of labetalol and metoprolol in patients with hypertension. *Am. J. Cardiol.*, 49:924. (abstr.)

32. Frishman, W. H., Schoenberger, J. A., Gorwit, J. I., Bedsole, G. D., Cubbon, J., and Poland, M. (1988): Multicenter comparison of dilevalol to placebo in patients with mild hypertension. *Am. J. Hypertens.*, 1:295S.

33. Frishman, W. H., and Silverman, R. (1979): Clinical pharmacology of the new beta-adrenergic blocking drugs. Part 3: Comparative clinical experience and new therapeutic applications. *Am. Heart. J.*, 98:119.

34. Frithz, G., and Weiner, L. (1987): Effects of bisoprolol on blood pressure, serum lipids and HDL-cholesterol in essential hypertension. *Eur. J. Clin. Pharmacol.*, 32:77.

35. Gallet, M., Kleinknecht, D., and Maurice, P. (1986): Antihypertensive effects of tertatolol: 3-month comparative study against acebutolol. *Am. J. Nephrol.* 6(2):83.

36. Granier, J., Amoretti, R., and Abastado, M. (1985): Relationship of tertatolol in the treatment of essential hypertension. 2nd European Meet Hypertension, Milan 1985. *Ric. Scient. Educaz. Perm.*, Suppl. 49:212.

37. Gretzer, I., and Rossner, S. (1986): Long-term effects of pindolol on serum lipoproteins in hypertensive patients. *Acta Med. Scand.*, 219:367.

38. Heber, M. E., Brigden, G. S., Caruana, M. P., Lahiri, A., and Raftery, E. B. (1987): Carvedilol for systemic hypertension. *Am. J. Cardiol.*, 59:400.

39. Hoffmann, W., and Hoffmann, II. (1986): Results of the Austrian celiprolol postmarketing surveillance study. *J. Cardiovasc. Pharmacol.*, 8 (Suppl 4):S88.

40. Hulthen, U. L., van Brummelen, P., Amann, F. W., and Buhler, F. R. (1983): Antihypertensive efficacy of the new long-acting β-blocker bopindolol as related to age. *J. Cardiovasc. Pharmacol.*, 5:426.

41. Ikeda, M., Inagaki, Y., Iimura, O., Kuramoto, K., and Takeda, T. (1986): Clinical evaluation of bisoprolol in patients with hypertension: In-

terim report. *J. Cardiovasc. Pharmacol.*, 8 (Suppl 11):S139.

42. The IPPPSH Collaborative Group. (1985): Cardiovascular risk and risk factors in a randomized trial of treatment based on the beta-blocker oxprenolol: The International Prospective Primary Prevention Study in Hypertension (IPPPSH). *J. Hypertens.*, 3:379.

43. Jain, A. (1986): Effectiveness of bevantolol in the treatment of hypertension: Once-daily versus twice-daily evaluation of home blood pressure measurements. *Angiology*, 239.

44. Johnson, B. F., Weiner, B., Marwaha, R., and Johnson, J. (1986): The influence of pindolol and hydrochlorothiazide on blood pressure, and plasma renin and plasma lipid levels. *J. Clin. Pharmacol.*, 26:258.

45. Khan, A. U. (1987): Comparison of a long-acting form of propranolol and conventional propranolol in the treatment of hypertension in elderly patients. *J. Int. Med. Res.*, 15:128.

46. Komajda, M., Genevray, B., and Grosgogeat, Y. (1986): Long-term experience with tertatolol in hypertension. *Am. J. Nephrol.*, 6 (2):106.

47. Labetalol/Hydrochlorothiazide Multicenter Study Group. (1985): Labetalol and hydrochlorothiazide in hypertension. *Clin. Pharmacol. Ther.*, 38:24.

48. Lange Andersen, K., Ottmann, W., Piatkowski, W., and Green, K. A. (1985): Working ability and exercise tolerance during treatment of mild hypertension. II: A comparison between atenolol and prazosin medication. *Int. Arch. Occup. Environ. Health*, 56(1):49.

49. Lardinois, C. K., and Neuman, S. L. (1988): The effects of antihypertensive agents on serum lipids and lipoproteins. *Arch. Intern. Med.*, 148:1280.

50. Lehtonen, A. A. P. O. (1984): The effect of acebutolol on plasma lipids, blood glucose and serum insulin levels. *Acta Med. Scand.*, 216:57.

51. Lehtonen, A., Hietanen, E., Marniemi, J., Peltonen, P., Niskanen, J. (1982): Effect of pindolol on serum lipids and lipid metabolizing enzymes. *Br. J. Clin. Pharmacol.*, 13:445S.

52. Leonetti, G., Mazzola, C., Boni, S., Guffanti, E., Meani, A., and Zanchetti, A. (1986): Comparison of the antihypertensive effect of urapidil and metoprolol in hypertension. *Eur. J. Clin. Pharmacol.*, 30:637.

53. Leren, P., Helgeland, A., Holme, I., Foss, P. O., Hjermann, I., Lund-Larsen, P. G. (1980): Effect of propranolol and prazosin on blood lipids. *Lancet*, 4.

54. Lindroos, M., and Lehtonen, A. (1984): Timolol and a hydrochlorothiazide-amiloride combination in the treatment of essential hypertension in young and middle-aged patients: A comparative study with once-daily administration. *Intern. J. Clin. Pharmacol.*, 12:643–645.

55. Lithell, H., Weiner, L., Selinus, I., and Vesby, B. (1986): A comparison of the effects of bisoprolol and atenolol on lipoprotein concentra-

tions and blood pressure. *J. Cardiovasc. Pharmacol.*, 8 (Suppl 11):S128.

56. Lucas, C. P., Morledge, J. H., and Tessman, D. K. (1985): Comparison of hydrochlorothiazide and hydrochlorothiazide plus bevantolol in hypertension. *Clin. Ther.*, 8:49.

57. Luomanmaki, K., and Hartikainen, M. (1986): A double-blind comparison of indoramin and pindolol added to hydrochlorothiazide for the treatment of mild to moderate hypertension. *J. Cardiovasc. Pharmacol.*, 8 (Suppl 2):S63.

58. Marks, A. D., Finestone, A., Sobel, E., and Lanzilotti, S. (1986): An office-based primary care trial of pindolol (Visken) in essential hypertension. *Curr. Med. Res. Opin.*, 10:296.

59. Marsh, B. T., Atkins, M. J., Talbot, D. J., and Fairey, I. T. (1987): A post-marketing acceptability study in 11,685 patients of the efficacy of timolol/bendroflumazide in the management of hypertension in general practice. *J. Int. Med. Res.*, 15:106.

60. Massie, B., MacCarthy, P., Ramanathan, K. B., et al. (1987): Diltiazem and propranolol in mild to moderate essential hypertension as monotherapy or with hydrochlorothiazide. *Ann. Intern. Med.*, 107:150.

61. M'Buyamba-Kabangu, J. R., Fagard, R., Lijnen, P., et al. (1987): Calcium entry blockade or beta-blockade in long-term management of hypertension in blacks. *Clin. Pharmacol. Ther.*, 41:45.

62. McGonigle, R. J. S., Williams, L., and Murphy, M. J. (1981): Labetalol and lipids (letter). *Lancet*, 1:163.

63. McGowan, G. K., and Baker, P. G. (1984): Treatment of essential hypertension with betablocker plus diuretic: A study of 1,402 patients treated by general practitioners with acebutolol 200 mg combined with hydrochlorothiazide 12.5 mg (Secadrex) once daily for 3 months. *J. Int. Med. Res.*, 12:87.

64. Medical Research Council Working Party. (1985): MRC trial of treatment of mild hypertension: Principal results. *Br. Med. J.*, 291:97.

65. Meyer-Sabellek, W., Schulte, K-L., Kloppenburg-Steinecke, F., Peters, P., and Gotzen, R. (1985): Effects of long-term treatment with carvedilol (BM 14190) versus metoprolol on haemodynamic parameters. *J. Hypertens.*, 3:422.

66. Middeke, M., Weisweiler, P., Schwandt, P., and Holzgreve, H. (1987): Serum lipoproteins during antihypertensive therapy with beta blockers and diuretics: A controlled long-term comparative trial. *Clin. Cardiol.*, 10:94.

67. Misson, R., Merkel, T., and Cutler, R. E. (1984): Comparison of blood pressure, plasma lipid and cardiac performance responses to prazosin versus propranolol in thiazide-treated hypertensive patients. *Am. J. Cardiol.*, 53:51A.

68. Mueller, J., Byrne, M. J., van Schalkwyk, J., and Opie, L. H. (1983): Renal impairment in hypertension not improved by nadolol when compared with atenolol. *Drugs*, 25 (Suppl 2):146.

69. Nash, D. T., Schoenfeld, G., Reeves, R. L.,

Black, H., and Weidler, D. J. (1987): A double-blind parallel trial to assess the efficacy of doxazosin, atenolol and placebo in patients with mild to moderate systemic hypertension. *Am. J. Cardiol.*, 59:87G.

70. Ohman, K. P., Weiner, L., von Schenck, H., and Karlberg, B. E. (1985): Antihypertensive and metabolic effects of nifedipine and labetalol alone and in combination in primary hypertension. *Eur. J. Clin. Pharmacol.*, 29:149.

71. Okawa, K. K. (1986): Dose response studies of bevantolol in hypertensive patients. *Angiology*, 233.

72. Okun, R., and Kraut, J. (1984): A comparison of prazosin versus nadolol in combination with a diuretic. *Am. J. Cardiol.*, 53:37A.

73. Pagnan, A., Pessina, A. C., and Hlede, M., et al. (1979): Effects of labetalol on lipid and carbohydrate metabolism. *Pharmacol. Res. Commun.*, 11:227.

74. Pasotti, C., Capra, A., Fiorella, G., Vibelli, C., and Chierichetti, S. M. (1982): Effects of pindolol and metoprolol on plasma lipids and lipoproteins. *Br. J. Clin. Pharmacol.*, 13:435S.

75. Ravid, M., Lang, R., and Jutrin, I. (1985): The relative antihypertensive potency of propranolol, oxprenolol, atenolol, and metoprolol given once daily: A double-blind, crossover, placebo-controlled study in ambulatory patients. *Arch. Intern. Med.*, 145:1321.

76. Rouffy, J., and Jaillard, J. (1984): Comparative effects of prazosin and atenolol on plasma lipids in hypertensive patients. *Am. J. Med.*, 105.

77. Rosendorff, C., Goodman, C., and Coull, A. (1985): Short- and long-term studies of bucindolol in mild to moderate hypertension: Efficacy, safety, and exercise responses. *J. Clin. Pharmacol.*, 25:223.

78. Rossner, S., and Weiner, L. (1983): A comparison of the effects of atenolol and metoprolol on serum lipoproteins. *Drugs*, 25(Suppl 2):322.

79. Rotmensch, H. H., Rocci, M. L., Vlasses, P. H., et al. (1984): Bucindolol, a beta-adrenoceptor blocker with vasodilatory action: Its effect in systemic hypertension. *Am. J. Cardiol.*, 54:353.

80. Ruddel, H., Schmieder, R., Langewitz, W., Neus, J., Wagner, O., and von Eiff, A. W. (1984): Efficacy of nitrendipine as baseline antihypertensive therapy. *J. Cardiovasc. Pharmacol.*, 6:S1049.

81. Salvetti, A., Lucchini, M., Airoldi, G., et al. (1985): Multicentre comparison of the antihypertensive effect of acebutolol and hydrochlorothiazide in uncomplicated mild-moderate hypertension in the elderly. *Eur. J. Clin. Pharmacol.*, 29:275.

82. Schiess, W., Welzel, D., and Gugler, R. (1984): Double-blind comparison of once-daily bopindolol, pindolol and atenolol in essential hypertension. *Eur. J. Clin. Pharmacol.*, 27:529.

83. Schmieder, R., Ruddel, H., Langewitz, W., Neus J., Wagner, O., and von Eiff, A. W. (1985): The influence of monotherapy with oxprenolol

and nitrendipine on ambulatory blood pressure in hypertensives. *Clin. Exper. Ther. Prac.*, A7 (2&3):445.

84. Silas, J. H., Freestone, S., Lennard, M. S., and Ramsay, L. E. (1985): Comparison of two slow-release formulations of metoprolol with conventional metoprolol and atenolol in hypertensive patients. *Br. J. Clin. Pharmacol.*, 20:387.

85. Soberman, J., Greenberg, S., and Frishman, W. (1987): The safety and efficacy of once-daily dilevalol in patients with mild hypertension: A placebo-controlled study. *J. Clin. Hypertens.*, 3:271.

86. Sommers, D. E. K., De Villiers, L. S., Van Wyk, M., Schoeman, H. S. (1981): The effects of labetalol and oxprenolol on blood lipids. *S. Afr. Med. J.*, 60:379.

87. Taylor, S. H., Beattie, A., and Silke, B. (1986): Celiprolol in the treatment of hypertension: A comparison with propranolol. *J. Cardiovasc. Pharmacol.*, 8 (Suppl 4):LS127.

88. Trimarco, B., DeLuca, N., Ricciardelli, B., et al. (1984): Diltiazem in the treatment of mild or moderate essential hypertension: Comparison with metoprolol in a crossover double-blind trial. *J. Clin. Pharmacol.*, 24:218.

89. Tsukiyama, H., Otsuka, K., and Yamamoto, Y. (1984): Effect of pindolol and nifedipine alone and in combination on haemodynamic parameters/variables in essential hypertension. *J. Int. Med. Res.*, 12:154.

90. Turner, A. S., and Brocklehurst, J. C. (1985): Once-daily acebutolol and atenolol in essential hypertension: Double-blind crossover comparison. *Am. Heart. J.*, 109:1178.

91. Van Brummelen, P. (1983): The relevance of intrinsic sympathomimetic activity for β-blocker-induced changes in plasma lipids. *J. Cardiovasc. Pharmacol.*, 5:51.

92. Van Brummelen, P., Bolli, P., Koolen, M. I., Staehelin, H. B., and Buhler, F. R. (1984): Plasma lipid fractions during long-term monotherapy with the ISA-containing β-adrenoceptor blocker bopindolol in hypertensive patients. *Br. J. Clin. Pharmacol.*, 17:86.

93. van der Veur, E., ten Berge, B. S., Donker, A. J. M., May, J. F., Schuurman, F. H., and Wesseling, H. (1985): A comparison of labetalol and prazosin combined with atenolol in non-responders to atenolol plus hydrochlorothiazide in uncomplicated hypertension. *Eur. J. Clin. Pharmacol.*, 28:507.

94. van Schaik, B. A. M., Geyskes, G. G., Kettner, N., Boer, P., and Dorhout Mees, E. J. (1986): Comparison of enalapril and propranolol in essential hypertension. *Eur. J. Clin. Pharmacol.*, 29:511.

95. Veterans Administration Cooperative Study Group on Antihypertensive Drugs. (1983): Efficacy of nadolol alone and combined with bendroflumethiazide and hydralazine for systemic hypertension. *Am. J. Cardiol.*, 52:1230.

96. Wahl, J., Singh, B. N., and Thoden, W. R. (1986): Comparative hypotensive effects of acebutolol and hydrochlorothiazide in patients with mild to moderate essential hypertension: A double-blind multicenter evaluation. *Am. Heart. J.*, 111:353.

97. Wahl, J., Turlapaty, P., and Singh, B. N. (1985): Comparison of acebutolol and propranolol in essential hypertension. *Am. Heart. J.*, 109:313.

98. Weber, M. A., and Drayer, J. I. M. (1985): Once-daily administration of acebutolol in treatment of hypertension. *Am. Heart. J.*, 109:1175.

99. Webster, J., Petrie, J. C., Robb, O. J., Jamieson, M., and Verschueren, J. (1985): A comparison of single doses of bucindolol and oxprenolol in hypertensive patients. *Br. J. Clin. Pharmacol.*, 20:393.

100. Weiner, L., and Frithz, G. (1986): Dose-effect relationship and long-term effects of bisoprolol in mild to moderate hypertension. *J. Cardiovasc. Pharmacol.*, 8 (Suppl 11):S106.

101. Wikstrand, J., Warnold, I., Olsson, G., et al. (1988): Primary prevention with metoprolol in patients with hypertension: Mortality results from the MAPPHY study. *JAMA*, 259:1976.

102. Wikstrand, J., Westergren, G., Berglund, G., et al. (1986): Antihypertensive treatment with metoprolol or hydrochlorothiazide in patients aged 60 to 75 years: Report from a double-blind international multicenter study. *JAMA*, 255:1304.

103. Wilhelmsen, L., Berglund, G., Elmfeldt, D., et al. (1987): Beta-blockers versus diuretics in hypertensive men: Main results from the HAPPHY trial. *J. Hypertens.*, 5:561.

104. Willimann, P., Peter, R., Siegenthaler, H., and the Swiss Bopindolol Cooperative Study Group (1986): Dose-finding study with bopindolol in arterial hypertension. *J. Cardiovasc. Pharmacol.*, 8 (Suppl 6):S25.

105. Witchitz, S., Moisson, P., and Kolsky, H. (1984): A comparative trial of ordinary metoprolol tablets and metoprolol sustained-release tablets in hypertensive patients at rest and on exercise. *Pharmacother.*, 3:566.

106. Zachariah, P. K., Bonnet, G., Chrysant, G., et al. (1987): Evaluation of antihypertensive efficacy of lisinopril compared to metoprolol in moderate to severe hypertension. *J. Cardiovasc. Pharmacol.*, 9 (Suppl 3):S53.

107. Zusman, R., Christensen, D., Federman, E., et al. (1987): Comparison of nifedipine and propranolol used in combination with diuretics for the treatment of hypertension. *Am. J. Med.*, 82 (3B):37.

New Therapeutic Strategies in Hypertension,
edited by Norman M. Kaplan,
Barry M. Brenner, and John H. Laragh.
Raven Press, Ltd., New York © 1989.

Angiotensin Converting Enzyme Inhibitors

Bernard Waeber, Jürg Nussberber, and Hans R. Brunner

Division of Hypertension, Centre Hospitalier Universitaire Vaudois, 1011 Lausanne, Switzerland

Increasing evidence suggests that the renin-angiotensin system plays an active role in the development and maintenance of high blood pressure in various forms of clinical hypertension. This information has been obtained mainly using angiotensin converting enzyme (ACE) inhibitors, i.e., agents which prevent the generation of the pressor hormone angiotensin II. Thus, it was found that blood pressure can be substantially reduced by blocking the renin-angiotensin system in a large fraction of hypertensive patients. The present chapter will review some of the experience accumulated during the last decade with the use of angiotensin converting enzyme inhibitors to treat hypertensive disorders.

THE RENIN-ANGIOTENSIN SYSTEM

Activation of the enzyme chain culminating in the generation of angiotensin II starts with renin secretion from the kidney (104) (Fig. 1). This proteolytic enzyme cleaves off the decapeptide angiotensin I from angiotensinogen, a protein substrate delivered into the circulation by the liver. Angiotensin I is devoid of any vasoactive effect; a converting enzyme splits it into two fragments of which the larger, an octapeptide, represents the final hormone angiotensin II. Most of the angiotensin I is transformed to angiotensin II during its passage through the pulmonary vascular bed. However, ACE is also known to be present in extrapulmonary endothelial cells. (46).

Angiotensin II can increase blood pressure by several mechanisms. By itself it is a potent vasoconstrictor peptide. In addition, it interacts with the sympathetic nervous system centrally and peripherally (105). Angiotensin II may gain access to the brain through areas which lack a tight blood-brain barrier and by this way raise sympathetic efferent nerve activity. At the sympathetic nerve ending, it enhances the release of norepinephrine by activating presynaptic receptors. Another well-established effect of angiotensin II is the stimulation of aldosterone secretion by the adrenal gland, which leads to renal sodium retention (66).

ACE INHIBITORS

Development

The first ACE inhibitors were a series of peptides found in the venom of the Brazilian viper, *Bothrops jararaca* (102). One of these, a nonapeptide, was synthetized to be evaluated in clinical trials (53). Although successful in lowering blood pressure of some hypertensive patients, this inhibitor, teprotide, had the shortcoming to be active only when administered parenterally. Based on the study of ACE and its interaction with angiotensin and various venom extracts, a hypothetical model of the active site of the enzyme was then developed. This made it possible to design several potent orally-active ACE inhibitors such as captopril, a compound containing a sulfhydril group (48,101), enalapril, and its lysine an-

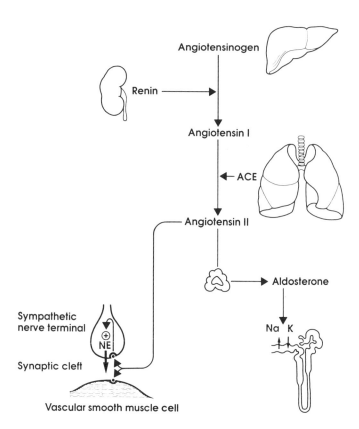

FIG. 1. Components of the renin-angiotensin system. Angiotensin II has a direct vasoconstrictor effect. It also enhances the release of norepinephrine (NE) from terminal nerve endings and increases aldosterone secretion.

alog lisinopril (8,105). These agents are currently available in most countries. A number of new inhibitors are in clinical development (benazepril, cilazapril, perindopril, ramipril, quinapril, fosinopril, spirapril, trandolapril, etc.) (17). The efficacy of these substances in inhibiting ACE in patients could be demonstrated by showing their ability to block the pressor effect of exogenous angiotensin I, to suppress plasma ACE activity, and to reduce circulating levels of angiotensin II (18).

Pharmacokinetics

Captopril is rapidly absorbed when administered orally. Maximal concentrations of the drug in the blood are reached between $\frac{1}{2}$ and $1\frac{1}{2}$ hours after intake. Bioavailability of an oral dose is around 60%. Approximately 30% of captopril is bound to plasma proteins. Almost 90% of circulating captopril is excreted in the urine, mostly in intact form. The mean elimination half-live averages 2 hours in patients with a normal renal function. Clinically it is very important that the elimination of captopril is prolonged when renal function is reduced. Adjustment of dose and/or dosing interval is thus required in the presence of renal failure (58).

Enalapril maleate is absorbed intact, achieving peak concentrations in the blood by 1 hour after intake, and disappearing completely from the circulation within the 4 hours after dosing. Enalapril maleate is the prodrug for the active metabolite, enalaprilat. Hydrolysis of the ester occurs in the liver. After oral administration of enalapril maleate, peak levels of enalaprilat are reached approximately 4 hours postdose. Bioavailability of an oral dose of enalapril is approximately 60%. The effective half-life of enalaprilat is 11 hours. Total drug (enalapril maleate and enalaprilat) is primarily excreted by the kidney. The doses of enalapril have therefore also to be adapted to the renal function. Theoretically, conversion of enalapril maleate to enalaprilat might be impaired in patients with hepatic dysfunction, although this seems rarely a clinically relevant problem (137).

Unlike enalapril maleate, lisinopril is not a prodrug. Peak serum concentrations of lisinopril occur about 6 to 8 hours after oral dosing. The average bioavailability of this agent is 25%. Lisinopril is not metabolized and is eliminated almost exclusively by the kidneys (56).

Captopril, enalapril, and lisinopril can be administered with food. Overall, aging has little influence on the pharmacokinetic characteristics of captopril and enalapril. Only the age-related decrease in renal function really has to be taken into account when prescribing these drugs to elderly patients. With respect to lisinopril, peak serum concentration is about twice as high in the elderly compared with the nonelderly subjects.

HEMODYNAMIC EFFECTS OF ACE INHIBITION

Effects on Blood Pressure, Heart Rate, and Cardiac Output

In response to ACE inhibition, one would expect a fall in blood pressure proportional to the preexisting level of activity of the renin-angiotensin system. The magnitude of the initial blood pressure reduction induced by ACE inhibitors is more or less closely related to pretreatment plasma-renin activity and plasma-angiotensin II levels (16,27,54,59). However, with long-term therapy, the relationship between the blood pressure fall and the pretreatment renin and angiotensin II status becomes very weak (2,28,144). In many patients, sustained ACE inhibition for several weeks lowers

blood pressure gradually to levels beyond those achieved at the beginning of treatment. Renin profiling appears therefore of relatively little practical value in predicting whether an ACE inhibitor is likely to normalize blood pressure of a particular patient. Nevertheless, good responders to acute ACE inhibition tend to remain well controlled during chronic therapy.

A hallmark of ACE inhibitors is that they lower blood pressure most of the time without inducing a reflex cardio-acceleration (30,47,76,89) (Fig. 2). Cardiac output also does not change when blood pressure is reduced by an ACE inhibitor (30,47,49,88, 122,148). During prolonged treatment, cardiac output may increase in some patients. This is most likely to occur in patients with malignant hypertension initially exhibiting a reduced cardiac output (122). Pulmonary vascular resistance is not affected by ACE inhibition (47).

ACE inhibitors interfere minimally with circulatory reflexes (76,89). In most hypertensive subjects, the blood pressure and heart rate response to changes in posture is not impaired. Both captopril and enalapril attenuate the blood pressure increase induced by physical exercise whereas the responses of heart rate and cardiac output are left intact (77,86).

Effects on Regional Blood Flow Distribution

ACE inhibitors, when lowering blood pressure, preserve the perfusion of "noble" organs intact. Renal blood flow is increased by both acute and chronic blockade of angiotensin II generation (4,44,60,80,110,126, 150). This effect is thought to be mediated by a preferential vasodilatation of the efferent arterioles of the glomeruli and is most pronounced in patients with an activated renin-angiotensin system. With regard to coronary perfusion, it may also be influenced by ACE inhibitors when the renin-angiotensin system is stimulated. Thus, di-

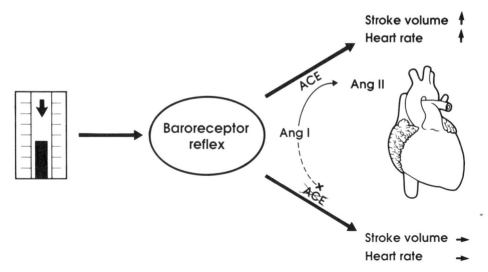

FIG. 2. Effect of ACE inhibition on the response of stroke volume and heart rate to arteriolar dilatation. Ang I and II = Angiotensin I and II; ACE = normally functioning enzyme; ~~ACE~~ = inhibited enzyme.

uretic therapy reduces coronary blood flow of hypertensives and acute ACE inhibition can reverse this effect despite the concurrent blood pressure fall (73). Finally, ACE inhibitors lower blood pressure of hypertensive patients without impairing cerebral blood flow (51). In one study, an increase in cerebral blood flow was observed after a few days of treatment (81). It appeared to be most pronounced in those patients who responded to ACE inhibition with the greatest blood pressure fall.

EFFECTS OF ACE INHIBITION ON THE COMPONENTS OF THE RENIN-ANGIOTENSIN SYSTEM

It is expected that ACE inhibitors reduce the circulating levels of angiotensin II. Clear-cut decreases in plasma angiotensin II could indeed be demonstrated following inhibition of the angiotensin I-processing enzyme (Fig. 3). Initially, however, investigators were faced with the problem that plasma angiotensin II did not fall to levels close to zero (59,94). The method for measurement of plasma angiotensin II then was

improved in order to specifically quantify the octapeptide. For this purpose, the different angiotensins and breakdown products of plasma extract were first separated by high performance liquid chromatogra-

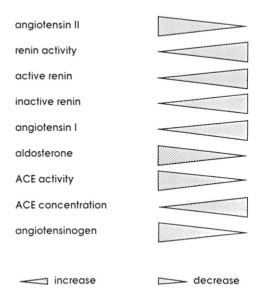

FIG. 3. Effect of ACE inhibition on the components of the renin-angiotensin-aldosterone system.

phy. The true angiotensin II fraction was then determined by radioimmunoassay. Using this technique, it became possible to demonstrate that angiotensin II virtually disappears from the circulation, at least during the peak effect of ACE inhibition (95–97).

Plasma-renin activity, which represents the amount of angiotensin I generated in plasma during a given incubation time, increases during ACE inhibition (16,27,54). This rise in plasma-renin activity has been generally attributed to the interruption of the negative feedback of angiotensin II on renin release (139). The active form of renin represents only one part of the total amount of renin found in the circulation. There indeed exists an inactive form of renin (often called prorenin) which is considered to be the precursor of active renin (68). The pattern of the changes in the two types of renin observed during ACE inhibition appears to differ with time. The active renin tends to rise during the acute phase at the expense of inactive renin, whereas during the chronic phase, active and inactive renin are both increased in parallel (55,74,98). The hyperreninemia resulting from ACE inhibition causes an increase in circulating levels of angiotensin I. There is no true accumulation of angiotensin I following ACE inhibition. Angiotensin I levels in the blood indeed remain proportionate to the rate of renin secretion even during administration of an ACE inhibitor (93). The renin response to ACE inhibition can be diminished by β-adrenoceptor blockade (128) as well as by cyclo-oxygenase inhibition (100,108).

Aldosterone production is decreased during short-term ACE inhibition (3,16,27). There has been concern whether aldosterone secretion still is suppressed during chronic treatment (9,57). However, careful evaluation has shown plasma levels of aldosterone to be reduced together with those of angiotensin II even during long-term ACE inhibition (20).

Plasma-ACE activity is frequently deter-mined to estimate the degree of blockade of angiotensin I conversion induced by ACE inhibitors. In the case of captopril, the enzyme activity has to be measured immediately following blood drawing because, *in vitro*, the captopril-ACE complex tends to dissociate and, therefore, the extent to which ACE is inhibited might be underestimated (114). There is an induction of ACE production during prolonged ACE inhibition (11,124). This adaptative increment passes completely unnoticed when ACE activity is assayed in the presence of an ACE inhibitor.

Therapy with ACE inhibitors decreases plasma levels of angiotensinogen (109). The consumption of this substrate is accelerated because of the high-plasma-renin concentrations achieved during ACE inhibition.

MECHANISMS OF ACTION OF ACE INHIBITORS

Angiotensin II

The blood pressure lowering effect of ACE inhibitors principally is due to the prevention of angiotensin II formation and therefore of the vasoconstriction induced by this circulating peptide. Recent observations suggest that angiotensin II may be generated directly in the blood vessel wall (24,45,82,132). Whether ACE inhibitors decrease blood pressure partly by virtue of inhibiting ACE in the vascular tissue is however still hypothetical.

Aldosterone

The decrease in aldosterone secretion occurring during ACE inhibition may lead to natriuresis in some patients, and probably accounts for the lack of sodium retention accompanying the blood pressure reduction (3,16). Total body sodium seems even to decrease in hypertensive patients treated chronically with an ACE inhibitor (39,120). To what extent this actively contributes to the antihypertensive effect of ACE inhibitors is difficult to determine.

Bradykinin

ACE is identical with kininase II, one of the enzymes physiologically involved in the breaking down of bradykinin, a vasodilator peptide (46). The antihypertensive effect of ACE inhibitors therefore could be heightened by an accumulation of bradykinin, either in the circulation or in the tissues. There is no univocal evidence for an increase in blood levels of bradykinin following ACE inhibition (35,61,64,133). Reduced destruction of bradykinin generated locally cannot be ruled out.

Prostaglandins

It also is conceivable that ACE inhibitors lower blood pressure through prostaglandins. Bradykinin is capable of activating phospholipase and thereby of stimulating the synthesis of arachidonic acid and prostaglandins (152). The vasodilatory prostaglandins may decrease arteriolar tone not only through their direct relaxant properties, but also through the attenuation of the vascular effect of pressor amines and hormones. Conflicting results have been reported with regard to the impact of ACE inhibitors on plasma levels of prostanoids (83,99,133,141). Cyclo-oxygenase inhibitors (such as nonsteroidal antiinflammatory drugs) block the generation of prostaglandins. They have been shown to blunt the antihypertensive effect of ACE inhibitors (83,99,100,118), possibly because they cause some sodium retention. This finding nevertheless does not necessarily indicate that the participation of prostaglandins in blood pressure regulation is intensified by ACE inhibition. It is well known that cyclo-oxygenase inhibitors attenuate the blood pressure lowering effect of various other antihypertensive agents.

Central and Peripheral Nervous System

The interplay between the renin-angiotensin and the sympathetic nervous system is of major importance to the mode of action of ACE inhibitors (104). The blood pressure lowering effect of these agents appears to be minimally counteracted by a reflex activation of sympathetic nerve activity. Plasma catecholamines essentially are not changed by ACE inhibition (12,89,91). The contribution of the sympathetic nervous system to the maintenance of blood pressure is probably reduced by ACE inhibitors because of the disappearance of angiotensin II both at the central and the peripheral level (Fig. 1). In addition, the pressor effect of norepinephrine also is lessened by ACE inhibition (62).

ACE inhibitors seem to exert a parasympathomimetic action (23,131). This property might be relevant for the absence of heart rate acceleration encountered habitually during ACE inhibition in the face of a blood pressure fall.

CLINICAL USE OF ACE INHIBITORS

Monotherapy

Given in monotherapy, ACE inhibitors normalize blood pressure in 40 to 60% of hypertensive patients (23,38,43,58,107,137, 140). These agents have been claimed to be more effective in younger than in older patients. This belief could, however, not be substantiated in recent trials comprising a large number of hypertensives treated either with captopril or enalapril (33,121, 142).

Co-Therapy

The most rational and efficacious combination therapy consists of an ACE inhibitor with a diuretic (15,38,58,87,107,137, 140,151). ACE inhibition prevents the reactive rise in circulating angiotensin II, which normally results from the diuretic-induced increase in renin release. During blockade of angiotensin II generation, the blood pressure lowering effect of diuretics is therefore not opposed by the pressor effect of the renin response to salt depletion (Fig. 4). This brings out the full antihypertensive action of the diuretic and allows the dose of the diuretic to be kept low (1).

Calcium channel blockers can also add a supplementary blood pressure reduction when administered together with an ACE inhibitor (14,42,78,119,127,129). The reflex increase in sympathetic nerve activity, induced particularly by calcium channel blockers of the dehydropyridin class, appears to be attenuated by inhibiting the ACE activity (6).

The co-administration of a β-adrenoceptor agent with an ACE inhibitor may be of help in some patients (50,78,128,151). This type of combination however appears not particularly appealing except if the β-blocker is indicated because of a concom-itant disease or in patients with a relatively high heart rate.

Multiple drug therapy may be needed in some patients. One advantage of ACE inhibitors is that they can be associated safely with all commonly-used antihypertensive agents, except the potassium-sparing diuretics (see p. 106, Metabolic Effects of ACE Inhibition).

ACE INHIBITORS IN RENOVASCULAR HYPERTENSION

Circulating angiotensin II may be critical to maintain a normal glomerular filtration rate. Thus, below a critical limit of renal perfusion pressure, glomerular filtration ceases if there is no angiotensin II available to induce efferent arteriolar vasoconstriction and thereby preserve an adequate glomerular filtration pressure (19). The presence of a stenosis in a renal artery may markedly reduce the glomerular perfusion pressure (Fig. 5). In such a case, ACE inhibition interrupts the principal mechanism

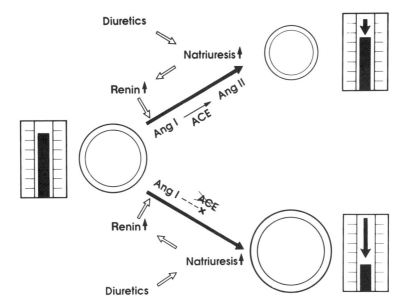

FIG. 4. Effect of ACE inhibition on the response of arteriolar tone and blood pressure to diuretic therapy. Ang I and II = angiotensin I and II; ACE = normally functioning enzyme; A̶C̶E̶ = inhibited enzyme.

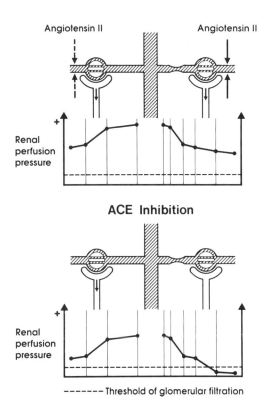

FIG. 5. Influence of angiotensin II-mediated posst-glomerular vasoconstriction on renal perfusion pressure and glomerular filtration rate in the absence or presence of a renal artery stenosis (See text for detailed explanation).

maintaining filtration of the kidney. It thus is not surprising that renal failure can be observed during treatment with an ACE inhibitor in patients with bilateral renal artery stenosis (as well as in patients with renal artery stenosis in a single kidney). In patients with unilateral renal artery stenosis and an intact contralateral kidney, however, the deterioration of ipsilateral renal function cannot be readily detected, since the contralateral kidney compensates for the loss in glomerular filtration (70,149).

Renovascular hypertension is usually a condition difficult to treat by conventional antihypertensive drugs. A good policy therefore would appear to check serum creatinine at the time blood pressure of these patients is successfully reduced by a drug

regimen including an ACE inhibitor. The experience available so far suggests that the impairment of renal function which may occur in patients with renovascular hypertension is reversible after withdrawal of the ACE inhibitor. Nevertheless, long-term ACE inhibition should, whenever possible, be avoided in patients with known renal artery stenosis, be it unilateral or bilateral.

ACE INHIBITION IN HYPERTENSION ASSOCIATED WITH OTHER DISORDERS

Chronic Renal Failure

In the presence of an underlying renal disease, ACE inhibitors given as monotherapy normalize blood pressure less frequently than in the face of an intact renal function. In patients with chronic renal failure, ACE inhibition has often to be combined with a loop diuretic in order to achieve a satisfactory blood pressure control (21,69). ACE inhibitors, like all antihypertensive agents, may cause a transient reduction in glomerular filtration rate during the first few days or weeks of therapy. Such behavior of renal function is due to the blood pressure drop *per se* and is most likely to be seen in patients already having some degree of renal insufficiency before introduction of the ACE inhibitor. The renal function of these patients is stabilized or even improved during long-term treatment (5,32). Urinary protein excretion decreases generally during chronic administration of an ACE inhibitor. This effect is probably accounted for by the reduction in systemic blood pressure and also by the changes in glomerular filtration pressure consecutive to the dilatation of the efferent arteriole.

Cardiac Hypertrophy

It is well established that ACE inhibition can reverse cardiac hypertrophy (40,44,49).

Congestive Heart Failure

ACE inhibitors undoubtedly represent an important advance in the treatment of patients with severe congestive heart failure and normal blood pressure (25,31,138). It therefore comes as no surprise that they can be very useful for the treatment of hypertensives with all degrees of heart failure.

Coronary Heart Disease

A main advantage of ACE inhibitors in patients with angina pectoris is the usual lack of a reflex increase in myocardial sympathetic tone in response to the blood pressure fall (37,79). As a consequence, oxygen consumption is expected to decrease. In one study, chronic ACE inhibition appeared to render less pronounced the ST-segment depression observed at the maximal double product (i.e., systolic blood pressure times heart rate) during ergometry (130). Recently, ACE inhibition has been shown to attenuate the development of ventricular dilatation and to improve exercise tolerance in normo- and hypertensive patients followed for one year after having experienced anterior myocardial infarction (107).

Cerebrovascular Disease

As already stated, ACE inhibitors lower blood pressure without diminishing cerebral blood flow. In hypertensive patients with unilateral cerebrovascular disease, blood flow to the affected hemisphere may actually rise in response to ACE inhibition (13).

Peripheral Vascular Disease

ACE inhibitors dilate both small and large arteries when lowering blood pressure (116). They have been shown to improve the pain-free interval and the maximal walking distance in hypertensive patients with claudication (71,112).

Pulmonary Disease

No deleterious effect of ACE inhibition on respiratory tests has been observed in hypertensive patients suffering from chronic obstructive pulmonary disease (7). Most important, antihypertensive therapy with ACE inhibitors was revealed to also be safe in asthmatic patients (41,111,117). Bronchial provocation testing was performed in asthmatics treated with an ACE inhibitor. The bronchial reactivity to metacholine (117) and bradykinin (41) was not enhanced by ACE inhibition.

Diabetes

The use of ACE inhibitors for the management of hypertensive diabetics appears especially attractive. These agents reduce glomerular capillary pressure, a pressure which is presumably abnormally increased in patients with diabetes mellitus, both in the presence and the absence of systemic hypertension. It is probably through this mechanism that ACE inhibitors decrease urinary protein excretion in patients with diabetic nephropathy (10,134) and seem to exert a beneficial action on renal function of diabetic patients (10).

ACE INHIBITORS AND PREGNANCY

At the present time, the use of ACE inhibitors in hypertensive pregnant women should be avoided. Neonatal anuria has been described after treatment with captopril or enalapril during pregnancy (113,125). In the latter case, peritoneal dialysis has proven life saving. ACE inhibition during pregnancy may impair closing of the ductus arteriosus. It should be said, however, that a number of pregnancies had a favorable outcome despite the administration of an ACE inhibitor (65).

METABOLIC EFFECTS OF ACE INHIBITION

In patients with a normal renal function, the suppression of aldosterone secretion mediated by ACE inhibitors generally does lead to a slight, not clinically relevant, increase in serum potassium (135,145,147). ACE inhibition however, may, precipitate the development of a frank hyperkalemia in patients with end-stage renal disease (135,145). ACE inhibitors reduce the renal loss of potassium induced by thiazides or loop diuretics (75,147). The addition of a potassium-sparing diuretic to an ACE inhibitor may be desirable in some patients with manifest hypokalemia. This can be done safely in patients with a normal renal function (84). Such a combination however, should, be avoided as soon as there is any evidence of renal failure. One should also be cautious when supplementing with potassium a patient treated with an ACE inhibitor (22).

Given as monotherapy, ACE inhibitors do not increase serum levels of cholesterol, very-low-density and low-density lipoprotein cholesterol, triglycerides, and glucose (75,123,147). These agents may partially prevent the hyperlipidemia and hyperglycemia induced by thiazide diuretics (75,147).

ACE inhibitors exert an uricosuric action (67). They reduce serum uric acid concentrations in patients with hyperuricemia. Diuretic-induced hyperuricemia is attenuated by ACE inhibition (75,147).

INITIATION OF TREATMENT WITH AN ACE INHIBITOR

An excessive and potentially harmful blood pressure drop may follow the administration of the first dose of an ACE inhibitor (59). The occurrence of hypotension has to be feared principally in patients already taking diuretics, in those who are dehydrated or hypovolemic, and in those with severe heart failure. To minimize the risk of developing hypotension, it is recommended to withdraw, or at least to reduce, the dose of diuretics for 24 to 48 hours before introducing an ACE inhibitor. When such a procedure is not practical, it is advised to give the first dose of the ACE inhibitor under surveillance. It then may be preferable to start therapy with a small dose of captopril (for instance 6.25 mg) rather than with enalapril (e.g., 2.5 mg). This is because captopril has a much faster onset of action and shorter duration of effect than enalapril. In cases of marked hypotension, infusion of isotonic saline solution usually suffices to restore normal blood pressure levels. In the vast majority of hypertensives, however, ACE inhibition can be initiated without any particular precaution.

DOSAGE OF ACE INHIBITORS

During chronic treatment, it is not necessary to suppress ACE activity throughout the day to obtain a satisfactory blood pressure control (143). Captopril, (25 mg to 50 mg b.i.d.), enalapril, (10 to 20 mg q.d.), or lisinopril, (10 to 40 mg q.d.), are sufficient in most patients. Captopril administered once a day (50 to 100 mg) may also be effective. It would seem reasonable to give half these doses when glomerular filtration rate falls below 30 to 40 ml/min.

SIDE-EFFECTS OF ACE INHIBITORS

Hypotension, hyperkalemia, and renal impairment are typically side-effects which are related to blockade of angiotensin II production and can be foreseen under certain circumstances already discussed. Development of renal insufficiency is very unlikely to occur unless there is a bilateral renal artery stenosis, a stenosis of the artery to a solitary kidney, or if blood pressure falls to very-low levels as in patients with severe congestive heart failure. Deterioration of renal function may be observed, however, in rare patients with wide-spread arteriolosclerosis (136). Dry, nonproductive cough has been recognized as a prominent side effect of the class of ACE inhibitors (29,34,115). The mechanisms responsible for this side-effect are still unclear but blockade of kinin inactivation is thought to play a role. ACE inhibition may render hypersensitive inhalation of substances releasing bradykinin (85). Inhalation of bradykinin is indeed known to induce cough (52). Of interest also is the observation that cyclo-oxygenase inhibition has been reported to reduce cough of patients receiving an ACE inhibitor. (92).

During the early phase of clinical development of captopril, excessively high doses were used. This was associated with a non-negligible incidence of side effects such as leucopenia, immune complex glomerulopathy, proteinuria, taste disturbance, and skin rash. With the reduction of the total daily dose, the troublesome hematologic and renal side effects of captopril have practically disappeared. The incidence of taste disturbance and skin rashes has also declined drastically. Cutaneous rashes and taste disturbances appear less frequent with enalapril and lisinopril. All 3 agents may cause angioneurotic edema. The overall incidence of unwanted effects of ACE inhibitors does not appear age dependent (26,63,90,146).

ACE INHIBITION AND QUALITY OF LIFE

The goal of antihypertensive therapy should be more and more to lower blood pressure without impairing the patient's enjoyment of life. There is now a large body of evidence indicating that ACE inhibitors often come close to satisfying this requirement. ACE inhibition does not alter memory function of hypertensive patients (72). It seems to improve the sense of well-being, work performance, and cognitive function while it has no influence on other indices of quality of life such as physical symptoms, sexual function, sleep, life satisfaction, and social participation (36).

CONCLUSIONS

An ideal antihypertensive drug should lower blood pressure without activating pressor mechanisms that oppose the blood pressure reduction. It should not impair the reflex responses to changes in posture or to physical exercise. It should be devoid of side-effects, should not affect adversely the well-being of patients, and have no deleterious metabolic effect. An ideal drug also ought to be easily combined with other agents and to be safely administered in hypertensives with concomitant diseases. ACE inhibitors often fulfill many of these criteria even if they cannot be considered perfect. They are therefore already used by many as first-line drugs for the treatment of hypertensive patients.

REFERENCES

1. Andren, L., Weiner, L., Svensson, A., and Hansson, L. (1983): Enalapril with either a "very low" or "low" dose of hydrochlorothiazide is equally effective in essential hypertension: A double-blind trial in 100 hypertensive patients. *J. Hypertens.* 1(Suppl.2):384–386.
2. Atkinson, A. B., Brown, J. J., Cumming, A. M. M., Fraser, R., Lever, A. F., Leckie, B. J., Morton, J. J., and Robertson, J. I. S. (1982): Captopril in renovascular hypertension: Long-term use in predicting surgical outcome. *Br. Med. J.*, 284:689–692.
3. Atlas, S. A., Case, D. B., Sealey, J. E., Laragh, J. H., and McKinstry, D. N. (1979): Interruption of the renin-angiotensin system in hypertensive patients by captopril induces sustained reduction in aldosterone secretion, potassium retention and natriuresis. *Hypertension*, 1:274–280.
4. Bauer, J. H., and Reams, G. P. (1986): Renal effects of angiotensin converting enzyme inhibitors in hypertension. *Am J. Med.*, 81 (Suppl.4C):19–27.
5. Bauer, J. H., Reams, G. P., and Lal, S. M. (1987): Renal protective effect of strict blood pressure control with enalapril therapy. *Arch. Intern. Med.*, 147:1397–1400.
6. Bellet, M., Sassano, P., Guyenne, T. T., Corvol, P., and Ménard, J. (1987): Sympatho-inhibitors effect of angiotensin converting enzyme inhibi-

tion during counter regulation induced by dihydropyridine. *J. Hypertens.*, 5(Suppl.5):583–585.

7. Bertoli, L., Fusco, M., Micallef, R. E., and Busnardo, I. (1985): Treatment of essential hypertension with captopril in patients with chronic obstructive pulmonary disease. *J. Hypertens.*, 3 (Suppl.2):153–154.

8. Biollaz, J., Burnier, M., Turini, G. A., Brunner, D. B., Porchet, M., Gomez, H. J., Jones, K. H., Ferber, F., Abrams, W. B., Gavras, H., and Brunner, H. R. (1981): Three new long-acting converting enzyme inhibitors: Relationship between plasma converting enzyme activity and response to angiotensin I. *Clin. Pharmacol. Ther.*, 29:665–670.

9. Biollaz, J., Brunner, H. R., Gavras, I., Waeber, B., and Gavras, H. (1982): Antihypertensive therapy with MK 421: Angiotensin II-renin relationships to evaluate efficacy of converting enzyme blockade. *J. Cardiovasc. Pharmacol.*, 4:966–972.

10. Björck, S., Nyberg, G., Mulec, H., Granems, G., Herlitz, H., and Aurell, M. (1986): Beneficial effects of angiotensin converting enzyme inhibition on renal function in patients with diabetic nephropathy. *Br. Med. J.*, 293:471–474.

11. Boomsma, F., De Bruyn, J. H. B., Derkx, F. H. M., and Schalekamp, M. A. D. H. (1981): Opposite effects of captopril on angiotensin I-converting enzyme "activity" and "concentration": Relation between enzyme inhibition and long-term blood pressure response. *Clin. Sci.*, 60:4911–4918.

12. Bravo, E. L., and Tarazi, R. C. (1979): Converting enzyme inhibition with an orally active compound in hypertensive man. *Hypertension*, 1:39–46.

13. Britton, K. E., Granowska, M., Nimmon, C. C., and Horne, T. (1985): Cerebral blood flow in hypertensive patients with cerebrovascular disease: Technique for measurement and effect of captopril. *Nuc. Med. Comm.*, 6:251–261.

14. Brouwer, R. M. L., Bolli, P., Erne, P., Conen, D., Kiowski, W., and Bühler, F. R. (1985): Antihypertensive treatment using calcium antagonists in combination with captopril rather than diuretics. *J. Cardiovasc. Pharmacol.*, 7(Suppl. 1):88–91.

15. Brunner, H. R., Gavras, H., and Waeber, B. (1980): Enhancement by diuretics of the antihypertensive action of long-term angiotensin converting enzyme blockade. *Clin. Exp. Hypertension*, 2:639–657.

16. Brunner, H. R., Gavras, H., Waeber, B., Kershaw, G. R., Turini, G. A., Vukovich, R. A., McKinstry, D. N., and Gavras, I. (1979): Oral angiotensin-converting enzyme inhibitor in long-term treatment of hypertensive patients. *Ann. Intern. Med.*, 90:19–23.

17. Brunner, H. R., Nussberger, J., and Waeber, B. (1985): The present molecules of converting enzyme inhibitors. *J. Cardiovasc. Pharmacol.*, 7(Suppl.1):2–11.

18. Brunner, H. R., Waeber, B., and Nussberger, J. (1983): Does pharmacological profiling of a new drug in normotensive volunteers provide a useful guideline to antihypertensive therapy. *Hypertension*, 5 (Suppl.III):101–107.

19. Brunner, H. R., Waeber, B., and Nussberger, J. (1987): Angiotensin converting enzyme inhibition and the normal kidney. *Kidney Int.*, 31 (Suppl.20):104–107.

20. Brunner, H. R., Waeber, B., Nussberger, J., Schaller, M. D., and Gomez, H. J. (1983): Long-term clinical experience with enalapril in essential hypertension. *J. Hypertens.*, 1 (Suppl.1):103–107.

21. Brunner, H. R., Waeber, B., Wauters, J. P., Turini, G. A., McKinstry, D. N., and Gavras, H. (1978): Inappropriate renin secretion unmasked by captopril (SQ 14,225) in hypertension or chronic renal failure. *Lancet*, ii:704–707.

22. Burnakis, T. G., and Mioderch, H. J. (1984): Combined therapy with captopril and potassium supplementation: A potential for hyperkalemia. *Arch. Intern. Med.*, 144:2371–2372.

23. Campbell, B. C., Sturani, A., and Reid, J. L. (1983): Parasympathomimetic activity of captopril in normotensive man. *J. Hypertens.*, 1 (Suppl.2):246–248.

24. Campbell, D. J. (1987): Tissue renin-angiotensin system: Sites of angiotensin formation. *J. Cardiovasc. Pharmacol.*, 10 (Suppl.7):1–8.

25. Captopril Multicenter Research Group. (1983): A placebo-controlled trial of captopril in refractory chronic congestive heart failure. *J. Am. Coll. Cardiol.*, 2:755–763.

26. Case, D. B. (1987): Angiotensin-converting enzyme inhibitors: Are they all alike? *J. Clin. Hypertension*, 3:243–256.

27. Case, D. B., Atlas, S. A., Laragh, J. H., Sealey, J. E., Sullivan, P. A., and McKinstry, D. N. (1978): Clinical experience with blockade of the renin-angiotensin-aldosterone system by an oral converting-enzyme inhibitor (SQ 14,225 or captopril) in hypertensive patients. *Progr. Cardiovasc. Dis.*, 21:195–206.

28. Case, D. B., Atlas, S. A., Laragh, J. H., Sullivan, P. A., and Sealey, J. E. (1980): Use of first dose response or plasma renin activity to predict the long-term effect of captopril: Identification of triphasic pattern of blood pressure response. *J. Cardiovasc. Pharmacol.*, 2:339–346.

29. Chalmers, D., Dombey, S. L., and Lawson, D. H. (1987): Post-marketing surveillance of captopril (for hypertension): A preliminary report. *Br. J. Clin. Pharmacol.*, 24:343–349.

30. Cody, R. J., Tarazi, R. C., Bravo, E. L., and Fouad, F. M. (1978): Hemodynamics of orally active converting enzyme inhibitor (SQ 14,225) in hypertensive patients. *Clin. Sci. Mol. Med.*, 55:453–459.

31. The Consensus Trial Study Group 1987. (1987): Effects of enalapril on mortality in severe congestive heart failure. *N. Engl. J. Med.*, 23:1429–1435.

32. Cooper, W. D., Doyle, G. D., Donohoe, J., Laher, M., Ledingham, J. G. G., Raine, A. E. G., Melinck, C., Unsworth, J., Raman, G. V., Van den Burg, M. J., Woollard, M. L., and Currie, W. J. C. (1985): Enalapril in the treatment of hypertension associated with impaired renal function. *J. Hypertens.*, 3 (Suppl.3):471–474.

33. Cooper, W. D., Glover, D. R., and Kimber, G. R. (1987): Influence of age on blood pressure response to enalapril. *Gerontology*, 33 (Suppl.1):48–54.

34. Cooper, W. D., Sheldon, D., Brown, D., Kimber, G. R., Isitt, V. L., and Currie, W. J. C. (1987): Post-marketing surveillance of enalapril: Experience in 11710 hypertensive patients in general practice. *J. Roy. Coll. Gen. Pract.*, 37:346–349.

35. Crantz, F. R., Swartz, S. L., Hollenberg, N. K., Moore, T. J., Dluhy, R. G., and Williams, G. H. (1980): Differences in response to the peptidyl-dipeptidase hydrolase inhibitors SQ 20,881 and SQ 14,225 in normal-renin essential hypertension. *Hypertension*, 2:604–609.

36. Croog, S. H., Levine, S., Testa, M. A., Brown, G., Bulpitt, C., Jenkins, C. D., Klerman, G. L., and Williams, G. H. (1986): The effects of antihypertensive therapy on the quality of life. *N. Engl. J. Med.*, 314:1657–1664.

37. Daly, P., Mettauer, B., Rouleau, J. L., Cousineau, D., and Burgess, J. H. (1985): Lack of reflex increase in myocardial sympathetic tone after captopril: Potential antianginal effect. *Circulation*, 71:317–325.

38. Davies, R. O., Irvin, J. D., Kramsch, D. K., Walker, J. F., and Moncloa, F. (1984): Enalapril worldwide experience. *Am. J. Med.*, 77 (2A):23–25.

39. De Zeeuw, D., Navis, G. J., Donker, A. J. M., and De Jong, P. E. (1983): The angiotensin converting enzyme inhibitor enalapril and its effects on renal function. *J. Hypertens.*, 1 (Suppl.I):93–97.

40. Devereux, R. B., Pickering, T. G., Cody, R. J., and Laragh, J. H. (1987): Relation of renin-angiotensin system activity to left ventricular hypertrophy and function in experimental and human hypertension. *J. Clin. Hypertension*, 3:87–103.

41. Dixon, C. M. S., Fuller, R. W., and Barnes, P. J. (1987): The effect of an angiotensin-converting enzyme inhibitor, ramipril, on bronchial responses in asthmatic subjects. *Br. J. Clin. Pharmacol.*, 23:91–93.

42. Donnelly, R., Elliott, H. L., and Reid, J. L. (1986): Nicardipine combined with enalapril in patients with essential hypertension. *Br. J. Clin. Pharmacol.*, 22:283s–287s.

43. Drayer, J. I. M., and Weber, M. A. (1983): Monotherapy of essential hypertension with a converting enzyme inhibitor. *Hypertension*, 5 (Suppl.3):108–113.

44. Dunn, F. G., Oigman, W., Ventura, H. O., Messerli, F. H., Kobrin, I., and Frohlich, E. D. (1984): Enalapril improves systemic and renal hemodynamics and allows regression of left ventricular mass in essential hypertension. *Am. J. Cardiol.*, 53:105–108.

45. Dzau, V. J. (1986): Significance of the vascular renin-angiotensin pathway. *Hypertension*, 8:553–559.

46. Erdös, E. G. (1976): Conversion of angiotensin I to angiotensin II. *Am. J. Med.*, 60:749–759.

47. Fagard, R., Amery, A., Reybrouck, T., Lijnen, P., and Billiet, L. (1980): Acute and chronic systemic and hemodynamic effects of angiotensin converting enzyme inhibition with captopril in hypertensive patients. *Am. J. Cardiol.*, 46:295–300.

48. Ferguson, R. K., Brunner, H. R., Turini, G. A., Gavras, H., and McKinstry, D. N., (1977): A specific orally active inhibitor of angiotensin converting enzyme in man. *Lancet*, i:775–778.

49. Fouad, F. M., Tarazi, R. C., and Bravo, E. L. (1983): Cardiac and haemodynamic effects of enalapril. *J. Hypertens.*, 1 (Suppl.1):135–142.

50. Franz, I. W., Behr, U., and Ketelhut, R (1987): Resting and exercise blood pressure with atenolol, enalapril and a low-dose combination. *J. Hypertens.*, 5(Suppl.3):37–41.

51. Frei, A., and Müller-Brand, J. (1986): Cerebral blood flow and antihypertensive treatment with enalapril. *J. Hypertens.*, 4:365–368.

52. Fuller, R. W. Dixon, C. M. S., Cuss, F. M. C., and Barnes, P. J. (1987): Bradykinin-induced bronchoconstriction in humans. *Ann. Rev. Respir. Dis.*, 135:176–180.

53. Gavras, H., Brunner, H. R., Laragh, J. H., Sealey, J. E., Gavras, I., and Vukovich, R. A. (1974): An angiotensin converting enzyme inhibitor to identify and treat vasoconstrictor and volume factors in hypertensive patients. *N. Engl. J. Med.*, 291:817–821.

54. Gavras, H., Brunner, H. R., Turini, G. A., Kershaw, G. R., Tifft, C. P., Cuttelod, S., Gavras, I., Vukovich, R. A., and McKinstry, D. N., (1978): Antihypertensive effect of oral angiotensin converting enzyme inhibitor SQ 14,225 in man. *N. Engl. J. Med.*, 298:991–995.

55. Goldstone, R., Horton, R., Carlson, E. J., and Hsueh, W. A. (1983): Reciprocal changes in active and inactive renin after converting enzyme inhibition in normal man. *J. Clin. Endocrinol. Metab.*, 56:264–268.

56. Gomez, H. J., Cirillo, V. J., and Moncloa, F. (1987): The clinical pharmacology of lisinopril. *J. Cardiovasc. Pharmacol.*, 9 (Suppl.3):27–34.

57. Griffing, G. T., Sindler, B. H., Aurecchia, S. A., and Melby, J. C. (1982): Temporal enhancement of renin-aldosterone blockade by enalapril, an angiotensin-converting enzyme inhibitor. *J. Clin. Pharmacol. Ther.*, 32:592–598.

58. Heel, R. C., Brogden, R. N., Speight, T. M., and Avery, G. S. (1980): Captopril: A preliminary review of its pharmacological properties and therapeutic efficacy. *Drugs*, 20:409–452.

59. Hodsman, G. P., Isles, C. G., Murray, G. D., Usherwood, T. P., Webb, D. J., and Robertson, J. I. S. (1983): Factors related to first dose hy-

potensive effect of captopril: Prediction and treatment. *Br. Med. J.*, 286:832–834.

60. Hollenberg, N. K., Meggs, L. G., Williams, G. H., Katz, J., Garnic, J. D., and Harrington, D. P. (1981): Sodium intake and renal responses to captopril in normal man and in essential hypertension. *Kidney Int.*, 20:240–245.

61. Hulthén, U. L., and Hökfelt, B. (1978): The effect of the converting enzyme inhibitor SQ 20,881 on kinins, renin-angiotensin-aldosterone and catecholamines in relation to blood pressure in hypertensive patients. *Acta Med. Scand.*, 204:497–502.

62. Imai, Y., Abe, K., Seino, M., Haruyama, T., Tajima, J., Sato, M., Goto, T., Hiwatari, M., Kasai, Y., Yoshinaga, K., and Sekino, H. (1982): Attenuation of pressor responses to norepinephrine and pitressin and potentiation of pressor response to angiotensin II by captopril in human subjects. *Hypertension*, 4:444–451.

63. Irvin, J. D., and Viau, J. M. (1986): Safety profiles of the angiotensin converting enzyme inhibitors captopril and enalapril. *Am. J. Med.*, 8(Suppl.4C):46–50.

64. Johnston, C. I., McGrath, B. P., Millar, J. A., and Matthews, P. G. (1979): Long-term effects of captopril (SQ 14,225) on blood pressure and hormone levels in essential hypertension. *Lancet*, 2:493–495.

65. Kreft-Joris, C., Plouin, P. F., and Tchobroutsky, C. (1987): Angiotensin converting enzyme inhibitors during pregnancy. *J. Hypertens.*, 5(Suppl.5):553–554.

66. Laragh, J. H., Angers, M., Kelly, W. G., and Lieberman, S. (1960): Hypotensive agents and pressor substances: The effect of epinephrine, norepinephrine, angiotensin II and others in the secretory rate of aldosterone in man. *JAMA*, 174:234–240.

67. Leary, W. P., and Reyes, A. J. (1987): Angiotensin I converting enzyme inhibitors and the renal excretion of urate. *Cardiovasc. Drugs Ther.*, 1:29–38.

68. Leckie, B. J. (1981): Inactive renin: An attempt at a perspective. *Clin. Sci.*, 60:119–130.

69. Ledingham, J. G. G. (1987): Effects of angiotensin II and angiotensin converting enzyme inhibitor in chronic renal failure. *Kidney Int.*, 31 (Suppl.20):112–116.

70. Levenson, D. J., and Dzau, V. J. (1987): Effects of angiotensin-converting enzyme inhibition on renal hemodynamics in renal artery stenosis. *Kidney Int.*, 31(Suppl.20):173–179.

71. Libretti, A., and Catalano, M. (1986): Captopril in the treatment of hypertension associated with claudication. *Postgrad. Med. J.*, 62(Suppl.I):34–37.

72. Lichter, I., Richardson, P. J., and Wyke, M. A. (1986): Differential effects of atenolol and enalapril on memory during treatment for essential hypertension. *Br. J. Clin. Pharmacol.*, 21:641–645.

73. Magrini, F., Shimizu, M., Roberts, N., Fouad, F. M., Tarazi, R. C., and Zanchetti, A. (1987):

Angiotensin converting enzyme inhibition and coronary blood flow. *Circulation*, 75(Suppl.I): I168–I173.

74. Malatino, L. S., Manhem, P., Ball, S. G., Leckie, B. J., Morton, J. J., Murray, G. D., and Robertson, J. I. S. (1986): Twenty-four hour changes in active and inactive renin after various oral doses of the converting enzyme inhibitor ramipril (HOE 498) in normal man. *J. Clin. Hypertens.*, 3:231–237.

75. Malini, P. L., Strochi, E., Ambrosioni, E., and Magnani, B. (1984): Long-term antihypertensive, metabolic and cellular effects of enalapril. *J. Hypertension*, 2 (Suppl.2):101–105.

76. Mancia, G., Parati, G., Pomidossi, G., Grassi, G., Bertinieri, G., Buccino, N., Ferrari, A., Gregorini, L., Rupoli, L., and Zanchetti, A. (1982): Modification of arterial baroreflexes by captopril in essential hypertension. *Am. J. Cardiol.*, 49:1415–1419.

77. Manhem, P., Bramnert, M., Hulthén, U. L., and Hökfelt, B., (1981): The effect of captopril on catecholamines, renin activity, angiotensin II and aldosterone in plasma during physical exercise in hypertensive patients. *Eur. J. Clin. Invest.*, 11:389–395.

78. McGregor, G. A., Markandu, N. D., Smith, S. J., and Sagnella, G. A. (1985): Captopril: Contrasting effects of adding hydrochlorothiazide, propranolol, or nifedipine. *J. Cardiovasc. Pharmacol.*, 7(Suppl.1):82–87.

79. Mettauer, B., Rouleau, J. L., and Daly, P. (1986): The effect of captopril in hypertensive patients with stable angina. *Postgrad. Med. J.*, 2 (Suppl.1):54–58.

80. Mimran, A., Brunner, H. R., Turini, G. A., Waeber, B., and Brunner, D. B. (1979): Effect of captopril on renal vascular tone in patients with essential hypertension. *Clin. Sci.*, 57:421s–423s.

81. Minematsu, K., Yamagushi, Y., Tsuchiya, M., Ito, K., Ikeda, M., and Omae T. (1987): Effect of angiotensin converting enzyme inhibitor (captopril) on cerebral blood flow in hypertensive patients without a history of stroke. *Clin. Exp. Hypertens.*, A9:551–557.

82. Mizuno, K., Nakamura, M., Higashimori, K., and Inagami, T. (1988): Local generation and release of angiotensin II in peripheral vascular tissue. *Hypertension*, 11:223–229.

83. Moore, T. J., Crantz, F. R., Hollenberg, N. K., Kolctsky, R. J., Leboff, M. S., Swartz, S. L., Levine, L., Podolsky, S., Dluhy, R. G., and Williams, G. H. (1981): Contribution of prostaglandins to the antihypertensive action of captopril in essential hypertension. *Hypertension*, 3:168–173.

84. Mooser, V., Waeber, G., Bidiville, J., Waeber, B., Nussberger, J., and Brunner, H. R. (1987): Kalemia during combined therapy with an angiotensin converting enzyme inhibitor and a potassium-sparing diuretic. *J. Clin. Hypertens.*, 3:510–513.

85. Morice, A. H., Lowry, R., Brown, M. J., and

Higenbottam, T. (1987): Angiotensin-converting enzyme and the cough reflex. *Lancet*, ii:1116–1118.

86. Morioka, S., Simon, G., and Cohn, J. N. (1988): Cardiac and hormonal effects of enalapril in hypertension. *Clin. Pharmacol. Ther.*, 34:583–589.

87. Muiesan, G., Agabiti-Rosei, E., Buoninconti, R., Cagli, V., Carotti, A., Corea, L., Innocenti, P., Malerba, M., Paciaroni, E., Pirrelli, A., Toso, M., and Botta, G. (1987): Antihypertensive efficacy and tolerability of captopril in the elderly: Comparison with hydrochlorothiazide and placebo in a multicenter, double-blind study. *J. Hypertens.*, 5 (Suppl.5):599–602.

88. Muiesan, G., Alicandri, C. L., Agabiti-Rosei, E., Fariello, R., Beschi, M., Boni, E., Castellano, M., Moniti, E., Muiesan, M. L., Romanelli, G., and Zanielli, A. (1982): Angiotensin-converting enzyme inhibition, catecholamines and hemodynamics in essential hypertension. *Am. J. Cardiol.*, 49:1420–1424.

89. Niarchos, A. P., Pickering, T. G., Morganti, A., and Laragh, J. H. (1982): Plasma catecholamines and cardiovascular responses during converting enzyme inhibition in normotensive and hypertensive man. *Clin. Exp. Hypertens.*, A4:761–789.

90. Nicholls, M. G. (1987): Side-effects and metabolic effects of converting-enzyme inhibitors. *Clin. Exp. Hypertens.*, A:653–664.

91. Nicholls, M. G., Espiner, E. A., Miles, K. D., Zweifler, A. J., and Julius, S. (1981): Evidence against an interaction of angiotensin II with the sympathetic nervous system in man. *Clin. Endocrinol.*, 15:423–430.

92. Nicholls, M. G., and Gilchrist, N. L. (1987): Sulindac and cough induced by converting enzyme inhibitors. *Lancet*, i:872.

93. Nussberger, J., Brunner, D. B., Waeber, B., Biollaz, J., and Brunner, H. R. (1987): Lack of angiotensin II accumulation after converting enzyme blockade by enalapril or lisinopril in man. *Clin. Sci.*, 72:387–389.

94. Nussberger, J., Brunner, D. B., Waeber, B., and Brunner, H. R. (1984): Measurement of low angiotensin concentrations after ethanol and Dowex extraction procedures. *J. Lab. Clin. Med.*, 103:304–312.

95. Nussberger, J., Brunner, D. B., Waeber, B., and Brunner, H. R. (1985): True versus immunoreactive angiotensin II in human plasma. *Hypertension*, 7(Suppl.I):I1–I7.

96. Nussberger, J., Brunner, D. B., Waeber, B., and Brunner, H. R. (1986): Specific measurement of angiotensin metabolites and in vitro generated angiotensin II in plasma. *Hypertension*, 8:476–482.

97. Nussberger, J., Brunner, D. B., Waeber, B., and Brunner, H. R. (1988): In vitro renin inhibition to prevent generation of angiotensins during determination of angiotensin I and II. *Life Sci.*, 42:1683–1688.

98. Nussberger, J., De Gasparo, M., Juillerat, L., Guyenne, T. T., Mooser, V., Waeber, B., and

Brunner, H. R. (1987): Rapid measurement of total and active renin: Plasma concentrations during acute and sustained converting enzyme inhibition with CGS 14,824A. *Clin. Exp. Hypertens.*, A9:1353–1366.

99. Ogihara, T., Maruyama, A., Hata, T., Mikami, H., Nakamaru, M., Naka, T., Ohde, H., and Kumahara, Y. (1981): Hormonal responses to long-term converting enzyme inhibition in hypertensive patients. *Clin. Pharmacol. Ther.*, 30:328–335.

100. Omato, K., Abe, K., Tsunoda, K., Yasujima, M., Chiba, S., Kundo, K., and Yoshinaga, K. (1987): Role of endogenous angiotensin II and prostaglandins in the antihypertensive mechanism of angiotensin converting enzyme inhibitor in hypertension. *Clin. Exp. Hypertens.*, A9:569–574.

101. Ondetti, M. A., Rubin, B., and Cushman, D. W. (1977): Design of specific inhibitors of angiotensin converting enzyme: New class of orally active antihypertensive agents. *Science*, 196:441–444.

102. Ondetti, M. A., Williams, N. J., Sabo, E. F., Pluscec, J., Cleaver, E. R., and Kocy, O. (1971): Angiotensin converting enzyme inhibitors from the venom of Bothrops jararaca: Isolation, elucidation of structure and synthesis. *Biochemistry*, 10:4033–4039.

103. Oparil, S., and Haber, E. (1974): The renin-angiotensin system. *N. Engl. J. Med.*, 291:389–401.

104. Zimmerman, B. G., Sybert, E. G., and Wong, P. C. (1984): Interaction between sympathetic and renin-angiotensin system. *J. Hypertens.*, 2:581–588.

105. Patchett, A. A., Harris, E., Tristram, E. W., Wyvratt, M., Wu, M. T., Taub, D., Peterson, E., Ikeler, T., Broeke, J., Payne, L., Ondeyka, D., Thorsett, E., Greenlee, W., Lohn, N., Maycock, A., Hoffsommer, R., Joshua, R., Ruyle, W., Roghrock, J., Itster, S., Robinson, F. M., Sweet, C. S., Ulm, E. H., Gross, D. M., Vassil, T. C., and Stone, C. A. (1980): A new class of angiotensin-converting enzyme inhibitors. *Nature*, 288:280–283.

106. Pfeffer, M. A., Lamas, G. A., Vaughan, E. D. Jr., Parisi, A. F., and Braunwald, E. (1988): Effect of captopril on progressive ventricular dilatation after arterior myocardial infarction. *N. Engl. J. Med.*, 319:80–86.

107. Pool, J. L., Gennari, J., Goldstein, R., Kochar, M. S., Lewin, A. J., Maxwell, M. H., McChesney, J. A., Mehta, J., Nash, D. T., Nelson, E. B., Rastogi, S., Rofman, B., and Weinberger, M. (1987): Controlled multicenter study of the antihypertensive effects of lisinopril, hydrochlorothiazide, and lisinopril plus hydrochlorothiazide in the treatment of 394 patients with mild to moderate essential hypertension. *J. Cardiovasc. Pharmacol.*, 9(Suppl.1):36–42.

108. Quilley, J., Duchin, K. L., Hudes, E. M., and McGiff, J. C. (1987): The antihypertensive effect of captopril in essential hypertension: Relation-

ship to prostaglandins and the kallikrein-kinin system. *J. Hypertens.*, 5:121–128.

109. Rasmussen, S., Nielson, M. D., and Giese, J. (1981): Captopril combined with thiazide lowers renin substrate concentration: Implications for methodology in renin assays. *Clin. Sci.*, 60:591–593.

110. Redgrave, J., Rabinowe, S., Hollenberg, N. K., and Williams, G. H. (1985): Correction of the abnormal renal blood flow response to angiotensin II by converting enzyme inhibition in essential hypertensives. *J. Clin. Invest.*, 75:1285–1290.

111. Riska, H., Stenius-Aarniala, B., and Sovijärvi, A. R. A. (1986): Comparison of the efficacy of an ACE inhibitor and a calcium channel blocker in hypertensive asthmatics: A preliminary report. *Postgrad. Med. J.*, 62(Suppl.I):76–77.

112. Roberts, D. H., Tsao, Y., McLoughlin, G. A., and Breckenridge, A. M. (1987): Placebo-controlled comparison of captopril, atenolol, labetolol, and pindolol in hypertension complicated by intermittent claudication. *Lancet*, ii:650–653.

113. Rothberg, A. D., and Lorenz, R. (1984): Can captopril cause fetal and neonatal renal failure? *Pediatric Pharmacology*, 4:189–192.

114. Roulston, J. E., McGregor, G. A., and Bind, R. (1980): The measurement of angiotensin-converting enzyme in subjects receiving captopril. *N. Engl. J. Med.*, 303:397.

115. Rush, J. E., and Merrill, D. D. (1987): The safety and tolerability of lisinopril in clinical trials. *J. Cardiovasc. Pharmacol.*, 9(Suppl.3):99–107.

116. Safar, M. E., Bouthier, J. A., Levenson, J., and Simon, A. (1983): Peripheral large arteries and the response to antihypertensive treatment. *Hypertension*, 5 (Suppl.III):63–68.

117. Sala, H., Abad, J., Juanmiguel, L., Plans, C., Ruiz, J., Roig, J., and Moura, J. (1986): Captopril and bronchial reactivity. *Postgrad. Med. J.*, 62(Suppl.1):76–77.

118. Salvetti, A., Abdel-Hag, B., Magagna, A., and Pedrinelli, R. (1987): Indomethacin reduces the antihypertensive action of enalapril. *Clin. Exp. Hypertens.*, A9:559–567.

119. Salvetti, A., Innocenti, P. F., Iardella, M., Pambianco, F., Saba, G. C., Rossetti, M., and Botta, G. (1987): Captopril and nifedipine interactions in the treatment of essential hypertensives: A crossover study. *J. Hypertens.*, 5(Suppl.4):139–142.

120. Sanchez, R. A., Marco, E., Gilbert, H. B., Raffaele, G. P., Brito, M., Gimenez, M., and Moledo, L. I. (1985): Natriuretic effect and changes in renal hemodynamics induced by enalapril in essential hypertension. *Drugs*, 30 (Suppl.I):49–58.

121. Saner, H., and Brunner, H. R. (1988): Antihypertensive Wirksamkeit und Verträglichkeit von Captopril. *Ergebnisse einer Schweizer Feldstudie. Therapei Woche Schweiz*, 2:157–165.

122. Saragoça, M. A., Homsi, E., Ribeiro, A. B., Ferreira-Filho, S. R., and Ramos, O. L. (1983): Hemodynamic mechanism of blood pressure re-

sponse to captopril in human malignant hypertension. *Hypertension*, 5 (Suppl. I):53–58.

123. Sasaki, J., and Arakawa, K. (1986): Effect of captopril on serum lipids, lipoproteins, and apolipoproteins in patients with mild essential hypertension. *Curr. Ther. Res.*, 40:898–902.

124. Sassano, P., Chatellier, G., Billaud, E., Alhenc-Gelas, F., Corvol, P., and Ménard, J. (1987): Treatment of mild to moderate hypertension with or without the converting enzyme inhibitor enalapril: Results of a six-month double-blind trial. *Am. J. Med.*, 83:227–235.

125. Schubiger, G., Flury, G., and Nussberger, J. (1988): Enalapril for pregnancy-induced hypertension: Acute renal failure in a neonate. *Ann. Intern. Med.*, 108:215–216.

126. Simon, G., Morioka, S., Snyder, D. K., and Cohn, J. N. (1983): Increased renal plasma flow in long-term enalapril treatment of hypertension. *Clin. Pharmacol. Ther.*, 34:459–465.

127. Singer, D. R. J., Markandu, N. D., Shore, A. C., and McGregor, G. A. (1987): Captopril and nifedipine in combination for moderate to severe essential hypertension. *Hypertension*, 9:629–633.

128. Staessen, J., Fagard, R., Lijnen, P., Verschueren, L. J., and Amery, A. (1981): The hypotensive effect of propranolol in captopril-treated patients does not involve the plasma renin-angiotensin-aldosterone system. *Clin. Sci.*, 61:441s–444s.

129. Stornello, M., Di Rao, G., Iachello, M., Pisani, R., Scapellato, L., Pedrinelli, R., and Salvetti, A. (1983): Hemodynamic and humoral interactions between captopril and nifedipine. *Hypertension*, 5(Suppl.III):154–156.

130. Strozzi, C., Cocco, G., Portaluppi, F., Padula, A., Urso, L., Alfiero, R., Rizzo, A., and Tasini, M. T. (1985): Ergometric evaluation of the effects of captopril in hypertensive patients with stable angina. *J. Hypertens.*, 3 (Suppl.2):147–148.

131. Sturani, A., Chiarini, C., Degli-Esposito, E., Santoro, A., Zuccala, A., and Zuchelli, P. (1982): Heart rate control in hypertensive patients treated by captopril. *Br. J. Clin. Pharmacol.*, 14:849–855.

132. Swales, J. D., and Heagerty, A. M. (1987): Vascular renin-angiotensin system: The unanswered questions. *J. Hypertens.*, 5 (Suppl.2):1–5.

133. Swartz, S. L., Williams, G. H., Hollenberg, N. K., Levine, L., Dluhy, R. G., and Moore, T. J. (1980): Captopril-induced changes in prostaglandin production. Relationship to vascular responses in normal man. *J. Clin. Invest.*, 65:1257–1264.

134. Taguma, Y., Kitamoto, Y., Futaki, G., Ueda, H., Monma, H., Ishizaki, M., Takanashi, H., Sekino, H., and Sasaki, Y. (1985): Effect of captopril on heavy proteinuria in azotemic diabetics. *N. Engl. J. Med.*, 313:1617–1620.

135. Textor, S. C., Bravo, E. L., Fouad, F. M., and Tarazi, R. C. (1982): Hyperkalemia in azotemic patients during angiotensin converting enzyme

inhibition and aldosterone reduction with captopril. *Am. J. Med.*, 73:719–725.

136. Thind, G. S. (1985): Renal insufficiency during angiotensin-converting enzyme inhibitor therapy in hypertensive patients with no renal artery stenosis. *J. Clin. Hypertens.*, 4:337–343.

137. Tood, P. A., and Heel, R. C. (1986): Enalapril: A review of its pharmacodynamic and pharmacokinetic properties, and therapeutic use in hypertension and congestive heart failure. *Drugs*, 31:198–248.

138. Turini, G. A., Brunner, H. R., Gribic, M., Waeber, B., and Gavras, H. (1979): Improvement of chronic congestive heart failure by oral captopril. *Lancet*, 1:1213–1215.

139. Vander, A. J., and Geelhoed, G. W. (1965): Inhibition of renin secretion by angiotensin II. *Proc. Soc. Exp. Biol. Med.*, 120:399–403.

140. Veterans Administration Cooperative Study Group on Antihypertensive Agents. (1983): Low-dose captopril for the treatment of mild to moderate hypertension. *Hypertension*, 5 (Suppl. 3):139–144.

141. Vinci, J. M., Horowitz, D., Zusman, R. M., Pisano, J. J., Catt, K. J., and Keiser, H. R. (1979): The effect of converting enzyme inhibition with SQ 20,881 on plasma urinary kinins, prostaglandin E and angiotensin II in hypertensive man. *Hypertension*, 1:416–426.

142. Waeber, B., Bornand, E., Vuichard, P., Nussberger, J., and Brunner, H. R. (1987): Enalapril: Ergebnisse einer multizentrischen Studie in der Schweiz unter besonderer Berücksichtigung von älteren Hypertonikern. In: *Enalapril in der Behandlung der Hypertonie,* edited by H. R. Brunner, and K. Lehmann, pp. 69–73. Georg Thieme, Stuttgart.

143. Waeber, B., Brunner, H. R., Brunner, D. B., Curtet, A. L., Turini, G. A., and Gavras, H. (1980): Discrepancy between antihypertensive effect and angiotensin converting enzyme inhibition by captopril. *Hypertension*, 2:236–242.

144. Waeber, B., Gavras, I., Brunner, H. R., Cook, C. A., Characopos, F., and Gavras, H. (1982): Prediction of sustained antihypertensive efficacy of chronic captopril therapy: Relationships to immediate blood pressure response and control plasma renin activity. *Am. Heart J.*, 103:384–390.

145. Waeber, B., Gavras, I., Brunner, H. R., and Gavras, H. (1981): Safety and efficacy of chronic therapy with captopril in hypertensive patients: An update. *J. Cardiovasc. Pharmacol.*, 21:508–516.

146. Weber, M. A. (1988): Safety issues during antihypertensive treatment with angiotensin converting enzyme inhibitors. *Am. J. Med.*, 84 (Suppl.4A):16–23.

147. Weinberger, M. H. (1985): Blood pressure and metabolic responses to hydrochlorothiazide, captopril, and the combination in black and white mild-to-moderate hypertensive patients. *J. Cardiovasc. Pharmacol.*, 7 (Suppl.1):52–55.

148. Wenting, G. J., De Bruyn, J. H. B., Man in't Veld, A. J., Woittiez, A. J. J., Derkx, F. H. M., and Schalekamp, M. A. D. H. (1982): Hemodynamic effects of captopril in essential hypertension, renovascular hypertension and cardiac failure: Correlations with short- and long-term effects on plasma renin. *Am. J. Cardiol.*, 49:1453–1459.

149. Wenting, G. J., Derkx, F. H. M., Tan-Tjiong, L. H., Van Seyen, A. J., Man in't Veld, A. J., and Schalekamp, M. A. D. H. (1987): Risks of angiotensin converting enzyme inhibition in renal artery stenosis. *Kidney Int.*, 31(Suppl. 20):180–183.

150. Williams, G. H., and Hollenberg, N. K. (1977): Accentuated vascular and endocrine response to SQ 20,881 in hypertension. *N. Engl. J. Med.*, 297:184–188.

151. Wing, L. M. H., Chalmers, J. P., West, M. J., Bune, A. J. C., Russel, A. E., Elliot, J. M., and Morris, M. J. (1987): Treatment of hypertension with enalapril and hydrochlorothiazide or enalapril and atenolol: Contrasts in hypotensive interactions. *J. Hypertens.*, 5(Suppl.5):603–606.

152. Zusman, R. M., and Keiser, H. R. (1977): Prostaglandin biosynthesis by rabbit renomedullary interstitial cells in culture: Stimulation by angiotensin II, bradykinin and arginine vasopressin. *J. Clin. Invest.*, 60:215–223.

New Therapeutic Strategies in Hypertension,
edited by Norman M. Kaplan,
Barry M. Brenner, and John H. Laragh.
Raven Press, Ltd., New York © 1989.

Calcium Blockers

Fritz R. Bühler

Department of Research, University Hospital, 4031 Basel, Switzerland

Aging is associated with pathophysiological adaptive changes in cardiovascular regulation including reduced baroreflex sensitivity and beta-adrenoceptor-mediated cardiac and renal responses. Accordingly, owing to such blunted counter-regulation, older patients gain a greater fall in blood pressure for a given peripheral vasodilation, e.g., with a calcium antagonist. Such age-related efficacy may be helped by the calcium antagonists' renal and antialdosterone effects resulting in natriuresis. In open and double-blind treatment trials, calcium antagonists in monotherapy proved more effective in reducing blood pressure to normal in older patients with hypertension and, for the same reasons, to those with a low-plasma-renin activity, or black patients. Pretreatment blood pressure was another independent predictor. Age, renin, and race are factors to be considered when planning antihypertensive treatment strategies with better blood pressure control and better well-being of the patient in mind.

Twenty-five years ago, the calcium antagonist verapamil was shown to lower blood pressure acutely in patients with high blood pressure and renal disease, while no effect was seen in normotensive patients with renal parenchymal disease or normal subjects following the intravenous administration of the drug (43). In the late 1960s and early 1970s the antihypertensive effectiveness of both verapamil (14,41) and nifedipine (5,75) was documented, and a greater fall in blood pressure was found when the pretreatment pressure was higher.

In 1979 one study already detected better antihypertensive efficacy of calcium antagonists in black patients (52) who were known to have a high proportion of low-plasma-renin activity (15). It was only in the late 1970s that long-term administration of calcium antagonists in hypertension was studied (53,55,65). In the last 5 to 7 years convincing evidence for the usefulness of calcium antagonists in long-term antihypertensive therapy has been provided (4,21,40). This coincided with the development of new concepts linking derangements in transmembrane sodium and calcium transport to the pathophysiology of essential hypertension (10,37).

Prognosticators for antihypertensive response to calcium antagonists have been sought for a number of years. The concept of age determining blood pressure response to antihypertensive therapy was introduced in 1975 when decreasing effectiveness of beta blockers was related to older age of the patients (20). This chapter reviews present data for the reasons and evidence that antihypertensive responses to calcium antagonists increase with old age.

Pathophysiological Logic for Antihypertensive Response

Different developmental phases characterize essential hypertension. In an early phase (or with younger age), beta-adrenoceptor-mediated cardiovascular responses, i.e., heart rate (9,22), exercise tachycardia (9), cardiac output as well as plasma renin activity (20), and renin responsiveness (25,33,79), are enhanced; renovascular resistance is practically normal (44).

In a later phase of hypertension or with older age, beta-adrenoceptor-mediated effects tend to be blunted (Fig. 1). Accordingly, exercise-induced tachycardia and heart rate responses to isoproterenol are reduced (6,9,57), plasma-renin activity is normal or low (15,20) and hyperresponsive to sympathetic stimuli (25,60), and peripheral vasodilator responses to beta-adrenoceptor

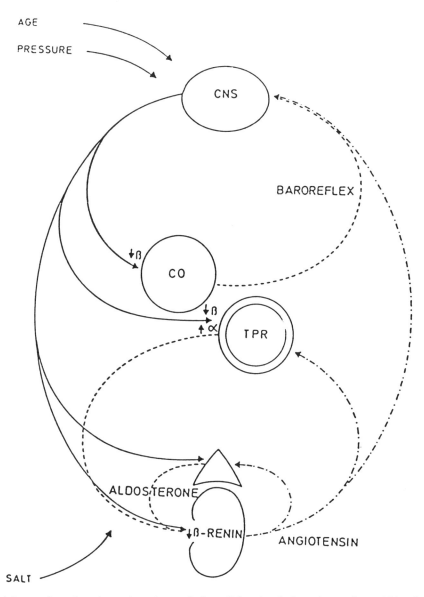

FIG. 1. Adrenergic and angiotensinergic regulation of the circulation. Age, salt, and blood pressure per se contribute to the transition from a predominantly hyper-beta-adrenoceptor-mediated cardiovascular regulation in younger patients to a later maintenance phase (older patients) where beta-effects and renin are blunted and alpha-adrenoceptor-mediated vasoconstriction prevails.

stimulation are diminished (34,90). Similarly, isoproterenol causes a lesser increase in renal blood flow of older patients or patients with low-renin hypertension (7). With blunting of beta-adrenoceptor-mediated functions, alpha-adrenoceptor-mediated vasoconstriction relatively prevails. Hence, the established phase of essential hypertension is characterized by an elevated peripheral vascular resistance to which enhanced postjunctional alpha-1- and alpha-2-adrenoceptor-mediated (2,11) and calcium-influx-dependent (45) vasoconstriction contribute. Enhanced calcium-influx-dependent vasoconstriction may operate to a great extent through postjunctional alpha-1- and alpha-2-adrenoceptors; this will eventually lead to increased intracellular-free calcium concentration in vascular smooth muscle cells. This appears to be reflected by an increased calcium concentration in platelets of patients with essential hypertension and its correlation with the height of blood pressure (32).

Cardiovascular and renal regulatory, as well as counter-regulatory mechanisms, have to be borne in mind when discussing the mode of action and place of calcium antagonists in treating patients with different forms of hypertension.

Mode of Action of Calcium Antagonists

Increased systemic vascular resistance in essential hypertension depends on increased calcium influx (45,83). Calcium antagonists lower cytosolic-free calcium concentrations mainly through a reduction of transmembranous calcium-influx and are potent arteriolar vasodilators. The maximal vasodilator responses of the forearm circulation to verapamil were inversely related to the patients' plasma-renin activity and angiotensin II concentration (45). This suggests greater calcium influx-dependent vasoconstriction when the renin-angiotensin pressor system is suppressed.

Acute and chronic antihypertensive drug effects differ with respect to the underlying pathophysiological mechanisms. When nifedipine was given sublingually to patients with essential hypertension there was an acute reduction of systolic and diastolic blood pressure (46). This decrease was associated with increases in heart rate, cardiac index, plasma norepinephrine concentrations and plasma-renin activity, while calculated systemic vascular resistance decreased. These findings suggest reflexly mediated sympathoneural activation due to arterial vasodilation. For a given stimulus, sympathetic stimulation will be greater in subjects with normally functioning baroreflexes.

The sensitivity of the arterial baroreflexes is blunted with high blood pressure (13) or with older age (39); each effect seems to be independent of the other (81). Accordingly, elderly hypertensive patients will have less counterregulatory reflex activation and sympathetically mediated vasoconstriction than younger and high-renin patients and the latter more than normotensive controls. Indirect evidence is derived from the observation that normotensive subjects have either no, or only a small, decrease of pressure after administration of calcium antagonists (45,64). More direct evidence comes from a study where arterial baroreflex sensitivity was related to the acute fall in blood pressure after nifedipine given sublingually (48). Baroreflex sensitivity was inversely related to age, and subjects with low sensitivities had the greatest acute falls in blood pressure. Subjects with the greatest increase in plasma-norepinephrine levels as a marker of changes of sympathetic activity had the greatest increase in cardiac output, a hemodynamic response pattern which would tend to counteract the decrease of pressure the most.

Other mechanisms probably also contribute to the antihypertensive effects of calcium antagonists but their quantitative importance remains to be precisely defined. Vasoconstriction due to adrenergic stimulation is markedly reduced during therapy, but it has been debated whether this inhibition applies to both alpha-1- and alpha-2-adrenoceptor-mediated vasoconstriction (26,29,91). The latter system is effectively blocked by calcium antagonists (86). Some interference with alpha-1-adrenoceptor-mediated vasoconstriction also seems likely since nifedipine reduced the blood pressure increases produced by the alpha-1-adrenoceptor agonist phenylephrine in patients with hypertension (87). Calcium antagonists reduce angiotensin's stimulatory effect on aldosterone biosynthesis and secretion (66), an effect which may be particularly pertinent when aldosterone is inappropriately high, e.g., low-renin-essential hypertension (23).

Blunted Cardiovascular Counter-Regulation with Old Age

The clinical investigation of calcium antagonists in hypertension has taught us a principle lesson on responses to antihypertensive drugs. On one hand, calcium antagonists eliminate excess calcium influx-dependent vasoconstriction and thereby tend to normalize elevated peripheral vascular resistance. On the other hand, peripheral vasodilation is countered by baroreflex-induced sympathetic nervous system activation that results in alpha-1- and alpha-2-adrenoceptor- and angiotensin-mediated vasoconstriction, as well as cardiac and renal stimulation. The more blunted the baroreflex, the greater the fall in blood pressure in beta-adrenoceptor and renin compensatory baroflex (Fig. 1). At the level of the vascular smooth muscle cell, calcium antagonists block slow channel calcium entry but other mechanisms, e.g., alpha-1-adrenoceptor- or angiotensin receptor-activated and inositol trisphosphate-mediated superficial sarcoplasmic calcium release may sustain vascular contraction (89). This logic helps to understand the efficacious

combination of a calcium entry blocker with a (renin suppression) beta blocker or angiotensin-converting enzyme inhibitor.

Unlike other vasodilating agents, calcium antagonists do not cause sodium volume retention, and no changes in blood volume have been observed by us (21,46) and by other investigators with nifedipine and verapamil (8,16). Renal vascular-dilating effects of calcium antagonists have been known since the early days (43,50) but their natriuretic effect of 6 to 10 g salt in the first few days of treatment only recently have been appreciated (38,54,61,85). Their common and perhaps prominent renal effect is to reduce elevated preglomerular resistance, and to maintain or increase glomerular filtration rate (58,59,62). It is conceivable that changes occurring in the aging kidney as well as the slightly elevated aldosterone with older age contribute significantly to the calcium antagonist action.

Age as an Indicator of Antihypertensive Response

The above (renal-) pathophysiological view of essential hypertension and the mechanisms of action have been tested in several pharmacotherapeutic studies. In the early phase of high blood pressure development, in younger patients, or in those with a high or normal renin ("normal" being too high for the elevated pressure), beta blockers and converting enzyme inhibitors were found to be more effective than in older or low-renin patients (19). Approximately 80% of the patients under the age of 40 years normalize their diastolic blood pressure to below 95 mm Hg with a beta blocker (18,20) (Fig. 2) or converting enzyme inhibitor (56). The response rates in the age group 40 to 60 years are about 50% and an age-relationship with beta blocker monotherapy was found in this subgroup as well (20). Over the age of 60 years, beta blockers and converting enzyme inhibitors

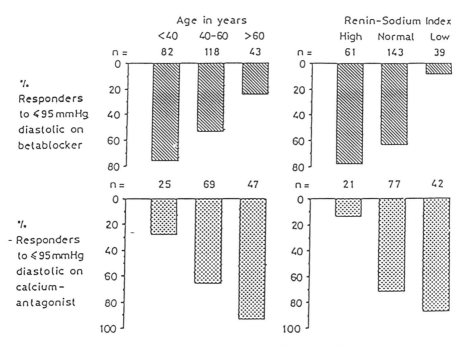

FIG. 2. Blood pressure normalization (≤ 95 mm Hg diastolic) to beta blockers (**upper panel**) occurs more often in younger (**left**) and high-renin (**right**) patients than with calcium antagonists (**lower panel**); and more often with calcium antagonists in older patients and those patients with lower plasma-renin activity.

normalize blood pressure in approximately 20% of the patients, and a combination therapy frequently is required for pressure control. A similar picture emerges for the renin subgroups with a response rate to beta blockers of about 80% in high, 50% in normal, and 20% in low renin essential hypertension. These response rates are comparable to those found with converting enzyme inhibitors (74). Although such an age- and renin-related response pattern has not been found in every beta blocker or converting enzyme inhibitor study, there is a substantial body of supportive information from investigators around the world (12,17,35,77).

Diuretic drugs were shown to be more effective than beta blockers in older patients (35) and low-renin patients (28,77,92). Blood pressure normalization with diuretics has been interpreted as normalization of

pretreatment volume-overfilling (28,92). In addition to some elevation of cardiopulmonary volume (49,72) there are two other important cardiovascular characteristics in old and low-renin patients: enhanced calcium influx-dependent vasoconstriction and blunted cardiovascular reflex regulation.

Calcium antagonists were found to have a response pattern similar to that seen with diuretics (21). Calcium antagonists normalize blood pressure in approximately 80% of patients older than 60 years or those with low-renin (Fig. 2); in 50% of patients between 40 to 60 years, or those with normal renin, and in approximately 20% of patients under 40 years or those with high-renin (21,31,47,71). Some of the more recent studies are in keeping with this view (Table 1) (3,27,30,36,51,63,69,70,71,76,78,80,82, 84,88,94,95). By using calcium antagonists

Table 1. *Greater antihypertensive effectiveness of calcium antagonists in older, low-renin, and black patients*

		Older	Low-renin	Black
Verapamil	Leary (52)			+
	Bühler (21)	+	+	
	Müller (71)	+		
Nifedipine	Erne (31)	+	+	
	Kiowski/Fadayomi (47)	+	+	+
	Landmark (51)	+		
	Nicholson (76)		+	
	Ribstein (82)	+		
	Ueda (88)	+		
Nitrendipine	Müller (71)	+	+	
	Moser (70)			+
	Dustan (30)		+	+
	Pedrinelli (78)	+	+	
	Fritschka (36)	X		
	Zachariah (95)		+	
	Weinberger (94)	+		
	M'Buyamba-Kabangu (63)	+	+	+
Nicardipine	Cluzel (27)	+		
Diltiazem	Moser (69)			+
	Amodeo (3)		+	
	Pool (80)	+		
	Schwartz (84)	+		

in a slow-release formulation (73) or with the newer longer-acting dihydropyridine types, e.g., nitrendipine (71) or amlodipine (24), antihypertensive care may be as simple as that with diuretic drugs.

Black hypertensive patients have a great prevalence of low renin, and diuretics are considered drugs of first choice (42,93). Beta blockers (67) and converting enzyme inhibitors (68) were less effective in black than in white patients. As a new alternative to diuretics, calcium antagonists have proven most efficacious in black hypertensives (Table 1) and in a recent double-blind, randomized comparison with atenolol a significant relationship between the patient's age and the antihypertensive response was found (63).

Independent Prediction of Age in a Multiple Regression Analysis

In another effort to evaluate the impact of possible indicators, placebo-controlled, prospective but single-blind studies in 138 patients with essential hypertension were treated with a calcium antagonist (47) and were subjected to a multiple linear regression analysis (Table 2).

Age, pretreatment blood pressure, and plasma-renin activity emerged as independent variables, and the fall of mean blood pressure during long-term therapy showed a multiple linear correlation ($r = 0.49$, $p < 0.001$). All three variables had independent

Table 2. *Linear correlations between factors influencing the antihypertensive response to calcium antagonists*

	Age	MBP	PRA	ΔMBP
Age	1.00	–	–	–
MBP	0.13 NS	1.00	–	–
PRA	-0.44^b	-0.25^a	100	–
ΔMBP	-0.36^b	-0.55^b	0.49^b	1.00

n, 138 (verapamil = 43, nifedipine = 66, nitrendipine = 29); MBP, pretreatment mean blood pressure; PRA, pretreatment plasma renin activity; ΔMBP, change of mean blood pressure during therapy; NS, not significant.
[a] $p < 0.01$, [b] $p < 0.001$.

and significant effects on antihypertensive response to calcium antagonists, with pretreatment blood pressure exhibiting the strongest influence ($F = 62.7$, $p < 0.1$) and plasma-renin activity the weakest influence ($F = 18.2$, $p < 0.05$). When considering a diastolic target pressure of <95 mm Hg during therapy, 94% of patients older than 60 years normalized their blood pressure, compared with 50% of middle-aged patients and 28% of younger patients ($p < 0.01$, X^2).

Why is it that an age, renin, or race-response relationship is not found in all the trials? There seem to be some common problems with drug testing relative to possible predictors. The impacts of these predictors, although highly significant, are not overwhelmingly strong. Analyses of these predictors have helped in the degree of treatment strategies but they are not mandatory criteria for drug selection in an individual patient. Correlations are usually found only with relatively sizeable study populations and in studies with a high degree of standardization. Daytime variation, quality of blood pressure recording, renin assay variability, and dose adjustment may be of importance here. Recognition of drug kinetics may yet be another age-related factor; a decrease in clearance of verapamil (1) and diltiazem (84) in elderly hypertensives has been shown. For these reasons, and because of the background noise in data collection, multicenter trials often fail to show these relationships in spite of a large study population. What is obviously needed are more double-blind trials which take into account the aforementioned problems and serve as proof for those not yet convinced by logic and available evidence.

REFERENCES

1. Abermethy, D. R., Schwartz, J. B., Todd, E. L., Luchi, R., and Snow, E. (1986): Verapamil pharmacodynamics and disposition in young and elderly hypertensive patients. *Ann. Intern. Med.,* 105:329–336.
2. Amann, F. W., Bolli, P., Kiowski, W., and Bühler, F. R. (1981): Enhanced alpha-adrenoceptor-mediated vasoconstriction in essential hypertension. *Hypertension,* 3(Suppl. I):119–123.
3. Amodeo, C., Kobrin, I., Ventura, H. O., Messerli, F. H., and Fröhlich, E. D. (1986): Immediate and short-term hemodynamic effects of diltiazem in patients with hypertension. *Circulation,* 73:108–113.
4. Anavekar, S. N., Christophidis, N., Louis, W. J., Doyle, A. E. (1981): Verapamil in the treatment of hypertension. *J. Cardiovasc. Pharmacol.,* 3:287–291.
5. Aoki, K., Kondo, S., and Mochizuki, A. (1978): Antihypertensive effects of cardiovascular Ca^{2+}-antagonists in hypertensive patients in the absence and presence of beta-adrenergic blockade. *Am. Heart. J.,* 96:218–227.
6. Astrand, P. O., and Rodahl, K. (1970): *Textbook of Work Physiology.* McGraw Hill, New York.
7. Bauer, J. H., Brooks, C. S., and Burch, R. N. (1982): Renal function and hemodynamic studies in low and normal renin hypertension. *Arch. Int. Med.,* 142:1317–1325.
8. Bayley, S., Dobbs, R. J., and Robinson, B. F. (1982): Nifedipine in the treatment of hypertension: Report of a double blind controlled trial. *Br. J. Clin. Pharmacol.,* 14:509–514.
9. Bertel, O., Bühler, F. R., Kiowski, W., and Lütold, B. E. (1980): Decreased beta-adrenoreceptor responsiveness as related to age, blood pressure and plasma catecholamines in patients with essential hypertension. *Hypertens.,* 2:130–138.
10. Blaustein, M. P. (1977): Sodium ions, calcium ions, blood pressure regulation and hypertension: A reassessment and a hypothesis. *Am. J. Physiol.,* 232:C165–C173.
11. Bolli, P., Erne, P., Ji, B. H., Block, L. H., Kiowski, W., and Bühler, F. R. (1983): Adrenaline induces vasoconstriction through postjunctional alpha-2-adrenoceptors and this response is enhanced in patients with essential hypertension. *J. Hypertens.,* 1:(Suppl. 2)257–259.
12. Breckenridge, A. (1985): MRC trial of mild hypertension: Principal results. *Br. Med. J.,* 291:89–90.
13. Bristow, J. D., Honour, A. J., Pickering, G. W., Sleight, P., and Peti, R. (1969): Diminished baroreflex sensitivity in high blood pressure. *Circulation,* 39:48–55.
14. Brittinger, W. C., Schwarzbeck, A., Wittenmeier, K. W., Twittenhoff, W. D., Stegaru, B., Huber, W., Ewald, R. W., von Henning, G. E., Fabricius, M., and Stauch, M. (1970): Klinisch-experimentelle Untersuchungen über die blutdrucksenkende Wirkung von Verapamil. *Deutsche Med. Wschr.,* 37:1871–1837.
15. Brunner, H. R., Sealey, J. E., and Laragh, J. H. (1973): Renin subgroups in essential hypertension. *Circ. Res.,* 32:(Suppl. I)99–104.
16. Bruun, N. E., Ibsen, H., Nielsen, F., Nielsen, M. D., Moelbak, A. G., and Hartling, O. J. (1986): Lack of effect of nifendipine on counterregulatory mechanisms in essential hypertension. *Hypertension,* 8:655–661.

17. Bühler, F. R. (1981): Antihypertensive action of beta-blockers. In: *Frontiers in Hypertension Research,* edited by Laragh, J. H., Bühler, F. R., and Seldin, D. W., pp. 423–436. Springer-Verlag, New York.

18. Bühler, F. R., Bertel, O., and Lütold, B. E. (1978): Simplified and age-stratified antihypertensive therapy based on betablockers. *Cardiovasc. Med.,* 3:135–148.

19. Bühler, F. R., Bolli, P., Kiowski, W., Erne, P., Hulthén, U. L., and Block, L. H. (1984): Renin profiling to select antihypertensive baseline drugs. *Am. J. Med.,* 20:36–42.

20. Bühler, F. R., Burkart, F., Lütold, B. E., Küng, M., Marbet, G., and Pfisterer, M. (1975): Antihypertensive betablocking action as related to renin and age: A pharmacological tool to identify pathogenic mechanisms in essential hypertension. *Am. J. Cardiol.,* 36:653–669.

21. Bühler, F. R., Hulthén, U. L., Kiowski, W., and Bolli, P. (1982): Greater antihypertensive efficacy of the calcium channel inhibitor verapamil in older and low renin patients. *Clin. Sci.,* 63:439–442.

22. Bühler, F. R., Kiowski, W., van Brummelen, P., Amann, F. W., Bertel, O., Landmann, R., Lütold, B. E., and Bolli, P. (1980): Plasma adrenoceptor-mediated and cardiac, renal and peripheral vascular adrenoceptor-mediated responses in different age groups of normal and hypertensive subjects. *Clin. Exp. Hypertens.,* 2:409–426.

23. Bühler, F. R., Laragh, J. H., Sealey, J. E., and Brunner, H. R. (1973): Plasma aldosterone-renin interrelationships in various forms of essential hypertension: Studies using a rapid assay of plasma aldosterone. *Am. J. Cardiol.,* 32:554–561.

24. Burger, R. A., Carter, D. G., Gardiner, D. G., and Higgins, A. J. (1985): Amlodipine: A new dihydropyridine calcium channel blocker with slow onset and long duration of action. *Br. J. Pharmacol.,* 85:281P.

25. Burkart, F., Bühler, F. R., Pfisterer, M., Lütold, B. E., and Küng, M. (1976): Hemodynamic responses to exercise and acute betablockade in renin subtypes of essential hypertension. *Clin. Sci.,* 51.

26. Cavero, I., Shepperson, N. B., Lefevre-Borg, F., and Langer, S. Z. (1983): Differential inhibition of vascular smooth muscle responses to alpha-1 and alpha-2-adrenoceptor agonists by diltiazem and verapamil. *Circ. Res.,* 52:169–176.

27. Cluzel, F. A., Muller, F. B., Bolli, P., Erne, P., Block, L. H., Kiowski, W., and Buhler, F. R. (1984): Antihypertensive therapy with the long-acting calcium antagonist nitrendipine. *Pharmacology,* 6:S1073–S1076.

28. Crane, M. G., Harris, J. J., and Johus, V. J. (1972): Hyporeninemic hypertension. *J Cardiovasc. Pharmacol.,* 52:457–466.

29. De Mey, J., and Vanhoutte, P. (1981): Uneven distribution of postjunctional alpha-1 and alpha-2-like adrenoceptors in canine arterial and venous smooth muscle. *Circ. Res.,* 48:875–884.

30. Dustan, H. P. (1987): Nitrendipine in Black U.S.

patients. *J. Cardiovasc. Pharmacol.,* 9:(Suppl. 4)267–271.

31. Erne, P., Bolli, P., Bertel, O., Hulthén, U. L., Kiowski, W., Müller, F., and Bühler, F. R. (1983): Factors influencing the hypotensive effects of calcium antagonists. *Hypertension,* 5:(Suppl. II)97–102.

32. Erne, P., Bolli, P., Bürgisser, E., and Bühler, F. R. (1984): Correlation of platelet calcium with blood pressure: Effect of antihypertensive therapy. *N. Engl. J. Med.,* 310:1084–1088.

33. Esler, M., Julius, S., Sweifler, A., Randall, O., Harburg, E., Gardiner, H., and de Quattro, V. (1977): Mild high renin essential hypertension: A neurogenic human hypertension? *N. Engl. J. Med.,* 296:405–411.

34. Fleisch, J. H. (1980): Age-related changes in the sensitivity of blood vessels to drugs. *Pharmacol. Therap.,* 8:477–487.

35. Fries, E. D. (1988): Age and antihypertensive drugs (hydrochlorothiazide, bendroflumethiazide, nadolol and captopril). *Am. J. Cardiol.,* 61:117–121.

36. Fritschka, E. (1984): Crossover comparison of nitrendipine with propranolol in patients with essential hypertension. *J. Cardiolvasc. Pharmacol.,* 6:(Suppl. 7)1100–1108.

37. Garay, R. P., and Meyer, P. H. (1979): A new test showing abnormal net Na^+ and K^+ fluxes in erythrocytes of essential hypertensive patients. *Lancet,* 17:349–353.

38. Garthoff, B., Kazda, S., Knoor, A., and Thomas, G. (1982): Factors involved in the antihypertensive action of calcium antagonists. *Hypertension,* 225:263–270.

39. Gribbin, B., Pickering, T. G., Sleight, P., and Peti, R. (1971): Effect of age and high blood pressure on baroreflex sensitivity in man. *Circ. Res.,* 29:424–431.

40. Guazzi, M. D., Fiorentini, C., Olivari, M. T., Bartorelli, A., Necchi, G., and Polese, A. (1980): Short- and long-term efficacy of a calcium antagonist agent (Nifedipine) combined with methyldopa in the treatment of severe hypertension. *Circulation,* 61:913–919.

41. Hagino, D. (1968): Application of ipoveratril in the pharmacotherapy of hypertension. *Jpn. J. Clin. Exper. Med.,* 45:208–242.

42. Hall, W. D. (1985): Pharmacologic therapy of hypertension in blacks. In: *Epidemiology, pathophysiology and treatment,* edited by Hall, W. D., Saunders, E., and Shulman, N. B. Year Book Medical Publishers, Chicago.

43. Heidland, A., Klütsch, K., and Oebeck, A. (1962): Myogenbedingte Vasodilatation bei Nierenischämie. *Münch. Med. Wsch.,* 35:1636.

44. Hollenberg, N. K., Borucki, L. J., and Adams, D. F. (1978): The renal vasculature in early essential hypertension: Evidence for a pathogenic role. *Medicine,* 37:167–178.

45. Hulthén, U. L., Bolli, P., Amann, F. W., Kiowski, W., and Bühler, F. R. (1982): Enhanced vasodilatation in essential hypertension by cal-

cium channel blockade with verapamil. *Hypertension,* 4:(Suppl. II)26–31.

46. Kiowski, W., Bertel, O., Erne, P., Hulthén, U. L., Bolli, P., Ritz, R., and Bühler, F. R. (1983): Haemodynamic and reflex mechanisms of acute and chronic antihypertensive therapy with the calcium channel blocker nifedipine. *Hypertension,* 5:(Suppl. 1)170–174.

47. Kiowski, W., Bühler, F. R., Fadayomi, M. O., Erne, P., Müller, F. B., Hulthén, U. L., and Bolli, P. (1985): Age, race, blood pressure and renin: Predictors for antihypertensive treatment with calcium antagonists. *Am. J. Cardiol.,* 56:81H–85H.

48. Kiowski, W., Erne, P., Bertel, O., Bolli, P., and Bühler, F. R. (1986): Acute and chronic sympathetic reflex activation and antihypertensive response to nifedipine. *J. Am. Coll. Cardiol.,* 7:344–348.

49. Kiowski, W., and Julius, S. (1978): Renin response to stimulation of cardiopulmonary mechanoreceptors in man. *J. Clin. Invest.,* 62:656–663.

50. Kluetsch, K., Schmidt, P., and Grosswendt, J. (1972): Der Einfluss von Bay a 1040 auf die Nierenbunktion des Hypertonikers. *Arzneim. Forsch.* 22:377–380.

51. Landmark, K. (1985): Antihypertensive and metabolic effects of long-term therapy with nifedipine slow-release tablets. *J. Cardiovasc. Pharmacol.,* 7:12–17.

52. Leary, W. P., Phil, D., and Asmal, A. C. (1979): Treatment of hypertension with verapamil. *Curr. Ther. Res.,* 25:747–752.

53. Lederballe-Pederson, O., Mikkelsen, E., Christensen, N. J., Kornerup, H. J., and Pedersen, E. B. (1979): Effect of nifedipine on plasma renin, aldosterone and catecholamines in arterial hypertension. *Eur. J. Clin. Pharmacol.,* 15:235–240.

54. Leonetti, G., Sala, C., Bianchini, C., Terzoli, L., and Zanchetti, A. (1980): Antihypertensive and renal effects of orally administered verapamil. *Eur. J. Clin. Pharmacol.,* 18:375–382.

55. Lewis, G. R. J., Morley, K. D., Lewis, B. M., and Bones, P. J. (1978): The treatment of hypertension with verapamil. *N. Zealand. Med. J.,* 84:351–354.

56. Lijnen, P., M'Buyamba, J. R., Fagard, R., Staessen, J., and Amergy, A. (1983): Age-related hypotensive response to captopril in hypertensive patients. *Meth. and Find. Exp. Clin. Pharmacol.,* 5(9):655–660.

57. London, G. M., Safar, M. E., Weiss, Y. A., and Milliez, P. L. (1976): Isoproterenol sensitivity and total body clearance of propranolol in hypertensive patients. *J. Clin. Pharmacol.,* 16:174–178.

58. Loutzenhiser, R., Epstein, M., Horton, C., and Sonke, P. (1984): Reversal by the calcium antagonist nisoldipine of norepinephrine-induced reduction of GFR: Evidence for preferential antagonism of preglomerular vasoconstriction. *J. Pharmacol. Exp. Ther.,* 232:382–387.

59. Loutzenhiser, R., Horton, C., and Epsetin, M. (1985): Effects of diltiazem and manganese renal hemodynamics: Studies in the isolated perfused rat kidney. *Nephron,* 39:382–388.

60. Lowder, S. C., Hamet, P., and Liddle, G. W. (1976): Contrasting effects of hypoglycemia on plasma renin activity and cyclic adenosine 3',5'-mono-phosphate (cyclic AMP) in low renin and normal renin essential hypertension. *Circ. Res.,* 38:105–109.

61. Luft, F. C., Aronoff, G., Sloan, R., Fineberg, N., and Weinberger, M. (1985): Calcium channel blockade with nitrendipine. *Hypertension,* 7:438–443.

62. Marre, M., Misumi, J., Raensch, K. D., Corvol, P., and Ménard, J. (1982): Diuretic and natriuretic effects of nifedipine on isolated perfused rat kidneys. *J. Pharmacol. Exp. Ther.,* 223:263–267.

63. M'Buyamba-Kabangu, J. R., Lepira, B., Lijnen, P., Tshiani, K., Fagard, R., and Amery, A. (1988): Intracellular sodium and the response to nitrendipine and acebutolol in African blacks. *Hypertension,* 11:100–105.

64. McGregor, G. A., Rotellar, C., Markander, N. D., and Sagnella, G. A. (1982): Contrasting effects of nifedipine, captopril and propranolol in normotensive and hypertensive subjects. *J. Cardiovasc. Pharmacol.,* 4:(Suppl. 3)358–361.

65. Midtbø, K., and Hals, O. (1980): Verapamil in the treatment of hypertension. *Curr. Ther. Res.,* 27:830–835.

66. Millar, J. A., McLean, K., and Reid, J. L. (1981): Calcium antagonists decrease adrenal and vascular responsiveness to angiotensin II in normal man. *Clin. Sci.,* 61:65s–69s.

67. Moser, M., and Cunn, J. (1981): Comparative effects of pindolol and hydrochlorothiazide in black hypertensive patients. *Angiology,* 32:561.

68. Moser, M., and Cunn, J. (1982): Responses to captopril and hydrochlorothiazide in black patients with hypertension. *Clin. Pharmacol. Ther.,* 32:307.

69. Moser, M., Cunn, J., and Materson, B. J. (1985): Comparative effects of diltiazem and hydrochlorothiazide in Blacks with systemic hypertension. *Am. J. Cardiol.,* 56:101H–104H.

70. Moser, M., Cunn, J., Nash, D. T., Burris, J. F., Winer, N., Simon, G., and Vlachakis, N. D. (1984): Nitrendipine in the treatment of mild to moderate hypertension. *J. Cardiovasc. Pharmacol.,* 6:(Suppl. 7)S1085–S1089.

71. Müller, F. B., Bolli, P., Erne, P., Block, L. H., Kiowski, W., and Bühler, F. R. (1984): Antihypertensive therapy with the long-acting calcium antagonist nitrendipine. *J. Cardiovasc. Pharmacol.,* 6:(Suppl. 7)1073–1076.

72. Müller, F. B., Bolli, P., Kiowski, W., Erne, P., Resink, T. J., Raine, A. E. G., and Bühler, F. R. (1986): Atrial natriuretic peptide is elevated in low renin essential hypertension. *J. Hypertens.,* 4:(Suppl. 6)S489–S491.

73. Müller, F. B., Ha, H. R., Hotz, H., Schmidlin, O., Follath, F., and Bühler, F. R. (1986): Once a day verapamil in essential hypertension. *Br. J. Clin. Pharmacol.* (in press).

74. Müller, F. B., Sealey, J. E., Case, D. B., Atlas, S. A., Pickering, T. G., Pecker, M., Preibisz, J. J., and Laragh, J. H. (1986): The captopril-test for identifying renovascular disease in hypertensive patients. *Am. J. Med.*, 80:633–644.

75. Murakami, M., Murakami, E., Takekoshi, N., Tsuchiya, M., Kin, T., Onoe, T., Takeuchi, N., Funatsu, T., Hars, S., Ishise, S., Mifune, J., and Maede, M. (1972): Antihypertensive effect of 4-(2′-Nitrophenyl)-2,6-dimethyl, 4-dihydropyridine-3,5-dicarbonic acid dimethylester (Nifedipine, Bay-a 1040), a new coronary dilator. *Jpn. Heart. J.*, 13:128–133.

76. Nicholson, J. P., Resnick, L. M., and Laragh, J. H. (1987): The antihypertensive effect of verapamil at extremes of sodium intake. *Ann. Int. Med.*, 107:329–334.

77. Niulla, E., Cusi, D., Colombo, R., Alberghini, E., and Bianchi, G. (1988): Which drugs work and which don't work in the same patients? A cross over study. *Abstract*, Third Annual Meeting of the American Society of Hypertension, New York.

78. Pedrinelli, R., Fonad, F. M., Tarazi, R. C., Bravo, E. L., and Textor, S. C. (1986): Nitrendipine, a calcium-entry blocker: Renal and humoral effects in human arterial hypertension. *Arch. Intern. Med.*, 146:62–65.

79. Perini, C., Müller, F. B., Rauchfleisch, U., Battegay, R., and Bühler, F. R. (1986): Hyperadrenergic borderline hypertension is characterized by suppressed aggression. *J. Cardiovasc. Pharmacol.*, 8:(Suppl. 5)S53–S56.

80. Pool, P. E., Massie, B. M., and Venkararaman, K. (1986): Diltiazem as monotherapy for systemic hypertension: A multicenter, randomized, placebo-controlled trial. *Am. J. Cardiol.*, 57:212–217.

81. Randall, O. S., Esler, M., Culp, B., Julius, S., and Zweifler, A. (1978): Determinants of baroreflex sensitivity in man. *J. Lab. Clin. Med.*, 91:514–519.

82. Ribstein, J., de Treglode, D., and Mimran, A. (1985): Acute effect of nifedipine on arterial pressure in healthy subjects and hypertensives. *Arch. Mal. Coeur*, 78:29–32.

83. Robinson, B. F., Dobbs, B. J., and Bayley, S. (1982): Response of forearm resistance vessels to verapamil and sodium nitroprusside in normotensive and hypertensive men: Evidence for a functional abnormality of vascular smooth muscle in primary hypertension. *Clin. Sci.*, 63:33–37.

84. Schwartz, J. B., and Abermethy, D. R. (1987): Responses to intravenous and oral diltiazem in elderly and younger patients with systemic hypertension. *Am. J. Cardiol.*, 59:1111–1117.

85. Thananoparvan, C., Golub, M. S., Eggena, P.,

Barrett, J. D., and Sambhi, M. P. (1985): Renal effects of nitrendipine monotherapy in essential hypertension. *J. Cardiovasc. Pharmacol.*, 6:(Suppl. 7)S1040–1044.

86. Timmermans, P. B. M. W. M., Mathy, M. J., Thoolen, M. J. M. C., DeJonge, A., Wilffert, B., and van Zwieten, P. A. (1984): Invariable susceptibility to blockade by nifedipine of vasoconstriction to various alpha-2 adrenoceptor agonists in pithed rats. *J. Pharm. Pharmacol.*, 36:772–775.

87. Timmermans, P. B. M. W. M., Mathy, M. J., Wilffert, B., et al. (1983): Differential effect of calcium entry blockers on alpha-1-adrenoceptor-mediated vasoconstriction in vivo. *Naunyn-Schmiedeberg's Arch. Pharmacol.*, 324:239–245.

88. Ueda, K. (1986): The efficacy and safety of long-term antihypertensive therapy with nifedipine. *Jpn. Heart J.*, 27:55–70.

89. van Breemen, C., and Bühler, F. R. (1988): Vascular smooth muscle superficial calcium barrier and its role in antihypertensive drug therapy. *J. Cardiovasc. Pharmacol.*, (in press).

90. van Brummelen, P., Bühler, F. R., Kiowski, W., and Amann, F. W. (1981): Age-related decrease in cardiac and peripheral vascular responsiveness to isoproterenol. *Clin. Sci.*, 60:571–577.

91. Van Meel, K. A., DeJonge, A., Kalkmann, H. O., Wilffert, B., Timmermans, P. B. M. W. M., and van Zwieten, P. A. (1981): Vascular smooth muscle contraction initiated by postsynaptic-adrenoceptor activation is induced by an influx of extracellular calcium. *Eur. J. Pharmacol.*, 69:205–208.

92. Vaughan, E. D. Jr, Laragh, J. H., Gavras, I., Bühler, F. R., Gavras, H., and Brunner, H. R. (1973): The volume factor in low and normal renin essential hypertsion: Its treatment with either spironolactone or chlorthalidone. *Am. J. Cardiol.*, 32:523–532.

93. Veterans Administration Cooperative Study Group on Antihypertensive Agents (1982): Comparison of propranolol and hydrochlorothiazide for the initial treatment of hypertension: I. Results of short-term titration with emphasis on racial differences in response. II. Results of long-term therapy. *JAMA*, 248:1996–2011.

94. Weinberger, M. H. (1987): The role of age, race and plasma renin activity in influencing the blood pressure response to nitrendipine or hydrochlorothiazide. *J. Cardiovasc. Pharmacol.*, 9:(Suppl. 4)272–275.

95. Zachariah, P. K., Schwartz, G. L., Ritter, S. G., and Strong, C. G. (1986): Plasma predictors of calcium channel blocker efficacy in hypertension. *J. Cardiovasc. Pharmacol.*, (in press).

New Therapeutic Strategies in Hypertension,
edited by Norman M. Kaplan,
Barry M. Brenner, and John H. Laragh.
Raven Press, Ltd., New York © 1989.

New Antihypertensive Drugs

D. G. Taylor and H. R. Kaplan

Department of Pharmacology, Parke-Davis Research Division, Warner-Lambert Company, Ann Arbor, Michigan 48105

Several reviews from this and other institutions have focused on cataloging new antihypertensive drugs from the worldwide literature (43,44,70). These agents have been categorized according to their proposed sites and mechanisms of action. It is not the intent of the authors to systematically update this list even though many, and eventually most, of these new compounds might prove unfit for further development because of adverse side effects, toxicity, undesirable pharmaceutical or pharmacokinetic properties, lack of clinical efficacy, or, perhaps, for commercial reasons. The focus of this chapter is on new antihypertensive drugs that are prototypes of future drugs or drugs at very early stages of development not dealt with in other chapters in this volume. These new agents have a high therapeutic potential and collectively represent promising new targets for selective pharmacologic intervention for the prevention and treatment of hypertension.

RENIN-ANGIOTENSIN SYSTEM

Renin Inhibitors

With the success of the angiotensin converting enzyme (ACE) inhibitors in hypertension (82) and heart failure (22), efforts have focused on inhibition of the renin-angiotensin system at other sites in the cascade, namely renin. For a number of reasons, renin is considered an attractive therapeutic target: 1) renin is the rate limiting step in angiotension II synthesis; 2) angiotensinogen is the only substrate for renin, thus, unlike ACE inhibitors, bradykinin should not be elevated; 3) molecular modeling information is available for renin; and 4) the proven therapeutic benefit and low-side-effect potential following inhibition of the renin-angiotensin system.

Renin has two aspartic acid residues in the active site which are essential for the catalytic activity. Other enzymes belonging to the aspartic proteinase family include pepsin, cathepsin D, cathepsin E, penicillipepsin, gastricsin, chymosin, and endothiapepsin. Renin crystalline structure and molecular modeling information are based on data from endothiapepsin.

Human renin is less selective than renin from other lower species in that it hydrolyzes angiotensinogen from species other than primate. This is in contrast to renin from lower species which poorly hydrolyze human angiotensinogen (78). These differences between primate and subprimate renin make it essential that renin inhibitors are tested against nonhuman primate or human renin, rather than other species usually employed in cardiovascular studies (i.e., dog and rat).

Inhibitors include poly- and monoclonal antirenin antibodies which are very potent and have been studied in preclinical animal models and in humans (28). One of the first natural inhibitors was pepstatin, a microbial peptide (79). Pepstatin is a weak renin inhibitor and interacts with other aspartic proteinases (Table 1).

Table 1. *Renin inhibitors*

Compound	Structure	IC$_{50}$ (nM)
Pepstatin	Iva-Val-Val-Sta-Ala-Sta	22 × 10^3
RIP	Pro-His-Pro-Phe-His-Phe-Phe-Val-Tyr-Lys	
SR 42,128	Iva-Phe-Nle-Sta-Ala-Sta	28
SCRIP	Iva-His-Pro-Phe-His-Sta-Leu-Phe-NH$_2$	16
	R	
H-142	Pro-His-Pro-Phe-His-Leu-Val-Ile-His-Lys	10
ES-305	BNMA-His-Sta-NH-2(S)-methylbutyl	9.2
	OH	
U71,038	Boc-Pro-Phe-(N-Me)His-Leu-Val-Ile-NH-CH$_2$(2-pyr)	0.39
CGP 38560		1.0

A-64,662		0.26

Synthetic renin inhibitors have evolved by replacing natural peptides at the sissile bond in angiotensinogen with stable amino acid analogs (34,63,84). The most potent of these are believed to act as transition-state mimetics. That is, agents which resemble the natural substrate at the sissile bond after they have bound to renin and have been activated for hydrolysis.

Statine, an unusual amino acid derived from pepstatin, or statine derivatives form an essential moiety for the transition-state analogs statine-containing renin inhibitory peptide (SCRIP), CGP 38,560, SR 42,128, and ES-305. Other potent transition-state inhibitors not containing statine include U71,038 and A-64,662.

As shown by the IC$_{50}$ values, all of these agents are potent in vitro inhibitors of non-human primate or human renin (Table 1). Additionally, all inhibitors when given intravenously lower blood pressure without tachycardia in high-renin normotensive monkeys (i.e., sodium deplete, diuretic treated). The reduction in blood pressure ranges between 15 and 30 mm Hg. U71,038 is reported to be orally active although the bioavailability is low (34).

Studies with renin inhibitors have revealed interesting information on plasma renin activity (PRA) and blood pressure control. In some studies the fall in plasma-renin activity is paralleled by a reduction in blood pressure (40,61,84). However, in other studies using SCRIP, the maximal fall in blood pressure occurred at doses far in excess of those causing maximal inhibition of PRA (6). Upon cessation of SCRIP, the recovery of blood pressure occurred more rapidly than the recovery of PRA. These data indicate that either SCRIP exerts a hypotensive action unrelated to renin or that SCRIP is acting on renin outside of the plasma compartment. The latter hypothesis is supported by the fact that similar dissociation between blood pressure and plasma-renin activity has been observed for agents unrelated chemically to SCRIP (46) and the presence of tissue renin-angiotensin systems (27).

Results in humans have been reported for H-142 (83) and RIP (88), and A64,662, CGP 38,560, and U71,038 are in early clinical trials. These trials have confirmed that a fall in blood pressure can be produced by renin inhibitors in normal volunteers and in hypertensive patients.

Angiotensin Converting Enzyme (ACE) Inhibitors

A number of ACE inhibitors are under development and comprehensive reviews are provided in other chapters in this volume (chapter by Waeber et al.) and elsewhere (49).

ACE inhibitors having other properties are less well known but these may yield a future generation of agents having benefits over currently available members of this class. SQ 27,786 and SQ 28,853 are ACE inhibitors which possess diuretic actions (25) (Fig. 1). They are orally active and studies in dog have revealed natriuretic and modest kaliuretic actions.

BW A575C combines ACE inhibition with β-adrenoceptor antagonism (3). At equivalent doses in rat and dog, the ACE inhibitor component of BW A575C is favored 2- to 10-fold over β-adrenoceptor blockade. The duration of action for ACE inhibition is similar to enalapril (i.e., 8 hr).

BW A575C is a mixture which has been resolved to a single diastereomer BW A385C. BW A385C is a potent ACE inhibitor with an IC_{50} value of 1.2 nM against rabbit lung ACE. The β-adrenoceptor blocking potency of BW A385C is approximately 150-fold less than pindolol. Considering the structural similarity of these agents and pindolol (2), there is little partial agonist activity that could be of concern. It is proposed that agents having a dual action of ACE inhibition and β-adrenoceptor blockade would combine the benefits of each mechanism. The ACE inhibition would result in lower angiotensin II and pre- and afterload reduction, while the β-adrenoceptor blockade could blunt the compensatory increase in renin release, as well as reduce the cardiac response to sympathetic stimulation.

Angiotensin II Receptor Antagonists

An angiotensin II receptor antagonist is considered a very attractive target for antihypertensive therapy. A receptor antagonist could interfere with angiotensin II which is generated by alternative synthetic pathways which circumvent renin and ACE; for example, tonin or cathepsin G under certain conditions (29).

Angiotensin II receptor antagonists have consisted primarily of angiotensin II analogs or smaller peptide fragments, with Sar^1 Ala^8 angiotensin (saralasin) representing the most-studied agent (60). It is not orally active and exhibits partial agonist properties when basal plasma renin activity is reduced. These properties have limited the clinical use of saralasin, but it remains an essential preclinical tool.

Recently, nonpeptide angiotensin II re-

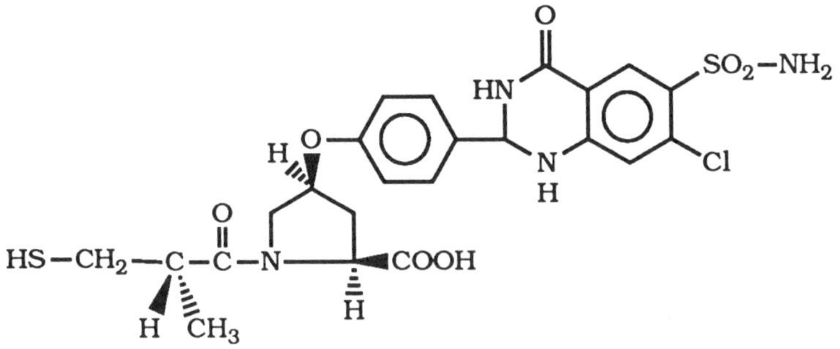

SQ 27,786

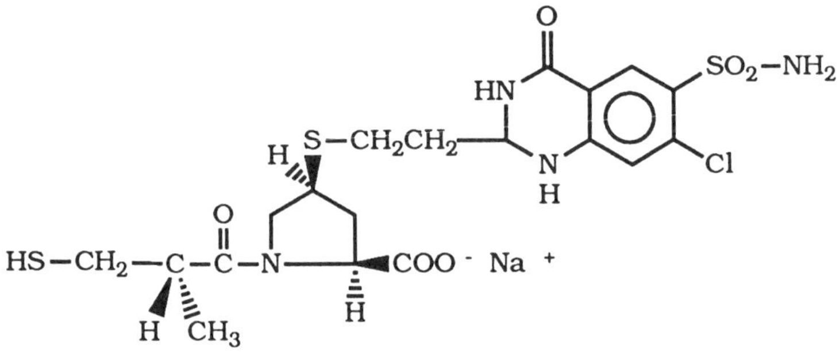

SQ 28,853

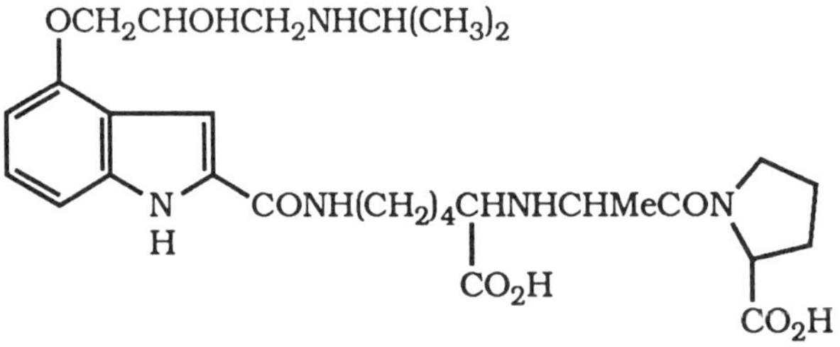

BW A575C

FIG. 1. Angiotensin I converting enzyme inhibitors with additional actions.

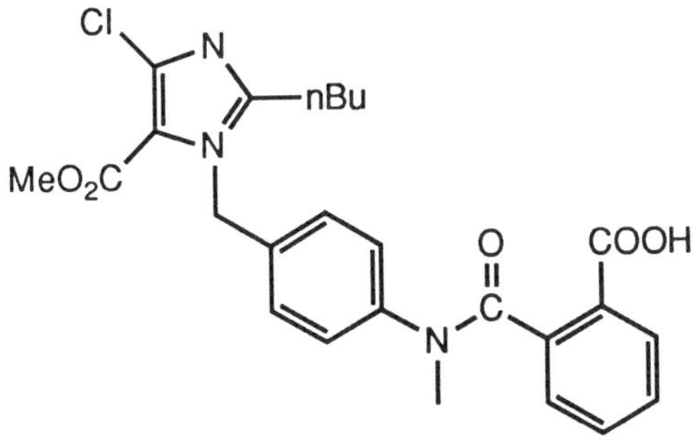

FIG. 2. Angiotensin II receptor antagonists.

ceptor antagonists have been disclosed (14). These are tetrasubstituted imidazole derivatives (Fig. 2), which inhibit angiotensin II binding in rat adrenal membranes and lower blood pressure in renal hypertensive rat.

ATRIAL NATRIURETIC PEPTIDE MODULATORS

Atrial natriuretic peptide (ANP) possesses many attractive properties which make it useful for the treatment of hypertension. The well-known diuretic, natriuretic, and vasodilatory actions are complimented by other beneficial effects, such as inhibition of release of renin, aldosterone, and vasopressin (31,51).

In spontaneously hypertensive rats ANP causes a reduction in arterial blood pressure and little tachycardia. The hemodynamic responses to ANP are dependent on the mode of administration. Whereas, bolus injections cause an increase in renal, mesenteric, and hindquarter blood flow, slow infusions cause a reduction in these regional blood flows (52). In dogs, infusion of ANP resulted in a drop in cardiac output and stroke volume (47). The fall in cardiac output is probably caused by venodilatation, a reduction in venous return (9), and possibly rapid volume contraction as indicated by an increase in hematocrit (51).

In normotensive humans, the infusion of ANP causes a prompt diuresis and natriuresis, a fall in systolic blood pressure, and a decrease in pulmonary wedge pressure (17). In congestive heart failure (CHF) patients, the renal responses were far less marked than those observed in normotensive humans. However, in most human studies, ANP has been given in doses which elevate plasma ANP concentrations to those observed in pathological states (51). Possibly, infusion at lower concentrations for longer duration would be more indicative of the responses attainable with chronic ANP administration.

ANP is a relatively large peptide (Fig. 3) and is not orally active. Efforts to synthesize smaller molecular weight peptides or peptides which are metabolically stable, have been relatively unsuccessful because of the tight structure activity relationships (SAR) of ANP (30).

ANP receptors have been identified primarily in kidney, brain, blood vessels, adrenal gland, and intestine. Two receptor subtypes have been identified and characterized: the so-called B-ANP receptor accounts for the biological actions of ANP involving elevation in cyclic GMP; the C-ANP receptor appears to function in the clearance of ANP from the circulation (56,72) (Fig. 4). The SAR is less constrained for the C-ANP receptor, and peptides (e.g., SC 46,542) have been synthesized that can interfere with the C-ANP receptor (48,71). Although unknown at this time, it is possible that orally active C-ANP receptor antagonists could be found which elevate ANP by preventing its plasma clearance.

In addition to clearing of ANP by receptor internalization, it is known that ANP is metabolized by circulating endopeptidases. One endopeptidase inhibitor, SQ 29,072, has been revealed (73). SQ 29,072 causes renal and cardiovascular actions which are consistent with an increase in plasma ANP. Generally, it exhibits little activity when

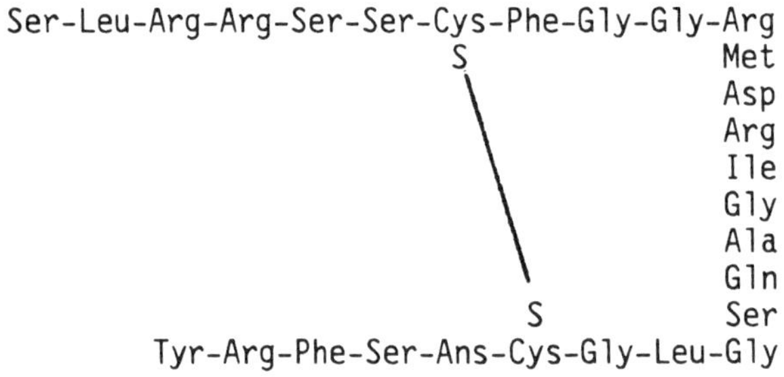

```
Ser-Leu-Arg-Arg-Ser-Ser-Cys-Phe-Gly-Gly-Arg
                       S              Met
                        \             Asp
                         \            Arg
                          \           Ile
                           \          Gly
                            \         Ala
                             \        Gln
                       S              Ser
        Tyr-Arg-Phe-Ser-Ans-Cys-Gly-Leu-Gly
```

Human ANP

[(des Phe[106], Gly[107], Ala[115], Gln[116])AP(103-126)]

SC 46542

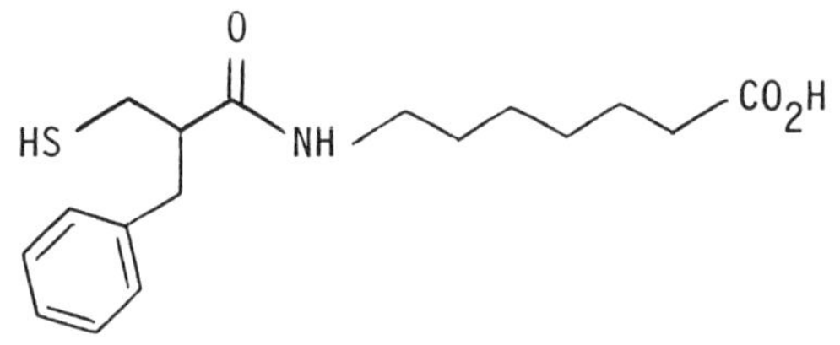

SQ 29,072

FIG. 3. Atrial natriuretic peptide (ANP) and modulators.

given alone and has to be coadministered with ANP.

POTASSIUM EFFLUX STIMULATORS

Agents which enhance potassium conductance are potent vasodilators. Newer antihypertensive agents representative of this class are pinacidil and BRL 34,915 (cro-makalim) (Fig. 5), but minoxidil sulfate is also believed to be acting by a mechanism involving increased potassium conductance (20). Efflux of ^{86}Rb from vascular smooth muscle cells is increased by these agents (8,39,64). Electrophysiological studies have revealed that the agents increase potassium current in single ventricular cells (21). Pinacidil and BRL 34,915 are generally poor

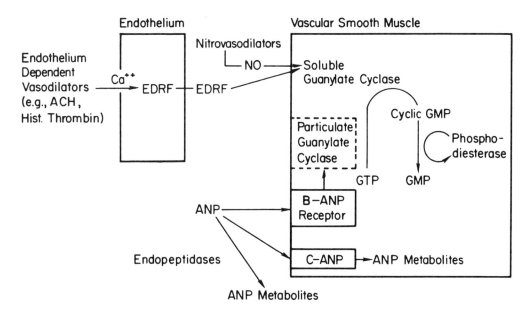

FIG. 4. Schematic depicting mechanism of action for ANP and cGMP modulators.

inhibitors of contractile responses produced by KCl or angiotensin II, but potent inhibitors of those responses produced by norepinephrine and phenylephrine (12,20,23). Effects of BRL 34,915 are reversed by the potassium channel antagonists, tetraethylaminonium (TEA) or 3,4 diaminopyridine, but not by the calcium channel antagonist, isradipine, or by apamin (8,64).

In animal studies, the antihypertensive effects are due to a decrease in total peripheral resistance and are usually accompanied by reflex tachycardia and increased cardiac output (20,23,39). Preferential vasodilatation is observed in coronary, gastrointestinal, and cerebral beds, but not in kidney or skeletal muscle beds (39). The tachycardia is sensitive to β-adrenoceptor blockade (20). Hormonal changes include elevations in plasma renin activity and catecholamines (20). In a canine occlusion-reperfusion model of myocardial ischemia, pinacidil failed to affect coronary blood flow to the ischemic zone or infarct size (41).

Pinacidil and BRL 34,915 are clinically ef-fective antihypertensive agents (13,42,80). However, in most patients monotherapy appears unlikely because of the fluid retention and/or reflex tachycardia. Most effective blood pressure control is attained by coadministration of a diuretic and/or a β-adrenoceptor antagonist.

SEROTONERGIC RECEPTOR ANTAGONIST AND AGONISTS

Agents that interact with serotonergic (5HT) receptors continue to be of interest because of the proven effects on vascular smooth muscle, platelet aggregation, and the sympathetic nervous system. Receptors gaining the most attention are the $5HT_2$ receptors which are involved in vascular smooth muscle contraction and platelet aggregation, and $5HT_{1A}$ receptors which affect smooth muscle and inhibit neurotransmitter release.

Ketanserin is a potent $5HT_2$ antagonist which exhibits antihypertensive efficacy in humans (81) (Fig. 6). Ketanserin is not only a $5HT_2$ antagonist but also a potent α_1-ad-

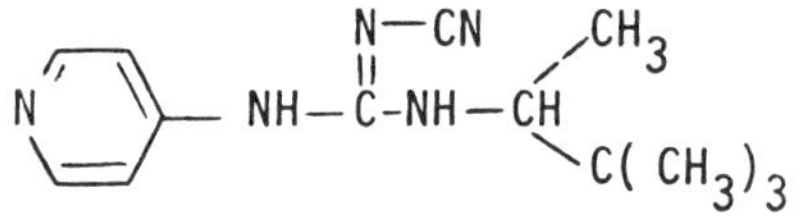

Pinacidil

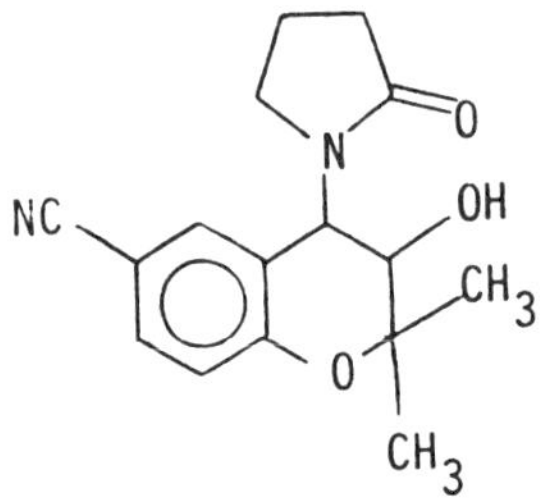

BRL-34915
(Cromakalim)

FIG. 5. Potassium efflux stimulators.

renoceptor antagonist. Recent studies have revealed that selective $5HT_2$ antagonists are virtually inactive as antihypertensives (18,19). Thus, the mechanism of ketanserin is probably related to inhibition of α_1-adrenoceptors. Although the mechanism is not completely understood it could possibly involve a cooperative interaction of $5HT_2$ and α_1-adrenoceptors (81).

Urapidil, flesinoxan (DU 29,373), and R28935 are $5HT_{1A}$ receptor agonists which exert antihypertensive activity (Fig. 6). Generally the decrease in blood pressure is not accompanied by reflex tachycardia (58,69). The absence of tachycardia could be related to an observed increase in cardiac vagal tone (65,68). ($-$)Pindolol and

($-$)propranolol are potent $5HT_{1A}$ receptor antagonists (26,75). It was reported that ($-$)pindolol could totally reverse the depressor effects of R28935 but not those produced by urapidil (26). Thus, urapidil's mechanism of action may not be related to $5HT_{1A}$ receptor stimulation, but rather to its known α_1-adrenoceptor blocking capabilities (54,69).

DOPAMINE RECEPTOR AGONISTS

Dopamine receptors have been classified into two subtypes (DA_1 and DA_2). The DA_1 receptors are predominantly postjunctional and are found on vascular smooth muscle of a number of vascular beds. The DA_2 receptors are found on presynaptic sympathetic nerve terminals and modulate catecholamine release (38). Fenoldopam (SKF 82526) is a selective DA_1 receptor agonist without β-adrenoceptor agonist properties (1) and quinpirole is a DA_2 receptor agonist (Fig. 7).

Although both agents lower arterial blood pressure and total peripheral resistance, the mechanism of action of each can be clearly differentiated (15,37). For example, fenoldopam behaves as a direct-acting vasodilator. It increases heart rate and plasma renin activity in baroreflex-intact animals, exerts vasodilatation in the absence of sympathetic tone (i.e., ganglionic blockade), and antagonizes pressor responses to norepinephrine and angiotensin II. The cardiovascular actions of fenoldopam are blocked by the DA_1 receptor antagonist SC 23390.

In contrast, quinpirole behaves like an indirect-acting vasodilator. The fall in blood pressure is accompanied by a bradycardia, decreased plasma renin activity, and is dependent on preexisting sympathetic tone (i.e., responses are abolished by ganglionic blockade). Quinpirole reduces the pressor response evoked by spinal cord stimulation, but does not affect pressor responses to exogenously administered pressor agents. The

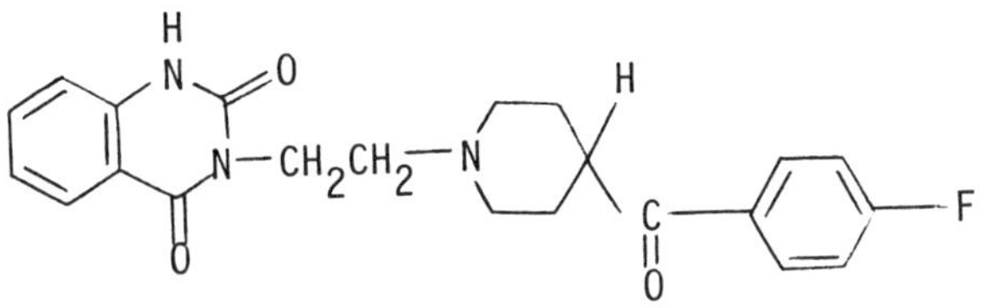

Ketanserin

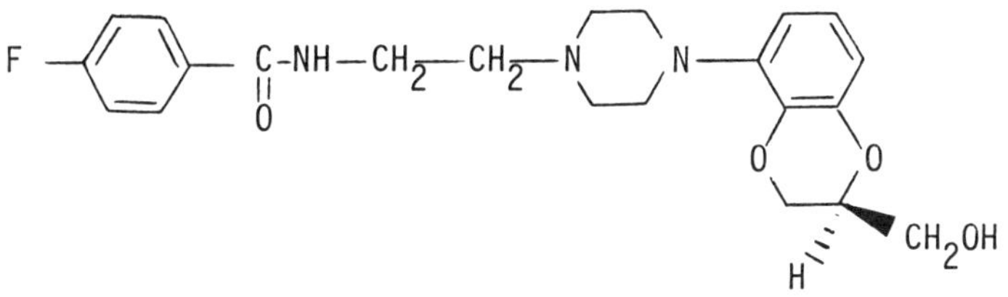

Flesinoxan
(DU 29373)

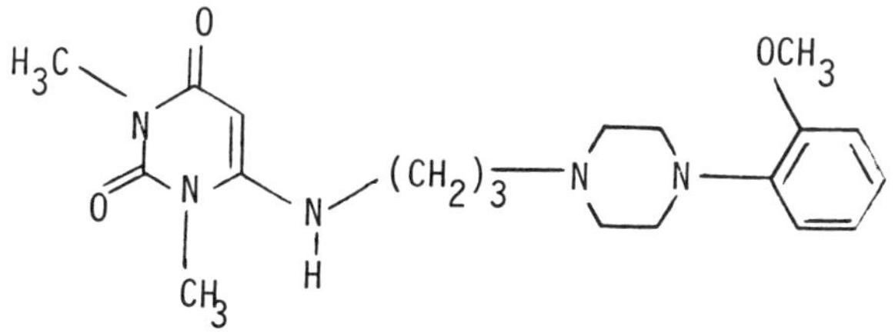

Urapidil

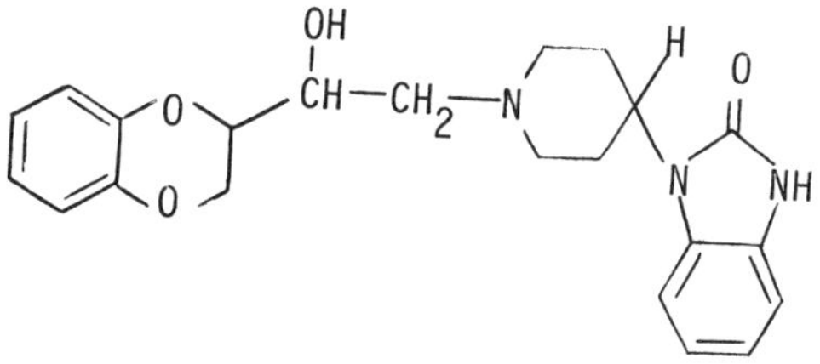

R 28935

FIG. 6. Serotonergic receptor antagonists and agonists.

effects of quinpirole are selectively antag- onized by the DA_2 receptor blocker, sul- piride (15).

In clinical studies, fenoldopam exerts an- tihypertensive effects, along with renal va- sodilatation (32,33). The bioavailability is poor and some tolerance development has been observed with fenoldopam (53). How- ever, intravenous fenoldopam is under de- velopment since it can adequately reduce blood pressure while maintaining renal function.

In contrast, quinpirole exerts a paradox- ical elevation in blood pressure in hyper-

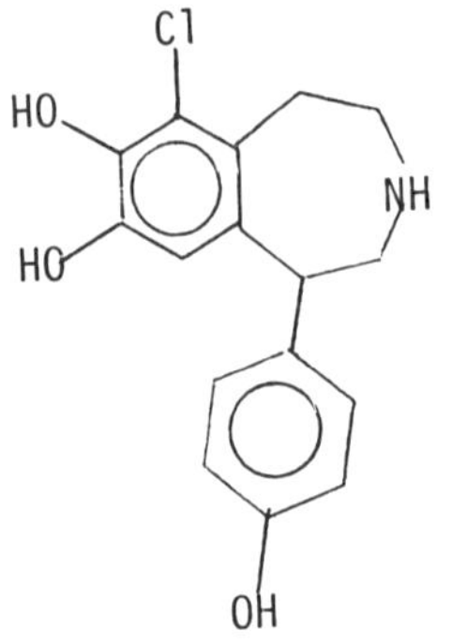

Fenoldopam

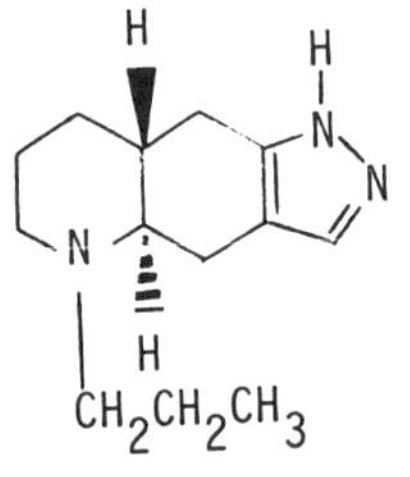

Quinpirole

FIG. 7. Dopamine receptor agonists.

tensive patients (55), quite possibly by a central DA_2 receptor mechanism (59).

ADENOSINE RECEPTOR AGONISTS

Adenosine and analogs of adenosine interact with specific receptors affecting the cardiovascular system. Burnstock and others have divided adenosine receptors into functionally distinct subclasses based upon responsiveness to various purine analogs (10,11). P_1-purinergic receptors selectively bind adenosine over its phosphorylated analogs, and their responses can be antagonized by methylxanthines such as theophylline (11). The P_2-purinergic receptors selectively bind ATP over adenosine and

their actions cannot be blocked by the methylxanthines. The P_1-purinergic receptor can be further subdivided into two additional subclasses; adenosine$_1$-receptors, which are negatively coupled to adenylate cyclase, and adenosine$_2$-receptors, which are positively coupled to adenylate cyclase (10). In addition to exerting opposing effects on cyclic AMP metabolism, adenosine$_1$- and adenosine$_2$-receptors differ in their sensitivity to different adenosine agonists, such as N^6-cyclohexyladenosine (CHA) and 2-(phenylamino)adenosine (CV-1808) (10).

Adenosine can modulate smooth muscle contractile function through a direct vasorelaxant effect, and also an inhibitory effect on neurotransmitter release (4,62). Recent studies have suggested that the direct effect of adenosine on smooth muscle is mediated by the adenosine$_2$-receptor (36) and that inhibition of neurogenic contractions by adenosine is mediated by the adenosine$_1$-receptor (62).

Two agonists, PD 117,519 and SC 32,796 (Fig. 8), have been studied quite extensively in hypertensive animal models (5,67,77). Both agents are relatively A_1 selective. PD 117,519 lowers blood pressure without causing tachycardia in a number of hypertensive animal models (e.g., spontaneously hypertensive rat, renal hypertensive rat, perinephritic hypertensive dog). Both agents are more potent in animal models in which plasma renin activity is elevated by diuretic coadministration and sodium restriction. This enhanced activity is consistent with the documented inhibitory action of adenosine and analogs, such as SC 32,796 on renin release (35,50,87).

Adenosine agonists are also very effective in deoxycorticosterone acetate hypertensive rat which exhibit very low plasma renin activity. Therefore the mechanism of action of adenosine agonists involves direct vasodilatation, renin release inhibition, catecholamine release inhibition and possibly natriuretic and diuretic actions

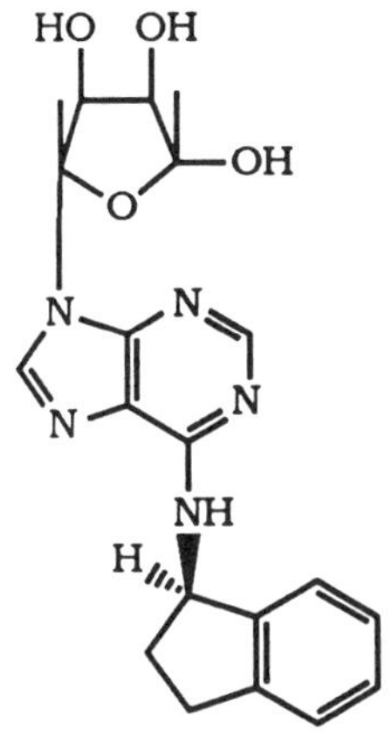

PD 117519

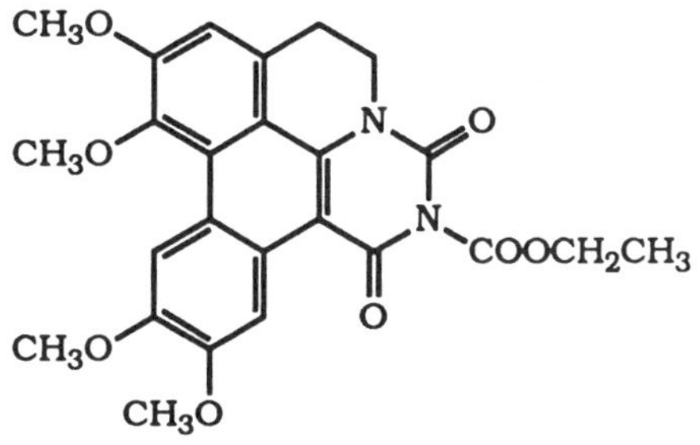

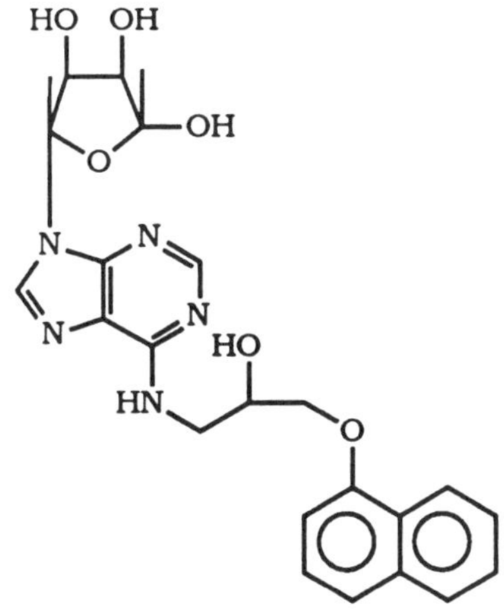

SC 32796

FIG. 8. Adenosine receptor agonists.

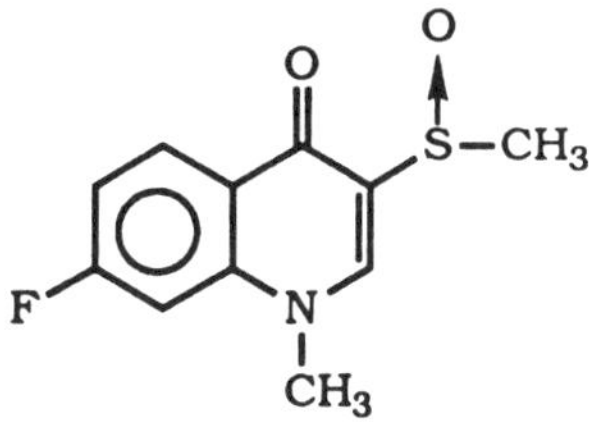

(16,67). Functionally these actions are very attractive and may well address the multifactorial nature of hypertensive disease.

CYCLIC GUANOSINE 3′,5′-MONOPHOSPHATE PHOSPHODIESTERASE INHIBITION

Cyclic guanosine 3′,5′-monophosphate phosphodiesterase (cGMP) is involved in

Compound 9

Flosequinan
(BTS-49465)

FIG. 9. Dibenzoquinazoline dione derivative (Compound 9) and flosequinan (BTS-49465).

regulation of vascular smooth muscle contraction (58). Naturally-occurring vasorelaxants, such as ANP and endothelium-derived relaxing factor (EDRF), and synthetic drugs, such as glyceryl trinitrate and sodium nitroprusside, are believed to cause vasorelaxation by elevating cGMP (57,66,76). The mechanism of action of these agents is believed to involve stimulation of particulate or soluble forms of guanylate cyclase (Fig. 4).

More recently, efforts have focused on elevation of cGMP by inhibition of phosphodiesterase metabolic enzymes. The benz[f]isoquinoquinazoline dione derivative, Compound 9, is a selective cGMP phosphodiesterase inhibitor (7) (Fig. 9). It lowers blood pressure in spontaneously hypertensive rats upon intravenous dosing; information is not available on oral dosing.

FLOSEQUINAN—DIRECT VASODILATOR

Flosequinan (BTS-49465) is a direct acting vasodilator with an undefined mechanism of action (Fig. 9). In preclinical studies, it was particularly effective in attenuation of pulmonary vasoconstriction induced by hypoxia (74). Clinically in normal volunteers, flosequinan caused arterial and venous dilatation (24) and in patients with severe congestive heart failure it produced sustained beneficial actions with once-daily dosing (45). The sustained hemodynamic changes are believed to be caused by the sulphone metabolite (86).

CONCLUSION

This chapter has focused on several targets for new antihypertensive drugs and has identified specific drugs and/or, prototypes in areas in which there is intensive research activity. The chapter is neither complete nor does it prioritize agents according to probability for success. Attention is not focused on the multifactorial nature of hypertension, i.e., differences in the disease from its onset, evolution or background of associated risk factors such as the effects of new antihypertensive drugs on plasma lipoproteins. These issues have been dealt with in other chapters. While no single drug or mechanism will accommodate the diverse needs of the hypertensive population, we believe new and better rationally designed antihypertensive drugs will emerge in the future consistent with our better understanding of the pathophysiology of hypertension and the availability of new technologies to define their mechanisms of action.

REFERENCES

1. Ackerman, D. M., Weinstock, J., Wiebelhaus, V. D., and Berkowitz, B. (1982): Renal vasodilators and hypertension. *Drug Dev. Res.*, 2:283–297.
2. Allan, G., Cambridge, D., Follenfant, M. J., and Hardy, G. W. (1988): Preclinical pharmacology of a novel dual acting angiotensin converting enzyme inhibitor with β-adrenoceptor blocking properties. *Cardiovascular Drug Rev.*, 6:84–96.
3. Allan, G., Cambridge, D., Hardy, G. W., and Follenfant, M. J. (1987): BW A575C, a chemically novel agent with angiotensin converting enzyme inhibitor and β-adrenoceptor-blocking properties. *Br. J. Pharmac.*, 90:609–615.
4. Allgaier, C., Hertting, G., Kügelgen, O. U. (1987): The adenosine receptor-mediated inhibition of norepinephrine release possibly in a N-protein and is increased by α_2-autoreceptor blockade. *Br. J. Pharmacol.*, 90:403–412.
5. Bittner, S. E., Thomsen, C. J., Salyers, A., Yang, P-C., Papaioannou, A., and Walsh, G. M. (1988): A differential antihypertensive action of SC-32796, an adenosine analogue, in normotensive, hypertensive, and salt-depleted hypertensive beagles. *FASEB J.*, 2:A362.
6. Blaine, E. H., Schorn, T. W., and Boger, J. (1984): Statine-containing renin inhibitor: Dissociation of blood pressure lowering and renin inhibition in sodium-deficient dogs. *Hypertension*, 6(suppl 1):I-III-I-118.
7. Booth, R. F. G., Buckham, S. P., Lung, D. O., Manley, P. W., and Porter, R. A. (1987): Dibenzoquinazoline diones as antihypertensive cyclic guanosine monophosphate phosphodiesterase inhibitors. *Biochem. Pharmacol.*, 36:3517–3521.
8. Bray, K. M., Newgreen, D. T., Small, R. C., Southerton, J. R., Taylor, S. G., Weir, S. W., and Weston, A. H. (1987): Evidence that the mechanism of the inhibitory action of pinacidil in rat and guinea pig smooth muscle differs from that of glyceryl trinitrate. *Br. J. Pharmac.*, 91:421–429.
9. Breuhaus, B. A., Saneii, H. H., Brandt, M. A., and Chimoskey, J. E. (1985): Atriopeptin II lowers cardiac output in conscious sheep. *Am. J. Physiol.*, 249:R776–R780.
10. Bruns, R. F., Lu, G. H., and Pugsley, T. A. (1986): Characterization of the A_2 adenosine receptor labeled by [^{3}H]NECA in rat striatal membranes. *Molecular Pharmacol.*, 29:331–346.
11. Burnstock, G. (1978): A basis for distinguishing two types of purinergic receptors. In: *Cell Membrane Receptors for Drugs and Hormones: A Multidisciplinary Approach*, edited by Straub, R. W. and Bolis, L., Raven Press, New York.
12. Buckingham, R. E. (1988): Studies on the antivasoconstrictor activity of BRL 34915 in spontaneously hypertensive rats. A comparison with nifedipine. *Br. J. Pharmacol.*, 93:541–552.
13. Byyny, R. L., Nies, A. S., LoVerde, M. E., and Mitchell, W. D. (1987): A double-blind, randomized, controlled trial comparing pinacidil to hy-

dralazine in essential hypertension. *Clin. Pharmacol. Ther.*, 42:50–57.

14. Carini, D. J., and Duncia, J. J. V. (1988): European Patent 0253310.

15. Cavero, I. Thiry, C., Pratz, J., and Lawson, K. (1987): Cardiovascular characterization of DA_1 and DA_2 dopamine receptor agonists in anesthetized rats. *Clin. and Exper. Hyper.*, A(5–6):931–952.

16. Churchill, P. C., and Bidani, A. K. (1989): *Adenosine and Renal Function* (in press).

17. Cody, R. J., Atlas, S. A., Laragh, J. H., Kubo, S. H., Covit, A. B., Ryman, K. S., Shaknovitch, A., Pondolfino, K., Clark, M., Camargo, M. J. F., Scarborough, R. M., and Lewicki, J. A. (1986): Atrial natriuretic factor in normal subjects and heart failure patients: Plasma levels and renal, hormonal, and hemodynamic responses to peptide infusion. *J. Clin. Invest.*, 78:1362.

18. Cohen, M. L., Fuller, R. W., and Kurz, K. D. (1983): Evidence that blood pressure reduction by serotonin antagonists is related to alpha receptor blockade in spontaneously hypertensive rats. *Hypertension*, 5:676–681.

19. Cohen, M. L., Kurz, K. D., and Fuller, R. W. (1987): Effects of meta-chlorophenyl-piperazine (mCPP), a central serotonin agonist and vascular serotonin receptor antagonist, on blood pressure in SHR. *Clin. Exp. Hyper.*, A9:1549–1565.

20. Cohen, M. L. (1986): Pinacidil monohydrate-novel vasdilator: Review of preclinical pharmacology and mechanism of action. *Drug Dev. Res.*, 9:249–258.

21. Conder, M. L., and McCullough, J. R. (1987): Purported K^+ channel opener, BRL 34915, blocks inwardly rectifying K^+ current in isolated guinea pig ventricular myocytes. *Biophys. J.*, 51:258a.

22. The Consensus Trial Study Group (1987): Effects of enalapril on mortality in severe congestive heart failure. *N. Engl. J. Med.*, 316:1429–1435.

23. Cook, N. S., Quast, U., Hof, R. P., Baumlin, Y., and Pally, C. (1988): Similarities in the mechanism of action of two new vasodilator drugs: Pinacidil and BRL 34915. *J. Cardiovasc. Pharmacol.*, 11:90–99.

24. Cowley, A. J., Wynne, R. D., Hampton, J. R. (1984): The effects of BTS 49465 on blood pressure and peripheral arteriolar and venous tone in normal volunteers. *J. Hypertens.*, 2(suppl 3):547–549.

25. DeForrest, J. M., Waldron, T. L., Powell, J. R., Floyd, D. M., and Sundeen, J. E. (1987): SQ 27,786 and SQ 28,853: Two angiotensin converting enzyme inhibitors with potent diuretic activity. *J. Cardiovasc. Pharmacol.*, 9:154–159.

26. Dodds, H. N., Boddeke, W. G. M., Kalkman, H. O., Hoyer, D., Mathy, M. R., and VanZwieten, P. A. (1988): Central $5-HT_{1A}$ receptors and the mechanism of the central hypotensive effect of (+)8-OH-DPAT, DP-5-CT, R 28935, and urapidil. *J. Cardiovasc. Pharmacol.*, 11:432–437.

27. Dzau, V. J. (1986): Significance of the vascular

renin-angiotensin pathway. *Hypertension*, 8:553–559.

28. Dzau, V. J. (1985): In vivo inhibition of renin by antirenin antibodies: Potential experimental and clinical applications. *J. Cardiovasc. Pharmacol.*, A53–A57.

29. Dzau, V. J. (1987): Possible prorenin activating mechanisms in the blood vessel wall. *J. Hypertens.*, 5(suppl 2):S15–S18.

30. Garcia, R., Thibault, G., Seidah, N. G., Lazure, C., Cantin, M., Genest, J., and Chrétien M. (1985): Structure-activity relationship of atrial natriuretic factor (ANF). II. Effect of chain-length modifications on vascular reactivity. *Biochem. Biophys. Res. Comm.*, 126:178–184.

31. Genent, J., Larochelle, P., Cusson, J. R., Gotkowska, J., and Cantin, M. (1988): The atrial natriuretic factor in hypertensive-state of the art lecture. *Hypertension*, 11(suppl 1):I-3–I-7.

32. Glück, Z., Jossen, L., Weidmann, P., Gnädinger, M. P., and Peheim, E. (1987): Cardiovascular and renal profile of acute peripheral dopamine$_1$-receptor agonism with fenoldopam. *Hypertension*, 10:43–54.

33. Goldberg, L. I., and Murphy, M. B. (1987): Potential use of DA_1 and DA_2 receptor agonists in the treatment of hypertension. *Clin. and Exp. Hyper.*, A9(5–6)1023–1035.

34. Greenlee, W. J. (1987): Renin inhibitors. *Pharmac. Res.*, 4:364–374.

35. Henrich, W. L., and Campbell, W. B. (1986): Importance of calcium in renal renin release. *Am. J. Physiol.*, 251:E98–E103.

36. Herlihy, J. T., Bockman, E. L., Berne, R. M., and Rubio, R. (1976): Adenosine relaxation of isolated vascular smooth muscle. *Am. J. Physiol.*, 230(5):1239–1243.

37. Hieble, J. P., Owen, D. A. A., Harvey, C. A., Blumberg, A. L., Valocik, R. E., and DeMarinis, R. M. (1987): Hemodynamic effects of selective dopamine receptor agonist in the rat and dog. *Clin. Exp. Hyper.*, A9(5–6):889–912.

38. Hilditch, A., and Drew, G. M. (1987): Subclassification of peripheral dopamine receptors. *Clin. and Exper. Hyper.*, A9(5–6):853–872.

39. Hof, R. P., Quast, U., Cook, N. S., and Blaser, S. (1988): Mechanism of action and systemic and regional hemodynamics of the potassium channel activator, BRL 34915, and its enantiomers. *Circ. Res.*, 62:679–686.

40. Hofbauer, K. G., Gulati, N., Michel, J-B., and Wood, J. M. (1987): Inhibition of renin or converting enzyme in salt depletion and experimental hypertension. In: *Proceedings of the International Symposium on Renovascular Hypertension*, edited by Glorioso, N., Laragh, J. H., and Rappelli, A., pp. 41–52. Raven Press, New York.

41. Imai, N., Liang, C-S., Stone, C. K., Sakamoto, S., and Hood, W. B. (1988): Comparative effects of nitroprusside and pinacidil on myocardial blood flow and infarct size in awake dogs with acute myocardial infarction. *Circulation*, 77:705–711.

42. Izzo, J. L., Licht, M. R., Smith, R. J., Larrabee,

P. S., Radke, K. J., and Kallay, M. C. (1987):
Chronic effects of direct vasodilation (pinacidil),
alpha-adrenergic blockade (prazosin) and angiotensin-converting enzyme inhibition (captopril) in
systemic hypertension. *Am. J. Cardiol.*, 60:303–
308.

43. Kaplan, H. R., and Ryan, M. J. (1986): Antihypertensive drugs: Current and future therapies.
In: *Central and Peripheral Mechanisms of Cardiovascular Regulation*, edited by Magro, A., Os-
wald, W., Reis, D., and Vanhoutte, P. pp. 197–
217. Plenum Publishing Corp., New York.

44. Kaplan, N. M. (1986): Treatment of hypertension: Drug therapy. In: *Clinical Hypertension*
(fourth edition), pp. 180–272. Williams and Wilkins, Baltimore.

45. Kessler, P. D., and Packer, M. (1987): Hemodynamic effects of BTS 49465, a new long-acting
systemic vasodilator drug, in patients with severe
congestive heart failure. *Am. Heart. J.*, 113:137–
143.

46. Kleinert, H. D., Martin, D., Chekal, M. A.,
Kadam, J., Luly, J. R., Plattner, J. J., Purun, T.
J., and Luther, R. R. (1989): Effects of renin inhibitor, A-64662 in monkeys with varying base-
line plasma renin activity (PRA). *Hypertension*,
(in press).

47. Kleinert, H. D., Volpe, M., Odell, G., Marion,
D., Atlas, S. A., Camargo, M. J., Laragh, J. H.,
and Maack, T. (1986): Cardiovascular effects of
atrial natriuretic factor in anesthetized and conscious dogs. *Hypertension*, 8:312–316.

48. Koepke, J., Tyler, L., Trapani, A., Bovy, P.,
Spear, K., Olins, G., and Blaine, E. (1988): Non-
vasorelaxant atriopeptin (AP) ligand and endopeptidase inhibitor on urine flow rate (V) and urinary sodium excretion (UNaV) in conscious rats.
FASEB J., 2:A527.

49. Kostis, J. B., and DeFelice E. A. (eds.) (1987):
Angiotensin Converting Enzyme Inhibitors. Alan
R. Liss, Inc., New York.

50. Kurtz, A., Bruna, R. D., Pfeilschifter, J., and
Bauer, C. (1988): Role of cGMP as second mes-
senger of adenosine in the inhibition of renin release. *Kidney Intl.*, 33:798–803.

51. Lang, R. E., Unger, T., and Ganten, D. (1987):
Atrial natriuretic peptide: A new factor in blood
pressure control. *J. Hypertension*, 5:255–271.

52. Lappe, R. W., Todt, J. A., and Wendt, R. L.
(1986): Hemodynamic effects of infusion versus
bolus administration of atrial natriuretic factor.
Hypertension, 8:866–873.

53. LeFeure-Brog, F., Lorrain, J., Lechaire, J.,
Thiry, C., Hicks, P. E., and Cavaro, I. (1988):
Studies on the mechanism of the development of
tolerance to the hypotensive effects of fenoldopam in rats. *J. Cardiovasc. Pharmacol.*, 11:444–
455.

54. Luft, F. C., Veelken, R., Becker, H., Ganten,
D., Lang, R. E., and Unger, T. (1986): Effect of
urapidil, clonidine, and prazosin on sympathetic
tone in conscious rats. *Hypertension*, 8:303–311.

55. McNay, J. L., Henry, D. P., DeLong, A., and
Crabtree, R. (1986): Paradoxical effect of LY

171555, a selective dopamine$_2$ agonist on blood
pressure in hypertensive subjects. *Clin. Pharmacol. Ther.*, 39:210.

56. Maack, T., Suzuki, M., Almeida, F. A., Nus-
senzveig, D., Scarborough, R. M., McEnroe, G.
A., and Lewicki, J. A. (1987): Physiological role
of silent receptors of atrial natriuretic factor. *Science*, 238:675–678.

57. Martin, W., Furchgott, R. F., Villani, G. M., and
Jothianandan, D. (1986): Phosphodiesterase inhibitors induce endothelium-dependent relaxation of rat and rabbit aorta by potentiating the
effects of spontaneously released endothelium-
derived relaxing factor. *J. Pharmacol. Exp.
Ther.*, 237:539–547.

58. Murad, F. (1986): Cyclic guanosine monophosphate as a mediator of vasodilation. *J. Clin. Invest.* 78:1–5.

59. Nagahama, S., Chen, Y. F., Lindheimer, M. D.,
and Oparil, S. (1986): Mechanism of the pressor
action of LY 171,555, a specific dopamine D$_2$ receptor agonist, in the conscious rat. *J. Pharmacol. Exp. Ther.*, 236:735–742.

60. Page, I. H. (1987): Blockade of angiotensin by
competitive peptide antagonists (Saralasin) in humans. In: *Hypertension Mechanisms*, pp. 433–
437. Grune and Stratton, Inc., New York.

61. Pals, D. T., Thaisrivong, S., Lawson, J. A., Kati,
W. M., Turner, S. R., DeGraaf, G. L., Harris,
D. W., and Johnson, G. A. (1986): An orally active inhibition of renin. *Hypertension*, 8:1105–
1112.

62. Paton, D. M. (1981): Structure-activity relations
for presynaptic inhibition of noradenergic and
cholinergic transmission by adenosine: Evidence
for action on A$_1$ receptors. *J. Auton. Pharmacol.*,
1:287–290.

63. Plattner, J. J., and Kleinert, H. D. (1987): Antihypertensive agents. In: *Annual Reports in Me-
dicinal Chemistry, Vol. 22*, edited by Bailey, D.
M., pp. 63–72. Academic Press, Inc., New York.

64. Quast, U. (1987): Effects of the K$^+$ efflux stimulating vasodilator BRL 34915 on ^{86}Rb efflux and
spontaneous activity in guinea pig portal vein. *Br.
J. Pharmacol.*, 9:569–578.

65. Ramage, A. G., and Fozard, J. R. (1987): Evidence that the putative 5-HT$_{1A}$ receptor agonist,
8-OH-DPAT and ipsapirone, have a central hypotensive action that differs from that of choline
in anesthetized cats. *Eur. J. Pharmacol.*,
138:179–191.

66. Rapoport, R. M., Waldman, S. A., Ginsburg, R.,
Molina, C. R., and Murad, F. (1987): Effects of
glyceryl trinitrate on endothelium-dependent and
-independent relaxation and cyclic GMP levels in
rat aorta and human coronary artery. *J. Cardiovasc. Pharmacol.*, 10:82–89.

67. Ryan, M. J., Mertz, T., Potoczak, R., Taylor, D.,
and Kaplan, H. R. (1988): PD 117,519 effects on
total peripheral resistance (TPR), plasma renin
activity (PRA), and urine flow. *FASEB J.*,
2:A606.

68. Sanders, K. H., and Jurna, I. (1985): Effects of
urapidil, clonidine, prazosin and propranolol on

autonomic nerve activity, blood pressure, and heart rate in anesthetized rats and cats. *Eur. J. Pharmacol.*, 110:181–190.

69. Schoetensack, W., Bruckscheu, E. G., and Zeck, K. (1983): Urapidil. In: *New Drugs Annual: Cardiovascular Drugs*, edited by Scriabine, A., pp. 19–48. Raven Press, New York.

70. Scriabine, A., and Taylor, D. G. (1985): Blood pressure lowering agents. In: *Ullmann's Encyclopedia of Industrial Chemistry, Vol. A4*, pp. 235–261. VCH Verlagsgesellschaft mbH, Weinheim.

71. Scarborough, R. M., Schenk, D. B., McEnroe, G. A., Arfsten, A., Kang, L. L., Schwartz, K., and Lewicki, J. A. (1986): Truncated atrial natriuretic peptide analogs. *J. Biol. Chem.*, 261:12960–12964.

72. Schenk, D. B., Phelps, M. N., Porter, J. G., Fuller, F., Cordell, B., Lewicki, J. A. (1987): Purification and subunit composition of atrial natriuretic peptide receptor. *Proc. Natl. Acad. Sci.*, 84:1521–1525.

73. Seymour, A. A., Delaney, N. G., Swerdel, J. N., Fennel, S. A., Neubeck, R., Druckman, S. P., Cushman, D. W., and DeForrest, J. M. (1988): Potentiation of atrial natriuretic peptides (ANP) by an inhibitor of neutral endopeptidase (NEP). *FASEB J.*, 2:A936.

74. Smith, J. G., and Kinasewitz, G. T. (1986): Effect of BTS 49465 on hypoxic pulmonary vasoconstriction. *J. Cardiovasc. Pharmacol.*, 8:878–884.

75. Sprouse, J. S., and Aghajanian, G. K. (1986): (−)-Propranolol blocks the inhibition of serotonin dorsal raphe cell firing by 5-HT$_{1A}$ selective agonists. *Eur. J. Pharmacol.*, 128:295–298.

76. Takayanagi, R., Imada, T., Grammer, R. T., Misono, K. S., Naruse, M., and Inagami, T. (1986): Atrial natriuretic factor in spontaneously hypertensive rats: Concentration changes with the progression of hypertension and elevated formation of cyclic GMP. *J. Hypertens.*, 4(suppl 3):S303–S307.

77. Taylor, D. G., Bruns, F., Bjork, F., Cohen, D., Singer, R., Olszewski, B. J., Ryan, M. J., Trivedi, B., and Kaplan, H. R. (1988): Antihypertensive profile of an adenosine analog, PD 117,519. *FASEB J.*, 2:A606.

78. Tewksbury, D. A., and Soffer, R. L. (ed) (1981): *Biochemical Regulation of Blood Pressure*. John Wiley and Sons, New York.

79. Umezawa, H., Aoyagi, T., Morishima, H., Matsuzaki, M., Hamada, M., and Takeuchi, T. (1970): Pepstatin: A new pepsin inhibitor produced by actinomycetes. *J. Antibiot.*, (Tokyo), 23:259–262.

80. VandenBurg, M. J., Woodward, S. M. A., Stewart-Long, P., Tasker, T., Pilgrim, A. J., Dews, I. M., and Fairhurst, G. (1987): Potassium channel activators: Antihypertensive activity and adverse effect profile of BRL 34915. *J. Hypertension*, 5(suppl 5):S193–S195.

81. Vanhoutte, P., Amery, A., and Birkenhäger, A., et al. (1988): Serotoninergic mechanisms in hypertension-focus on the effects of ketanserin. *Hypertension*, 11:111–133.

82. Veterans Administration Cooperative Study Group on Antihypertensive Agents. (1982): *JAMA*, 248:1996–2003.

83. Webb, D. J., Manhem, P. J. O., Ball, S. G., Inglis, G., Leckie, B. J., Lever, A. F., Morton, J. J., Robertson, J. I. S., Murray, G. D., Menard, J., Hallett, A., Jones, D. M., and Szelke, M. (1985): A study of the renin inhibitor H-142 in man. *J. Hypertens.*, 3:653–658.

84. Wood, J. M., Stanton, J. L., and Hofbauer, K. G. (1987): Inhibitors of renin as potential therapeutic agents. *J. Enzyme Inhibition*, 1:169–185.

85. Wouters, W., Hartog, J., and Bevan, P. (1988): Flesinoxan. *Cardiovasc. Drug Rev.*, 6:71–83.

86. Wynne, R. D., Crampton, E. L., and Hind, I. D. (1985): The pharmacokinetics and hemodynamics of BTS 49465 and its major metabolite in healthy volunteers. *Eur. J. Pharmacol.*, 28:659–664.

87. Yang, P. C., Babler, A. M., DalCorobbo, M. D., Bittner, S. E., Papaioannou, A., and Walsh, G. M. (1988): Effects of SC-32796, an adenosine agonist on renin release. *FASEB J.*, 2:A363.

88. Zusman, R. M., Burton, J., Christensen, D., Dodds, A., and Haber, E. (1983): Hemodynamic effects of a competitive renin inhibitory peptide in man: Evidence for multiple mechanisms of action. *Trans. Assoc. Am. Physicians*, 96:365–374.

New Therapeutic Strategies in Hypertension,
edited by Norman M. Kaplan,
Barry M. Brenner, and John H. Laragh.
Raven Press, Ltd., New York © 1989.

Strategies in Choosing Therapy for Hypertension

John H. Laragh

Cardiovascular Center, The New York Hospital-Cornell Medical Center, New York, New York 10021

The strategy for choosing therapy for hypertension has been changing at an exponential rate and is now radically different from what it was just a few years ago. Powering this change is the proof and realization of hypertension's heterogeneity: heterogeneity of etiology, of pathophysiologic mechanisms, of patient risk and prognosis. All this is coupled in both cause and effect with the growing heterogeneity and specificity in therapeutic agents and procedures. Hypertension is not a single disease process, and as a result it has no blanket treatment. Differential diagnosis is as germane to the phenomenon of hypertension as it is to that of fever or weight loss, and it is the starting point of therapeutic strategy. Such a strategy no longer confronts an invisible, unknown enemy.

The first part of this chapter addresses what is now known or what may be usefully (if sometimes tentatively) assumed about the various mechanisms that share the common marker of high blood pressure, and the diagnostic findings by which these mechanisms may be assessed and discriminated. Therapeutic strategies appropriate to these findings and to the patient's well-being and safety are then discussed.

HETEROGENEITY OF HYPERTENSION

Clinical Heterogeneity

There is scarcely a physician in primary practice who does not know that essential hypertension is heterogeneous in its clinical course and outcome. Clinical evidence demonstrates over and over again that the height of the blood pressure reading is an unreliable indicator of the type of hypertension, its severity, or its prognosis. Only in general statistical terms can it be said that the higher the blood pressure the higher the expected organ damage, the more severe the illness, and the shorter the survival; there are too many exceptions to make this more than a broad rule of thumb. Some patients with severe hypertension, even in the region of 250/130 mm Hg, live what appears to be a normal life span without serious health problems. Some patients with relatively mild hypertension succumb prematurely to heart attack, stroke, or other cardiovascular incident.

Statistics show that whereas about 10 to 15% of hypertensive persons are at risk of coronary disease or stroke, perhaps only 1 to 2% of normotensive persons are in such danger (40). However, the corollary of this is that 85% or more of hypertensives, particularly those with mild elevations, are at little or no more risk than anyone else. In mild hypertension, very often the blood pressure will return spontaneously to normal. It is quite possibly the case that only 1% of patients with mild hypertension are at risk. For 99% of the group, the treatment itself may introduce more risk than that posed by the untreated disease if long-term therapy is uncritically applied to the group as a whole.

Undoubtedly, patients with severe disease, i.e., those with diastolic pressures of

110 or more or with target organ damage, need drug therapy. Treatment can protect significant numbers of these patients from cardiovascular trauma (19). Nevertheless, even in this group it has been shown that the large majority are not at greater risk: most patients in the untreated portion of the original Veteran's Administration trial suffered no added morbidity during the five years of observation (19).

Most current antihypertensive drugs have some toxicity and unpleasant side effects. It is inefficient, to say the very least, to subject large numbers of patients to the risks, intrusions, and costs of a lifetime of single or multiple drug therapy from which they can derive no real benefit. The best medical practice places the highest urgency on the goals of identifying those patients who are truly at cardiovascular risk and treating them appropriately, at the same time reducing or even withholding therapy for many patients with essential hypertension. The goals of antihypertensive therapy must be to give each patient the fewest number of drugs in the smallest amount and in the lowest possible frequency for the long-term or lifetime commitment that antihypertensive therapy may involve. To accomplish this requires not merely a general acknowledgment that hypertension is heterogeneous but the careful application of that knowledge to evaluation and treatment.

Pharmacologic Heterogeneity

It is also an inevitable clinical observation that essential hypertension surely demonstrates its heterogeneity in the response or lack of response to specific types of drug therapy. For example, dietary sodium deprivation is effective only in a minority of patients, actually raising blood pressure in some as it may in animal models (37). Even a low-salt diet is not always risk-free, a fact that is sometimes forgotten. Where there is significant renal involvement, as in malig-

nant or renovascular hypertension, such a diet can be overtly harmful (37).

Even more germane is the fact that available antihypertensive drugs elicit widely varying responses among equally hypertensive patients. Any one type of drug is, at best, fully effective in only 30 to 50% of patients. Significantly, the response is highly individual: for example, those who respond to a beta blocker alone are not those who respond to a diuretic alone, and vice versa. This phenomenon is widely recognized among clinicians but has yet to be critically addressed in clinical trials. In over 1,000 clinical trials of antihypertensive drugs, practically no effort was made to quantify and analyze nonresponders and to study their subsequent response to other types of agents given alone (35).

Endocrinologic Heterogeneity

Patients with untreated essential hypertension exhibit an abnormally wide splay in their plasma renin activity values when these values are indexed against the concurrent 24-hr rate of urinary sodium excretion determined by means of the renin-sodium profile (5). About 30% have low-renin and 20% have high-renin profiles (see Fig. 1). A large body of evidence strongly suggests that these different renin patterns among equally hypertensive patients reflect differences in pathophysiology (28,29).

Increased plasma renin levels mean increased blood levels of the powerful vasoconstrictor, angiotensin II. That this could be the cause (or at least an important factor) in the sustained hypertension of high-renin patients is strongly suggested by the dramatic success, in high-renin patients, of pharmacologic probes whose mechanism of action is demonstrably anti-renin (30).

As for low-renin patients, other, nonrenin mechanisms may be implicated. Low-renin patients are often as hypertensive as patients with high-renin disease (5). Low-renin patients' vasoconstriction, however,

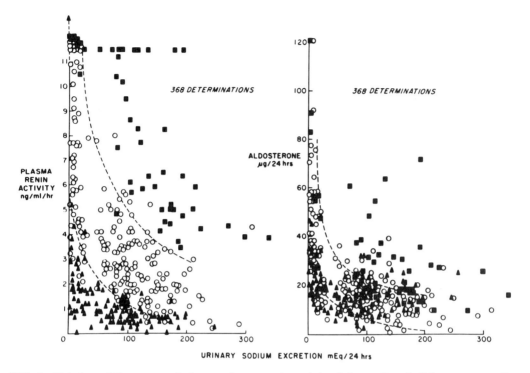

FIG. 1. Relation of the noon ambulatory plasma renin activity (**left panel**) and of the corresponding daily urinary aldosterone excretion (**right panel**) to the concurrent daily rate of urinary sodium excretion. The **broken lines** define the normal channel derived from the study of normotensive people. A total of 219 patients with untreated essential hypertension were studied, some on several occasions at different levels of sodium intake. ▲ = low renin, ○ = normal renin, ■ = high renin essential hypertension. Three major subgroups are defined by the appropriateness or normalcy of the plasma renin activity to the rate of sodium excretion which is used as an index of dietary intake and of sodium balance. Additional abnormal subgroups are defined when aldosterone (**right**) is included in the analysis. (From Laragh, ref. 30, with permission.)

appears to be mediated not by renin activity but by abnormal sodium retention (26,39), for these individuals often respond to dietary sodium depletion or to diuretics with a full correction of their blood pressure. Also, the fact that ingestion of extra amounts of salt regularly lowers plasma renin levels in normal subjects supports the idea that low-renin patients may be retaining sodium.

Thus, two identifiable patterns of heterogeneity are suggested, opening the door to a modern bipolar analysis of vasoconstrictive mechanisms. The analysis allows us to stratify and treat hypertensive patients according to demonstrable specific pathogenic mechanisms.

ROLE OF THE RENIN SYSTEM

The common factor in all essential hypertension is diastolic hypertension. All such hypertensive patients display increased total peripheral resistance, usually due to arteriolar vasoconstriction that may sometimes be complicated by secondary, structural changes. This vasoconstriction, however, like the disease process it informs, is heterogeneous in nature. It is becoming increasingly apparent that there are two different types of vasoconstriction (26,39) and that these are associated with two distinct patterns of abnormal renal functioning. In one pattern, the kidneys secrete an excess of renin, leading to commensurate vasoconstrictive effect and an increased peripheral resistance. In the other pattern, an abnormally low plasma renin level suggests that the kidneys have failed to excrete enough salt, leading to sodium-volume expansion. This, in turn, lowers plasma renin and, in some undefined manner, induces arteriolar vasoconstriction, with a rise in peripheral resistance. Thus, in both cases the kidneys play a central, albeit, different role in arranging the increased vasoconstriction.

The crucial role of the kidneys in both types of vasoconstriction is played out, either causally or reactively, via the activation or suppression of the renal endocrine system that appears to be the major long-term physiological regulator of blood pressure and electrolyte homeostasis. An understanding of this system's operations is vital to the diagnostic process and to therapeutic strategy.

Normally, the kidneys respond to reduced renal arterial pressure or to reduced sodium supply in the renal distal tubule by secreting renin, which then triggers the release of angiotensin I from a plasma substrate; then, in a first pass through the lungs angiotensin I is converted by pulmonary enzymes to the powerful vasoconstrictor angiotensin II (34,38). Angiotensin not only constricts the arterioles but it acts on the renal tubules to promote increases in renal sodium retention and it stimulates the adrenals to secrete aldosterone (1). These actions restore or increase renal perfusion: the first raises blood pressure; the second and third, by promoting sodium retention in exchange for potassium, create volume expansion and improve circulatory flow (see Fig. 2) (31). These pressure and volume effects, under normal circumstances, restore pressure and flow and thereby turn off the initial signals for renin release.

In responding to ambient conditions of flow and pressure, in the classic feedback operation of hormones, the renin system exhibits a rise or decline in activity relative to the current state of sodium balance or to any other force, such as posture, that affects flow and pressure at the kidney. Study of this system as it is functioning is reflected in shifting levels of renin activity that can reveal much about the nature of the hypertensive process.

There is direct evidence that small increases in renin activity can induce and sustain hypertension in normal subjects (1). For example, a normal woman was given a continuous infusion of angiotensin for 11 days (see Fig. 3), keeping her mildly hypertensive, 135/86 mm Hg compared to her normal reading of 110/60 mm Hg (1,39). Her urinary sodium excretion was shut off almost entirely for the first three to five days, undoubtedly because of the concurrent aldosterone secretion (she gained 2 kilos in weight). After this point, she "escaped" from further sodium retention and established a new balance. A large natriuresis occurred when the infusion was stopped.

The key finding is that less and less angiotensin, ultimately reduced to one-fifth of the starting dose, was required to keep the subject hypertensive as the experiment proceeded. This is because renal sodium retention, resulting from the action of angiotensin, both direct and by way of aldosterone stimulation, progressively reduced the need for angiotensin to support blood pressure. It could be seen that serial sodium-volume accumulation turns off the need for angiotensin-induced vasoconstriction either by amplifying the pressor response to it or by displacing it with another pressor mechanism. In this way, as the renin system defends blood pressure over the long term, an initial vasoconstrictor mechanism is increasingly enhanced or replaced as sodium balance becomes more positive. Vasoconstriction is the initial defense, but it is a poor one because it induces ischemia. Accordingly, it is gradually displaced by a volume-pressor mechanism proceeding from aldosterone-induced so-

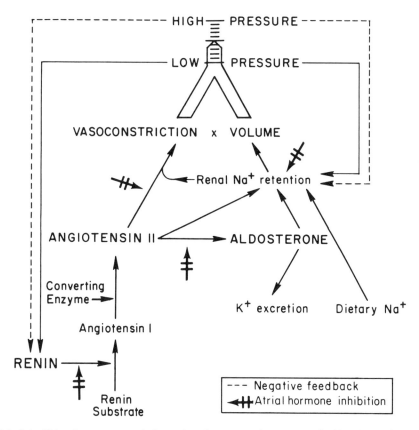

FIG. 2. Model of blood pressure and electrolyte homeostasis as controlled by the renin-angiotensin-aldosterone system and atrial natriuretic peptide. Renin, secreted in response to a decrease either in arterial pressure or in sodium supply to the renal distal tubule, acts to release angiotensin II, a potent vasoconstrictor that immediately raises blood pressure, increases renal sodium retention, and stimulates aldosterone secretion, thereby promoting both sodium and water retention and improving blood flow. The increased arterial pressure and blood volume turn off further renin release (indicated by **broken lines**). Atrial natriuretic hormone (ANH), it is thought, opposes the renin system at the 4 points indicated by **crossed arrows**. In the kidney, ANH's natriuretic effect antagonizes aldosterone action and stops renin secretion. ANH antagonizes angiotensin-stimulated vasoconstriction in the vasculature and, in the adrenal cortex, it blocks angiotensin stimulation of aldosterone release. Note that, although renin system functioning as depicted here is well established, the role of ANH has yet to be confirmed. (Adapted from Laragh, ref. 32, with permission.)

dium retention and associated with improved tissue flow.

In pathological hypertension, however, a lesion in the system's lines of communication interferes with these reciprocating feedback responses. The kidneys may relentlessly churn out renin (perhaps feedback control is damaged), as in medium- or high-renin disorders, or, as in the low-renin defects, they may be unable to get rid of excess sodium. The hypertensive state is thus sustained by either a sodium-mediated or a renin-mediated mechanism of vasoconstriction.

TWO FORMS OF VASOCONSTRICTION THAT OPERATE INAPPROPRIATELY TO SUSTAIN HYPERTENSION

As already noted above, the existence of the reciprocal polar opposites of high-renin

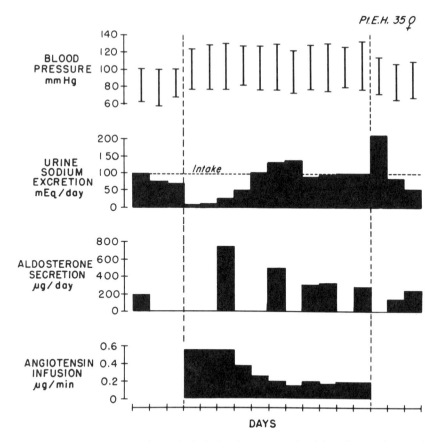

FIG. 3. Prolonged continuous angiotensin infusion in a normal subject for 11 days. The dose of angiotensin was adjusted to keep a mildly pressor response. Angiotensin II induced a marked and selective increase in the adrenal cortical secretion of aldosterone together with consequent sodium retention. As sodium was retained, angiotensin became more pressor. Because of this increasing pressor sensitivity to angiotensin, the dose was serially reduced to a point where aldosterone secretion returned to control levels. Thus, the pressor sensitivity to angiotensin increased as sodium retention progressed. The results indicate that angiotensin, unlike norepinephrine, can produce and thus sustain hypertension in diminishingly small amounts as sodium-volume gain turns off the need for angiotensin. (From Laragh et al., ref. 32, with permission.)

and low-renin hypertensions within the context of the common phenomenon of increased peripheral resistance suggests two forms of vasoconstriction, one associated with low-renin and the other with high-renin values. A comparison of the prototypical pathologic characteristics of the two forms of vasoconstriction is presented in Figure 4 (32). As the model indicates, high-renin vasoconstriction is characterized by intensely vasoconstricted arterioles, a very high peripheral resistance, high levels of aldoster-one resulting from angiotensin II stimulation, reduced plasma volume and cardiac output, a higher hematocrit, and higher blood urea and viscosity, all of which predispose to poorer tissue perfusion. Hypertensive patients with this type of vasoconstriction in its full expression are on the brink of ischemia. They tend to experience hypotension on standing, as a result of the foregoing, particularly the hypovolemia. Patients with malignant hypertension and renovascular disease exemplify this model.

HIGH RENIN
(dry vasoconstriction)   LOW RENIN
                                                   (wet vasoconstriction)

PATHOPHYSIOLOGIC DIFFERENCES

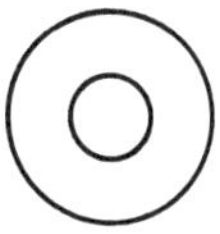

Arterioles

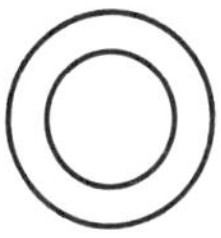

High Renin		Low Renin
Higher	Peripheral resistance	High
High	Aldosterone	Low to High
Low	Plasma volume	High
Low	Cardiac output	High
High	Hematocrit	Low
High	Blood urea	Low
High	Blood viscosity	Low
Low	Tissue perfusion	High
Yes	Postural hypotension	No

CLINICAL EXAMPLES

High-renin essential hypertension	Low-renin essential hypertension
Renovascular & malignant hypertension	Primary aldosteronism

VASCULAR SEQUELAE

(+)	Stroke	(−)
(+)	Heart attack	(−)
(+)	Renal damage	(−)
(+)	Retinopathy-encephalopathy	(−)

TREATMENTS

(+)	Converting enzyme inhibitors	(−)
(+)	Beta blockers	(−)
(−)	Calcium channel blockers	(+)
(−)	Diuretics	(+)
(−)	Alpha blockers	(+)

FIG. 4. High blood pressure mechanisms. (Adapted from ref. 41.)

In very severe malignant hypertension, such as that of malignant scleroderma, there may be acrocyanosis. This picture can be dramatically reversed by a converting enzyme inhibitor (41).

On the right side of the figure an equally hypertensive subject with low-renin values is profiled. Here, too, peripheral resistance is increased, though not usually as markedly as in the very high-renin state. Here, however, the similarities stop. In low-renin people there is instead considerable evidence for hypervolemia and hemodilution. Thus, plasma volume and cardiac output are relatively higher (36), and there is he-modilution indicated by lower hematocrit, protein, urea, and blood viscosity values (6). Extracellular volumes also tend to be higher. With this relatively high-volume state, microcirculatory flow is well maintained. There is no postural hypotension, and there is much less risk of tissue ischemia. This second type of vasoconstriction may be called "wet," or hypervolemic, as opposed to the "dry," or hypovolemic vasoconstriction seen in a high-renin patient (26,39). The low-renin form of hypertension finds its most florid expression in primary aldosteronism, where there is a massive sodium-volume excess, with hypervolemia and with plasma renin values close to zero.

The sodium-volume excess characteristic of the low-renin state (36) makes this type of hypertension the most responsive to diuretics (27,67). Sodium depletion by means of diuretics, hemodialysis, or a low-salt diet can correct blood pressure in these patients, often to normal levels. In contrast, sodium depletion is contraindicated in the high-renin, dry forms of hypertension, for such a strategy will serve only to intensify the renin-mediated vasoconstriction factor. Restricting dietary salt intake or administering diuretics have been shown to worsen the situation in both animals (29,37) and humans (27,37). It is important to note, however, that both in animals (29,37,46) and in patients with renovascular or malignant hypertension (25,29) sodium administration may correct a hypovolemic, ischemic condition and improve blood pressure.

The two types of long-term vasoconstriction have been demonstrated and defined both in the laboratory and in the clinic. In a series of studies, anti-renin-system pharmacologic probes were given to untreated patients: oral propranolol to block renin secretion (8), intravenous saralasin to block angiotensin II (3), intravenous teprotide to block conversion of angiotensin I to angiotensin II (11,12,21), and captopril, the first oral analog of teprotide (10). The antihypertensive action of each of these different probes was highly correlated with the base-line plasma renin level, demonstrating beyond reasonable doubt that the plasma renin activity accurately reflects the degree of renin's participation in the hypertensive (or normal) state (30).

Just as meaningfully, all four antirenin agents were either significantly less effective or totally ineffective in low-renin states, depending on how low the renin values were. These states include low-renin essential hypertension, primary aldosteronism, and loss of both kidneys. Indeed, beta

blockers are often *pressor* in these situations because, with no renin to block, their main action creates unopposed alpha tone.

The angiotensin II antagonist, saralasin, also is pressor in low-renin states but for a different reason. It is a partial weak agonist whose small pressor effect is uncovered when vascular angiotensin receptors are wholly unoccupied (11,68). It is for this reason that saralasin, initially thought to be a useful probe, grossly underestimated the true renin dependency of hypertensive patients in the medium- or slightly low-renin categories. Its blockade action here was only partial, being counteracted by the agent's agonism.

However, the experience with converting enzyme inhibitors (CEIs), which inhibit the conversion of angiotensin I to active angiotensin II, was unambiguous. This can be seen in Figure 5 (9–12) which summarizes an extensive experience with the acute administration of either intravenous teprotide or oral captopril. The depressor action of both agents was remarkably predictable by the height of the base-line renin values. Significantly, these agents had little or no effect when base-line plasma renin levels were below 1.0 ng/ml/hr; in such patients a sodium-mediated rather than a renin-mediated vasoconstriction may be postulated.

The vasoconstriction associated with a low-renin profile is apparently salt-mediated or at least dependent on prior sodium retention; a low-salt diet or a diuretic regularly corrects it in humans and animals (30). In an experimental prototype of one such form of hypertension, the DOC-salt animal model, which is an analog to human primary aldosteronism, the continued administration of sodium-retaining steroid results in massive sodium retention with volume expansion and very low-renin levels. As in human forms of low-renin hypertension, this condition is preventable or reversible by dietary sodium deprivation or diu-

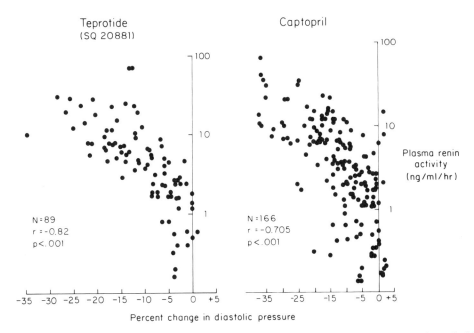

FIG. 5. The acute effects (at 90 min) of intravenous converting enzyme inhibitors on diastolic blood pressure (DBP). With both drugs, the percentage fall in blood pressure is closely related to the pretreatment levels of plasma renin activity in quietly seated, untreated hypertensive patients. The **left panel** illustrates the effects of administering the nonapeptide isolated from snake venom, teprotide (SW 20881), intravenously to 89 patients; data are replotted from refs 11 and 12. The **right panel** shows changes in seated DBP 90 minutes after a single oral dose of captopril, 25 mg, to 166 patients; data are replotted from ref. 10. Setting aside the errors in cuff pressure measurements, the data reveal remarkable and extremely similar correlations between the height of the pretreatment plasma renin value and the degree of induced fall in blood pressure. Note that patients with plasma renin values below 1.0 ng/ml/hr usually exhibited no change in pressure. The data in both panels also provide strong indirect evidence that a plasma renin value closely reflects that active role of renin in supporting arterial pressure in hypertensive individuals.

retics. In its early stages, increased cardiac output may occur, but this eventually gives way to increased peripheral resistance (45).

The Two Forms of Vasoconstriction in Goldblatt Hypertension

Two classic forms of experimental hypertension are analogous to variants of human hypertension (4). One form, with one kidney clipped and the other kidney intact, is associated with high-renin levels and relatively reduced blood volumes; it is analogous to classical, unilateral, surgically curable human renovascular disease. The second model, with one kidney clipped and the other removed, is associated with a reduced glomerular filtration rate, higher blood and extracellular volume and, consequently, lower plasma renin values. It resembles the hypertension of chronic bilateral renal insufficiency, where sodium retention is impaired and resultant sodium-volume retention suppresses renin secretion. It is not difficult to demonstrate that these two forms of experimental renovascular hypertension are sustained by two different vasoconstrictor mechanisms. An infusion either of angiotensin antibodies or of saralasin shows that the vasoconstriction of the two-kidney, one-clip model is renin-dependent (4) (See Fig. 6) whereas the vasoconstriction of the one-kidney model is renin-independent and volume-dependent (22). In the two-kidney model, because the opposite kidney is in chronic "pressure natriuresis," there is little or no volume component.

One might assume that the vasoconstriction of the one-kidney Goldblatt model, shown to be renin-independent, is sodium-dependent. Nevertheless, several weeks of stringent dietary sodium deprivation failed to reduce the blood pressure in these animals. But when this one-kidney model was again challenged with angiotensin blockade, blood pressure promptly decreased to normal. The hypertension of these animals had become renin-dependent (22).

These findings reveal the dynamic reciprocation of sodium-mediated and renin-mediated forms of vasoconstriction, both working to maintain hypertension. With free access to salt, the vasoconstriction of the one-kidney model is volume-dependent (22) and renin-independent, but when the volume support is removed by sodium deprivation, the animal defends its hypertension by turning on renin. This was demonstrated by showing that only after sodium depletion was this hypertension correctable by angiotensin blockade (22). After sodium repletion, however, the angiotensin-blocking drug again becomes totally ineffective.

Accordingly, there are two forms of vasoconstriction operating in experimental renovascular hypertension: one is renin-mediated, and the other is sodium-volume-mediated and renin independent. The two can operate reciprocally to maintain hypertension in the same animal. The physiological goal in these experimental animals seems to be the achievement of enough systemic hypertension to maintain intrarenal artery normotension downstream from the

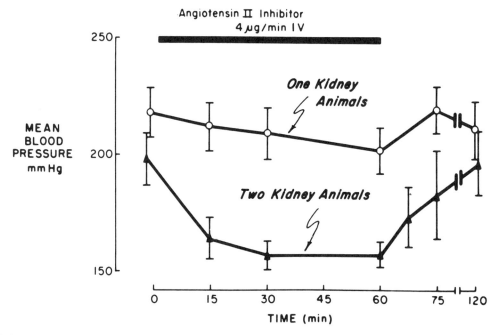

FIG. 6. The renin factor in the two-kidney form of experimental renovascular hypertension. Infusion of an angiotensin II antibody or inhibitor produced an immediate progressive fall in blood pressure. In sharp contrast, antirenin-system agents produced no significant effect on blood pressure in the one-kidney form of hypertension. (From Brunner et al., ref. 4, with permission.)

STRATEGIES IN CHOOSING THERAPY FOR HYPERTENSION   *151*

clamp. However, the one-kidney renovascular model differs from low-renin-essential hypertension because in the former the renin secretory response to a low-sodium diet is always strong enough to sustain the hypertension.

One might predict from these studies that if we could completely block both the renin-mediated and the sodium-volume-induced mchanisms of vasoconstriction, renovascular hypertension could be totally corrected or even prevented. If we could demonstrate this, then the equation

$$BP = renin \times aldo\ (Na)$$

or, more simply,

$$BP = renin \times volume$$

might be applied to analyze the active components of renovascular hypertension. Indeed, Davis and colleagues (18) have verified this equation by showing that the deletion of both the renin and the sodium-volume factors can totally prevent development of experimental renovascular hypertension in the dog.

The Two Forms of Vasoconstriction in Malignant and Renovascular Hypertension

Under balance ward conditions, in both malignant and renovascular forms of hypertension it has been possible to demonstrate reciprocation of the renin-mediated and sodium-volume-dependent mechanisms of vasoconstriction. In malignant hypertension, blood pressure can be instantly corrected by the continuous infusion of the angiotensin antagonist saralasin (3). Then, while maintaining this angiotensin blockade, the infusion of sodium chloride over several days can restore the hypertension, but on a volume-dependent rather than a renin-dependent basis. This hypertension is then promptly correctable by a furosemide diuresis (see Fig. 7).

In bilateral renovascular disease, too, we have found that a saralasin infusion only partly corrects the hypertension. An additional pressor component can be attributed to the sodium-volume mechanism because it is promptly corrected by superimposing a furosemide-induced sodium diuresis. The

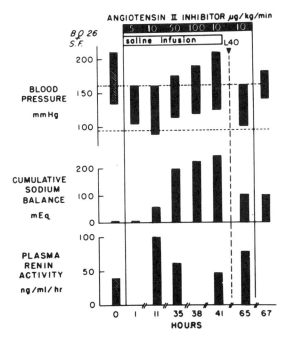

FIG. 7. A patient with malignant hypertension studied under balance ward conditions. First vasoconstriction and then volume support to the hypertension are demonstrated. Angiotensin blockade produced dramatic improvement in the blood pressure. However, as the blockade was maintained, when sodium chloride was infused over the next 40 hr, the blood pressure returned to the high control value, and volume replaced vasoconstriction in the support of blood pressure. (From Brunner et al., ref. 3, with permission.)

hypertension of this disorder, too, can be analyzed in terms of the operation of two reciprocating vasoconstrictor mechanisms.

The Two Forms of Vasoconstriction in Uncomplicated Essential Hypertension

The response of blood pressure to tilting to 60 degrees on a tilt table has been tested in subjects maintained on either a high-salt or a low-salt diet. In patients with mild hypertension ingesting a high-salt diet (300 mEq/day for 5 days), blood pressure was well maintained in response to tilt but renin secretion rose, possibly to help defend the arterial pressure (48). To address the latter question, on the same day each subject was given 1 mg of intravenous propranolol to block renin secretion, and the tilt study was then repeated. The usual plasma renin response to tilt was blocked by the propranolol, but blood presure still did not change. Thus, on a high-salt diet, maintenance of arteriolar tone in response to a tilt challenge is apparently renin-independent.

The same patients were restudied after ingestion of a low-salt diet (10 mEq/day) for 5 days. The new diet raised their plasma renin levels considerably and, upon tilting, plasma renin jumped even higher (from about 3 to 7 ng/ml/hr). Thus, on a low-salt diet, the blood pressure defense in response to tilt is associated with a sharp further rise in plasma renin. Then, on the same day, 1 mg of propranolol was again administered to each patient to block the renin-secretory response and the response to tilting was again studied. During propranolol blockade, renin did not rise in response to tilt, the blood pressure fell to near 0, and all four patients fainted.

This was not an exercise in cruelty. What we wanted to show was that on a high-salt diet, some function of that diet provides the means to maintain arteriolar tone and to defend blood pressure in response to a defined challenge. The low-salt diet renders this vasoconstrictor mechanism inoperative but

causes it to be replaced with a renin-mediated mechanism that instead accomplishes the defense of blood pressure. In the sodium-depleted state, when this renin defense mechanism is also removed by acute administration of an antirenin drug such as propranolol or captopril, both mechanisms that could support arteriolar tone are eliminated. Again the data indicate that blood pressure defense is accomplished by two vasoconstrictor mechanisms that operate reciprocally, depending on dietary salt. One mechanism is renin-mediated; the other operates in the absence of renin and is activated by a higher dietary sodium intake.

The Two Forms of Vasoconstriction in the Edematous State of Congestive Heart Failure

In their abnormally wide range of renin patterns, patients with congestive heart failure resemble hypertensive patients (14). Even when the degree of heart failure appears, renin levels are very high in some patients and markedly reduced in others. However, in all of these patients excessive or inappropriate arteriolar vasoconstriction is associated with marked reductions in cardiac output.

To elucidate the mechanisms of arteriolar vasoconstriction that participate in chronic congestive heart failure, Cody and colleagues studied the effects of changing dietary sodium intake under controlled, metabolic ward conditions (13). Ten heart failure patients, removed from diuretics or vasodilators, were given a constant diet of sodium, either 10 mEq or 100 mEq daily for periods of one week, in alternate sequences. The daily administration of this modest amount of sodium in the second period led to weight gain unaccompanied by any increase in either blood volume or cardiac output, indicating that the retained sodium was largely extravascular.

The exquisite sensitivity of the renin system to these modest changes in salt intake was surprising. Just 4 g (68 mEq) daily of sodium were sufficient to suppress plasma renin values consistently, at times to very low values, resembling those found in overt low-renin essential hypertension or even in primary aldosteronism. Moreover, these changes were closely correlated with a companion suppression in urinary aldosterone excretion and with concurrent increases in 24-hr urinary sodium excretion. Thus, it is probably safe to conclude that both of these hormones were actively involved in determining renal sodium excretion and sodium balance during both dietary periods.

To analyze the arteriolar vasoconstrictor mechanisms operating after one week of each diet, hemodynamic patterns were studied by right heart catheterization. For the group studied, mild sodium repletion produced no significant changes in cardiac output nor in systemic vascular resistance. However, the mechanism of the vasoconstriction was changed. Thus, on the higher-sodium diet, when plasma renin activity values were suppressed, administration of 25 mg of captopril had little or no effect. On the low-salt diet, however, when plasma renin was increased, captopril administration significantly and sharply reduced both blood pressure and systemic vascular resistance. Accordingly, on a high-salt diet these patients, by means of a renin-independent mechanism, maintained the same degree of arteriolar tone that they sustained on a low-salt diet by means of a renin-governed mechanism.

This study is thus in keeping with the concept of two different and reciprocating mechanisms of vasoconstriction, one renin-mediated, the other renin-independent and related to some function of the body salt content. A further demonstration of these two mechanisms working in heart failure (See Fig. 8) (15) was made with the finding that the intravenous converting enzyme inhibitor enalaprilat could dramatically "unload" systemic and pulmonary vascular resistance in high-renin congestive heart failure but was quite ineffective in this regard when given to patients with similarly advanced heart failure in whom plasma renin levels were low. In the latter situation, the calcium antagonist nifedipine was instead dramatically effective, suggesting that the low-renin type of vasoconstriction may involve abnormal calcium transport.

The Two Forms of Vasoconstriction in the Nephrotic Syndrome

In patients with nephrotic syndrome, plasma-renin values may also be either markedly increased or suppressed (43). Patients in the low-renin group exhibit larger blood and extracellular fluid volumes and reduced glomerular filtration rates, indicating renal sodium retention. This group has membranous nephritis by biopsy. Conversely, the high-renin group has normal renal function, less expansion of body sodium, and little or no blood volume expansion. Patients in this latter group exhibit minimal lesion disease by biopsy; they characteristically respond to steroid therapy. Accordingly, it is likely that in these two different types of nephrotic syndrome, as in the other hypertensive states discussed here, sodium-mediated and renin-mediated types of vasoconstriction are operating.

STRATEGIC ISSUES: VASOCONSTRICTION AND THE SODIUM-CALCIUM LINK

It is common knowledge now that the action of most hormones is linked to subtle changes in cytosolic calcium, as is the activation of cardiac and smooth muscle contraction. Resnick has shown that patients with high-renin hypertension have the highest serum ionized calcium values, whereas low-renin patients exhibit the lowest serum ionized calcium values (58). Similar deviations have been demonstrated in prototypical low- and high-renin experimental models of hypertension (62). Also, the clin-

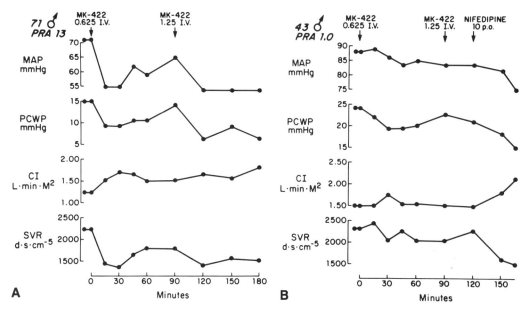

FIG. 8. Response to intravenous converting enzyme inhibition (MK-422), based on specific mechanisms of vasoconstriction. **(A)** A high-renin heart failure patient had prompt hemodynamic improvement following a small dose of i.v. MKL-422, with further improvement in repeat challenge. **(B)** A low-renin patient with comparable heart failure did not respond to i.v. MK-422, but had a prompt response to the oral calcium-channel inhibitor nifedipine (10 mg). These findings are representative of the relative selectivity of response based on the mechanism of vasoconstriction. MAP, mean arterial pressure; PCWP, pulmonary capillary wedge pressure; CI, cardiac index; SVR, systemic vascular resistance. (From Cody et al., ref. 15, with permission.)

ical low-renin hypertensive states of primary aldosteronism and chronic renal disease have been known to be associated with relatively lower serum ionized calcium levels (16,57).

A link has been shown between these deviations and the ingestion of sodium. A metabolic ward study of 12 patients with essential hypertension alternately fed high- and low-salt diets showed that those patients who had a pressor response to dietary salt also exhibited significant companion suppressions in serum ionized calcium (59). Moreover, the greatest pressor responses were associated with the highest increase in calciotropic hormones. This was not seen among the salt-insensitive patients.

The findings suggest that the capacity of dietary salt to raise blood pressure is related to its ability to alter calcium metabolism,

perhaps by inducing an abnormal influx of calcium into cells and so activating vasoconstriction. Here are a few other observations that support this concept:

1. Calcium feeding can correct the low-renin form of hypertension but is of no value or even pressor in high-renin patients (55,61). This has been verified in experimental models.

2. The pressor effect of sodium feeding observed in salt-sensitive hypertensive patients can be blocked by concurrently feeding calcium to these patients (56).

3. The antihypertensive calcium channel antagonist drugs nifedipine, verapamil, and nitrendipine are most effective in lowering pressure in the low-renin, lower-calcium hypertensive individuals, and they are least effective in the high-renin, higher-calcemic

type of hypertension. Furthermore, when these drugs correct the hypertension, serum calcium and plasma renin values tend to rise.

In a recent study, patients were maintained on constant diets of either low (10 mEq/day) or high (200 mEq/day) sodium for a week before receiving verapamil or nitrendipine. Both drugs were at least as effective, perhaps even more so, when patients ingested the high-salt diet (which lowered renin values) as when they were on the low-salt diet (51,52). In other words, these calcium-blocking agents are the first antihypertensive drug species in which sodium depletion does not add to effectiveness and may actually retard it.

Similar results have been obtained with dietary or diuretic sodium depletion in combination with a calcium antagonist (24,42,47). Here, too, calcium channel antagonists were most effective against the abnormal vasoconstriction of the nonrenin, sodium-sensitive type, identifiable in low-renin patients, and least effective in renin-mediated vasoconstriction. It appears that sodium depletion, by turning off the sodium factor and simultaneously activating renin secretion, actually reduces the antivasoconstrictor effectiveness of this type of agent.

Such results further implicate abnormal calcium influx in the pathogenesis of vasoconstriction consequent to dietary sodium. Practically, *and very germane to a correct therapeutic strategy,* the advantages of a more liberal sodium intake—improved tissue perfusion, exercise tolerance, and resistance to infections—can be exploited by using this type of antihypertensive therapy.

Yet it is known that higher blood pressures are uniformly associated with commensurately higher levels of free intracellular calcium (17). This poses a puzzle: how do low-renin, lower-calcemic vasoconstriction and high-renin, higher-calcemic vaso-constriction both activate a similar final common pathway in which cytosolic calcium is increased?

Figure 9 illustrates a hypothesis, consistent with a number of clinical and pharmacological observations, that reconciles this postulated intracellular uniformity in the face of different extracellular environments. Let us assume that in all vasoconstriction there is increased cytosolic-free calcium in vascular smooth muscle, proportionate to the increased blood pressure. In the low-renin, sodium-related form of vasoconstriction, extracellular ionized calcium levels are reduced. Thus, the intracellular abnormality is opposite to the extracellular deviation. For this lesion, we propose a Type I defect in the plasma membrane, which normally maintains a gradient of 10,000:1 between extra- and intracellular calcium concentrations. The membrane has become slightly more permeable to calcium, with more calcium accumulating inside the cell from outside sources. This results in the metabolic pattern observed in the low-renin state, where lower extracellular calcium values are associated with an accumulation of higher calcium levels inside the cell. This hypothesis may be consistent with a number of possible membrane defects in hypertension, many already postulated. The situation might come about from any membrane abnormality if calcium entry is increased or if the removal of calcium by active transport is impaired.

Recent research supports the concept of increased calcium influx in this Type I defect (20,23,52,60). Thus, we have found that this type of vasoconstriction is exquisitely sensitive to correction by calcium-channel blocking drugs that reduce calcium entry through voltage-operated channels in the cell membrane. In this correction the low-extracellular-calcium levels are restored. As discussed earlier, this form of vasoconstriction is "salt sensitive," that is, induced or amplified by sodium administration.

In high-renin vasoconstriction a final

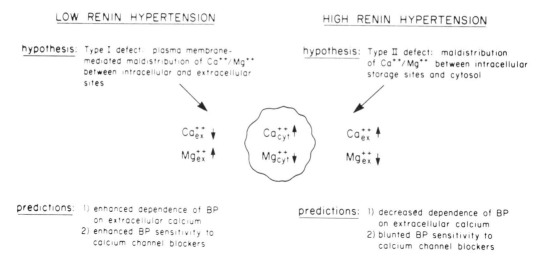

FIG. 9. Cellular calcium hypothesis of hypertension that reconciles observed heterogeneous extracellular divalent cation measurements among hypertensive individuals with their presumed uniformly abnormal intracellular concentrations. $Ca^{++}ex$ = extracellular calcium; $Ca^{++}cyt$ = cytosolic free calcium; $Mg^{++}ex$ = extracellular magnesium; $Mg^{++}cyt$ = cytosolic free magnesium; BP = blood pressure. (From Resnick, ref. 55, with permission.)

common pathway in which intracellular calcium ions are increased may also be assumed. However, in this type of vasoconstriction, levels of ionized calcium are also increased *outside* the cell. This relationship may be called the Type II defect. Here, the higher intracellular calcium apparently comes not from the outside plasma source but from intracellular sites. With such a change in intracellular partitioning of calcium, one would expect an otherwise normal plasma membrane to pump out the excess-free cytosolic calcium, resulting in the observed increases in extracellular calcium. In this situation, a primary increase in mobilized intracellular calcium becomes the cause of the higher observed serum ionized calcium levels.

The following chain of events may occur. Increased plasma angiotensin II may engage specific angiotensin-receptor-operated channels in the cell membrane of vascular smooth muscle. This receptor engagement would then trigger, via the IP³ pathway, the intracellular mobilization of calcium stores

from the sarcoplasmic reticulum and thus trigger more vasoconstriction. In this process, a number of other downstream molecular abnormalities might possibly be involved, including changes in sarcoplasmic reticulum or mitochondrial function and abnormal calcium-protein partitioning.

Whatever the final intracellular pathways, patients with renin-mediated vasoconstriction, as would be predicted, are less sensitive to the depressor effects of calcium channel blockade because the increased intracellular calcium is not primarily dependent on influx from outside. The pressor effect of salt feeding and the depressor effect of salt depletion is not observed in the high-renin state, presumably because such maneuvers work by modifying calcium influx from outside sources. Further, the preexisting increase in intracellular calcium could operate to gate its own calcium channels. Finally, as also would be required, this vasoconstrictor mechanism is supremely sensitive to deletion of angiotensin II by a converting enzyme inhibitor.

STRATEGIC ISSUES: VASOCONSTRICTION AND THE SYMPATHETIC NERVOUS SYSTEM

The nervous system has long been recognized to play a role in vasopressor phenomena, especially for mediating acute short-term stimuli. The neural pathway is most heavily traveled in reactions to emotion and stress, but its complicity in chronic forms of hypertension, other than pheochromocytoma, has been harder to show. Nevertheless, alpha-adrenergic mediation of neuronal norepinephrine release is a recognized pathway for arteriolar vasoconstriction, and blockade of this pathway with the older, less selective ganglionic blocking drugs and with more modern, selective alpha-blockers (2,53) can in fact lower arterial blood pressure in hypertensive patients, especially in the upright position.

Furthermore, it has been demonstrated (2) and verified (53) that the antihypertensive effectiveness of the specific alpha-1 postsynaptic blocker, prazosin, is greatest in low-renin and least in high-renin hypertensive patients. The degree of the first-dose depressor response to prazosin is also inversely correlated with the base-line plasma renin value. Moreover, this alpha blockade, when it does lower pressure, stimulates reactive renin secretion. Thus, the spectrum of effectiveness of alpha blockade resembles that for diuretics and calcium antagonists.

Therefore it is apparent that an alpha-adrenergic mechanism participates in the low-renin sodium-volume form of vasoconstriction. Whatever the mechanism, it is clear that alpha-adrenergic blockers, like calcium-channel blockers, are most effective at the low-renin region of the hypertensive spectrum, where diuretics exert their greatest therapeutic effect. The exact interrelationships between sodium-volume changes and calcium transport in low-renin vasoconstriction are still unclear, but the effectiveness of calcium blockers, alpha blockers, and diuretics in this hypertensive subgroup suggests a functional link between sodium and calcium metabolism and alpha-adrenergic receptor activity.

Another large body of evidence links beta-adrenergic activity to the renin-mediated type of arteriolar vasoconstriction (25,64). The renal adrenergic receptor governing renin secretion is apparently a beta-1 receptor. Beta-receptor blocking drugs have a consistent and impressive ability to block renal renin secretion and plasma renin activity (7). They are increasingly effective for reducing blood pressure in medium- and high-renin hypertensive states (25,64).

Activation of each of these two long-term vasoconstrictor mechanisms may involve their twin control by alpha- and beta-receptor-mediated channels, respectively. At present, these neural pathways appear to be modulators rather than initiators because both vasoconstrictor mechanisms seem to operate, albeit to a lesser degree, in the absence or blockade of these neural influences.

A MODERN THERAPEUTIC STRATEGY

Clearly, hypertension covers a heterogeneity of causes and effects in which the level of hypertension *per se* provides little diagnostic clue. The evidence for this has been compiled in the clinic, where it is abundantly evident that patients with comparable degrees of hypertension differ significantly in their endocrinologic profiles, in their response or lack of response to particular drugs, and in their prognosis and outcome. Confirming this evidence, indeed, making some of it possible, is a battery of new antihypertensive drugs targeted against separate and specific hypertensive mechanisms.

Sustained arteriolar vasoconstriction is the basis for all diastolic hypertension; two long-term mechanisms have been identified to account for major portions of this vaso-constriction. One is due largely to an excess of the vasoconstrictive hormone angiotensin II, generated by plasma renin consequent to excessive renal secretion of renin; it can be addressed by antirenin or antiangiotensin agents. The other long-term mechanism is marked by a low plasma renin value; it produces arteriolar vasoconstriction related to antecedent excessive renal retention of sodium. The vasoconstrictive pathway of the sodium-related mechanism is not entirely clear but appears now to be associated, at least partly, with an imbalance between intracellular and extracellular calcium. This form of vasoconstriction may be addressed by diuretics, calcium-channel blockade, or alpha-adrenergic blockade.

The meaning of all this is that we are at last able to mount a modern, realistic evaluation and management program for hypertensive patients that is several important steps removed from the blind empiricism of the past.

Overall Goals of Evaluation and Treatment

A rational method for selecting drugs for the individual hypertensive patient must be based on an individual pathophysiologic evaluation. The diagnostic workup, aside from the routine blood count and urinalysis, includes serum potassium, blood urea nitrogen, serum creatinine, a base-line echocardiogram for evaluation of left ventricular mass, and the renin-sodium profile. The first goal of this process (see Table 1) is to identify or exclude definable and curable causes for the hypertensive disorder (33). To do so may spare many patients a lifetime of needless, costly, and intrusive drug therapy; often a cure can be effected by relatively simple, nonsurgical techniques.

The remaining 90% or so of patients, for whom no definable cause for the hypertension can be found but who can be stratified

Table 1. *Overall goals for evaluating and treating hypertensive patients*

Goals of Evaluation
1. To identify all curable and definable forms of hypertension.
2. To stratify all other forms, based on their underlying pathophysiologic mechanisms.

Goals of Long-term Drug Therapy
1. To give the minimum number of drugs,
2. In the minimum effective amounts,
3. With the minimum frequency possible, thus minimizing both short- and long-term side effects.

pathophysiologically by the renin-sodium test, are candidates for long-term drug therapy. This assumes that their hypertension is significant (>150/95 mm Hg) and sustained, is possibly causing target organ strain, and is not responsive to simple non-pharmacologic therapies (weight reduction, exercise, low-salt diet, alcohol and tobacco withdrawal). For these individual patients the base-line evaluation process informs the selection of the most effective and least counterproductive drug or drug regimen from the diverse modern antihypertensive agents available.

With the initial workup in hand, today's practitioner can arrive more directly at the primary goal in applying any long-term drug therapy: to give each patient the fewest number of drugs in the smallest effective amounts and with the lowest possible frequency. This goal is particularly important in hypertension, considering that every antihypertensive drug presents a problem of toxicity of one degree or another and that the commitment to such a drug is sure to be long-term and possibly lifelong. Effective monotherapy for hypertension is now more possible than many physicians are aware, and this is a significant advance in a field so characterized in the past by additive and multiple drug therapy.

Identifying Curable Forms of Hypertension

Curable forms of hypertension should be identified before contemplating long-term drug therapy. Barring the rarer causes of chronic hypertension, the base-line evaluation has much to offer in detecting the presence or absence of kidney disease, including such surgically curable forms of hypertension as renovascular hypertension, coarctation, pheochromocytoma, and primary aldosteronism.

The renin-sodium profile, which often shows increased renin levels in curable renovascular disease or coarctation and suppressed levels in primary aldosteronism, is a valuable primary screen in this endeavor. It is no more expensive or complicated than the cholesterol assays so common nowadays, and it is potentially far more relevant, not only because it can enable the absolute diagnosis of curable forms but also because it can be used for evaluating pathophysiology and planning treatment (36). The test involves the collection of a 24-hr urine for sodium measurement and a venous blood sample for renin measurement, the latter collected while the patient is seated quietly in the office. The plasma-renin activity level is plotted against the 24-hr urinary sodium level, thus correcting for the fact that renin, as a regulatory hormone, rises normally in response to a low-salt diet and declines in response to a high-salt diet. As with most laboratory tests, the renin-sodium profile is most powerful when its deviations from normal are great. Very low- or very high-values lead one to suspect, respectively, adrenocortical or curable renovascular disease. Indeed, the base-line plasma renin and serum potassium measurements are essential tools for the exclusion or diagnosis of these types of hypertension.

The matter of excluding curable hypertension has a special meaning and urgency these days, for the possibilities of cure of renovascular disease have multiplied dramatically with the advent of balloon angioplasty, and the number of cases being detected by the simple and inexpensive captopril test (described later) has increased. In the last three years at The New York Hospital-Cornell Medical Center we have successfully employed balloon dilatation in treating over 400 patients. More than two-thirds of these individuals are now completely off drugs and fully corrected. If not for today's advanced testing protocols, a very large proportion of these patients would be on a lifetime regimen of drugs, incorrectly thought to have "essential hypertension."

It is no longer admissible to commit a new patient to long-term drug therapy before the diagnosis of curable renovascular disease has been duly considered and excluded. The steps necessary to accomplish this goal are now simple and precise. Previously the intravenous pyelogram proved neither sensitive nor specific, and renin assays frequently were technically inadequate. But today, peripheral blood-renin assays are uncomplicated and reliable.

Any untreated hypertensive patient with an ambulatory plasma renin over 2.5 ng/ml/ hr is a candidate for further evaluation for unilateral renal artery stenosis. So far, in 52 consecutive patients, we have not seen a patient with proven unilateral renal disease whose renin level was below that value. Any patient with an abnormal serum-creatinine value, regardless of plasma renin values, is also a candidate for further workup, because renin is not always elevated in bilateral renal artery stenosis. Moreover, renin levels may be reduced in reaction to impaired sodium excretion. Even in this group, however, a renin value under 1 ng/ml/hr is unusual.

Patients with ambulatory plasma renin values over 2.5 ng/ml/hr or with an abnormal serum creatinine are given the diagnostically powerful "captopril test." This test, best performed in untreated patients (patients receiving only a beta blocker can also be considered), is based on the remarkable specificity of captopril to wipe out the angiotensin II effect and induce a reactive increase in renin secretion from the kidney. Patients who are salt-depleted because of either a low-salt diet or a diuretic are ineligible for the test because they start with high-renin levels and may show a falsely positive increase (50). Other false positives may occur (i.e., patients with renal diseases), but the test has great value as a screening device because false negatives are extremely rare (50).

In this test, a single dose of 25 mg of oral captopril is given to a quietly seated patient (Fig. 10). Captopril is rapidly absorbed, producing blockade of the renin system within one hour. Patients with renovascular hypertension react to this blockade with an unusually vigorous rise in renin secretion from the ischemic kidney, whereas those hypertensive patients without renal artery obstruction show little or no plasma-renin response. With the angiotensin effect wiped out by the captopril, the kidney with renovascular disease abruptly loses its intense efferent constriction and its filtration is threatened. In reaction, renin secretion from the stenotic kidney soars in the attempt to restore the situation.

Table 2 lists the procedures for performing the captopril test, and Table 3 displays the criteria for interpreting the test (50). It must be emphasized that the 60-min plasma renin response rather than the blood pressure response is the discriminator for the diagnosis of renovascular hypertension. Although a substantial blood pressure fall usually, but not always, accompanies the plasma-renin fling, this is not altogether a reliable indicator of renin dependency or of renovascular hypertension because other, transient defenses of the blood pressure level may operate acutely.

A positive test meeting the criteria listed in Table 3 strongly implies renovascular disease (50). In a series comparing 56 patients with proven renovascular disease against 112 with essential hypertension, the test was found to be 95% sensitive and 95% specific for renin-dependent hypertension related to renal artery stenosis (50).

A positive captopril test establishes dependency but does not discriminate between unilateral or bilateral kidney disease, nor among parenchymal, arteriolar, or vascular lesions. In patients with a positive captopril test these questions can be definitively resolved by digital subtraction angiography or arteriography of the renal vessels and by a renal vein renin study. In typical renovascular disease, renin is secreted from only one kidney; a simple arithmetical analysis of the concentration of renin in each renal vein can be used to identify the renin-secreting kidney and assess its degree of ischemia. At the same time, the peripheral blood level reflects the secretion rate of renin from that kidney (54,66).

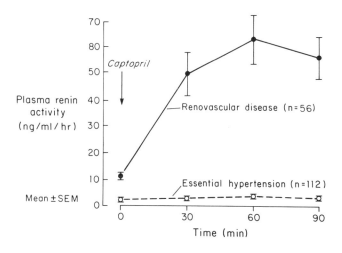

FIG. 10. Increase in plasma renin activity after a single oral dose of captopril (25 mg) in 112 patients with essential hypertension and 56 patients with renovascular disease. (Redrawn from Müller et al., ref. 50.)

Table 2. *How to do a captopril test*

1. Maintain the patient on normal salt intake; give no diuretics.
2. If possible, withdraw all antihypertensive medications 3 weeks prior to the test.
3. Allow the patient to sit quietly for at least 30 minutes.
4. Measure blood pressure at 20, 25, and 30 min (average the three readings to obtain base-line).
5. Draw a venous blood sample for measurement of base-line renin activity.
6. Administer captopril, 25 mg, orally.
7. Measure blood pressure 15, 30, 40, 45, 50, 55, and 60 min after captopril.
8. At 60 min, draw a second venous blood sample for measurement of stimulated plasma renin activity.

Curable primary aldosteronism is characterized typically by the diagnostic triad of (1) serum potassium below 3.5 mEq/L; (2) markedly-suppressed plasma renin activity—plasma renin levels are typically below 0.5 ng/ml/hr but occasionally may be as high as 1.3; and (3) hyperaldosteronism, revealed by urine or plasma aldosterone measurements. These aldosterone values may not be very high, but they should be assessed in relation to the degree of hypokalemia, which markedly suppresses aldosterone secretion, even in primary aldosteronism. Special radiographic studies, a CT scan, and in some instances, adrenal vein hormone measurements then enable definitive diagnosis of either adenoma or bilateral hyperplasia.

Chronic bilateral renal disease or bilateral

Table 3. *Criteria for the captopril test that together distinguish patients with renovascular hypertension from those with essential hypertension*

1. Stimulated plasma renin activity of 12 ng/ml/hr or more

   AND

2. Absolute increase in plasma renin activity of 10 ng/ml/hr or more

   AND

3. Percentage increase in plasma renin activity of 150% or more, or 400% or more if base-line plasma renin activity is less than 3 ng/ml/hr.

renal artery stenosis is possible when the creatinine value is over 1.2 mg%. In the former hypertensive state, plasma-potassium values tend to be high, and renin is often suppressed because of impaired sodium excretion and volume expansion. Proteinuria may also be present. In bilateral renovascular disease, however, parenchymal function is less impaired, proteinuria is absent or mild, and sodium-volume expansion will dampen activation of the renin system.

To complete the initial pretreatment evaluation, special tests for other uncommon curable forms such as pheochromocytoma, Cushing's syndrome, and thyroid disease should also be performed whenever the clinical picture is suggestive.

Determining Drug Therapy: The Renin Profile

After the initial evaluation in which the diagnosis or exclusion of curable renovascular disease has been accomplished, the clinician will find the same base-line renin data of additional use in deciding which treatment to give the patients whose hypertension is not curable but rather, "essential." With the renin participation already well defined, the pathway to simpler and more specific drug treatments can be considerably clearer for patients without renovascular disease; especially, too, for those in whom balloon dilatation is either impractical or technically unsuccessful.

Numerous experimental studies reveal that renin secretion from a normal kidney approaches zero in the presence either of high blood pressure or a high-salt diet. Thus, *any* renin secretion in the face of high arterial pressure is probably abnormal, implying a nephric lesion of either global or regional proportions (63).

When plasma-renin values are very low (below 1.0 ng/ml/hr), converting enzyme inhibitors usually are ineffective or produce very little depressor effect (39). When plasma renin values are very high (>10/ng/

ml/hr), converting enzyme inhibitors are almost always effective in lowering pressure. However, base-line renin measurements in the middle ranges are less consistently predictive for choosing the first-line drug in therapy for patients in whom curable disease has been excluded. This is because (Fig. 5) there is considerable overlap of blood pressure responses in the middle region (between 1 and 10 ng/ml/hr) of the plasma renin spectrum (36). Some patients in this range will exhibit little or no depressor response to antirenin system agents while others will respond impressively. In this region the renin test is like many other commonly used and valuable tests, such as the electrocardiogram and blood sugar assay. In all of these, normal values or near normal values may not be helpful or conclusive, but as deviations become more extreme they can often redirect therapeutic strategy.

Possibly, those hypertensive patients with mid-zone renin values have a mixed vasoconstrictive signal involving both renin and sodium factors. In some, for reasons still unclear, the sodium-related vasoconstriction mechanism may have displaced the renin mechanism. In either case, the frequent success of combination therapy indicates that one or both of the two mechanisms are still involved in some reciprocal manner.

In any event, the renin test's lack of real predictive power in the middle ranges should not detract from its usefulness in the high- and low-regions of the spectrum where, in a considerable number of cases, it clearly identifies two different vasoconstrictive mechanisms. One of these mechanisms will most likely respond to monotherapy with antirenin agents, and the other generally responds to monotherapy with diuretics or calcium antagonists.

A few other general guidelines for selecting drugs, some so well known or obvious as to appear trivial, should be mentioned here because of their practical value.

Elderly, black, or obese patients are prone to lower renin levels; these individuals are somewhat more likely to respond to diuretics or calcium antagonists. Diabetic patients should not be given thiazide diuretics or beta blockers, which should also be avoided when there is bradycardia, airway disease, or peripheral vascular disease. In addition, converting enzyme inhibitors and calcium antagonists, because of their putative positive effects on the renal circulation, may be preferred in hypertensive patients with diabetes or with chronic renal disease. Beta blockers and calcium antagonists may be preferred in the setting of coronary insufficiency.

Drug Therapy for the High-Renin Patient

For those patients with a medium- to high-renin profile (>2.5 ng/ml/hr) in whom the captopril test confirms renin dependency but who turn out not to have curable renovascular disease, the modern choice for first-line therapy is most certainly a converting enzyme inhibitor (CEI), either captopril or enalapril. It is so because of the specificity of these drugs: there is no longer any doubt that the overwhelming portion of their depressor effect is due to their inhibition of angiotensin II formation (10–12). The effectiveness of converting enzyme inhibition is illustrated in Figure 5, where it can be seen that the higher the base-line renin, the more dramatic the blood pressure correction and vice versa. Not illustrated in this plot of the acute response to the drug is the additional long-term effect achieved by the accompanying blockade of aldosterone's sodium retention.

A reasonable alternative for first-drug therapy in the high-renin group is a beta blocker. Though not as potent as converting enzyme inhibitors, beta blockers are extremely effective in lowering renal-renin secretion, and in certain subgroups (e.g., those with tachycardia or coronary disease). They have the added value of reducing cardiac work and perhaps protecting the patient from future coronary events.

Drug Therapy for the Low-Renin Patient

A low-renin profile suggests a nonrenin, sodium-dependent factor in the hypertension, and here the choice of first-line therapy is somewhat broader. Historically the first choice for this group, a strict low-sodium diet or a diuretic has been the cornerstone of an empirical approach to treating essential hypertension. This treatment mode was necessary in the past because all of the older drugs caused reactive fluid retention. Now, even in low-renin patients, the ground occupied by diuretics is under sharp challenge by the newer calcium-channel antagonists and alpha-1-adrenergic blockers. The latter agents appear to be most effective in low-renin patients, many of whom have the sodium-dependent type of vasoconstriction.

The specificity of calcium antagonists for this group is by no means absolute: these drugs may also produce significant depressor responses in medium- and even high-renin patients, possibly because increased cytosolic calcium may be the final pathway for all forms of vasoconstriction. However, their greater effectiveness against low-renin hypertension may be exploited in an interesting way. We have shown that sodium administration, surprisingly and paradoxically, actually does not impair, and may even slightly enhance, the antihypertensive action of these agents (51). Feeding salt reduces renin and shifts the patient to the sodium-dependent type of vasoconstriction, against which calcium antagonists are most effective. On the other hand, verifying the same principle, sodium depletion and high-renin secretion induced by diet or diuretic therapy may rob these agents of their depressor power while enhancing the antihypertensive effect of converting enzyme inhibitors. This relationship is of practical interest because patients can liberalize their

sodium intake and thereby improve volume and flow without adverse effect on blood pressure.

The calcium-channel blockers are theoretically more attractive than diuretics because, in the same manner as the converting enzyme inhibitors, as they reduce blood pressure they actually improve blood flow to the heart, brain, and kidneys. They are not associated, as the diuretics are, with dehydration, hemoconcentration, impotence, abnormal lipid profiles, hyperuricemia, and azotemia. Indeed, it may be for these reasons that long-term clinical trials utilizing a diuretic-based regimen have failed to show protection against coronary artery disease. Quite possibly, converting enzyme inhibitors and calcium-channel blockers might demonstrate cardioprotection in long-term controlled trials.

All this suggests that the effect of antirenin therapy with either converting enzyme inhibitors or beta blockers might be significantly enhanced (when such enhancement appears to be needed) by adding a calcium antagonist instead of a diuretic. This has been shown to be the case (49). Such a two-pronged approach, when necessary, is likely to be effective in a large majority of patients.

It would be prudent here to insert some cautionary considerations. When combination therapy is indicated, the foregoing suggests combining antirenin and antisodium agents. However, the data that provide the rational basis for such combinations also indicate that hypotension and possible renal failure may occur when full dosage antirenin therapy is given in states that already involves excessive sodium depletion. In fact, both in animal models and humans, prior sodium depletion with high-renin activity can set the stage for converting enzyme inhibitors to produce marked hypotension and acute renal failure (44). For this reason converting enzyme inhibitors should probably always be commenced in sodium-replete patients, and sodium depletion should be gradually superimposed only in resistant patients. Such precautionary guidelines are not applicable when beta blockers are used as the antirenin agent, for their antirenin effect is less complete.

Another flow-conserving alternative is provided by such alpha blockers as prazosin. As with calcium-channel blockade, the best responders to prazosin are those patients with low-renin (2,53). The new alpha-1 blockers and calcium-channel blockers appear to address the same vasoconstrictor mechanism, perhaps because of the close proximity of alpha and calcium receptors on the cell wall (65).

Drug Therapy for the Medium-Renin Patient

As can be seen in Figure 5, plasma renin activity values above 8 to 10 ng/ml/hr and under 1.0 point reliably to selective and effective monotherapy, but intermediate values may be ambiguous. In this range renin-mediated and sodium-mediated mechanisms of vasoconstriction possibly may overlap or function reciprocally. Unfortunately, this is where the majority of patients with essential hypertension are to be found, and the clinician must rely on the empiric techniques of what Alderman calls *diagnosis ex juvantibus* (35). As shown in Figure 11, five major drug types are now available for this exercise.

The process need not be as blind as previously, however, and it most surely is not as limited in its alternatives. For one thing, the renin profile may be available to add its weight to other tests in the base-line evaluation: values on the high-medium or low-medium side are suggestive of which type of drug should be tried first. In general, unless the renin profile is very low or at the edges between low and medium, it is best to begin the trial-and-error strategy with a converting enzyme inhibitor.

The rationale for this choice is that the converting enzyme inhibitor, of all the

medications available, is the most specific, so a negative result is as informative as a positive one. The strongest effect of converting enzyme inhibition is against angiotensin's direct vasoconstriction. Over the long term, however, converting enzyme inhibitors also block aldosterone secretion, thus working on the sodium-related side as well, albeit more slowly. If after a few weeks they fail, the next alternatives—now seeking a purely sodium-related solution, are, in sequence, the calcium-channel blockers, alpha-1-adrenergic blockers, and diuretics. The reason for this ranking is that the first three kinds of agent, when bringing about a successful depressor result, do so without affecting the blood flow so vital to cardiovascular health (and that may be compromised by diuretics). There are, of course, exceptions to this sequence. Diuretics may be a first choice in patients with overt hemodilution or fluid retention, phenomena that are often present in obese and low-renin hypertensive subjects.

Perhaps the most efficient and conceptually attractive approach for patients in whom converting enzyme or calcium antagonist monotherapy fails is to combine the two agents, thereby blocking both major vasoconstrictive mechanisms. With a liberalized salt intake, this strategy may maintain or improve tissue blood flow as blood pressure is reduced.

There is also a rational basis for combining an antirenin drug with a diuretic in order to block both vasoconstrictor mechanisms. In low-renin and some medium-renin patients with an underlying sodium excess in whom converting enzyme inhibitors alone are ineffective, diuretic therapy may arouse a reactive renin release, iatrogenically introducing an element of renin-dependent vasoconstriction, and thus enabling the converting enzyme inhibitor to work to achieve full control However, as indicated above, the full exploitation of this dual blockade of both vasoconstrictor mechanisms can be hazardous in the more severely sodium-depleted patients.

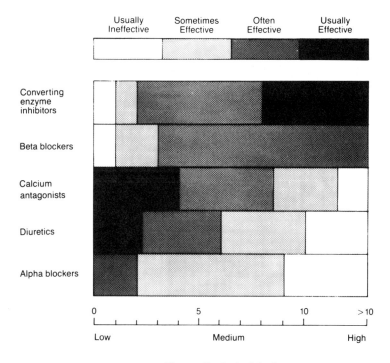

FIG. 11. A schematized representation of the selective action of major types of antihypertensive drugs. Research that has defined two fundamentally different mechanisms of long-term vasoconstriction, one renin-dependent, the other mediated by sodium and volume factors—is supported by assessments of the level of activity of renin in the blood. It is estimated that some 30% of people with essential hypertension have low levels of renin activity, about 50% have medium levels, and about 20% have high levels. The plasma renin activity (PRA) measurement is an aid in predicting the potential effectiveness of antihypertensive drug treatment. Converting enzyme inhibitors (CEIs) and beta-receptor blockers are most useful in people whose hypertension is renin-mediated. CEIs also lower blood pressure in many patients with intermediate or even somewhat low levels of plasma renin. They are ineffective when plasma renin is near zero. Beta blockers resemble CEIs in their spectrum of effectiveness but are less useful when high-renin levels are brought about by sodium depletion. Calcium antagonists, diuretics, and alpha-receptor blockers are most useful in people with the renin-independent, sodium-volume-mediated type of vasoconstriction. Alpha blockers may be effective in low-renin patients but, more often than calcium antagonists or diuretics, they fail to fully control blood pressure in such patients. (From Laragh, ref. 33, with permission.)

Two important caveats should be observed in applying the empiric process to patients in the medium-renin range. First, the clinician should restrain the temptation to begin adding other drugs when at first converting enzyme monotherapy seems inadequate. Converting enzyme inhibitors also wipe out aldosterone secretion, but since the effect of this reaches its full expression slowly (endogenous aldosterone activity accounts for only 1 to 2% of the daily renal sodium reabsorption), it may be several weeks before the full benefits of converting enzyme inhibitors are felt in patients in whom a sodium-dependency shares culpability with renin-dependency. This component of the converting enzyme inhibitor's antihypertensive action resembles that of spironolactone in the delayed onset of what eventually can be a considerable depressor force, often greater than full dose thiazides.

Second, the clinician must be willing to pursue the objective of monotherapy and to try only one drug at a time. Additive therapy, unless a rigorous, systematic trial of monotherapies make it the last resort, is no trial at all. It provides few clues to the nature of the basic hypertensive lesion, little advance in our understanding of the pathophysiology of hypertension, and less than optimal service to the patient. Superimposing one drug upon the other, as is so often done in the stepped-care regimen, makes the entire pursuit impossible to analyze and leaves many patients taking nontherapeutic (and possibly detrimental) drug agents for life. As a recent review of 1,486 clinical trials shows, the finding that a greater number of patients were controlled by combination therapy than by monotherapy most likely represents a summing of patients, not of drug effectiveness (35). These patients, responding separately and specifically to the effective components in their antihypertensive recipe, would have been better served had there been an orderly effort to discover to which component of the combination they were responding.

A word might be said about other possible combinations of the five major drug types that work against either the renin- or sodium-related type of vasoconstriction. The addition of a beta blocker can counter the reflex tachycardia and headache that sometimes accompanies the use of the dihydropyridine types of calcium antagonists and alpha blockers. Caution should be exercised, however, in combining beta blockade with verapamil or diltiazem, drugs that slow A-V nodal conduction; in this case converting enzyme inhibition is the safer anti-renin additive.

Using Older Agents

What about the role of the older antihypertensive agents, hydralazine, minoxidil, and guanethidine? These agents can often be very effective. However, the reflex tachycardia and reactive fluid retention of hydralazine and minoxidil make it almost impossible to use them except in combination with two other types of drugs, a beta blocker and a diuretic. Today, this type of triple therapy is rarely needed, inasmuch as converting enzyme inhibitors or calcium blockers, even given alone, are usually simpler alternatives. Similarly, guanethidine is a most potent agent but is too often associated with an array of unpleasant side effects consequent to broad autonomic blockade. Accordingly, this group of agents now serve only in a backup role.

Furthermore, drugs that lower pressure by acting on the brain should be the last choice for treating hypertension. This is because these drug types (e.g., reserpine, methyldopa, clonidine, guanabenz) interfere with mood, mentation, and sexual function. There are surely situations, however, when these side effects do not occur or when they are not an issue. And there are indeed still special but rare situations where these drugs can be useful as primary agents or adjuvants.

REFERENCES

1. Ames, R. P., Borkowski, A. J., Sicinski, A. M., and Laragh, J. H. (1965): Prolonged infusions of angiotensin II and norepinephrine and blood pressure, electrolyte balance, aldosterone and cortisol secretion in normal man and in cirrhosis with ascites. *J. Clin. Invest.*, 44:1171–1186.
2. Bolli, P., Amann, F. W., and Bühler, F. R. (1980): Antihypertensive response to post-synaptic alpha-blockade with prazosin in low and normal renin hypertension. *J. Cardiovasc. Pharm.*, 2(Suppl. 3):S399–S405.
3. Brunner, H. R., Gavras, H., Laragh, J. H., and Keenan, R. (1974): Hypertension in man: Exposure of the renin and sodium components using angiotensin II blockade. *Circ. Res.*, 34(Suppl. I):35–43.
4. Brunner, H. R., Kirshman, J. D., Sealey, J. E., and Laragh, J. H. (1971): Hypertension of renal origin: Evidence for two different mechanisms. *Science*, 174:1344–1346.
5. Brunner, H. R., Laragh, J. H., Baer, L., Newton, M. A., Goodwin, F. T., Krakoff, L. R., Bard, R.

H., and Bühler, F. R. (1972): Essential hypertension: Renin and aldosterone, heart attack and stroke. *N. Engl. J. Med.,* 286:441–449.

6. Brunner, H. R., Sealey, J. E., and Laragh, J. H. (1973): Renin as a risk factor in essential hypertension: More evidence. *Am. J. Med.,* 55:295–302.

7. Bühler, F. R. (1981): Antihypertensive actions of beta blockers. In: *Frontiers in Hypertension Research,* edited by Laragh, J. H., Bühler, F. R., and Seldin, D. W., pp. 423–435. Springer-Verlag, New York.

8. Bühler, F. R., Laragh, J. H., Baer, L., Vaughan, E. D., Jr., and Brunner, H. R. (1972): Propranolol inhibition of renin secretion. A specific approach to diagnosis and treatment of renin-dependent hypertensive diseases. *N. Engl. J. Med.,* 287:1209–1214.

9. Case, D. B., Atlas, S. A., and Laragh, J. H. (1981): Physiologic effects and diagnostic relevance of acute converting enzyme blockade. In: *Frontiers of Hypertension Research,* edited by Laragh, J. H., Bühler, F. R., and Seldin, D. W., pp. 541–550. Springer-Verlag, New York.

10. Case, D. B., Atlas, S. A., Laragh, J. H., Sealey, J. E., Sullivan, P. A., and McKinstry, D. N. (1978): Clinical experience with blockade of the renin-angiotensin-aldosterone system by an oral converting-enzyme inhibitor (SQ 14,225, Captopril) in hypertensive patients. *Prog. Cardiovasc. Dis.,* 21:195–206.

11. Case, D. B., Wallace, J. M., Keim, H. J., Weber, M. A., Drayer, J. I. M., White, R. P., Sealey, J. E., and Laragh, J. H. (1976): Estimating renin participation in hypertension: Superiority of converting enzyme inhibitor over saralasin. *Am. J. Med.,* 61:790–796.

12. Case, D. B., Wallace, J. M., Keim, H. J., Weber, M. A., Sealey, J. E., and Laragh, J. H. (1977): Possible role of renin in hypertension as suggested by renin-sodium profiling and inhibition of converting enzyme. *N. Engl. J. Med.,* 296:641–646.

13. Cody, R. J., Covit, A. B., Schaer, G. L., Laragh, J. H., Sealey, J. E., and Feldschuh, J. (1986): Sodium and water balance in chronic congestive heart failure. *J. Clin. Invest.,* 77:1441–1452.

14. Cody, R. J., and Laragh, J. H. (1983): The role of the renin-angiotensin-aldosterone system in the pathophysiology of chronic heart failure. In: *Drug Treatment of Heart Failure,* edited by Cohn, J., pp. 35–51. Yorke Medical Books, New York.

15. Cody, R. J., Laragh, J. H., Atlas, S. A., and Case, D. B. (1983): Converting enzyme inhibition to identify and treat renin-mediated or sodium-volume related forms of increased peripheral resistance in hypertension and in congestive heart failure. *J. Hypertens.,* 1(Suppl. 1):77–84.

16. Conn, J. W., Knopf, R. F., and Nesbit, R. M. (1964): Clinical characteristics of primary aldosteronism from an analysis of 145 cases. *Am. J. Surg.,* 107:159.

17. Erne, P., Bolli, P., Burgisser, E., and Bühler, F.

R. (1984): Correlation of platelet calcium with blood pressure: Effect of antihypertensive therapy. *N. Engl. J. Med.,* 310:1084–1088.

18. Freeman, R. H., Davis, J. O., and Seymour, A. A. (1982): Volume and vasoconstriction in experimental renovascular hypertension. *Fed. Proc.,* 41:2409–2414.

19. Freis, E. D. (1967): Effects of treatment on morbidity in hypertension: Results in patients with diastolic blood pressure averaged 115–129 mmHg. Veterans Administration Cooperative Study Group on Antihypertensive Agents. *JAMA,* 202:1028–1034.

20. Garthoff, B., and Bellemann, P. (1987): Effects of salt loading and nitrendipine treatment on dihydropyridine receptors in hypertensive rats. *J. Cardiovasc. Pharm.,* 10(Suppl.):S36–S38.

21. Gavras, H., Brunner, H. R., Laragh, J. H., Sealey, J. E., Gavras, I., and Vukovitch, R. A. (1974): An angiotensin converting enzyme inhibitor to identify and treat vasoconstrictor and volume factors in hypertensive patients. *N. Engl. J. Med.,* 291:817–821.

22. Gavras, H., Brunner, H. R., Vaughan, E. D., Jr., and Laragh, J. H. (1973): Angiotensin-sodium interaction in blood pressure maintenance of renal hypertensive and normotensive rats. *Science,* 180:1369–1371.

23. Hall, C. E., and Hungerford, S. (1983): Prevention of DOCA-salt hypertension with the calcium blocker nitrendipine. *Clin. Exp. Hypertens.,* A5:721–728.

24. Hallin, L., Andren, L., and Hansson, L. (1983): Controlled trial of nifedipine and budroflumenthiazide in hypertension. *J. Cardiovasc. Pharm.,* 5:1083–1085.

25. Kincaid-Smith, P., Fang, P., and Laver, M. C. (1973): A new look at the treatment of severe hypertension. *Clin. Sci. Mol. Med.,* 43(1):75–87.

26. Laragh, J. H. (1973): Vasoconstriction-volume analysis for understanding and treating hypertension: The use of renin and aldosterone profiles. *Am. J. Med.,* 55:261–274.

27. Laragh, J. H. (1978): The renin system in high blood pressure, from disbelief to reality: Converting-enzyme blockade for analysis and treatment. *Prog. Cardiovasc. Dis.,* 21:159–166.

28. Laragh, J. H. (1981): The renin-angiotensin-aldosterone system for blood pressure regulation and for subdividing patients to reveal and analyze different forms of hypertension. In: *Frontiers in Hypertension Research,* edited by Laragh, J. H., Bühler, F. R., and Seldin, D. W., pp. 183–194. Springer-Verlag, New York.

29. Laragh, J. H. (1981): Hypertension, vasoconstriction, and the causation of cardiovascular injury: The renin-sodium profile as an indicator of risk. In: *Frontiers in Hypertension Research,* edited by Laragh, J. H., Bühler, F. R., and Seldin, D. W., pp. 383–385. Springer-Verlag, New York.

30. Laragh, J. H. (1984): The meaning of plasma renin measurements: Renin and sodium volume-mediated (low-renin) forms of vasoconstriction in experimental and human hypertension and in the

oedematous states of nephrosis and heart failure. *J. Hypertension,* 2(Suppl. 1):141–150.

31. Laragh, J. H. (1985): Atrial natriuretic hormone, the renin-aldosterone axis, and blood pressure-electrolyte homeostasis. *N. Engl. J. Med.,* 313(21):1330–1340.

32. Laragh, J. H. (1987): Role of the renin-angiotensin-aldosterone axis in human hypertensive disorders. In: *Perspectives in Hypertension: The Kidney in Hypertension,* edited by Kaplan, N. M., Brenner, B. M., and Laragh, J. H., pp. 35–51. Raven Press, New York.

33. Laragh, J. H. (1988): Issues and goals in the selection of first-line drug therapy for hypertension. *Hypertension,* (in press).

34. Laragh, J. H., Baer, L., Brunner, H. R., Bühler, F. R., Sealey, J. E., and Vaughan, E. D., Jr. (1972): Renin, angiotensin and aldosterone system in pathogenesis and management of hypertensive vascular disease. *Am. J. Med.,* 52:633–652.

35. Laragh, J. H., Lamport, B., Sealey, J. E., and Alderman, M. H. (1988): Diagnosis ex juvantibus: Individual response patterns to drugs reveal hypertensive mechanisms and simplify treatment (editorial). *Hypertension,* 12:223–226.

36. Laragh, J. H., Letcher, R. L., and Pickering, T. G. (1979): Renin profiling for diagnosis and treatment of hypertension. *JAMA,* 241:151–156.

37. Laragh, J. H., and Pecker, M. S. (1983): Dietary sodium and essential hypertension: Some myths, hopes and truths. *Ann. Intern. Med.,* 98:735–743.

38. Laragh, J. H., and Sealey, J. E. (1973): The renin-angiotensin-aldosterone hormonal system and regulation of sodium, potassium, and blood pressure homeostasis. In: *Handbook of Physiology—Renal Physiology,* 2nd ed. edited by Orloff, J., and Berliner, R. W., pp. 831–908. Waverly Press, Inc., Baltimore, Maryland.

39. Laragh, J. H., Sealey, J. E., Niarchos, A. P., and Pickering, T. G. (1982): The vasoconstriction-volume spectrum in normotension and pathogenesis of hypertension. *Fed. Proc.,* 41:2415–2423.

40. Lew, E. A. (1973): High blood pressure, other risk factors, and longevity: The insurance viewpoint. *Am. J. Med.,* 55:281–294.

41. Lopez-Ovejero, J. A., Saal, S. D., D'Angelo, W. A., Cheigh, J. S., Stenzel, H., and Laragh, J. H. (1979): Reversal of vascular and renal crises of scleroderma by oral angiotensin converting enzyme blockade. *N. Engl. J. Med.,* 300:1417–1418.

42. MacGregor, G. A., Markandu, N. D., Smith, S. J., and Sagnella, G. A. (1985): Does nitrendipine reveal a functional abnormality of arteriolar smooth muscle cell in essential hypertension: The effect of altering sodium balance. *J. Cardiovasc. Pharm.,* 7(Suppl. 6):S178–S181.

43. Meltzer, J. I., Keim, H. J., Laragh, J. H., Sealey, J. E., Jan, K. M., and Chien, S. (1979): Nephrotic syndrome: Vasoconstrictive and hypervolemic forms suggested by renin profiling. *Ann. Intern. Med.,* 91:688–696.

44. Ménard, J., Michel, J. B., Corman, B., et al. (1987): Les effets rénaux benefiques et nefastes

de l'inhibition de l'enzyme de conversion. In: *Seminaires du uro-nephrologie,* edited by Legrain, M., pp. 157–169. Masson, Paris.

45. Miller, A. W., II, Bohr, D. R., Schork, A. M., and Terris, J. M. (1979): Hemodynamic responses to DOCA in young pigs. *Hypertension,* 1:591–597.

46. Mohring, J., Petri, M., Szokol, M., Haack, D., and Mohring, B. (1976): Effects of saline drinking on malignant course of renal hypertension in rats. *Am. J. Physiol.,* 230:849–857.

47. Morgan, T., Anderson, A., Wilson, D., Myers, J., and Murphy, J. (1986): Paradoxical effect of sodium restriction on blood pressure in people on slow-channel blocking drugs. *Lancet,* 1(8484):793.

48. Morganti, A., Lopez-Ovejero, J. A., Pickering, T. G., and Laragh, J. H. (1979): Role of the sympathetic nervous system in mediating the renin response to head-up tilt: Their possible synergism in defending blood pressure against postural change during sodium deprivation. *Am. J. Cardiol.,* 43:600–604.

49. Müller, F. B., Bolli, P., Linder, L., Kiowski, K., Erne, P., and Bühler, F. R. (1986): Calcium antagonists and the second drug for hypotensive therapy. *Am. J. Med.,* 81(Suppl. 6A):25–29.

50. Müller, F. B., Sealey, J. E., Case, D. B., Atlas, S. A., Pickering, T. G., Pecker, M. S., Preibisz, J. J., and Laragh, J. H. (1986): The captopril test for identifying renovascular disease in hypertensive patients. *Am. J. Med.,* 80:633–644.

51. Nicholson, J. P., Resnick, L. M., James, G. D., Jennis, R., and Laragh, J. H. (1986): Sodium restriction and the antihypertensive effects of nitrendipine. *Clin. Res.,* 34:404. (abstr.).

52. Nicholson, J. P., Resnick, L. M., and Laragh, J. H. (1987): The antihypertensive effects of verapamil at extremes of dietary sodium intake. *Ann. Intern. Med.,* 107:329–334.

53. Nicholson, J. P., Resnick, L. M., Pickering, T. G., Marion, R. M., Sullivan, P., and Laragh, J. H. (1985): Relationship of blood pressure response and the renin-angiotensin system to first-dose prazosin. *Am. J. Med.,* 78:241–244.

54. Pickering, T. G., Sos, T. A., Vaughan, E. D., Jr., Case, D. B., Sealey, J. E., Harshfield, G. A., and Laragh, J. H. (1984): Predictive value and changes of renin secretion in hypertensive patients with unilateral renovascular disease undergoing successful renal angioplasty. *Am. J. Med.,* 76:398–404.

55. Resnick, L. M. (1987): Uniformity and diversity of calcium metabolism in hypertension: A conceptual framework. *Am. J. Med.,* 82(Suppl. 1B):16–26.

56. Resnick, L. M., DiFabio, B., Marion, R. M., James, G. D., and Laragh, J. H. (1986): Dietary calcium modifies the pressor effects of dietary salt intake in essential hypertension. *J. Hypertension,* 4(Suppl. 6):S679–S681.

57. Resnick, L. M., and Laragh, J. H. (1985): Calcium metabolism and parathyroid function in primary aldosteronism. *Am. J. Med.,* 78:385–390.

58. Resnick, L. M., Laragh, J. H., Sealey, J. E., and Alderman, M. H. (1983): Divalent cations in essential hypertension: Relations between serum ionized calcium, magnesium, and plasma renin activity. *N. Engl. J. Med.*, 309:888–891.

59. Resnick, L. M., Nicholson, J. P., and Laragh, J. H. (1985): Alterations in calcium metabolism mediate dietary salt sensitivity in essential hypertension. *Trans. Assoc. Am. Physicians*, 98:313–321.

60. Resnick, L. M., Nicholson, J. P., and Laragh, J. H. (1987): Calcium, the renin-aldosterone system, and the hypotensive response to nifedipine. *Hypertension*, 10:254–258.

61. Resnick, L. M., Sealey, J. E., and Laragh, J. H. (1983): Short and long-term oral calcium alters blood pressure (BP) in essential hypertension. *Fed. Proc.*, 42:300. (Abstr.).

62. Resnick, L. M., Sosa, R. E., Corbett, M. L., Gertner, J. M., Sealey, J. E., and Laragh, J. H. (1987): Effects of dietary calcium on sodium volume vs. renin-dependent forms of experimental hypertension. *Trans. Assoc. Am. Physicians*, 99:172–179.

63. Sealey, J. E., Blumenfeld, J. D., Bell, G. M., Pecker, M. S., Sommers, S. C., and Laragh, J. H. (1988): Presidential address on the renal basis for essential hypertension: Nephron heterogeneity with discordant renin secretion and sodium excretion causing a hypertensive vasoconstric-tion-volume relationship. *J. Hypertension*, 6:763–777.

64. Van Breeman, C., Leijten, P., Yamamoto, H., Aaronson, P., and Cauvin, C. (1986): Ca^{2+} activation of vascular smooth muscle. *Hypertension*, 8(Suppl. II):II89–II95.

65. Van Zwieten, P. A., van Meel, J. A. C., and Timmermans, P. B. M. W. M. (1983): Pharmacology of calcium entry blockers interaction with vascular alpha-adrenoceptors. *Hypertension*, 5(Suppl. II):II-8–II-17.

66. Vaughan, E. D., Jr., Bühler, F. R., Laragh, J. H., Sealey, J. E., Baer, L., and Bard, R. H. (1973): Renovascular hypertension: Renin measurements to indicate hypersecretion and contralateral suppression, estimate renal plasma flow and score for surgical curability. *Am. J. Med.*, 55:402–414.

67. Vaughan, E. D., Jr., Laragh, J. H., Gavras, I., Bühler, F. R., Gavras, H., Brunner, H. R., and Baer, L. (1973): Volume factor in low and normal renin essential hypertension: Treatment with either spironolactone or chlorthalidone. *Am. J. Cardiol.*, 32:523–532.

68. Wallace, J. M., Case, D. B., Laragh, J. H., Sealey, J. E., Keim, H. J., and Drayer, J. I. M. (1977): The immediate pressor response to saralasin: A measure of the degree of angiotensin II vascular receptor vacancy. *Trans. Assoc. Am. Physicians*, 90:300–312.

New Therapeutic Strategies in Hypertension,
edited by Norman M. Kaplan,
Barry M. Brenner, and John H. Laragh.
Raven Press, Ltd., New York © 1989.

Withdrawal of Drug Therapy in the Treatment of Hypertension

Michael H. Alderman and Bernard Lamport

Department of Epidemiology and Social Medicine, Albert Einstein College of Medicine, Bronx, New York 10461

Soon after orally effective antihypertensive therapy became available, the question of whether successful treatment could be followed by sustained blood pressure control was raised. In 1962, Page and Dustan reported that 9 (33%) of 27 controlled hypertensive patients remained normotensive for more than 1 year following drug withdrawal (27). They (7,27), and other early observers (40), chose to focus primarily upon the recidivism that characterized the course of most patients whose pharmacological intervention had been interrupted. But it was also clear that the return of high blood pressure was gradual in virtually all patients, and, for a minority of subjects, normotension was maintained for periods in excess of a year.

The stimulus to withdraw drugs derives from several facts. The first relates to the admonition "primum non nocere." Virtually all medication carries the potential of adverse and sometimes unanticipated consequences. Some unwanted effects of aspirin, for example, were first noted only decades after this seemingly innocuous drug was introduced. The prospect of lifelong commitment to recently discovered and rather nonspecific therapy is particularly frightening. The second reason for physicians to resist unnecessary therapy is based upon the realization that the available drugs were not aimed at the "cause" of stroke or heart attack, but rather at an apparently predisposing "risk" factor. Not all hypertensives are candidates for stroke or heart attack. In fact, most hypertensive persons would live a long and happy life without benefit of therapeutic intervention. Since the benefit of drugs is realized by only a minority of hypertensive persons, avoidance of unnecessary drug therapy certainly makes sense. To these considerations can be added the urge not to "medicalize" so large a segment of the population and thereby further escalate health care costs. Quite appropriately, therefore, the 1988 Joint National Committee Report on the "Detection, Evaluation, and Treatment of High Blood Pressure" (31) has recommended that all successfully treated hypertensives be exposed to the possibility of drug withdrawal.

The goal of this chapter is to review the available data regarding the consequences of drug withdrawal in successfully treated patients and suggest guidelines for clinical practice. Systematic study of drug withdrawal from hypertensive patients is relatively new and, not surprisingly, sufficient information has not yet accumulated to make precise recommendations suitable for each clinical situation. General principles do, however, appear to be supportable on the basis of available evidence.

STUDIES OF DRUG WITHDRAWAL

Since the first report of Page and Dustan (27), there have been 18 studies of drug

Table 1. *Drug withdrawal after treatment of hypertension*

Reference	Number of patients	BP at withdrawal	Normotensive patients (%) ≥1 year
(27)	27	<95	33
(7)	34	<95	6
	9[a]	<95	0
(40)	69	<90	23
(41)	60[a]	<95	15
(3)	20	<100	5
(22)	24[a]	<90	5
(24)	31[a]	<90	74
(10)	59	<85	64
(20)A	70	<180/95	45
B	89[b]	<180/95	35
(37)	44[c]	<90	50
(1)	66	<140/85[d]	44
		<150/90[e]	
(26)	N/A[a]	<90	52
(6)	95	<140/90	28
	1647		32

[a] Placebo controlled.
[b] Patients were ≥120% above ideal weight.
[c] Alcohol intake <26 g/day.
[d] For patients <65.
[e] For patients ≥65.

withdrawal as part of the course of hypertensive treatment (1,3,6–8,10,18,20,22,24, 26,27,28,34,35,37,40,41). Four (18,28,34, 35) will not be further considered because of small numbers of participants, or short periods of observation. One study (8) was not included because it involved subjects on a low-salt diet <100 mEq/day. The remaining 13 studies included 1,647 patients (Table 1). Most patients had essential hypertension, although 25 patients with malignant hypertension, renal arterial stenosis, and/or renal parenchymal disease were included in several studies (7,27). The average age of patients was 54 years, and 60% were men. In most of the studies, the majority of patients were white. The "known" duration of hypertension varied from 0.5 to 22 years. The time of drug treatment before withdrawal varied from 0.5 to 10 years with a mean of 3.8 years. All classes of antihypertensive drugs in a variety of combinations were used. Levels of BP control believed sufficient for a trial of withdrawal

varied from 160/100 to 140/80 mmHg. In the Medical Research Council (MRC) study (26), withdrawal was arbitrarily undertaken after a specific period of treatment, regardless of BP level. The time of controlled BP on drugs before withdrawal varied from 0.5 to 5 years. Six studies were controlled (7,20,22,24,26,41) and in 5, the withdrawn drugs were replaced by placebo. The longest observed duration of normotension following withdrawal was 10 years (7). In 2 studies (20,37) drug withdrawal was accompanied by nutritional intervention (weight reduction and/or sodium restriction), and some studies were extensions of large scale intervention trials (26,41).

After completion of the Veterans Administration study (41), in which the pretreatment average BP was 171/112 mmHg, 86 patients whose treated DBP had been ≤95 mmHg for two years or longer were entered into a study to determine the effect of drug withdrawal. These 86 patients were assigned by stratified randomization so that 60 received placebo double blind and 26 were continued on active medication. During the 72 weeks of follow-up, 51 of the 60 placebo-treated patients had to terminate the trial. Of this number, 42 experienced return of increased arterial pressure, 6 had major cardiovascular complications, and 3 were removed for unrelated reasons to their BP. Among the 26 who were actively treated there were no morbid events and only one patient had a gradually rising DBP. Nevertheless, at the end of the 18-month period, 15% of 60 patients whose pretreatment BP averaged 171/109 mmHg were still normotensive without active drug therapy.

A similar study followed completion of the MRC trial (26). Of 4,286 early entrants who had completed 5½ years of follow-up (active and placebo groups) before the end of the study, 2,765 agreed to participate in a study of drug withdrawal. Patients who had been receiving bendrofluazide, propranolol, or a placebo were randomly assigned to continue their regimens or be

Table 2. *MRC study, patients withdrawn from therapy with diastolic pressure <90 mmHg 1 year later (%)*

		Men	Women
Bendrofluazide	Continued	73	83
	Withdrawn	57	56
Propranolol	Continued	79	77
	Withdrawn	48	45
Placebos	Continued	53	52
	Withdrawn	52	53

Adapted from ref. 26.

withdrawn. The report described 2,332 patients who completed three months of follow-up, 1,422 for 12 months, and 650 for 24 months.

The results are presented in Table 2. It can be seen that controlled pressure (DBP<90) was as likely to be maintained in patients withdrawn from active drugs as by those withdrawn from placebo. Thus, among these mildly hypertensive patients, withdrawal of active treatment for 9 to 12 months produced the same result in terms of blood pressure control as was reached by those withdrawn from placebo (Table 2). The authors reasonably concluded that long-term active drug use conferred no particular benefit. But, from the perspective of those interested in the consequences of drug withdrawal, it is important that 45 to 56% of those withdrawn from drugs were still normotensive 12 months later, as was realized also by those withdrawn from placebo (Table 2). This suggests that the explanation for prolonged drug-free normotension may have little to do with any effect produced by the active drug.

The effect of repeated withdrawal of antihypertensive drugs has not been studied. In patients who have had more than one period without drug treatment, the course of arterial pressure was reported to be similar each time (7). If this is confirmed, then the process of drug withdrawal can and must be repeated. The overall potential of drug withdrawal will then be substantially increased.

DEGREE OF SUCCESSFUL WITHDRAWAL OF DRUG TREATMENT

In the reported studies (Table 1), the percentage of successful withdrawal of drug treatment (maintenance of normal blood pressure for more than 1 year) varied from 0 to 74% with an average of 32%. Since all but one of these studies included selected patients and were not denominator based, they should not be used to estimate the percentage of all persons receiving BP medications who could manage without drugs.

One study (1) was, however, denominator based (Fig. 1). All 196 patients in a work-site-based hypertension control program were studied. To be eligible for the study, participants had to: 1) be taking BP medication at the time of initial screening, or 2) have an average of BP readings on at least two separate pretreatment occasions of ≥160/95 mmHg or higher; and have 3) a 6-month period of medication use, and 4) no contraindication to drug withdrawal such as angina or peripheral edema. The population investigated was predominantly female, and white, with a mean age of 55.7 years. The BP criteria for drug withdrawal were at least two readings in 6 months ≤140/85 mmHg for those younger than 65 years old, and ≤150/90 mmHg for those 65 and older. Of the 157 patients who met entry criteria, 88 (56.1%) met BP control criteria for withdrawal. It must be noted that if the criterion for BP control had been relaxed to ≤160/90 mmHg, then 98.6% of the entire group of patients would have been eligible for withdrawal. Sixty-six of these 88 patients actually had drugs withdrawn. Of these, 44 (70%) remained drug-free for more than one year; and at the end of the second year, 18 (54.5%) of the available 35 patients were still controlled. In sum, more than one-quarter of all patients in this general hypertensive population remained normotensive without drugs for at least one year.

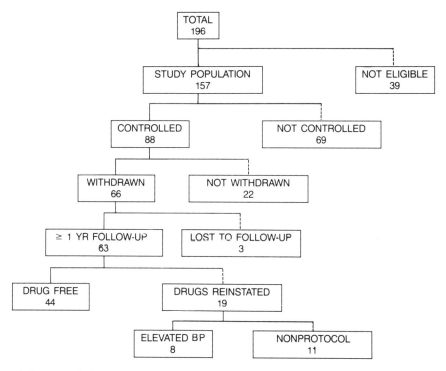

FIG. 1. Follow-up of withdrawal study population. (From Alderman et al., ref. 1, with permission.)

FACTORS INFLUENCING THE SUCCESS OF WITHDRAWAL

No studies have been specifically designed to determine whether there are demographic, constitutional, or clinical features of hypertensive patients, or aspects of process of treatment, or characteristics of the process of drug withdrawal, that determine the success or failure of drug withdrawal. However, assessment of the available data suggests that some general rules may apply.

Demographic Factors

Age

In the VA study, the 25 patients under age 50 experienced a rise in BP sooner after drug withdrawal than did 35 patients above age 50 (41). Several other observers also found that younger patients were less able to sustain posttreatment normotension than were older subjects (34,35). In one study however, just the reverse occurred (22). Thus, on the basis of the data, it is not possible to determine what, if any, impact age has on the likelihood of successful withdrawal. What is clear, however, is that even older subjects, whose vascular systems might be expected to condone less variability and whose hypertension is more established are able to interrupt medication and maintain normotension.

Race

In the VA study (41), after drug withdrawal BP rose more quickly in 30 black than in 30 white patients. The authors suggest that this probably related to the level of pretreatment BP, which was higher in black than white patients (DBP 112 and 106 mmHg, respectively).

Clinical Characteristics

Pretreatment BP Level

Not surprisingly, the likelihood of successful drug withdrawal and the mean duration of sustained normotension is strongly related to pretreatment levels. In virtually all studies, those with milder levels maintained normotension longer than did those with higher levels. For example, in the VA study (41), pretreatment BP in successfully withdrawn patients was 153/102 mmHg, while those who relapsed had prestudy levels of 174/110 mmHg.

This observation is clearly consistent with the view that blood pressure varies widely and, therefore, those closest to normal may have the best chance of achieving normality, at least on some occasions. In other words, regression toward the mean may account for some of the success observed after drugs are interrupted.

The Duration of Antihypertensive Therapy

This is of considerable importance since it would be of considerable value to know how soon an attempt to discontinue drugs could be made. Page and Dustan found that in 8 hypertensive patients treated for less than 2 years, 2 (25%) remained controlled for 1 year after drug withdrawal, while of 10 patients treated for 2 to 6 years, 8 (80%) remained normotensive, and in 12 patients treated for 5 to 9 years, 9 (76%) remained normotensive (27). It has more recently been suggested that withdrawal of drugs in hypertension could be attempted after six months of control (11). Others have suggested that the period of treatment should be longer than six months, but less than five

years (21). In the absence of more precise data, there appears to be no contraindication to attempting to remove drugs at any time. Moreover, despite the variety of their modes of action, there is no evidence that any particular drug treatment produces an important difference in posttreatment effect.

POSTWITHDRAWAL ACTIONS THAT MAY EXTEND NORMOTENSION (Table 3)

Nutritional interventions have been tested as means to extend the normotensive period after drugs. Since both sodium restriction and weight loss have been touted as effective means to reduce blood pressure, it is natural that they have also been recommended as adjuvants in the postwithdrawal phase.

In one uncontrolled study, it was suggested that sodium restriction was useful (8), since 75% of patients with salt restriction (<100 mEq/day) remained normotensive for one year after drug withdrawal, which appears to be higher than in studies not accompanied by salt restriction (see Table 1). In two controlled studies, the issue of nonpharmacological augmentation of drug withdrawal has been assessed (20,37). In one (37), 141 drug-withdrawn subjects were allocated to either alcohol restriction alone, or in association with weight reduction and sodium restriction. It was found that the more comprehensively advised group did better (69 versus 50%, $p<0.03$) than the alcohol alone restricted group at one year (Table 3).

A more discrete model was assessed among graduates of the Hypertension Detection and Follow-Up Program (HDFP) study (20) (Table 3). Participants were stratified into overweight and normal weight categories. Normal weight subjects were randomized to sodium restricted or control groups after drug withdrawal. Of note is the

Table 3. *Influence of nutritional intervention on blood pressure after drug withdrawal—%*
normotensive[a] at 1 year

Reference	Weight status[b]	Intervention	Experimental % (#)	Control % (#)	Significance
(20)	Normal	Na[c] <40 mEq/day	53(68)	45(70)	n.s.
	20% overweight	Na[c] <40 mEq/day	45(101)	35(89)	n.s.
	20% overweight	4.5 kg weight loss[d]	59(87)	35(89)	<0.05
(37)	10 to 49% overweight	Na+ <78 mEq/day +1.8 kg[d] weight loss	69(97)	50(44)	<0.03 chi-square = 4.73

[a] <180/95 mmHg in (20): and <90 in (37).
[b] By 1959 Metropolitan Life Insurance Tables for Desirable Body Weights.
[c] Alcohol <26 g/day.
[d] Group mean.

fact that, overall, persons of normal weight had greater success than thse who were obese. The overweight subjects were further randomized to either sodium restriction, weight loss, or control groups. Sodium restriction conferred no important advantage, but weight loss substantially increased the likelihood of success at one year.

The potential contribution to blood pressure containment that calcium, potassium, and/or fat intake might make has not been specifically evaluated. The value of physical exercise had not been assessed either.

WHAT IS THE MECHANISM OF POSTWITHDRAWAL NORMOTENSION?

Resetting the Baroreceptor

The notion that a change in carotid sinus barorcccptor setting could be responsible for postwithdrawal normotension was first suggested by Page and Dustan in 1962 (27). It had been previously shown that the carotid sinus of a Goldblatt dog lost the capacity to react by electric discharge to a further elevation of BP. Page and Dustan suggested that prolonged artificial normotension restored the ability of carotid baroreceptor to react to increased BP by lowering it. While attractive, this hypothesis lacks experimental validation.

Structural Regression

Vascular wall thickening (2) and left ventricular hypertrophy (LVH) (14) have long been recognized as consequences of sustained high blood pressure, although these morphological findings may sometimes preceed the discovery of hypertension. Both these structural changes are also believed to play a role in sustaining hypertension. Following discovery of effective antihypertensive therapy, it was demonstrated that prolonged artificial reduction of blood pressure could reverse these structural changes (13,15,17). It was then noted, first in rats (4) and then in men (18,19), that the maintenance of normotension after drug therapy withdrawal was related to the regression of the heart and blood vessel enlargement. There was, however, a study involving 24 patients in which it was discovered that left ventricular mass did not differ between patients whose pressure remained normal and those whose pressure rose after drug withdrawal (22).

On balance, the weight of evidence supports the logical notion that some hypertrophy of vessels and heart play a role in the maintenance of blood pressure elevation.

Table 4. *Spontaneous remission among persons with initial BP >160/95 mmHg*

Reference	Number of patients	Follow-up (years)	% <160/95 mmHg
(32)	1,963	3	48
(23)	865	5	40

When corrected by therapy, this might contribute to sustained normotension. The "structural-regression" hypothesis suggests a potentially predictive sign of what might happen after drug withdrawal. Patients with pronounced regression, or absence of LVH, and/or elevated total peripheral resistance index would be promising candidates for successful withdrawal of drug treatment.

The Natural History of Blood Pressure Hypothesis

Blood pressure varies each day and over time in all persons, both hypertensive and normotensive. Moreover, long-term studies of representative populations demonstrate that not all persons experience a rise in pressure over time. In fact, pressure often actually falls (23,32) (Table 4). Of 865 control subjects with initial DBP >160/95 mmHg 40% had, after 5 years, BP <160/95 mmHg despite no treatment (23). In the Australian National Trial of Antihypertensive therapy (32) 48% of mild hypertensives who had been randomized to the control-placebo group experienced a fall in pressure that persisted up to three years (32).

POTENTIAL AND REAL HAZARDS OF DRUG WITHDRAWAL

No studies of drug withdrawal in hypertension have reported any substantial adverse consequences. However, there are three possible areas of reasonable concern:

loss to follow-up, withdrawal syndrome, and increased risk of CVD after withdrawal of drugs even by normotensive subjects.

Loss to Follow-Up

Loss of follow-up has plagued hypertension control efforts since the dawn of the modern treatment era. Attrition is high even in regular drug treatment programs and its increase after drug withdrawal seems a reasonable project (36). But, to our knowledge, no study has shown that dropouts increase after drugs are withdrawn. In fact, among patients withdrawn from drugs in one study (1) it was specifically noted that there was no increase in patient loss. Nevertheless, it is reasonable to be concerned that in this asymptomatic condition, some patients, lacking the need to refill a prescription, would permit their adherence to lapse. We believe, however, that patient adherence is central to all antihypertensive treatment and must be vigorously addressed in drug treated as well as withdrawn patients.

Withdrawal Syndrome

Three kinds of withdrawal syndrome have been noted to follow cessation of antihypertensive therapy (29): (1) BP remains relatively controlled or rises comparatively slowly, but the patient experiences signs and symptoms of sympathetic overactivity, or the occurrence of some morbid CVD event in predisposed patients, such as unstable angina, arrhythmias, AMI, or sudden death; (2) a rapid return of BP to pretreatment levels with symptoms and signs of sympathetic overactivity and sometimes encephalopathy, cerebrovascular accidents, or other catastrophic CV events; and (3) "overshoot" of hypertension—a rapid rise of BP above pretreatment levels associated with subjective symptoms and signs of sympathetic overactivity and/or morbid CV events. These forms of withdrawal syndrome presumably may develop after cessation of treatment with all classes of antihypertensive drugs, but have actually been seen to develop in only a few situations, i.e., after withdrawal of the central alpha-adrenoceptors clonidine and methyldopa (29). Happily, in studies designed specifically to assess the impact of drug withdrawal, there has been no notice of any form of withdrawal syndrome. However, it certainly might occur and is a strong argument for continuing surveillance. Sufficient experience now exists, however, to make it exceedingly unlikely that an immediate catastrophic clinical event will immediately follow drug withdrawal. If reasonable precautions of gradual withdrawal are followed, risks should be minimal, particularly in mild or moderate hypertension.

Unanticipated Loss of Cardioprotective Effect

Some antihypertensive agents have cardioprotective effects beyond their hypotensive capacity, i.e., beta blockers (5). Perhaps their withdrawal could increase risk of myocardial infarction. In view of the fact that in clinical trials of therapy for mild hypertension there was no cardioprotective effect of treatment, this seems more a theoretical than a practical concern.

By contrast, however, in the withdrawal study following the VA trial (41) which involved patients with average entry BP of 171/112 mmHg, of 60 patients withdrawn from drug treatment, 6 developed severe cardiovascular complications (fatal MI, nonfatal congestive heart failure, atrial fibrillation, and right bundle branch block), while none of 26 patients continuing drug treatment had such serious CVD complications. Although this difference did not attain significance, in view of the small sample size its importance remains. It should be noted that these patients were severely hypertensive before treatment, and after withdrawal were premitted to have pressures well above normal. Clearly, the conditions of drug reintroduction that characterized current practice were not applied in that study.

ADVANTAGES OF DRUG WITHDRAWAL

Medical

Antihypertensive drugs can adversely effect electrolyte, carbohydrate, and lipid metabolism (12,33,38). Withdrawal of drugs have been shown to normalize these metabolic shifts. Patients treated with diuretics have been shown to experience hyperuricemia, hyperglycemia, hyperlipidemia, and hypokalemia (33). It is hard to imagine that these metabolic dearrangements offer any particular medical benefit, although the actual extent of their adverse consequences is unknown. In a variety of studies (10,33,41), it has been shown that most metabolic alterations disappear or, at the very least, tend to regress toward pretreatment levels after drugs are withdrawn. Other adverse reactions to bendrofluazide and/or propranolol such as impotence, dizziness, Raynaud's phenomenon, dyspnea, rash, lethagy, nausea, and headaches, also were rapidly reversible after withdrawal of these drugs (33). Moreover, drug discontinuation has a substantial psychological effect by providing patients with objective evidence of improvement (9).

Economic

About 33% of 60 million hypertensive patients in the United States, or about 20 million patients, are taking antihypertensive medication (30). Extrapolation from the small denominator-based experience available (1) suggests that it may be possible to interrupt, for periods as long as one year, the drugs of one-quarter of these patients. This would translate into 5 million persons free of drugs and still normotensive.

The annual cost of drug treatment is about $200 ($140 for drugs and $60 for laboratory tests to detect drug complications) (39). Elimination of this cost for 5 million patients would mean an annual savings of $1 billion.

CONCLUSION

What then are reasonable recommendations for clinical practice that derive from the accumulated experience reviewed here? We believe that the data sustain several important conclusions. First, that discontinuation of antihypertensive drugs in successfully treated hypertensive patients is safe. In fact, there is little credible evidence that, even in patients whose pretreatment blood pressure levels were very high, that there was any risk of dramatic adverse effects. Second, although blood pressure tends to rise in most patients after drug withdrawal so by the end of one year, the majority again require pharmacological intervention, the return is gradual, and a substantial minority remain normotensive for at least one year. Third, only pretreatment level of pressure predicts the likelihood of successful withdrawal and, not surprisingly, milder patients tend to do better than more severe hypertensives. Nevertheless, patients with higher pressures do have the capacity, sometimes, to maintain normotension for prolonged periods of time. They also deserve an attempt at withdrawal. The promising observation that regression of heart and blood vessel hypertrophy may predict successful withdrawal requires further assessment. Fourth, nonpharmacological measures may, in some patients, improve the chances for extending the period of normotension. This appears more likely when weight loss rather than sodium restriction is prescribed. Fifth, treatment-associated metabolic arrangements disappear in most patients following drug withdrawal. Finally (and disappointingly), it is not possible to explain why normotension persists in some patients whose drugs are removed, or why it fails in others. This should hardly be surprising since neither the explanation for blood pressure elevation nor the determinants of its natural history are known.

In sum, the withdrawal of antihypertensive drug therapy deserves to become a standard dimension in the care of patients with high blood pressure. The notion that all hypertensive patients must remain on drugs for the rest of their lives is no longer consistent with available medical knowledge. Indeed, the regular attempt to reduce and, when possible, discontinue all medication should become a routine component of good medical practice for each and every patient. The goal of care is blood pressure control purchased with the least possible therapeutic intrusion. While the exact duration of successful control that should preceed an attempt to discontinue drugs is unknown, it is generally felt that perhaps six months, or certainly one year, is a sufficient period to preceed withdrawal of drug therapy with safety and some chance of success. It should be done gradually and in combination with regular patient follow-up to ensure timely reintroduction of drug therapy.

If interrupted treatment becomes standard therapy, perhaps one-quarter of all treated hypertensives may be successfully managed without drugs for periods in excess of one year. Society will benefit through reduced drug costs, but more importantly, the real gains will be to large numbers of individual patients freed of the discomfort, potential hazards, and expense of drug dependence without sacrificing the benefits of normal blood pressure.

REFERENCES

1. Alderman, M. H., David, T. K., Gerber, L. M., and Robb, M. (1986): Antihypertensive drug therapy withdrawal in a general population. *Arch. Intern. Med.*, 148:1309–1311.
2. Berry, C. (1985): Mechanical vascular changes and hypertension: Pathological consequences. *Path. Res. Pract.*, 180:336–337.

3. Boyle, R. M., Price, M. L., and Hamilton, M. (1979): Thiazide withdrawal in hypertension. *J. Royal Coll. Physicians Lond.*, 13:172–173.
4. Cadilhac, M., and Giudicelli, J. F. (1986): Myocardial and vascular effects of perindopril, a new converting enzyme inhibitor, during hypertension development in spontaneously hypertensive rats. *Arch. Int. Pharmacodyn.*, 284:114–126.
5. Cohn, J. N. (1987): Role of drugs for systemic hypertension and their effect on the heart. *Am. J. Cardiol.*, 60:72G–74G.
6. Dannenberg, A. L., and Kannel, W. B. (1987): Remission of hypertension: The 'natural' history of blood pressure treatment in the Framingham study. *JAMA*, 257:1177–1183.
7. Dustan, H. P., Page, I. H., Tarazi, R. C., and Frolich, E. D. (1968): Arterial pressure responses to discontinuing antihypertensive drugs. *Circulation*, 37:370–379.
8. Fernandez, P. G., Galway, A. B., Kim, B. K., and Granter, S. (1982): Prolonged normotension following cessation of therapy in uncomplicated essential hypertension. *Clin. Investigative Med.*, 5:31–37.
9. Finnerty, F. A. (1981): Step-down therapy in hypertension: Importance in long-term management. *JAMA*, 246:2593–2596.
10. Finnerty, F. A. (1984): Step-down treatment of mild systemtic hypertension. *Am. J. Cardiol.*, 53:1304–1307.
11. Finnerty, F. A. (1985): Slowing the return of hypertension after stopping medication: A letter. *JAMA*, 254:503.
12. Flamenbaum, W. (1983): Metabolic consequences of antihypertensive therapy. *Arch. Intern. Med.*, 98(part 2):875–880.
13. Folkow, B. (1987): The structual factor in primary hypertension: Its relevance for future principles of treatment. *J. Hypertens.*, 5(Suppl 5):5611–5613.
14. Frolich, E. D. (1988): The heart in hypertension: Unresolved conceptual challenges. *Hypertension*, 11(Suppl 1):1-19–1-24.
15. Hartford, M., Wendelhag, I., and Berglund, G., et al. (1988): Cardiovascular and renal effects of long-term antihypertensive treatment. *JAMA*, 259:2553–2557.
16. Houston, M. C. (1981): Abrupt cessation of treatment in hypertension: Considerations of clinical features, mechanisms, prevention and management of the discontinuation syndrome. *Am. Heart J.*, 102:415–430.
17. Jennings, G. L., Esler, M. D., and Korner, P. H. (1980): Effect of prolonged treatment on haemodynamics of essential hypertension before and after autonomic block. *Lancet*, 11:166–169.
18. Jennings, G. L., Korner, P., Esler, M., and Restall, R. (1984): Redevelopment of essential hypertension after cessation of long term therapy: Preliminary findings. *Clin. and Exp. Hyper-Theory Pract.*, A6(1&2):493–505.
19. Korner, P. I., Jennings, G. L., Esler, M. D., and Broughton, A. (1987): A new approach to the identification of pathogenetic factors and to therapy in human primary hypertension. *J. Clin. Hypertens.*, 3:187–196.
20. Langford, H. G., Blaufox, D., Oberman, A., et al. (1985): Dietary therapy slows the return of hypertension after stopping prolonged medication. *JAMA*, 253:657–664.
21. Langford, H. G., Blaufox, M. D., Oberman, A., and Hawkins, C. M. (1985): A letter. *JAMA*, 254:503.
22. Levinson, P. D., Khatri, I. M., and Freis, E. D. (1982): Persistence of normal BP after withdrawal of drug treatment in mild hypertension. *Arch. Intern. Med.* 142:2265–2268.
23. Liu, L., Ling, Y., and Jao, S. (1979): A five year follow-up study of hypertension in 10,450 steel workers. *Chinese Med. J.*, 92:719–722.
24. Maland, L. J., Lutz, L. J., and Castle, H. (1983): Effect of withdrawing diuretic therapy on blood pressure in mild hypertension. *Hypertension*, 5:539–544.
25. McCubbin, J. W., Green, J. H., and Page, I. H. (1956): Baroreceptor function in chronic renal hypertension. *Circulation Res.*, 4:205–210.
26. Medical Research Council Working Party on Mild Hypertension. (1986): Course of blood pressure in mild hypertensives after withdrawal of long term antihypertensive treatment. *Br. Med. J.*, 293:988–992.
27. Page, I. H., and Dustan, H. P. (1962): Persistence of normal blood pressure after discontinuing treatment in hypertensive patients. Editorial. *Circulation*, 25:433–436.
28. Perry, H. M., Schroeder, H. A., Catanzaro, F. J., Moore-Jones, D., and Camel, G. H. (1966): Studies on the control of hypertension, VIII: Mortality, morbidity, and remissions during twelve years of intensive therapy. *Circulation*, 33:958–972.
29. Reid, J. L. (1986): Alpha-adrenergic receptors and blood pressure control. *Am. J. Cardiol.*, 57:6E–12E.
30. Report. (1985): Hypertension prevalence and the status of awareness, treatment, and control in the United States: Final Report of the Subcommittee on Definition and Prevalence of the 1984 Joint National Committee. *Hypertension*, 7:457–468.
31. Report. (1988): 1988 Joint National Committee. The 1988 Report of the Joint National Committee on detection, evaluation, and treatment of high blood pressure. *Arch. Intern. Med.*, 148:1023–1038.
32. Report by the Management Committee of the Australian Therapeutic Trial in Mild Hypertension. (1982): Untreated mild hypertension. *Lancet*, II:185–191.
33. Report of Medical Research Council Working Party on Mild to Moderate Hypertension. (1982): Adverse reactions to bendrofluazide and propranolol for the treatment of mild hypertension. *Lancet*, II:539–542.

34. Ruoff, G. (1986): Effect of withdrawal of tera-zosin therapy in patients with hypertension. *Am. J. Med.*, 80(Suppl 5B):35–41.
35. Smith, S. A., Mace, J. E., and Litter, W. A. (1986): Felodipine, blood pressure, and cardio-vascular reflexes in hypertensive humans. *Hypertension*, 8:1172–1178.
36. Smith, W. M. (1982): Resetting of barostat re-vised. *Arch. Intern. Med.*, 142:2263–2264.
37. Stamler, R., Stamler, J., Grimm, R., et al. (1987): Nutritionoal therapy for high blood pressure: Final report of a four-year randomized controlled trial—the hypertension control program. *JAMA*, 257:1184–1191.
38. Stark, R. M. (1988): The atherogenic risk of an-tihypertensive therapy. *Am. J. Med.*, 84(Suppl 1B):86–88.
39. Stason, W. B. (1986): Opportunities for improv-ing the cost-effectiveness of antihypertensive treatment. *Am. J. Med.*, 81(Suppl 6C):45–49.
40. Thurm, R. H., and Smith, W. M. (1967): On re-setting of "Barostats" in hypertensive patients. *JAMA*, 201:85–88.
41. Veteran Administration Cooperative Study Group on Antihypertensive Agents. (1975): Re-turn of elevated blood pressure after withdrawal of antihypertensive drugs. *Circulation*, 51:1107–1113.

New Therapeutic Strategies in Hypertension,
edited by Norman M. Kaplan,
Barry M. Brenner, and John H. Laragh.
Raven Press, Ltd., New York © 1989.

Treatment of Severe Hypertension

Lionel H. Opie

Department of Medicine and Hypertension Clinic, University of Cape Town Medical School and Groote Schuur Hospital, Observatory 7925, South Africa

True hypertensive emergencies are rare but require hospital admission, preferably to an Intensive Care Unit. Threatened acute impairment of vital end-organ function (brain, heart, kidney) may dominate the therapeutic requirements. In contrast, much more typical is urgent hypertension without acute life-threatening severe end-organ complications. Sublingual or oral nifedipine is frequently used in the latter situation. However, initiation of oral therapy with other standard agents such as oral atenolol or labetalol would probably be equally effective, although not as rapid in onset of action. Labetalol may be safer than atenolol in avoiding a reactive hypertension in inapparent cases of pheochromocytoma. Angiotensin enzyme inhibitors may also be used after exclusion of bilateral renal artery stenosis. The combination nifedipine-captopril seems promising. When intravenous (IV) therapy is deemed appropriate, the emphasis has swung away from agents previously used such as diazoxide and hydralazine to newer compounds such as labetalol. Other available IV agents include sodium nitroprusside, verapamil, and furosemide. Of these, verapamil especially deserves wider use. Throughout it is imperative to balance the benefits of acute blood pressure reduction versus the risks of end-organ ischemia caused by excess hypotension.

SIGNIFICANCE OF SEVERE HYPERTENSION

The therapy of mild to moderate hypertension remains desirable, however, in absolute terms the benefit may be modest. For example, Strasser of the World Health Organization in Geneva, estimates that the risk of mild hypertension might be somewhere between driving a car and smoking cigarettes (34). Likewise, the recent British Medical Research Council trial (24) suggested that the therapy of 850 patients with mild hypertension for one year might be required to prevent one stroke. Even in the case of severe hypertension the documented benefits of therapy are limited. Some of the earliest outcome trials in hypertension showed that patients in the malignant phase, but without severe renal impairment, had a good response to treatment (15); and even despite renal failure, therapy seemed to be effective (5,37). However, no properly controlled studies have ever been undertaken. In the case of acute therapy of severe hypertension there are likewise no correctly designed prospective trials. Clearly double-blind trials are ethically open to criticism, yet the problem remains that, unless firm end-points are measured, it is difficult to know what therapy of hypertension achieves apart from blood pressure reduction. Furthermore, there appear to be no data assessing the outcome of severe hypertension when a gradual drop of blood pressure is compared with a sudden drop. A start has now been made by a comparison of nifedipine and nitroprusside regarding cost-effectiveness and efficacy of blood pressure control in severe hypertensives (12). Therefore, while it is axiomatic that severe hypertension is dangerous for the patient, just how dangerous it really is remains a matter of conjecture. While no one would argue that severely hypertensive patients should be untreated, we remain severely handicapped by not knowing exactly what therapy can be expected to accomplish.

CLINICAL PICTURE

Severe hypertension is usually taken as a sustained diastolic level of above 120 mmHg (5th Korotkoff point, disappearance of heart sounds). The fear is that such levels may give rise to serious complications including stroke and other cerebrovascular complications, renal failure, and myocardial infarction. In assessing the patient, the first point to decide is whether the diastolic pressure is really that high; we have found that in some patients quiet bedrest for one hour results in much more acceptable diastolic levels. The process of an office or hospital visit seems falsely to elevate the blood pressure in many patients. Other patients may be seen early in the morning during a "therapeutic gap" between taking the drugs and their effect; especially during therapy with the vasodilator group including nifedipine that may have marked "pulsed" effects. Therefore, the ideal practice is to: recheck the initial blood pressure, elicit a full history and do a careful examination for end-organ damage, all the time not conveying any sense of emergency, and repeat blood pressure measurements over a period of time, including the end of the evaluation.

URGENCY RATHER THAN EMERGENCY

A critical point to decide is whether the patient has urgent hypertension requiring rapid evaluation and urgent (but not instant) therapy or whether the hypertension and its complications are truly sufficiently severe to constitute a genuine medical emergency. This distinction between "urgency" and "emergency" is critical and most patients, even with high diastolic blood pressures, fall into the "urgent" group. If the blood pressure elevation is not genuinely compelling and if there are no serious end-organ complications demanding specific therapy, a reasonable policy is to initiate a relatively simple "standard" oral therapy such as nifedipine (16) or atenolol (17) or labetalol (14). Thereafter, either bring the patient into hospital for full evaluation or, if already evaluated on the previous occasion, monitor the response to nifedipine (whether introduced as sole therapy in patients who have lapsed from their previous therapy, or whether brought in as additional agent) over 24 hr by ambulatory blood pressure monitoring. The patient should return the next day. We have been surprised at the number of patients with apparently frightening initial blood pressure values who, even without any therapy, show much lower values during the course of 24-hr monitoring.

Even some patients with high diastolic values and papilledema or fresh hemorrhages and exudates (= malignant hypertension) present with no other clinically detectable end-organ damage requiring emergency therapy and can initially be treated by monotherapy such as atenolol or nifedipine (17), so the problem remains one of urgency rather than of emergency. In our hospital, we emphasize the difference between full evaluation of the patient, which is urgent, and the institution of antihypertensive therapy, which may be less urgent.

TREATMENT OF URGENT HYPERTENSION

Nifedipine

In nonemergency, but urgent, hypertension, we have come to use nifedipine as an agent of first choice (Fig. 1). We have studied more than 200 patients (always after careful overall evaluation, including physical examination) and, with very few ex-

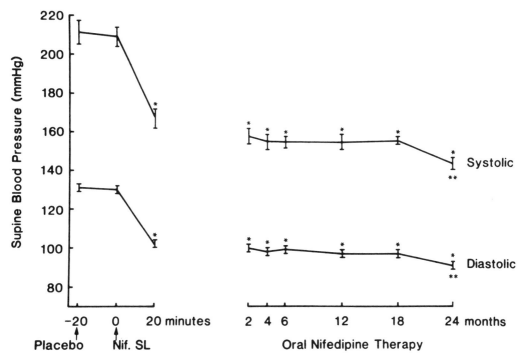

FIG. 1. Comparison of short- and long-term effects of nifedipine (Nif) on severe and apparently refractory hypertension. Note that placebo induces no change in the mean blood pressure values, but that short-term administration of nifedipine reduces the blood pressure. The effect at 20 min (10 mg sublingually) in 18 patients follow-up for 24 months is similar to the effect at 24 months (10 mg orally). Mean values ± SEM. * Difference from time zero with $p < 0.001$; ** difference from 20 min value with $p < 0.01$ (Reproduced from Jennings, et al., ref. 18, with permission of the *American Heart Journal*.)

ceptions, have achieved a substantial reduction in blood pressure. Our experience accords with that of others. It seems, in the absence of a clinically threatened end-organ, rapid reduction of blood pressure is safe, seemingly simple, and without obvious dangers (18).

Although usually given sublingually in severe hypertension, the most rapid absorption of nifedipine is found with the bite-and-swallow technique (35). Such a rapid onset of action suits the doctor but is not essential for the patient, so the use of ordinary oral capsules should be quite satisfactory (16).

There are, however, a few reservations. First, we believe it essential to evaluate the possible dangers of acute blood pressure reduction in the given patient. Thus, nifedi-

pine should not be given indiscriminantly to a patient who has not been examined and evaluated. It is not known whether the rapid rate of fall of blood pressure achieved with nifedipine is beneficial or harmful. The rarity of excess hypotension (not found in our studies, except in some patients in whom there was an interaction with prazosin or beta-blockade) and the limited fall of blood pressure in response to the relatively low dose used (Fig. 1), as well as the cerebral vasodilatory properties of nifedipine (4), may be of importance in avoiding cerebral side effects during the initial rapid hypotensive phase of action of nifedipine.

Second, in elderly patients where baroreflexes are depressed and cardiovascular reflexes may not be so effective, 5 mg nifedipine should be given as an initial test dose. In countries where 5 mg capsules are not available, such as the United States, the contents of a 10 mg capsule can be sucked into a syringe and half administered to the patient. Alternatively, the capsule can be cut approximately in half.

Third, the actual benefit of nifedipine is not proven, although acute blood pressure reduction can apparently be achieved without any harm. Oral nifedipine, however, is better than IV nitroprusside because it is simpler, requires less time in the Intensive Care Unit (12), and avoids the danger of rebound found after nitroprusside. Slow reduction of blood pressure (for example, by atenolol or presumably by other beta blockers; or by labetalol; or by other dihydropyridines with a slower onset of action, such as nifedipine tablets (17), should achieve the same effect. Of these alternative therapies, we prefer labetalol which carries with it less risk of precipitation of a crisis in patients with pheochromocytoma than does the use of a beta blocker such as atenolol. The major benefit of the rapid reduction with nifedipine is the knowledge that the lower blood pressure can be achieved within only 20 to 30 min. This is reassuring to both patient and doctor; furthermore, time and money are saved for the patient.

Nifedipine Resistance and Combination Oral Therapy

In a minority of patients, less than 10% of our population of severely hypertensives (18), one capsule of nifedipine has little or no effect on the blood pressure. If there is some, but inadequate, effect even after waiting 45 min after the first capsule, the next step is to administer another 10 mg and to wait a further 20 to 30 min. If there is still little or no response, in our experience a further increase of dose is unlikely to be effective. On first principles, the problem is likely to be that the acute vasodilation in-

duced by nifedipine has been limited by the baroreflex response which involves adrenergic alpha- and beta-stimulation, also with increased levels of renin and angiotensin-II. We have therefore added to prior nifedipine therapy, 2 mg prazosin and/or 25 mg captopril, the latter 30 min after a test dose of 6.25 mg chewed. The combination nifedipine-captopril especially is one that we have found to be very effective, although not uniformly successful in cases of nifedipine resistance (for follow-up we frequently use nifedipine-captopril-diuretic). We have no experience with nifedipine-labetalol, yet the latter agent combined with alpha-beta-blocking properties should logically combine well with nifedipine. Labetalol should inhibit all the efferent arcs of the baroreceptor reflex.

Other Calcium Antagonists

Oral Verapamil

Oral verapamil takes only 30 min for a hypotensive effect (8), but experience in severe hypertension is very limited.

Diltiazem

Intravenous diltiazem (investigational) as a bolus injection of 0.2 mg/kg followed by an infusion of 0.1 mg/kg for 25 min has been compared with dihydralazine 0.1 mg/kg for 25 min (30). Dihydralazine was more effective in reducing total peripheral resistance and blood pressure but increased the heart rate and cardiac index considerably, whereas diltiazem left both of these essentially unchanged. Furthermore, diltiazem increased the brachial artery diameter and the flow through it, whereas dihydralazine decreased the brachial artery diameter and left the flow unchanged. Intravenous diltiazem is not generally available, yet the oral form takes only about 60 min for a hemodynamic effect (8) and deserves wider testing. We have tested the acute hypotensive effect of *oral diltiazem* (average dose 90 mg) and found that blood pressure fell, ejection fraction rose, and diastolic function improved. All these effects were very similar to one nifedipine 10 mg capsule, except that the latter acted more rapidly.

Beta-blockade by Atenolol

Conventional therapy with an "ordinary" beta blocker without dilating qualities such as atenolol has also been shown to control even malignant hypertension (2,17). The atenolol study is important because it shows that simple therapy is effective even in malignant hypertension, although the blood pressure may come down less abruptly. It must be recalled that it is by no means certain that rapid blood pressure reduction is always safe or desirable. We do not routinely use beta-blockade in urgent hypertension because a small number of such patients will be suffering from pheochromocytoma with sustained blood pressure values, and beta blockade may precipitate a hypertensive crisis.

Oral Clonidine

If it is desired to sedate the patient and to treat hypertension rapidly, a standard oral dose of clonidine (because of its rapid absorption and high bioavailability) will act within $\frac{1}{2}$ to 2 hr. In some countries intramuscular (IM) clonidine is available; however, all IM agents should be avoided whenever possible in severe hypertension.

Other Regimes: Prazosin, Oral Labetalol, Sublingual Captopril

Other regimes that have been used for severe hypertension are the acute administration of oral prazosin or oral labetalol (14) or sublingual captopril (2) (Table 1). However, there is a reservation to the use of captopril. In severe hypertension, there always is the

possibility (however remote) that the disease may be caused by renal artery stenosis, in which case the high-circulating renin values may cause a dramatic response to ACE inhibition, including overshoot hypotension and potential renal failure. This risk is much more marked in the rare patient with bilateral renal artery stenosis. Therefore, when renal disease or renal artery stenosis cannot be excluded, and captopril is used for conditions such as severe hypertension and congestive heart failure combined, a very low, initial test dose (about 6.25 mg captopril sublingually) is mandatory. Thirty minutes later 25 mg captopril may be given. Enalapril with a much slower onset of action is not advisable because of the delay in assessing the results of a test dose.

Follow-up Therapy

The *combination beta-blockade-nifedipine* has been available as acebutolol-nifedipine in Europe for some time, and the new combination of atenolol-nifedipine is shortly to be marketed. Such combinations would be logical carry-on therapy after the acute phase of urgent blood pressure reduction with nifedipine is over. When the acute phase therapy has been nifedipine-captopril, we have continued this combination with success in the follow-up period. Frequently a diuretic is added to nifedipine-atenolol or nifedipine-captopril.

TRUE EMERGENCY CRISES

Sometimes, although increasingly less so, severe hypertension presents a true crisis situation. The clinical conditions causing the emergency can be threatened stroke, congestive cardiac failure, and accelerating renal failure.

Hypertensive Encephalopathy

This condition, frequently discussed and taught, may in reality be rather rare. By

Table 1. *Oral hypotensive agents for use in hypertensive urgencies*[a]

Agent	Usual dose	Side effects	Comments
Nifedipine	10–20 mg sublingually or orally; repeat within 2 hr if needed, then 10 mg every 6-hr. Alternatively, 1 tablet of 40 mg nifedipine slow-release preparation	Few unless excess hypotension. Theoretical risk of cerebral ischemia seems remote in practice, except in elderly	Simple therapy, usually effective; needs further evaluation in presence of papilledema and hypertensive encephalopathy. If no response after second dose, add prazosin or captopril
Labetalol	400 mg orally, then 100–200 mg every 6-hr	Few unless excess hypotension; exclude asthma, heart block	If no response within 2 hr, change drug
Atenolol	100 mg orally once daily	Exclude pheochromocytoma, asthma, sinus bradycardia, heart block	Slower onset of action than with nifedipine, lower heart rate
Captopril	25 mg chewed	Risk of renal failure	Exclude renal artery stenosis; not well-tested. Add furosemide if no response to captopril

[a] Caution, see text for reservations.

definition encephalopathy should be a generalized deterioration of the activity of the brain, responding to removal of the metabolic or similar diffuse cause and without an underlying focal neurological lesion. An analogy would be hepatic encephalopathy where there is no true cerebral damage but mental function is impaired by metabolic changes in the circulation. Logically, hypertensive encephalopathy should be found in conjunction with papilledema because of severely raised intracranial pressure. Some adult patients apparently having hypertensive encephalopathy probably have threatened strokes (23) or small hemorrhages.

In children, however, especially those with severe glomerular nephritis, the cerebral deterioration in association with excessively high blood pressure (sometimes only moderately elevated) is correctly termed "hypertensive encephalopathy". True hypertensive encephalopathy demands blood pressure reduction; however, the ideal rate of blood pressure reduction is not known nor are there any trials available about the agents used in the therapy of this condition. It is important clinically to differentiate hypertensive encephalopathy from threatened stroke.

Threatened Stroke

Threatened stroke presents a different situation where the possibility of antihypertensive therapy reducing flow through a carotid or vertebral artery stenosis must be considered (see Cerebral Autoregulation) so that considerable care in blood pressure reduction is required.

Threatened stroke may encompass two diverse clinical situations: severe hypertension with past transient ischemic attacks especially in the presence of carotid artery bruits and focal cerebral signs evolving during the physical examination of a patient with severe hypertension. The former is not an emergency and merely calls for avoidance of excess hypotension. In the latter sit-uation, the hypertension might either be contributing to the evolution of the stroke, or possibly helping to maintain blood pressure to the ischemic area. No clinical trials appear to be available. In a given patient, it is not possible to indicate whether the high blood pressure itself is helpful or harmful without a trial of therapy. Carefully controlled blood pressure reduction by a very slow infusion of labetalol or nitroprusside seems indicated, all the time reevaluating whether the progressive fall of pressure is beneficial or not. Of these two agents, labetalol might be easier to use than nitroprusside because the latter agent requires very tight hemodynamic control and carries the risk of rebound hypertension.

Hypertensive Heart Failure

Diastolic Dysfunction

In *compensated hypertrophy,* patients may present with radiologic cardiomegaly, hypertension, and exertional dyspnea. There may, in addition, be a fourth heart sound, the result of atrial hypertrophy. The combination may lead to the diagnosis of congestive heart failure. When, however, the ejection fraction is measured, it is usually high or high-normal. This apparent paradox may be explained as follows: the ejection fraction is essentially a reflection of the systolic function of the heart and its interaction with the peripheral vascular resistance and aortic impedance. As myocardial hypertrophy develops in response to sustained hypertension, there is diastolic dysfunction of the heart, which probably explains the dyspnea in the absence of pulmonary crepitations. Therapy with digoxin is not appropriate for this category of patient; rather, afterload reduction with an antihypertensive agent is required. In the present state of knowledge and in the absence of definite outcome trials, no preference can be given to any particular agent. However, an oral afterload reducer such as nifedipine or hydralazine would seem logical.

Systolic Dysfunction

In *myocardial dilation with congestive heart failure,* there is poor systolic function associated with some or all of the features of congestive heart failure such as pulmonary crepitations, an enlarged liver, an increased jugular venous pressure, and marked dyspnea. The ideal therapy is probably a loop diuretic combined with an ACE inhibitor such as captopril (36), or a loop diuretic with nifedipine. However, there are no well documented studies on therapy for severe hypertension combined with heart failure. It must be considered that furosemide sometimes exacerbates congestive heart failure (12). In the presence of severe hypertension, IV furosemide is very likely to have an antihypertensive effect, thereby in itself relieving congestive heart failure. Again, no controlled therapeutic trials are available.

If *acute pulmonary edema* caused by severe arterial hypertension is the presenting feature, sublingual nifedipine is proven therapy (29). The apparent reduction in the preload is explained as an indirect consequence of afterload reduction.

In severe myocardial failure, *IV load reduction* by nitrates or nitroprusside is sometimes required when the blood pressure level is very serious. It is also required when captopril or nifedipine fail to control the arterial pressure; nifedipine is contraindicated because of severe depression of the inotropic state of the myocardium; or IV furosemide fails.

Aortic Aneurysm, Threatened Rupture

When aortic aneurysm presents together with severe hypertension, it is conventional to use beta-blockade to control the hypertension and bring down the heart rate. In the past IV propranolol has been used as the agent of choice. At present, however, the newly available ultrashort-acting beta blocker esmolol should be used first although there are no detailed clinical studies yet reported.

Renal Failure

An important distinction must be made between *apparent renal failure* (sometimes the result of volume depletion caused by therapy with thiazide diuretics or poor renal perfusion from an excess of afterloading agents including nifedipine) and *true acute deterioration of renal function.* The latter condition is a rare but a severe problem when it arises on the basis of accelerating hypertension. Diuretics (especially furosemide) are of critical importance in volume overloaded patients. There is no firm evidence that any of the currently available antihypertensive agents genuinely "spare" renal function, although several, if not most, agents give a relative preservation of renal function, as measured by a maintained glomerular filtration rate despite a fall in blood pressure. Such apparent "renal sparing" can be explained on the basis of renal autoregulation. Some recent evidence argues for a true preservation of renal function by calcium antagonists, yet the blood pressure levels in those studies were generally not severe. Thus, the ideal agent for the management of severe hypertension combined with renal failure remains to be defined.

In some patients with malignant hypertension and renal failure, dialysis is required; the higher the initial serum creatinine level, the more likely is the requirement for dialysis (20).

In general, two important precautions are: not to drop the blood pressure excessively so as to avoid precipitation of renal failure and to avoid ACE inhibitors if bilateral renal artery stenosis is suspected.

DRUG-INDUCED HYPOTENSION AND MECHANISMS FOR CEREBRAL, RENAL, AND CORONARY AUTOREGULATION DURING ANTIHYPERTENSIVE THERAPY

Cerebral Autoregulation: How Much of a Blood Pressure Fall can be Tolerated?

In patients with untreated or ineffectively treated severe hypertension, a resting mean blood pressure could be reduced from 145 to 113 mmHg before the loss of cerebral autoregulation (33). That means that, for example, an initial blood pressure of 160/120 mmHg could be acutely and safely reduced to 120/105 mmHg. However, the situation regarding more severe hypertension with much higher initial values is not known. In one series (21), initial blood pressure values of about 237/152 mmHg (average of all patients) were acutely dropped to 113/71 mmHg, usually by IV diazoxide with or without IV hydralazine, with the disastrous precipitation of severe and sometimes fatal neurological symptoms. In another two patients (9), blindness was precipitated by therapeutic over-enthusiasm, when the blood pressure fell in one patient from 250/170 mmHg to 90/70 mmHg and from 270/175 mmHg to about 120/50 mmHg in the other patient. Clearly these values are below those required for cerebral autoregulation according to the data of Strandgaard (33). Yet in some individual patients (21), cerebral symptoms were sometimes found at blood pressure levels that should have been in the "safe" range.

The complexity of varying cerebral artery anatomy (unknown degree of arterial stenosis and/or atherosclerosis, variable degree and anatomy of collateral circulation), *makes it seem impossible to be dogmatic about the blood pressure reduction that will be tolerated in any given patient*. In patients with threatened stroke (see above), very careful blood pressure reduction is required. In other patients, the use of either nifedipine tablets, atenolol, or labetalol as

the sole initial agent should result in blood pressure reductions which do not overshoot (17). Initial, carefully-monitored monotherapy may be safest to avoid the hazards of drug interaction and excess hypotension.

Renal Autoregulation and Risk of Renal Failure

As in the case of the brain, complex factors govern the effects of blood pressure reduction on the kidneys. Normally autoregulation will cushion the effects of wide swings of blood pressure on the renal circulation. However, in patients with renal artery stenosis, the situation is complex, and blood pressure reduction may precipitate poststenotic ischemia to impair renal function. Most of the reported cases of deterioration in renal function following abrupt hypoperfusion have been after the use of the angiotensin converting enzyme inhibitors (3); some cases have followed other vasodilators (10). The complex and varying anatomy in renal artery stenosis or in diffuse renal atherosclerotic disease means it is difficult to predict the results of acute blood pressure reduction. In general, the principle would appear to be that the blood pressure reduction should not be excessive, especially in the presence of pretherapy impairment of renal function (10). It is very difficult to fully exclude bilateral renal artery stenosis before institution of angiotensin converting enzyme inhibition; careful auscultation for abdominal bruits is the only feasible bedside procedure, so that in practice a very low, initial test dose of an ACE inhibitor is safest (e.g., captopril 6.25 mg is better than enalapril 2.5 mg, because it is quicker acting and not so long-lasting in its hypotensive effect).

Coronary Autoregulation and Risk of Myocardial Ischemia

Abrupt hypotension may also precipitate myocardial ischemia. For example, hydralazine may induce angina pectoris by combination of reduced perfusion pressure and tachycardia. Recent evidence suggests that nifedipine also may adversely affect myocardial perfusion if given routinely to patients with threatened myocardial infarction (25); however, data regarding the possible effects of nifedipine on the clinical *combination of hypertension and threatened myocardial infarction* are not available. It would seem logical that such patients should be treated in a way similar to threatened stroke, dropping the blood pressure very cautiously. Nonetheless, well designed studies relating the rate of control of blood pressure to the outcome of threatened myocardial infarction are not available. The ultrashort-acting beta blocker, IV esmolol, may come to have a special role in threatened infarction, both bringing down the blood pressure and providing myocardial protection.

Autoregulation: Summary

The possible risk of cerebral, renal, or myocardial underperfusion cannot be extrapolated solely from the initial blood pressure value nor can a "safe" rate of fall of blood pressure or a "safe" range of blood pressures be anticipated because of the impossibility of knowing the exact arterial anatomy or collateral flow in the various circulations. The health of the autoregulatory systems may also vary, as in the case of the baroreceptor reflex. In a minority of patients, there will always be the added risk of arterial stenosis or diffuse atheroma, so no preconceived policy is likely to be perfect. Rather, *each patient needs separate evaluation of the possible risk of continued blood pressure elevation versus the benefit of reduction and the harm of excess reduction.* A suitable compromise may lie in the policy of Strandgaard (33): "Initial treatment of severely hypertensive patients should aim at some reduction but not a complete normalization of the blood pressure."

INTRAVENOUS AGENTS USED IN THE THERAPY OF TRUE HYPERTENSIVE EMERGENCIES

If the initial physical assessment reveals a true medical emergency, the patient must be hospitalized and a further, careful, detailed examination carried out specifically to evaluate end-organ effects. Pheochromocytoma must be considered and excluded as much as possible because it requires specific therapy. In all patients very careful regulation of the rate of fall of blood pressure is required so an abrupt drop of blood pressure should not precipitate end-organ damage and further exacerbate the problem. Intravenous labetalol is probably the agent of choice and, if contraindicated, then IV nitroprusside will probably be effective, but requires much stricter hemodynamic monitoring. Lesser-used IV agents are diazoxide and hydralazine. However, it must be stressed that many, if not the majority, of patients can satisfactorily be treated by oral therapy without requiring IV control.

Intravenous Beta-Alpha-Blockade by Labetalol

Labetalol, a combined beta-alpha-adrenoceptor blocking agent with vasodilatory properties, has been used as repeated IV bolus injections, or bolus injection plus infusion, or infusion alone (2 mg/kg to total of 1–2 mg/kg) in the reduction of blood pressure (27,28). Such administration is said to be safe without the need for hemodynamic monitoring. However, the hypotensive response is not always uniform and may vary. Side effects of high oral doses are well-known and include orthostatic hypotension and nausea (22). Labetalol, with its predominant beta-blocking qualities, is contraindicated in congestive heart failure, although studies on patients with hypertension and angina suggest that labetalol will lessen the inhibitory impact of beta-adrenergic blockade on the circulation by its added vasodilatory effect and by afterload reduction (13). The degree of alpha-blockade possessed by labetalol may not be sufficient to fully control the severe hypertension of pheochromocytoma or of clonidine withdrawal, although successful therapy is reported (1). Failure of labetalol in the therapy of these conditions should logically be followed by an added vasodilator acting through another mechanism; for example, nitrates, verapamil, or diazoxide (Table 2).

Agents Acting via an Elevation of Vascular Smooth Muscle Levels of Cyclic GMP

IV Sodium Nitroprusside

The advantages of an infusion of sodium nitroprusside (up to 40 to 75 μg/min) are its consistent benefit and very rapid action. However, because nitroprusside may drop the blood pressure so rapidly, it should be given only under hemodynamic monitoring in an Intensive Care Unit with very careful dose-titration. Furthermore, there is danger of rebound at the cessation of nitroprusside. A practical problem is that the agent is light-sensitive.

IV Nitrates

These agents are quite frequently used in some European countries for hypertensive emergencies and should theoretically be best suited for those with associated heart failure and pulmonary edema, or when myocardial ischemia is threatened. In practice, IV nitrates have been best studied in postcoronary bypass hypertension (11). The mean infusion rate was about 300 μg/min; the drug was initiated by a dose of 5 to 10 μg/min and increased every 3 to 5 min until the blood pressure was lowered by 10 to 40 mmHg. The mean initial blood pressure before therapy was 115 mmHg and after therapy was 90 mmHg. Nitroglycerin seemed better than nitroprusside because pulmonary gas exchange was more im-

paired by nitroprusside. Of interest is the reduced arterial stiffness resulting from brief infusions of nitroglycerin as the blood pressure falls (31,32). By this mechanism arterial impedance should be reduced so that myocardial oxygen demand is lessened both by preload and afterload reduction.

Direct-acting Vasodilators, Mechanism not Known

IV Diazoxide

Diazoxide used to be given in IV boluses to lower blood pressure. However, because of the danger of "overshoot," sudden excess hypotension may threaten damage to the myocardial or cerebral circulation. A proposed alternative is slow IV infusion (5 mg/kg at 15 mg/min or slower). Diazoxide (like nitroprusside) should not be given without careful and regular monitoring of blood pressure and pulse rate, ideally under Intensive Care Unit conditions.

IV or Intramuscular (IM) Hydralazine or Dihydralazine

Hydralazine or dihydralazine speed up the heart rate considerably (30) and may have a positive inotropic effect. Hence, it is not indicated for hypertensive crises because of the possible co-existence of silent myocardial ischemia which could be exaggerated by hydralazine. An exception may be in those groups in which myocardial ischemia is rare, for example, in pregnant women. The use of IM hydralazine or dihydralazine, still common in some hospitals, is mentioned only to be condemned. An IM agent can easily "overshoot" the mark and cause prolonged excess hypotension.

Calcium Antagonists: IV Verapamil

One of the earliest uses of IV verapamil was in severe renal failure when it was shown to be effective in blood pressure re-

Table 2. *Intravenous hypotensive agents for use in true hypertensive emergencies*[a]

Agent	Usual dose	Side effects	Comments
Verapamil	5 mg bolus; or infuse up to 25 mg at 2.5 mg/min	Exclude myocardial failure, sick sinus syndrome, or heart block	Do not use after nifedipine failure
Furosemide	80 mg IV	Hypokalemia, dehydration	Combined with oral captopril or enalapril to achieve optimal effects
Labetalol	Infuse at 2 mg/min to total of 1.2 mg/kg	May worsen cardiac failure yet vasodilation probably minimizes this risk.	Avoids tachycardia. Smooth and rapid dose-related fall in blood pressure
Nitroprusside	Infusion of 40–75 μg/min	Hypotension, must monitor constantly. Rebound hypertension	Especially useful if pulmonary edema or encephalopathy
Diazoxide	100–150 mg IV for 5 min to 300 mg Infusion: 5 mg/kg at 15 mg/min	Difficult to control hypotensive effect; risk of cerebral ischemia	Better than single bolus
Hydralazine	5–10 mg IV every 4–6 hr	Less danger of hypotension than diazoxide. Tachycardia, contraindicated in angina, ischemic strokes	Probably safer as infusion. Tachycardia can be countered by propranolol 1–2 mg IV
Dihydralazine	6.25–12.5 mg IV slowly or infuse IV as 0.1 mg/min to total of 25 mg	As above, prefer infusion	As above

[a] Caution, see text for reservations.
For further details, see ref. 39.

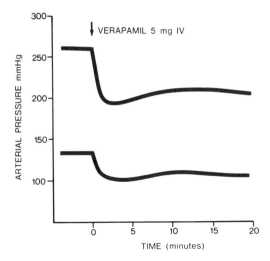

FIG. 2. Acute effects of IV verapamil in severe hypertension. (Modified from Brittinger, et al., ref. 6, with permission.)

duction, even in patients with an initial diastolic blood pressure of about 135 mmHg (6). Acting as a peripheral calcium antagonist, it is the only currently available calcium antagonist that can be given in a widely available IV form (dose: IV infusion of 1 mg/min to total of 10 mg, or IV bolus of 5 mg). Verapamil, with fewer contraindications than beta-blockade (labetalol, esmolol, propranolol), deserves wider use in severe hypertension (Fig. 2). Myocardial failure, AV nodal block, and sick sinus syndrome must be excluded before its use.

Acute IV Beta-Blockade: Esmolol or Propranolol

Esmolol is a new ultrashort-acting beta blocker (dose 50–400 μg/kg/min) which may be ideal in cases of threatened myocardial ischemia, infarction combined with severe hypertension, in perioperative hypertension, or for threatened aortic aneurysm rupture. As with other beta blockers, it is contraindicated in pheochromocytoma. It is likely that the indications for this agent, recently approved for use in the United States by the Food and Drug Administration, will

increase as experience is gained. Recovery from beta-blockade occurs within 30 min of drug cessation.

IV propranolol (0.1 mg/kg up to 10 mg given slowly) may likewise be used for the above indications, but the half-life is 1 to 6 hr.

In both cases the many contraindications to beta-blockade (including pheochromocytoma) need to be excluded. Neither agent is suited for the therapy of "standard" hypertensive emergencies because of the tendency for an acute increase in the peripheral vascular resistance. This increase compensates for the decreased cardiac output so that blood pressure does not fall in the first few hours of therapy.

IV Loop Diuretics: Furosemide

IV furosemide, acting as a vasodilator and as a diuretic, is particularly useful in "volume-loaded" severe hypertension; for example, in patients with severe renal failure. Furosemide may be combined with captopril (36); in standard cases of severe hypertension, IV furosemide 80 mg has been given alone (26), or IV furosemide 50 mg has been combined with 50 mg IM chlorpromazine (chlorpromazine has peripheral vasodilating properties) to give a smooth blood pressure reduction over 4 hr without tachycardia (38). However, in principle, I feel that any agent with a central sedative effect should be avoided in severe hypertension (see next).

Agents with a Central Action

IV or IM Reserpine

Although reserpine has been used, it cannot be recommended. IM reserpine may result in excess and uncontrolled hypotension, whereas both the IM and IV form cause severe cerebral depression and drowsiness, which makes difficult the evaluation of any possible cerebral complications directly resulting from the hypertension.

Clonidine

Clonidine may be given IV for the total dose of approximately 400 μg over ½ hour with side effects of dry mouth and drowsiness (22). Because the drowsiness may be confused with developing stoke, clonidine is best avoided. Hemodynamic effects include an increase in ejection fraction, a decreased end-diastolic volume, and a decreased end-systolic volume with a fall in the peripheral vascular resistance (22).

Urapidil

The investigational agent is similar to clonidine. The standard IV infusion dose is 2 mg/min. It is specifically used for controlled hypotension in neurosurgery because it does not increase the intracranial pressure.

Ketanserin

This investigational agent, currently being assessed for use in hypertension of all severities, is not suited for IV use because of the variable result and frequent drowsiness (19).

Emergencies: Summary

In the rare event of a true emergency hypertension, a judicious combination of IV hypotensive therapy and careful specific management of end-organ damage is required. It must be stressed that most patients with severe hypertension do not have a true emergency but rather have "urgent hypertension" which usually does *not* require IV therapy (see next). *Three essential rules* in the treatment of true emergency hypertension are: (1) excess hypotension or too rapid a fall in the pressure must be avoided; (2) all agents impairing the level of consciousness (reserpine, clonidine, chlorpromazine) should also be avoided, otherwise there may be confusion between the results of therapy and developing stroke or encephalopathy; and (3) IM administration of agents such as reserpine, hydralazine, and dihydralazine which cannot give the desired measure of fine control of the blood pressure and may "overshoot" with risk of hypotension, must also be avoided.

RECOMMENDATIONS

True hypertensive emergencies are rare and require hospital admission, preferably to an Intensive Care Unit; careful evaluation by an experienced physician is required. The optimal course of therapy and, indeed, the optimal agent is never clear, so that generalizations cannot be made. Threatened acute impairment of vital end-organ function (brain, heart, kidney) may dominate the therapeutic requirements.

In contrast, *more common is urgent hypertension without acute life-threatening severe end-organ complications*. In general, even very high diastolic blood pressure levels respond well to nifedipine 10 mg sublingually or orally. There is no evidence that such acute blood pressure reduction is either beneficial or harmful, although it is more cost-effective than is the use of nitroprusside. Failure to respond to nifedipine suggests use of the combination of this agent with an alpha₁-blocker such as prazosin, with captopril, or with an alpha-beta-blocker such as labetalol. A slower and apparently equally effective drop of blood pressure can usually be achieved over 24 hr by monotherapy with a standard cardioselective beta blocker such as atenolol. This, however, is not the therapy of choice for fear of pheochromocytoma; labetalol would be safer. In urgent hypertension, many other orally active agents can probably be used, including prazosin, verapamil, diltiazem, and captopril. To prevent excess hypotension, combined therapy should only begin when the effect of a single agent has leveled off. As in the case of hypertensive emergencies, every patient merits careful evaluation and individualized therapy.

In both emergency and in urgency hypertension, the benefits of acute blood pressure reduction must be balanced against the risks. Even in the case of seemingly severe "emergency" hypertension, the best advice is to "make haste slowly" unless there are cogent and specific reasons for acting otherwise.

ACKNOWLEDGMENTS

My colleagues, Dr. A. R. Daniels, Dr. A. A. Jennings, Dr. A. van Zyl, and Dr. L. D. Jee have provided critical help in running the Hypertension Clinic and in the treatment of patients with severe hypertension. Professor R. van Zyl Smit kindly reviewed the manuscript.

REFERENCES

1. Agabiti-Rosei, E., Brown, J. J., and Lever, A. F., et al. (1976): Treatment of phaeochromocytoma and of clonidine withdrawal hypertension with labetalol. *Br. J. Clin. Pharmacol.*, (Suppl.): 809–815.
2. Bannan, L. T., and Beevers, D. G. (1981): Emergency treatment of high blood pressure with oral atenolol. *Br. Med. J.*, 282:1757–1758.
3. Bender, W., La France, N., and Walker, W. G. (1984): Mechanism of deterioration in renal function in patients with renovascular hypertension treated with enalapril. *Hypertension,* 6(Suppl. 1):193–197.
4. Bertel, O., Conen, D., Radu, E. W., et al. (1983): Nifedipine in hypertensive emergencies. *Br. Med. J.*, 286:19–21.
5. Breckenridge, A., Dollery, C. T., and Parry, E. H. O. (1970): Prognosis of treated hypertension: Changes in life expectancy and causes of death between 1952 and 1967. *Quart. J. Med.*, 39:411–429.
6. Brittinger, W. D., Schwarzbeck, A., Wittenmeier, K. W., et al. (1970): Clinical trial of the hypotensive effect of verapamil. *Dtsch. Med. Wochenschr.*, 95:1871–1877.
7. Bussmann, W-D. (1986): Left-sided heart failure in hypertensive crisis. In: *Acute and Chronic Heart Failure: Diagnosis and Therapy,* edited by W-D. Bussman, pp. 155–159. Springer-Verlag, Berlin.
8. Chaffman, M., and Brogden, R. N. (1985): Diltiazem: A review of its pharmacological properties and therapeutic efficacy. *Drugs,* 29:387–454.
9. Cove, D. H., Seddon, M., and Fletcher, R. F., et al. (1979): Blindness after treatment for malignant hypertension. *Br. Med. J.*, 2:245–246.
10. Diamond, J. R., Cheung, J. Y., and Fang, L. S. T. (1984): Nifedipine-induced renal dysfunction: Alterations in renal hemodynamics. *Am. J. Med.*, 77:905–909.
11. Flaherty, J. T., Magee, P. A., Gardner, T. L., et al. (1982): Comparison of intravenous nitroglycerin and sodium nitroprusside for treatment of acute hypertension developing after coronary artery bypass surgery. *Circulation,* 65:1072–1077.
12. Francis, G. S., Siegel, R. M., Goldsmith, S. R., et al. (1985): Acute vasoconstrictor response to intravenous furosemide in patients with chronic congestive heart failure. *Ann. Intern. Med.*, 103:1–6.
13. Frishman, W. H., Strom, J. A., Kirschner, M., et al. (1981): Labetalol therapy in patients with systemic hypertension and angina pectoris: Effects of combined alpha- and beta-adrenoceptor blockade. *Am. J. Cardiol.*, 48:917–927.
14. Ghose, R. R., and Sampson, A. (1977): Rapid onset of oral labetalol in severe hypertension. *Curr. Med. Res. Opin.*, 5:147–151.
15. Harington, M., Kincaid-Smith, P., and McMichael, J. (1959): Results of treatment in malignant hypertension: A seven-year experience in 94 cases. *Br. Med. J.*, 2:969–980.
16. Houston, M. C. (1986): Treatment of hypertensive urgencies and emergencies with nifedipine. *Am. Heart. J.*, 111:963–969.
17. Isles, C. G., Johnson, A. D. C., Milne, F. J. (1986): Slow release nifedipine and atenolol as initial treatment in blacks with malignant hypertension. *Br. J. Pharmacol.*, 21:377–383.
18. Jennings, A. A., Jee, L. D., Smith, J. A., et al. (1986): Acute effect of nifedipine on blood pressure and left ventricular ejection fraction in severely hypertensive outpatients: Predictive effects of acute therapy and prolonged efficacy when added to existing therapy. *Am. Heart. J.*, 111:557.
19. Jennings, A. A., and Opie, L. H. (1987): Effects of intravenous ketanserin on severely hypertensive patients in a single-blind study. *J. Cardiovasc. Pharmacol.*, 9:120–124.
20. Lawton, W. J. (1982): The short-term course of renal function in malignant hypertensives with renal insufficiency. *Clin. Nephrol.*, 17:277–283.
21. Ledingham, J. G. G., and Rajagopalan, B. (1979): Cerebral complications in the treatment of accelerated hypertension. *Quart. J. Med.*, 48:25–41.
22. Masotti, G., Scarti, L., Poggesi, L., et al. (1986): Treatment of hypertensive emergencies: Classic and newer approaches. *J. Cardiovasc. Pharmacol.*, 8(Suppl. 3):S46–S50.
23. Matenga, J., Kitai, I., and Levy, L. (1986): Strokes among black people in Harare, Zim-

babwe: Results of computed tomography and associated risk factors. *Br. Med. J.,* 292:1649–1651.

24. Medical Research Council Working Party (1985):
MRC trial of treatment of mild hypertension:
Principal results. *Br. Med. J.,* 291:97–104.

25. Muller, J. E., Morrison, J., and Stone, P. H., et
al. (1984): Nifedipine therapy for patients with
threatened and acute myocardial infarction: A
randomized double-blind, placebo-controlled
comparison. *Curculation,* 69:740–747.

26. Nielsen, P. E., Krogsgaard, A., and McNair, A.,
et al. (1980): Emergency treatment of severe hypertension evaluated in a randomized study: Effect of rest and furosemide and a randomized
evaluation of chlorpromazine, dihydralazine and
diazoxide. *Acta Med. Scand.,* 208:473–480.

27. Pearson, R. M., and Havard, C. W. H. (1976):
Intravenous labetalol in hypertensive patients
treated with β-adrenoceptor-blocking drugs. *Br.
J. Clin. Pharmacol.,* 3:(Suppl.) 795–798.

28. Pearson, R. M., and Havard, C. W. H. (1978):
Intravenous labetalol in hypertensive patients
given by fast and slow injection. *Br. J. Clin. Pharmacol.,* 5:401–405.

29. Polese, A., Fiorentini, C., Olivari, M. T., et al.
(1979): Clinical use of a calcium antagonistic
agent (nifedipine) in acute pulmonary edema. *Am.
J. Med.,* 66:825–830.

30. Safar, M. E., Simon, A. C., Levenson, J. A., et
al. (1983): Hemodynamic effects of diltiazem in
hypertension. *Circ. Res.,* 52(Suppl. 1):169–173.

31. Simon, ACh., Levenson, J. A., Levy, B. Y., et
al. (1982): Effect of nitroglycerin on peripheral

large arteries in hypertension. *Br. J. Clin. Pharmacol.,* 14:241–246.

32. Smulyan, H., Mookherjee, S., and Warner, R. A.
(1986): The effect of nitroglycerin on forearm arterial distensibility. *Circulation,* 73:1264–1269.

33. Strandgaard, S. (1976): Autoregulation of cerebral blood flow in hypertensive patients: The
modifying influence of prolonged antihypertensive treatment on the tolerance to acute, drug-
induced hypotension. *Circulation,* 53:720–727.

34. Strasser, T. (1987): Inferences from drug trials:
Risks, probabilities, ethics, and decision taking.
In: *Mild Hypertension: From Drug Trials to Practice,* edited by T. Strasser, D. Ganten, pp. 77–
83. Raven Press, New York.

35. Van Harten, J., Burggraaf, K., Danhof, M., et al.
(1987): Negligible sublingual absorption of nifedipine. *Lancet,* ii:1363–1365.

36. White, N. J., Rajagopalan, H., and Yahaya, H.,
et al. (1980): Captopril and frusemide in severe
drug-resistant hypertension. *Lancet,* ii:108–110.

37. Woods, J. W., and Blythe, W. B. (1967): Management of malignant hypertension complicated
by renal insufficiency. *New Engl. J. Med.,*
277:57–61.

38. Young, R. J., Lawson, A. A. H., and Malone, D.
N. S. (1980): Treatment of severe hypertension
with chlorpromazine and furosemide. *Br. Med.
J.,* 280:1579.

39. Opie, L. H. (ed.) (1987): *Drugs for the Heart,*
Second expanded edition. Grune & Stratton, Or-
lando.

New Therapeutic Strategies in Hypertension,
edited by Norman M. Kaplan,
Barry M. Brenner, and John H. Laragh.
Raven Press, Ltd., New York © 1989.

Treatment of Hypertension in Patients with Cardiovascular Disorders

Robert J. Cody

Division of Cardiology, Department of Medicine, The Ohio State University Medical School and Hospital, Columbus, Ohio 443210

It is difficult to separate cardiovascular disorders from systemic hypertension, because of the considerable overlap of three key components: coronary artery disease, hypertension, and congestive heart failure. It has been clear from the outset, and supported by large population studies (14,18,22,24,27,32,47,48,57), that hypertension carries with it a considerable risk of death, myocardial infarction, stroke, and congestive heart failure. It has been particularly difficult to separate a cause and effect role for these various components, as it is quite likely that they are closely interrelated. Three findings in general population surveys point out the need for a recrystalization of treatment approaches of hypertension in these patients. First, the number of elderly people (defined as older than 65 years) is increasing progressively, such that one out of three subjects will be over age 65 by the year 2050. Second, the treatment of coronary artery disease has become more aggressive, with a greater likelihood of surviving an acute event and with a need for chronic medical therapy. Third, the number of patients with congestive heart failure is increasing, with current estimated incidence of 2.5 million subjects, and approximately 300,000 new cases diagnosed yearly.

With these factors in mind, the present chapter will review the cardiovascular characteristics of hypertension, identify disorders of the heart and circulation likely to be encountered in the treatment of hypertension, and highlight the treatment of the hypertensive patient as it relates to disorders of the heart and circulation. Finally, several issues that may be germane to the overall treatment of hypertension in individuals with cardiovascular disorders will be discussed.

CARDIOVASCULAR CHARACTERISTICS OF HYPERTENSION

It is reasonable to state that every patient with hypertension has a cardiovascular disorder. The spectrum and characteristics of ventricular remodeling in hypertension have been recently reviewed (33). Several factors, however, should be stressed. With the exception of labile hypertension, and certain subsets of hypertension, the majority of individuals with systemic hypertension have an inappropriate increase of vascular tone. This increase of vascular tone (systemic vascular resistance) may be mediated by a number of factors. These include enhanced sympathetic nervous system activity, activation of vasoconstrictor hormonal pathways, and excessive sodium content within the arterial wall and surrounding tissue. Evidence does exist that suggests the heart itself may be a causal factor under certain conditions (25,53). In most cases, the heart responds in an adaptive or maladaptive way to the increased wall stress resulting from increased vascular resistance and pressure in the arterial bed. Abnormalities of cardiac dysfunction in hypertension can be categorized into several groups. These are disorders of systolic function, diastolic function, chronotropic activity, and baroreceptor responsiveness. It can now be stated that there may be hormonally-mediated disorders of the heart given the presence of atrial natriuretic factor within secretory granules of atrial and ventricular myocytes.

Systolic abnormalities are the most readily appreciated. This is due to the fact that the heart must generate an enormous energy output in order to empty during systole against the increased resistance and pressure within the arterial bed. Ultimately, the persistence of this increased afterload will result in gross systolic dysfunction in hypertensive subjects. Hypertension, at one point, was one of the most common forms of congestive heart failure in the United States, and still remains a major determinant, or a prodrome, to the development of chronic congestive heart failure in many individuals.

The diastolic abnormalities of the heart are only receiving equal attention within the last decade, despite earlier reports that diastolic abnormalities could exist in the hypertensive population (29,58). There are both active and passive components to the relaxation of the ventricle in diastole. This is perhaps the pivotal portion of the cardiac cycle, in that compliance abnormalities may alter ventricular filling (stroke volume), and the majority of coronary blood flow occurs at this time. It is likely that diastolic abnormalities in hypertension are a direct reflection of abnormalities of coronary blood flow as well as abnormal ventricular mechanics. However, it is quite clear that these factors may contribute to the ischemic conditions identified in patients with hypertension, and absence of large vessel coronary disease (2–4,9,16,17,19,26,35,40, 41,46,48,52,54).

Baroreceptor abnormalities may be part of a large constellation of sympathetic nervous system changes that characterize the hypertensive process. If arterial and great vessel baroreceptors cannot respond appropriately to changes in arterial filling, this will produce an inappropriate enhancement of arterial tone, and lack of chronotropic and inotropic suppression of the ventricle, thereby producing an inappropriate mismatch of vascular reactivity and cardiac responsiveness with a net result of increased blood pressure in systole. This mismatch may contribute to the incidence of pure systolic hypertension in the elderly.

Atrial natriuretic factor (ANF) is primarily secreted by atrial myocytes (5,7), and ventricular myocytes can be recruited, particularly when the ventricle undergoes hypertrophy. One would anticipate that enhanced secretion of atrial natriuretic factor with its natriuretic and vasodilator properties (7) would actually be favorable in hypertension. However, most studies demonstrate that ANF levels in hypertension have an 80% overlap with the normal range (7). One can therefore reason that there is an inappropriately low production of atrial natriuretic factor in many patients with hypertension, particularly in view of the tendency for an increased circulatory volume and cardiac output in many hypertensive subjects. Inadequate secretion of atrial natriuretic factor would permissively contribute to the volume overload in hypertension that has necessitated the extensive use of diuretics in this population.

Relatively less attention has been given to the abnormal status of the systemic vasculature in patients with hypertension, where abnormal vascular reactivity and structural changes contribute to the hypertensive process by increasing arterial resistance. It is clear from studies performed under stress conditions, such as exercise, that the arterial bed in hypertensive subjects does not dilate to the same extent as that of normal subjects (8).

Abnormalities of the lesser circulation, i.e., the pulmonary circulation may also occur in patients with hypertension. Under resting conditions, pulmonary pressure and resistance can be increased in subsets of hypertensive subjects. This is not a uniform abnormality; some hypertensive subjects will demonstrate normal pulmonary reactivity where others do not. This abnormality of the pulmonary circulation is enhanced during low level and maximal exercise (8). The currently available literature does not establish the mechanism for abnormal pulmonary reactivity, nor does it address the issue of whether this represents a passive phenomenon due to left ventricular dysfunction. Irrespective of the mechanism(s), the right ventricle is placed under an inordinate stress as a result of increased pulmonary resistance and pressure. This may help to explain the development of independent right ventricular failure, or specific contribution to the biventricular failure pattern of long-term hypertension, particularly where treatment is inadequate.

HEART AND CIRCULATORY ABNORMALITIES FREQUENTLY ENCOUNTERED IN PATIENTS WITH HYPERTENSION (Table 1)

Perhaps the most common and important coexistent disorder in patients with hypertension is the spectrum of coronary artery disease, particularly in the aging adult population. Except under unusual circumstances, the presence of an asymptomatic

Table 1. *Heart and circulatory abnormalities frequently encountered in hypertension*

Coronary artery disease
Congestive heart failure
Vascular disease
Valvular heart disease
Arrhythmias

noncritical coronary lesion may not impose a considerable stress on the myocardium. However, when one combines this lesion with systemic arterial hypertension, it is easy to envision abnormal perfusion in the targeted region of the myocardium. The reduction of perfusion pressure across such a coronary lesion, particularly when left ventricular end-diastolic pressure (LVEDP) is increased, will result in diminished coronary flow (2–4,15,17,22,35,40,46,52). Myocardial ischemia is likely to be more profound when LVEDP increases with exercise in hypertensive subjects (8). It is therefore readily apparent that the risk of severe ischemia or infarction is even greater when there is coexistent critical obstruction of one or more coronary arteries. This may be more than a additive risk. Considering the potential of enhanced sympathetic activity, increase of angiotension II, and a propensity for vasospasm within the hypertensive population, the coexistence of hypertension and fixed coronary obstruction likely results in a synergistic progressive compromise of coronary perfusion. Ultimately, such patients may be more prone than their normotensive counterparts to a high incidence of myocardial infarction (9,22,27,46,47,48,57). Myocardial infarction therefore is an expected or predictable sequelae to these coexistent disease processes. One might predict that the presence of systemic hypertension may predispose to a myocardial infarction of greater severity or deleterious outcome when compared to normotensive subjects. Abnormalities of platelet function blood viscosity (12) may contribute to abnormal flow characteristics and hypertrophy within the hypertensive population. Such abnormalities contribute to the overall "resistance" to flow encountered in the hypertensive population, and may contribute to the thrombotic events that typify acute myocardial infarction. It has been documented that the extent of the infarct zone relates to the speed and extent with which the acute thrombotic lesion resolves. In the hyprtensive patient, underlying abnormalities of both platelet function and viscosity could impede clot resolution, resulting in myocardial infarction of much greater severity than in normotensive subjects. It is now well established that an infarcted myocardial segment may undergo a phase of expansion, contributing to overall deterioration of left ventricular function (16). In the spontaneously hypertensive rat, ligation of the left anterior descending coronary artery will produce myocardial infarction. However, treatment of these rats with a converting enzyme inhibitor resulted in improved survival compared to placebo (43). Thus, based on rheologic, hemodynamic, and structural phenomena, greater tendency for severe complicated myocardial infarction could be anticipated in hypertensive subjects, compared with normotensive subjects.

The occurrence of congestive heart failure is perhaps one of the best known and well described cardiovascular sequelae in patients with hypertension. However, it has always been assumed that the majority of heart failure symptomatology was due to systolic dysfunction. While this may be true, particularly in the era preceding the availability of vasodilator therapy (9), it is likely that a considerable amount of this "failure" is due to stiffness of the left ventricle, or impaired diastolic relaxation. This is based on several lines of evidence. It has been shown that abnormal diastolic filling characteristics occur frequently in patients with hypertension (29,33,37,39,40,52,54). While pulmonary wedge pressure is well within the normal range under resting conditions, marked increases of pulmonary wedge pressure occur during exercise (8). It is much more likely that ventricular diastolic abnormalities rather than systolic abnormalities will be encountered while a patient is actively hypertensive. By the time that systolic abnormalities are apparent, systolic blood pressure is often attenuated or even normal, due to left ventricular

power failure. This is supported by animal studies, demonstrating that the marked elevation of blood pressure in the spontaneously hypertensive rat (SHR) attenuates, and actually normalizes as the ventricle fails (16). This is analogous to the clinical observation that patients who have "hypertensive cardiomyopathy" are frequently normotensive at the time of symptomatic presentation. The distinction of systolic versus diastolic dysfunction is significant. With systolic dysfunction, one would likely treat with pharmacologic classes similar to those used to treat chronic congestive heart failure. With diastolic dysfunction one might be more prone to use alternate drug groups, such as beta-adrenergic blockers, or calcium channel antagonists.

Structural disease of the conduit and resistance vessels is also common in hypertension. There are several types of vascular ischemic events that have been well described in hypertension. Disease of the great vessels of the neck is a common accompaniment of hypertension. Prevention trials have demonstrated that treatment of hypertension is associated with a reduction of the incidence of stroke (10,13,21,27, 32,48). Furthermore, the tendency for intercranial hemorrhage from congenital or Charcot-Bouchard aneurysms (44) could be reduced when arterial shearing stresses are reduced with antihypertensive therapy. This effect is also germane to aortic dissection and aneurysmal aortic dilatation (49). An obvious, yet critical, association in many hypertensive patients is the presence of unilateral or bilateral renal arterial occlusive disease. One point regarding renal artery stenosis should be discussed here. Occasionally drug-resistant hypertension will occur in a patient whose blood pressure had previously been easy to control. Many of these patients may have developed secondary renal artery stenosis, superimposed upon essential hypertension, resulting in a combined disease process.

This section would be incomplete if two

additional aspects of cardiovascular disease were not discussed. Systemic arterial hypertension may be associated with valvular heart disease. The coexistence of regurgitant aortic or mitral lesions with arterial hypertension may produce a greater degree of eccentric ventricular hypertrophy and dilatation, thereby accelerating the progression to systolic ventricular dysfunction and failure. Stenotic aortic and mitral valve lesions will have a different impact. Aortic stenosis will accelerate concentric hypertrophy of the ventricle that may already be present as a result of hypertension. Both aortic and mitral stenosis will mechanically limit cardiac output, thereby reducing stroke volume. While regurgitant lesions will respond favorably to vasodilator therapy, the low-cardiac output associated with stenotic valvular lesions will be less responsive. Finally, conduction abnormalities must be considered in patients with hypertension. Bradycardia and functional or structural block at any of several points in the conduction system may have a profound influence on the choice of drugs to treat hypertension. Furthermore, it has been suggested that hypertensive patients may be prone to enhanced ventricular irritability (36). This could contribute to the mortality observed in large clinical trials of diuretic therapy, since the well-known electrolyte depleting effect of diuretics would accentuate the tendency for ventricular arrhythmias.

ANTIHYPERTENSIVE THERAPY IN PATIENTS WITH CARDIOVASCULAR DISORDERS

The purpose of this section is to consider the broad indications of the major antihypertensive drug classes for patients with associated cardiovascular disorders. The goal of treatment in this group of patients is effective blood pressure control and hopefully, co-treatment of other existing diseases. This is not meant to be an exhaustive

Table 2. *Specific cardiovascular indications for antihypertensive drug classes*

Diuretics
  congestive heart failure
Central sympatholytics
  aortic dissection
Beta-adrenergic blockers
  coronary artery disease
  aortic dissection
  some atrial/ventricular arrhythmias
Vasodilator agents
  congestive heart failure
  peripheral vascular disease
  some cases of coronary artery disease
ACE inhibitors
  congestive heart failure
  myocardial ischemia/infarction (probable)
  ventricular arrhythmias?
Calcium channel antagonists
  coronary artery disease
  peripheral vascular disease
  some atrial/ventricular arrhythmias

survey, as these drug classes are treated elsewhere in this text in greater detail. Specific indications for pharmacologic classes are summarized in Table 2.

Diuretics are perhaps the most widely used antihypertensive therapy (38). This is based on their low cost, ease of administration, and goal of counterbalancing the excessive sodium intake in the hypertensive population. However, in terms of their effectiveness in cardiovascular disorders, their primary role is two-fold: the rapid excretion of excess sodium and water, and the treatment of congestive heart failure. In many instances, these two goals are sought in the same individual. It is difficult otherwise to delineate a conceptual or pathophysiologic rationale for diuretic usage in the treatment of hypertension associated with cardiovascular disorders. That is, it is difficult to identify a specific favorable effect of diuretics that is germane to patients with associated coronary artery disease, myocardial infarction, or peripheral vascular disease. One can actually perceive several relative contraindications. For instance, induction of electrolyte depletion in this setting promotes ventricular arrhythmias (45) or activation of hormonal pathways (e.g., the renin system) that may adversely influence the outcome of the disease. The latter can be readily identified in congestive heart failure where sodium depletion activates the renin-angiotensin system and the sympathetic nervous system (6,31), which would be counterproductive in terms of the overall outcome of the heart failure patient. Similarly, in severe hypertension due to renal artery disease, diuretic therapy will further activate the already increased renin system activity. In contrast, the effects of diuretics, when used in moderate doses, are most readily apparent in the situation of hypertension associated with congestive heart failure. Here, diuretics are associated with a reduction of circulatory and tissue congestion, and ultimately, a reduction of symptomatology.

Central Sympatholytics

These agents generally consist of the central alpha agonists, which reduce general sympathetic outflow. Guanethidine is a prototypic agent in this class. Once used as the drug of choice for refractory hypertension, this drug is now used sparingly. While a similar role was established for alpha-methyldopa, this latter compound still enjoys wide utilization among practitioners. With the availability of potent peripherally acting vasodilators with relatively safe profiles, minimal side effects, and patient tolerance, use of the central alpha agonists becomes more questionable. In patients with heart and circulatory disorders, it is difficult to identify discrete indications for this class of drug. In fact, the bradycardia and orthostatic hypotension which central sympathetics produce may actually be detrimental in many patients with cardiovascular disorders. One persistent role for guanethidine, however, is the treatment of acute aortic dissection (49).

Beta-adrenergic Blockade

The number of drugs which now are available under this category has grown considerably (1,10,23,28,34). However, the general distinction that can be applied to all these agents is whether or not they are beta 1 selective and whether they exert any of the putative partial beta agonist effects that have resulted in the subclassification of intrinsic sympathomimetic activity. Beta-adrenergic blockers are readily effective in patients with any of several associated cardiovascular disorders.

These drugs are clearly effective in treating patients with coronary artery disease. Beta blockers limit symptomatology, maintain a protective effect against myocardial ischemia, and actually improve survival among patients with myocardial infarction, and indicate that these drugs should be particularly effective in the treatment of coexistent hypertension and coronary artery disease. Prior to converting enzyme inhibitors, propranolol was widely used in patients with renal artery disease, because beta-adrenergic blockade significantly reduces renin activity (1). Several of the beta-adrenergic blockers are available for parenteral administration. Certainly, beta-adrenergic blocking agents remain one of the drugs of choice for the treatment of aortic dissection (49), particularly during the acute phase of aortic leakage, as they lower ventricular dp/dt (thereby reducing shearing forces within the aorta), in addition to reducing systolic blood pressure. Beta blockade can be effective as an adjunct for controlling ventricular rate in those subjects with atrial fibrillation.

However, there are several disorders in which beta-adrenergic blockade may be detrimental. In patients with congestive heart failure, the predominant hemodynamic effect of beta-adrenergic blockade is a reduction of both chronotropy and inotropy, so that there is at least a moderate risk that congestive heart failure will be exacerbated in the course of therapy. Currently there is considerable debate in the heart failure field as to whether this class of drugs has a therapeutic role. However, practical clinical experience with currently recommended doses would not support this claim, and there is at least a moderate risk that heart failure will be intensified. In patients with peripheral vascular disease, beta-adrenergic blockade may produce limb ischemia by central and peripheral mechanisms. Because of the negative chronotropic and intropic effects of beta blocking agents, their use in valvular heart disease, particularly aortic or mitral stenosis, is limited.

Vasodilator Agents

There are several pharmaceutical classes with vasodilator properties that fall under this broad category. These include the direct acting vasodilators such as nitroprusside, hydralazine, and minoxidil. These drugs produce relaxation of vascular smooth muscle, and as typified by nitroprusside, the cellular mechanism is mediated by activation of soluble guanylate cyclase in vascular smooth muscle. These drugs are potent, rapidly acting vasodilators; nitroprusside and hydralazine can be administered parenterally. Their potent vasodilator properties makes these drugs particularly effective in hypertensive therapy that coexists with congestive heart failure, peripheral vascular disease, and in some instances, coronary artery disease.

Peripheral postsynaptic alpha-adrenergic blocking agents such as prazosin and terazosin are potent vasodilators that reduce alpha mediated vasoconstriction. As with the direct acting vasodilators, they are effective in the presence of a wide variety of cardiovascular disorders.

Angiotensin Converting Enzyme Inhibitors

The angiotensin converting enzyme inhibitors have elicited considerable enthu-siasm and have enjoyed a wide application since they became available approximately 10 years ago. They are effective in many patients with hypertension (13,28,39,48) particularly when combined with a diuretic. They are very effective in some of the more complicated forms of hypertension such as renovascular hypertension, and malignant-phase hypertension. The effectiveness of these agents is augmented by the fact that they are generally well tolerated in virtually all of the associated cardiovascular disorders discussed. Perhaps most notable is their efficacy, safety, and wide applicability in patients with congestive heart failure, irrespective of mild or severe symptomatology. As with severe renovascular hypertension, converting enzyme inhibitors can induce profound hypotension or progression of renal insufficiency in patients with coexistent heart failure. There is now an interesting body of data which would suggest that there may be a potential role for converting enzyme inhibitors for the stabilization of acute myocardial infarction, and prevention of subsequent infarct expansion and progressive left ventricular dysfunction (16,43). These issues, however, are the subject of ongoing clinical trials where data generation and analysis are pending.

Calcium Channel Antagonists

This chemically-diverse class of drugs antagonizes the influx of calcium through the slow channels of cardiac and vascular muscle cells, and decreases cytosolic calcium. Despite this common mechanism of action, there are considerable structural and physiological differences among the commonly-available calcium channel antagonists (28,30,41,55,56). Verapamil, for instance, may have more of a negative inotropic effect, and both verapamil and diltiazem tend to reduce cardiac electrical conduction; the dihydropyridines may have a greater action on vascular smooth muscle and tend to increase heart rate via sympathetic nervous system mechanisms. The prototypic compounds that comprise this class have been used in Europe for decades, yet have been used in the United States only in the last 5 to 10 years. Irrespective of the differences among these drugs, it is clear that they are all potent vasodilators, and in the coronary circulation, dilate large and small vessels, thereby reducing angina. More recent data in animal models of hypertension and heart failure demonstrate that these agents can reverse small vessel spasm and improve ventricular compliance. Their vasodilator properties make blood pressure reduction considerable, perhaps masking much of the real or potential negative inotropic effect in the hypertensive population. Therefore, the use of calcium channel antagonists for the treatment of hypertension, associated with all degrees of coronary artery disease, is quite logical. Perhaps one limitation would be the induction of excessive hypotension in the setting of acute myocardial infarction, with parenteral (intravenous or sublingual) drug administration. The favorable effect of these drugs can also be anticipated in the presence of peripheral vascular disease, through reversal of the vasospastic component of blood flow reduction, particularly in the arteries of resistance size. The use of these agents in congestive heart failure is quite controversial, and the majority of the current data would suggest that calcium channel antagonists should not be first-line vasodilator therapy in heart failure. However, in the hypertensive population where there is a range of systolic and diastolic ventricular abnormalities, use of calcium channel antagonists can be highly effective, particularly in patients with left ventricular hypertrophy and diastolic dysfunction. Thus, concerns regarding calcium channel antagonists may be less important in the hypertensive patient, except in cases where overt systolic dysfunction is present. Likewise, calcium channel antagonists could produce adverse effects in severe valvular heart disease by inducing a negative inotro-

pic effect, and slowing the heart rate to less than desirable levels. Verapamil and diltiazem particularly should be used with caution in the presence of conduction disease or when used in combination with a beta-adrenergic blocking agent. There continues to be little published data regarding a direct comparison of beta-adrenergic blocking agents and calcium channel antagonists.

ADDITIONAL CONSIDERATIONS OF ANTIHYPERTENSIVE TREATMENT IN PATIENTS WITH HEART AND CIRCULATORY DISORDERS

As with all therapies, there will be considerable patient-to-patient variability in responsiveness, despite the putative effects of individual antihypertensive therapies, and the use of combination drug therapy further obscures the interpretation of individual drug actions. Additional factors such as obesity, diabetes, and lipid disorders may also effect, and be effected by, drug treatment. Obesity is emerging as perhaps one of the most compromising factors on the circulatory system of the hypertensive patient (11). Volume overload and eccentric hypertrophy act in tandem with hypertension, further impairing ventricular performance (33,37). It has become popular to judge antihypertensive therapies by their effects on serum lipids. With few exceptions, however, the effect of antihypertensive agents on serum lipids is relatively small and one has to question the clinical significance of such changes (48). Thus, while diuretics and beta-adrenergic blocking agents will produce an increase of serum lipids, and while angiotensin converting enzyme inhibitors and calcium channel antagonists reduce serum lipids, it is obvious that a much greater impact would be observed by encouraging patients to strongly adhere to appropriate dietary measures directed at lipid reduction. It is not likely that the antihypertensive drugs would induce a significant increase in lipids if an appropriate dietary plan and weight reduction are instituted.

ANTIHYPERTENSIVE THERAPY AND MYOCARDIAL INFARCTION

In the last 20 years, it has been clear that antihypertensive therapy has provided effective control of blood pressure and a reduction of stroke, thus, fulfilling the hopes of generations of clinicians and researchers (13,20,21,32). However, a similar impact of antihypertensive therapy on the incidence of myocardial infarction has not been realized. The reasons for this are not clear. For instance, diuretics are the traditional first step in the standardized step care approach to therapy, and have been the most widely used class of drugs for treating hypertension (38). Yet, their mechanism of action does not produce a favorable direct physiologic effect on co-existent coronary artery disease. However, the problem is likely to be more complex and the lack of a greater impact of antihypertensive therapy on myocardial infarction may be the result of several characteristics of the hypertensive patient with coronary artery disease. First, there is a reduction of coronary blood flow, particularly with increased left ventricular filling pressures and hypertrophy, especially with fixed obstruction of the coronary arteries. Second, increased blood viscosity may be present, yielding a greater tendency for clot formation and coronary thrombosis. Third, relative dissociation of vascular stiffness and autonomic control of the heart emerges in the presence of hypertension. Fourth, increased neurohormonal activity exists, with a predominance of vasoconstriction/spasm. Fifth, there may be a greater proclivity to cardiac arrhythmias in this disease combination. Against this background, one would be hard-pressed to expect diuretics to have had a favorable impact, and diuretics might actually adversely effect these pathophysiologic events. These possibili-

ties carry several implications. First, the abnormalities of the heart in hypertension, particularly with coexistent coronary artery disease, must be more completely characterized. Second, the treatment of hypertension in the patient with coronary artery disease or ventricular dysfunction, must be targeted to more directly address the pathophysiologic abnormalities in the heart. Third, the design of large-scale antihypertensive treatment trials should identify *specific* cardiovascular markers to follow in order to judge safety and efficacy endpoints.

SUMMARY

This chapter has considered the treatment of hypertension in patients with cardiovascular disorders. Without establishing rigid formulae, the chapter has considered factors that may ultimately influence the clinical outcome of treatment strategies. The management of hypertension in patients who have associated cardiovascular disorders will always be complex and difficult. Treatment strategies must be structured not only to reduce the ambient blood pressure, but also to address the pathophysiologic abnormalities in this disease subset and the hemodynamic consequences of the antihypertensive treatment that is chosen.

REFERENCES

1. Bühler, F. R. (1981): Antihypertensive actions of beta-blockers. In: *Frontiers in Hypertension Research*, edited by J. H. Laragh, F. R. Bühler, and D. W. Seldin, pp. 423–435. Springer-Verlag, New York.
2. Cannon III, R. O., Bonow, R. O., Bacharach, S. L., Green, M. V., Rosing, D. R., Leon, M. B., Watson, M. R., and Epstein, S. E. (1985): Left ventricular dysfunction in patients with angina pectoris, normal epicardial coronary arteries, and abnormal vasodilator reserve. *Circulation*, 71:218–226.
3. Cannon III, R. O., Watson, R. M., Rosing, D. R., and Epstein, S. E. (1983): Angina caused by

reduced vasodilator reserve of the small coronary arteries. *J. Am. Coll. Cardiol.*, 1:1359–1373.

4. Cannon III, R. O., Cunnion, R. E., Parrillo, J. E., Palmeri, S. T., Tucker, E. E., Schenke, W. H., and Epstein, S. E. (1987): Dynamic limitation of coronary vasodilator reserve in patients with dilated cardiomyopathy and chest pain. *J. Am. Coll. Cardiol.*, 10:1190–1200.

5. Cody, R. J., Atlas, S. A., Laragh, J. H., Kubo, S. H., Covit, A. B., Ryman, K. S., Shaknovich, A., Pondolfino, K., Clark, M., Camargo, M. J. F., Scarborough, R. M., and Lewicki, J. A. (1986): Atrial natriuretic factor in normal subjects and heart failure patients: Plasma levels and renal, hormonal, and hemodynamic responses to peptide infusion. *J. Clin. Invest.*, 78:1362–1374.

6. Cody, R. J., Covit, A. B., Schaer, G. L., Laragh, J. H., Sealey, J. E., and Feldschuh, J. (1986): Sodium and water balance in chronic congestive heart failure. *J. Clin. Invest.*, 77:1441–1452.

7. Cody, R. J., Atlas, S. A., and Laragh, J. H. (1987): Physiological and pharmacological studies of atrial natriuretic factor, a natriuretic and vasoactive peptide. *J. Clin. Pharmacol.*, 27:927–936.

8. Cody, R. J., Kubo, S. H., Ryman, K. S., Shaknovich, A., and Laragh, J. H. (1987): Systemic and pulmonary hemodynamic responses to nicardipine during graded ergometric exercise in patients with moderate to severe essential hypertension. *J. Amer. Coll. Cardiol.*, 10:647–654.

9. Cohn, J. N. (1977): Heart disease in the hypertensive patients. *Med. Clin. N. Am.*, 61:581–591.

10. Cutler, J. A., and Furberg, C. D. (1985): Drug treatment trials in hypertension: A review. *Prevent. Med.*, 14:499–518.

11. de Divitiis, O., Fazio, S., Petitto, M., Maddalena, G., Contaldo, F., and Mancini, M. (1981): Obesity and cardiac function. *Circulation*, 64:477–482.

12. Devereux, R. B., Drayer, J. I. M., Chien, S., Pickering, T. G., Letcher, R. L., DeYoung, J., Sealey, J. E., and Laragh, J. H. (1984): Whole blood viscosity as a determinant of cardiac hypertrophy in systemic hypertension. *Am. J. Cardiol.*, 54:592–595.

13. Dollery, C. T. (1983): Hypertension and new antihypertensive drugs: Clinical perspectives. *Fed. Proc.*, 42:207–210.

14. Dollery, C. T. (1987): An update on the medical research council hypertension trial. *J. Hypertens.*, 5(suppl 3);S75–S78.

15. Epstein, S. E., Cannon III, R. O., Watson, R. M., Leon, M. B., Bonow, R. O., and Rosing, D. R. (1985): Dynamic coronary obstruction as a cause of angina pectoris: Implications regarding therapy. *Am. J. Cardiol.*, 55:61B–68B.

16. Fletcher, P. J., Pfeffer, J. M., Pfeffer, M. A., and Braunwald, E. (1982): Effects of hypertension on cardiac performance in rats with myocardial infarction. *Am. J. Cardiol.*, 50:488–496.

17. Fox, K. M., Levy, R. D., Mockus, L., and Wright, C. (1987): Hypertension and the ischaemic myocardium. *J. Hypertens.*, 5(suppl 3):S17–S18.

18. Froelicher, V. F., Jr. (1977): Review of epidemiology in clinical cardiology. *Aviat. Space Environ. Med.*, 48:659–664.

19. Frohlich, E. D. (1987): Coexistence of hypertensive and coronary arterial disease (editorial). *Hypertension*, 10:473–475.

20. Goodwin, J. F. (1974): Prospects and predictions for the cardiomyopathies. *Circulation*, 50:210–219.

21. Gordon, T., and Kannel, W. B. (1982): Multiple risk functions for predicting coronary heart disease: The concept, accuracy, and application. *Am. Heart J.*, 103:1031–1039.

22. Hansson, L., and Lundin, S. (1984): Hypertension and coronary heart disease: Cause and consequence or associated disease? *Am. J. Med.*, Feb 27:41–44.

23. Hansson, L. (1987): β-Blockers in hypertension. *J. Hypertens.*, 5(suppl 3):S61–S67.

24. Hollander, W. (1976): Role of hypertension in atherosclerosis and cardiovascular disease. *Am. J. Cardiol.*, 38:786–800.

25. James, T. N., Hagemann, G. R., and Urthaler, F. (1979): Anatomic and physiologic considerations of a cardiogenic hypertensive chemoreflex. *Am. J. Cardiol.*, 44:852–859.

26. James, T. N. (1974): Diseases of the large and small coronary arteries. *Arch. Intern. Med.*, 134:163–176.

27. Kannel, W. B. (1987): New perspectives on cardiovascular risk factors. *Am. Heart J.*, 114:213–219.

28. Kaplan, N. M. (1987): Antihypertensive drugs: How different classes can impact patients' coronary heart disease risk profile and quality of life. *Am. J. Med.*, 82(suppl 1A):9–14.

29. Karliner, J. S., Williams, D., Gorwit, J., Crawford, M. H., and O'Rourke, R. A. (1977): Left ventricular performance in patients with left ventricular hypertrophy caused by systemic arterial hypertension. *Br. Heart J.*, 39:1239–1245.

30. Klein, W. W. (1984): Treatment of hypertension with calcium channel blockers: European data. *Am. J. Med.*, 77:143–146.

31. Kubo, S. H., Clark, M., Laragh, J. H., Borer, J. S., and Cody, R. J. (1987): Identification of normal neurohormonal activity in mild congestive heart failure and the stimulating effect of upright posture and diuretics. *Am. J. Cardiol.*, 60:1322–1328.

32. Levy, R. I., and Moskowitz, J. (1982): Cardiovascular research: Decades of progress, a decade of promise. *Science*, 217:121–129.

33. Liebson, P. R., Devereux, R. B., and Horan, M. J. (1987): Hypertension research: Echocardiography in the measurement of left ventricular wall mass. *Hypertension*, 9(suppl II):II1–II104.

34. Lowenthal, D. T., Saris, S. D., Packer, J., Haratz, A., and Conry, K. (1984): Mechanisms of action and the clinical pharmacology of beta-adrenergic blocking drugs. *Am. J. Med.*, 77:119–127.

35. Maron, B. J., Wolfson, J. K., Epstein, S. E., and Roberts, W. C. (1986): Intramural ("small ves-

sel'') coronary artery disease in hypertrophic cardiomyopathy. *J. Am. Coll. Cardiol.*, 8:545–547.

36. Messerli, F. H., Ventura, H. O., Elizardi, D. J., Dunn, F. G., and Frohlich, E. D. (1984): Hypertension and sudden death: Increased ventricular ectopic activity in left ventricular hypertrophy. *Am. J. Med.*, 77:18–22.

37. Messerli, F. H. (1983): Clinical determinants and consequences of left ventricular hypertrophy. *Am. J. Med.*, 75:51–56.

38. Moser, M. (1987): Diuretics in the management of hypertension. *Med. Clin. N. Am.*, 71:935–946.

39. Motz, W., and Strauer, B. E. (1984): Regression of structural cardiovascular changes by antihypertensive therapy. *Hypertension*, 6(suppl III): III133–III139.

40. Nichols, A. B., Sciacca, R. R., Weiss, M. B., Blood, D. K., Brennan, D. L., and Cannon, P. I. (1980): Effect of left ventricular hypertrophy on myocardial blood flow and ventricular performance in systemic hypertension. *Circulation*, 62:329–340.

41. O'Rourke, R. A. (1985): Rationale for calcium entry-blocking drugs in systemic hypertension complicated by coronary artery disease. *Am. J. Cardiol.*, 56:34H–40H.

42. Oliver, M. F. (1984): Strategy of reducing coronary risk and the use of drugs. *J. Cardiovasc. Pharmacol.*, 6(suppl 6):S880–S887.

43. Pfeffer, J. M., Pfeffer, M. A., and Braunwald, E. (1985): Influence of chronic captopril therapy on the infarcted left ventricle of the rat. *Cir. Res.*, 57:84–95.

44. Pickering, G., Sir. (1972): Hypertension: Definitions, natural histories and consequences. *Am. J. Med.*, 52:570–583.

45. Poole-Wilson, P. A. (1987): Diuretics, hypokalaemia and arrhythmias in hypertensive patients: Still an unresolved problem. *J. Hypertens.*, 5(suppl 3):S51–S55.

46. Prisant, L. M., Frank, M. J., Carr, A. A., von Dohlen, T. W., and Abdulla, A. M. (1987): How can we diagnose coronary heart disease in hypertensive patients? *Hypertension*, 10:467–472.

47. Rose, G. (1987): Review of primary prevention trials. *Am. Heart. J.*, 114:1013–1017.

48. Shea, S., Cook, E. F., Kannel, W. B., and Goldman, L. (1985): Treatment of hypertension and its effect on cardiovascular risk factors: Data from the Framingham Heart Study. *Circulation*, 71:22–30.

49. Slater, E. E., and Desanctis, R. W. (1980): Diseases of the aorta. In: *Heart Disease: A Textbook of Cardiovascular Medicine*, edited by E. Braunwald, pp. 1597–1632. W. B. Saunders Co, Philadelphia.

50. Solberg, L. A., and Strong, J. P. (1983): Risk factors and atherosclerotic lesions: A review of autopsy studies. *Arteriosclerosis*, 3:187–198.

51. Stamler, J. (1973): Epidemiology of coronary heart disease. *Med. Clin. N. Am.*, 57:5–46.

52. Strauer, B. E. (1987): Structural and functional adaptation of the chronically overloaded heart in arterial hypertension. *Am. Heart J.*, 114:948–957.

53. Tarazi, R. C. (1985): The heart in hypertension. *N. Engl. J. Med.*, 312:308–309.

54. Topol, E. J., Traill, T. A., and Fortuin, N. J. (1985): Hypertensive hypertrophic cardiomyopathy of the elderly. *N. Engl. J. Med.*, 312:277–283.

55. Urquhart, J., Patterson, R. E., Bacharach, S. L., Green, M. V., Speir, E. H., Aamodt, R., and Epstein, S. E. (1980): Comparative effects of verapamil, diltiazem, and nifedipine on hemodynamics and left ventricular function during acute myocardial ischemia in dogs. *Circulation*, 69:382–390.

56. Urquhart, J., Epstein, S. E., and Patterson, R. E. (1985): Comparative effects of calcium-channel blocking agents on left ventricular function during acute ischemia in dogs with and without congestive heart failure. *Am. J. Cardiol.*, 55:10B–16B.

57. Wilhelmsen, L. (1984): Risk factors for coronary heart disease in perspective. *Am. J. Med.*, 77:37–40.

58. Wisneski, J. A., and Bristow, J. D. (1978): Left ventricular stiffness. *Ann. Rev. Med.*, 29:475–483.

New Therapeutic Strategies in Hypertension,
edited by Norman M. Kaplan,
Barry M. Brenner, and John H. Laragh.
Raven Press, Ltd., New York © 1989.

Treatment of Hypertension in the Elderly

Charles P. Tifft and Aram V. Chobanian

Cardiovascular Institute and the Evans Memorial Department of Clinical Research, Boston University, School of Medicine, Boston, Massachusetts 02118

Hypertension is one of the most common reasons older individuals seek health care as outpatients. Hypertension management requires follow-up at regular intervals and thus may be considered a facilitator of routine health care by encouraging regular interaction with a health-care provider. Although the clinician may focus on the blood pressure while seeing the hypertensive, questioning for side effects and other "quality of life" concerns opens a window for possible improved overall health care. It is this unmeasurable factor that has made some of the intervention trials difficult to interpret at face value.

It has been estimated that by the year 1990 almost thirty million Americans will be 65 years of age or older and of these, almost two-thirds will have elevated blood pressures of at least 140 mmHg systolic or 90 mmHg diastolic.

DEFINITION OF HYPERTENSION IN THE ELDERLY

Most definitions of hypertension in the elderly have used systolic blood pressure levels greater than or equal to 160 mmHg or diastolic blood pressures of greater than or equal to 90 mmHg or both. The prevalence of hypertension in the elderly obviously depends upon which definition is used. Borderline systolic hypertension may be defined as systolic blood pressure between 140 and 159 mmHg and definite systolic hypertension at 160 mmHg or greater.

Diastolic blood pressures of 90 mmHg or greater should be considered hypertensive. Diagnosis should be based on the 1988 Report of the Joint National Committee on Detection, Evaluation, and Treatment of High Blood Pressure (JNC IV) (37).

Pseudohypertension, in some elderly patients, may overestimate the prevalence of hypertension but does not negate any benefits that have been shown to occur with drug treatment since control groups have an equal prevalence of overdiagnosis (87). On the other hand, in some hypertensives overestimation of the blood pressure may help explain some of the drug intolerance that is seen with multiple attempts to lower blood pressure. Although direct intraarterial measurement of blood pressure may be the most definitive method of diagnosis, physical examination for the palpable and pulseless artery when the cuff is insufflated and careful clinical observation with cautious blood pressure reduction may be the most reasonable approach (56). Noninvasive measurement using infrasonic recorders may provide a more satisfactory approach to screening for pseudohypertension (29). This problem is not inconsequential since somewhere between 12 and 36% of the discrepancies of greater than 10 mmHg diastolic may be found between indirect and direct arterial reading in elderly patients who have risk factors for vascular disease (61,91).

Another cause of false blood pressure determination is the presence of an auscultatory gap which is larger than the usual few millimeters of mercury. When this gap is increased, the difference between the first Korotkoff sound, its disappearance, and its reappearance as the third Korotkoff sound may exceed 40 to 50 millimeters of mercury. If the cuff is then insufflated between the first and the third Korotkoff sounds, the third may be mistaken as the systolic blood pressure. To ensure that the true systolic blood pressure has been obtained, insufflation should vigorously elevate the cuff pressure to that level which causes the radial pulse to disappear before deflation is initiated (20).

Occasionally the diastolic blood pressure is unobtainable and the "tapping" sounds may be heard to extremely low levels. In this case, clinicians should listen for a muffling or fourth Korotkoff sound and consider that level to be the diastolic blood pressure.

One oversight that may have clinical consequences when measuuring the blood pressure in some older hypertensives is not measuring orthostatic changes, especially when antihypertensive agents are being utilized that may cause orthostatic hypotension. This could have obvious consequences in the patients so affected.

Finally, blood pressure should be initially determined in both arms in the elderly since obstruction to arterial flow may occur proximal to the brachial artery. The arm with the higher reading should be used to monitor the blood pressure and it is best to mark the chart and instruct the patient that only that arm be used. Failure to do this may result in unusually labile blood pressure readings and under- or over-treatment, depending upon the arm which is used for a given blood pressure reading.

Blood pressure may vary with the time of day but other influences such as food ingestion may be of more import in diagnosing as well as evaluating the effects of therapy since falls in systolic blood pressure of at least 25 mmHg may be seen in elderly subjects at approximately one-half hour after ingestion of a meal (50,97).

PREVALENCE OF VARIOUS LEVELS OF BLOOD PRESSURE IN THE ELDERLY

The National Health and Nutrition Examination Survey (NHANES II) screened 2,607 noninstitutionalized individuals aged 65 to 74 years regardless of their medication status (73). The blood pressure classification was based upon three determinations at one sitting, and thus may underestimate the true prevalence of hypertension, but this is lessened somewhat by the fact that individuals already taking medication were included in the screening. An approximation of the various subsets of hypertensives is depicted in Figure 1 (73). Four percent of the population were high normal (85–89 mmHg, diastolic), 22% were mild (90–104 mmHg, diastolic), 3% were moderate (105 to 114 mmHg, diastolic), and 1% was severe (greater than 114 mmHg, diastolic). Close to 30% had isolated systolic blood pressure greater than 140 mmHg but only 8% were greater than 160 mmHg systolic. Thus, hypertension appears to be common in this population but severe hypertension is uncommon.

More recently, the Systolic Hypertension in the Elderly Program (SHEP) pilot study screened 7,778 individuals aged 65 to 74 years and 5,566 individuals aged 75 years or older with repeated determinations at separate sittings (33). A systolic blood pressure greater than 160 mmHg was found in 68% of the younger age group and 75% in the older group. This prevalence may slightly overestimate the true prevalence since the subjects were probably self-selected for having hypertension (39% reported taking antihypertensive medication at the time of initial screening); nevertheless, it is apparent that systolic hyperten-

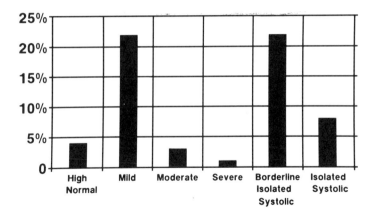

FIG. 1. Hypertension prevalence in Americans aged 65 to 74 years based upon the National Health and Nutrition Examination Survey (NHANES II). (Adapted from Rocella, ref. 73.)

sion is a common finding in the older individual.

CHARACTERISTICS FOUND WITH INCREASING AGE IN HYPERTENSION

Aging and hypertension have a number of similar findings in regards to the blood vessel wall. These findings have been recently reviewed and are summarized in Table 1 (6). Some hypertrophy of endothelial cells as well as an increase in endothelial permeability may be found with smooth muscle cell proliferation and increases in glycosaminoglycans and collagen. These changes account for the increase in rigidity that is found in both situations and lead to a decrease in vascular compliance in the older or hypertensive individual. The rise in systolic blood pressure with age probably is chiefly related to these changes. This increase in rigidity is accentuated when the process of atherosclerosis also involves the arterial conduit.

There are some differences between aging and the hypertensive state (6,77,92). For example, the older individual does not show the increased sensitivity to pressor substances that may be found in the hypertensive, nor is the hypertensives' increased beta-adrenoreceptor affinity to agonists found with aging. On the other hand, increased sympathetic response to posture and exercise may be found with aging (9,64).

Reduced elasticity and compliance are also associated with an increase in pulse pressure. Baroreceptor sensitivity is lessened with aging but is further reduced when the individual is also hypertensive (25). This reduced baroreceptor sensitivity probably inhibits the elderly individuals' ability to compensate for both increases as well as decreases in blood pressure.

At the same level of blood pressure

Table 1. *Comparisons between aging and hypertension in the arterial wall*

	Aging	Hypertension
Endothelium		
Changes in cell shape and intimal thickening	+	+
Increase in endothelial permeability	+	+
Smooth muscle cell proliferation	+	+
Glycosaminoglycans accumulation	+	+
Calcium deposition	+	+/0
Media		
Smooth muscle cell proliferation	+	+
Collagen	+	+
Increased sensitivity to pressor agents	0	+
Beta adrenoreceptor affinity to agonists	−	+

Adapted from Chobanian, ref. 6.

Table 2. *Cardiovascular hemodynamics in 60 young and old hypertensives with equal mean arterial blood pressure*

	Young	Old[b]
Age (years)	32	73
Systolic BP[a]	lower	higher
Diastolic BP[a]	higher	lower
Cardiac output	higher	lower
Stroke volume	higher	lower
Total peripheral resistance	lower	higher
Renal blood flow	lower	higher

Adapted from Messerli et al., ref. 55.
[a] BP = Blood pressure.
[b] $p < 0.05$, older versus younger.

younger patients tend to exhibit a higher cardiac output and lower peripheral resistance than that found in the older hypertensive (52,55). These findings are summarized in Table 2 (55). Resting stroke volume, exercise-induced maximum heart rate and cardiac index are reduced as well as ejection fraction. Lastly, the duration to complete diastolic relaxation is increased as well as the time to complete systolic contraction (44,45).

Left ventricular hypertrophy increases with age so that almost 40% of individuals over age 70 years in the Framingham cohort have demonstrated left ventricular hypertrophy by echographic examination (49). Obviously the presence of hypertension only serves to magnify these changes described above.

The previously described hemodynamic changes are accompanied by a reduction in plasma volume of approximately 8% in the face of the reduced renal reserve and renal blood flow that develops with aging (12,15,47,55). Thus, the older individual is less able to manage large swings in salt and water intake or loss. As a consequence the older hypertensive may have an altered distribution, bioavailability, and physiologic effect of a given dosage of many of the pharmacologic agents including the antihypertensive agents.

Older hypertensives show a lesser rise in catecholamines upon stimulation as well as a lessened tissue responsiveness to catecholamine stimulation. This in part may explain why plasma catecholamines may be increased in older hypertensives as well as the finding of reduced cellular receptors that has been described. Other factors such as decreased renal excretion or metabolism of the catecholamines themselves may also be important (16,46).

Basal renin and aldosterone levels are reduced in older hypertensives as compared to the younger hypertensives and these hormones show a reduced stimulation in response to upright posture as well as to furosemide stimulation. Thus, the older hypertensive individual is different in many ways from the younger. A summary of our findings from a group of hypertensives is summarized in Table 3 (21). It is presumed that these changes develop over time but one cannot be certain that the characteristics of systolic, diastolic, and combined systolic-diastolic hypertension are the same. In addition, those hypertensives who developed hypertension, say, in their late 60s and beyond, may possibly have different characteristics than those who have longer-standing hypertension. Finally, elderly hypertensives who have severe or abrupt onset hypertension may have a secondary form of hypertension and may have been

Table 3. *Humoral findings in unmedicated young and old hypertensives*

	Younger than 40 years	Older than 60 years
% High PRA[a]	14	2
% Low PRA[a]	2	48
Plasma aldosterone	normal	normal
Plasma norepinephrine	lower	higher
Response of PRA[a] and plasma aldosterone to oral furosemide stimulation	greater	lesser

Adapted from Gavras et al. ref. 21.
[a] PRA, Plasma renin activity.

excluded from analyses that have been performed to date.

RISK OF HYPERTENSION IN THE ELDERLY AND BENEFITS OF ITS TREATMENT

Systolic and/or diastolic hypertension is not benign. Data from a retirement community demonstrated a markedly higher prevalence of sudden death, diabetes, aortic calcification, and stroke among 72 elderly individuals with systolic elevations as compared to a 4-year follow-up of matched controls (7). The Chicago Stroke Study revealed that in individuals aged 65 to 74 years with diastolic blood pressures less than 95 mmHg, systolic blood pressures greater than 180 mmHg were associated with a 59% increase in mortality over 3 years of follow-up (78).

The Framingham Heart Study has shown that increasing systolic blood pressure increases cardiovascular risk and that this risk does not become attenuated with age; the curve actually becomes steeper (38). This is important since many practitioners still accept the rise in blood pressure with age as a normal consequence of aging. Although it is seen in salt-consuming, acculturated societies, hypertension must still be viewed as a marker and/or cause for subsequent cardiovascular events.

Individuals aged 60 to 69 years with untreated systolic blood pressure greater than 160 mmHg at the beginning of the Hypertension Detection and Follow-Up Program (HDFP) had close to twice the race-sex-adjusted mortality rates over an 8-year follow-up (34). For each millimeter of mercury increase in systolic blood pressure there was a 1% increase in all-cause mortality.

Epidemiologic data accumulated to date reinforce the fact that the presence of hypertension in an older individual is not benign but does this mean that treatment is of benefit? Unfortunately, sparse information is available to support the clinician in the decision to employ pharmacotherapy. The Veterans Administration Cooperative Study has been reevaluated and supports the drug treatment of the 81 (20% of total subjects) who were over 60 years of age. In this study, this age group suffered more than one-half of the morbid events in follow-up (93,94).

A double-blind prospective trial of antihypertensive treatment was performed in 91 Japanese hypertensives with an average age of 76 years who were followed up for four years (42). This very small study showed no difference in outcome in the treated group except that antihypertensive therapy prevented worsening of the blood pressure level since eight patients treated with placebo developed blood pressures in excess of 200/110 mmHg as compared to none in the actively-treated group.

The Australian National Blood Pressure Study treated hypertensives with diastolic blood pressures of at least 95 mmHg and included 582 hypertensives aged 60 to 69 years of which 293 received active drug treatment (71,72). No differences in morbidity or mortality were shown after almost three years of follow-up, but total trial endpoints were higher in the placebo (n=42) than in the actively-treated group (n=27), a reduction of 39% (p<0.025). The observed trends are parallel to the results of the study as a whole but the actual number of older hypertensives in the study is too small to make independent subgroup analysis valid.

Only two completed studies of reasonable size using diastolic blood pressure of 90 mmHg for treatment are available, the HDFP subgroups of individuals aged 60 to 69 years on entry and the European Working Party on High Blood Pressure in the Elderly (EWPE) trial of individuals over age 60 years (1,2,34,35). Both studies used diuretic-based therapy followed by the sympatholytic, methyldopa, as the primary treatment modality. A potassium-sparing diuretic, hydrochlorothiazide/triamterene, was used in the EWPE trial whereas specific attention to potassium was individualized in the HDFP trial. The 2 trials combined a total of only 3,216 hypertensive subjects.

Figure 2 depicts the HDFP's reduction in fatal plus nonfatal five-year stroke rate of 5.5% to 3.0% (a 46% reduction). A similar reduction in fatal stroke was also observed. In this study, the greatest reduction in stroke of usual referred care versus special care was found in the oldest subgroup of hypertensives. Overall, mortality rates were reduced from 15.2% to 12.7% (a 16% reduction) with special treatment for 5 years. This was achieved with reduction of slightly less than 5 mmHg diastolic blood pressure in the special-care group compared to the referred-care group. Thus, five-year treatment of 100 hypertensives aged 60 to 69 years with an intensive immersion into health care which included free medication, home visits when necessary, and, presumably, enhanced triage for other health problems results in 2.5 fewer deaths than occurred in a community-treated group of equally-aged hypertensives.

The EWPE trial is the only placebo-controlled, double-blind, randomized trial of antihypertensive therapy conducted in hypertensive subjects over 60 years of age. This study has limits to its interpretation because of the relatively small enrollment of only 840 hypertensives recruited at 18 centers. Entry criteria included both a sitting diastolic blood pressure on placebo treatment between 90 to 119 mmHg and a systolic blood pressure between 160 to 239 mmHg. Blinded active treatment was given to 416 subjects for 7 years as outlined in Figure 3. The combination capsule of 25 mg hydrochlorothiazide/50 mg triamterene was given in a dosage of 1 capsule daily to 51% of subjects and 2 or more capsules daily to 45% of the hypertensives at the end of the blinded portion of the trial; 4% of treated subjects were not taking diuretics. In the active-treatment group, 65% were on diuretic therapy only; 26% were taking between 250 mg and 1,000 mg daily of methyldopa; and 9% were taking greater than 1,000 mg of methyldopa daily. As expected, placebo-treated subjects received more tablets than actively-treated hypertensives.

Prerandomization blood pressures were the same, following a period of placebo treatment: *182/101 ± 16/7 versus 182/101 ± 17/7* mmHg. The hypertensives probably had slightly higher blood pressures than these since placebo therapy, even on a short-term basis, may reduce blood pressure to some extent. Thus, this study examined the results of therapy in a group of older hypertensives with moderate rather than mild hypertension. The large 1976–1980 NHANES II screening in the United States found that diastolic hypertension above 104 mmHg was present in no more than four percent of hypertensives aged 65 to 74 years. Thus, it appears that most of the hypertensives a practitioner will see

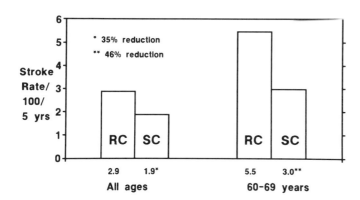

FIG. 2. Incidence of stroke by age and treatment group found in the Hypertension Detection and Follow-up Program (HDFP). Data adjusted for race, sex, entry DBP. (Adapted from ref. 35.)

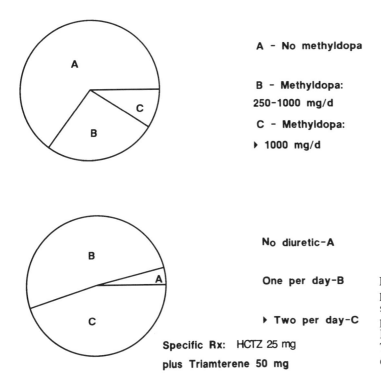

A - No methyldopa

B - Methyldopa:
250–1000 mg/d

C - Methyldopa:
▸ 1000 mg/d

No diuretic–A

One per day–B

▸ Two per day–C

Specific Rx: HCTZ 25 mg

plus Triamterene 50 mg

FIG. 3. Specific drug therapies used in treating hypertensives at the end of the European Working Party on High Blood Pressure in the Elderly Trial. (Adapted from Amery et al., ref. 1.)

may have lower blood pressure than those treated in this intervention trial.

The trial lasted 12 years; by the end of the trial only 35% of the subjects remained. As expected, because of the age of the participants, 19% of the subjects had died by the end of the trial but no difference in overall mortality was found between those treated with placebo and those on active medication (9% reduction in mortality with treatment, $p = 0.41$). Although stroke mortality was reduced by 32%, this did not reach statistical significance ($p = 0.16$). There were 29 fewer cardiovascular deaths overall and 14 fewer cardiovascular deaths per 1,000 patient years of active treatment during the double-blind phase of the trial.

A further analysis of the EWPE trial found that cardiovascular mortality increased with increasing systolic but not diastolic blood pressure at presentation (2). The effect of treatment was significant even when age, sex, baseline systolic and diastolic blood pressure were taken into ac-

count. The proportional reduction in cardiovascular mortality was similar in the 30% of subjects who had previous cardiovascular complications compared to those without complications. This study suggests that therapy is of benefit at least through 79 years of age. However, it is not clear how much benefit may be obtained after that age since only 155 subjects, of which 140 were female, were older than 79 years of age.

Individuals who have experienced a thrombotic stroke deserve good control of hypertension but overzealous control may not be helpful. Patients with multiinfarct dementia were followed for almost two years (57). Among those who were hypertensive, improved cognition and clinical course correlated with control of systolic blood pressure to levels between 135 and 150 mm Hg but, when blood pressures were reduced to lower levels, the dementia appeared to deteriorate. Poorer outcome is found after a stroke in those individuals who continue to have higher blood pressures (36,96). Stroke recurrence has not been reduced by anti-hypertensive treatment but no large long-term antihypertensive trials have been performed. One small study found a reduction in recurrence of stroke in hypertensive stroke patients who were less than 65 years of age and had blood pressures of 110 mmHg diastolic two weeks after the neurologic insult (5). This notwithstanding, most clinicians attempt to control blood pressure after the acute stroke with special attention to diastolic blood pressure since the HDFP results were encouraging for primary prevention of stroke (69,89). Caution and careful follow-up is always indicated since, for example, both carotid and lower extremity occlusive disease has been demonstrated by duplex scans in one-third to one-half of those with isolated systolic hypertension, and reduction in blood pressure may also impair circulation to other organs (75,84).

In summary, treatment of diastolic hypertension between ages 60 to 69 has the most supporting evidence for beneficial effects. Above this age, there is suggestive but not definitive evidence of benefit. There is no intervention trial data that conclusively demonstrates any benefit of treating systolic hypertension. Thus, a decision to treat should weigh the possible benefits and risks of therapy. A rough guide for decision-making in regards to antihypertensive treatment is outlined in Table 4.

Treatment of any persistent diastolic hypertension over 90 mmHg may be indicated and therapy above 180 mmHg systolic seems reasonable due to the marked increase in risk above this level demonstrated in epidemiologic studies. Levels of systolic blood pressure between 140 and 180 mmHg require a more individualized approach except when hypertensive complications, such as congestive heart failure, angina pectoris, and previous stroke, are already present.

Table 4. *Relative indications and contraindications to antihypertensive therapy in the older hypertensive*

Indications	Contraindications
Diastolic blood pressure ≥90 mmHg	True pseudohypertension
Systolic blood pressure >180 mmHg[a]	Systolic blood pressure between 140–180 mmHg[b]
Hypertension with target organ damage: retinopathy, congestive heart failure, renal failure, cerebral hemorrhage, coronary artery disease, aortic aneurysm	Worsening peripheral vascular disease symptoms with treatment
	Poor response to multiple therapies and worsening of quality of life with therapy[b]
Risk factors: smoking, diabetes, dyslipidemia	

[a] Based upon epidemiologic risk.
[b] Individualized approach suggested.

EVALUATION

Evaluation of the elderly individual with hypertension should be no different than in the younger individual, except that examination and laboratory tests may be more likely to show target organ damage or glucose intolerance. Recent onset of moderate or severe hypertension should at least raise the suspicion of a secondary cause of the elevated blood pressure, especially since it is uncommon to see severe hypertension in the elderly. On the other hand, it may not be reasonable to pursue evaluation of secondary causes of hypertension if the clinician or the patient is unwilling to alter the therapeutic strategy based upon the acquired information. Age and other cardiovascular disease is not necessarily a reason to avoid aggressive therapeutic approaches since these individuals seem to tolerate renovascular surgery better today than in the past and the benefits of improving blood pressure control and sometimes renal function can outweigh the risks involved (17,18,31,32,63,79). Each older hypertensive requires an individualized approach since the evaluation, for example, arteriography even with digital enhancement, is not innocuous (27,88). Recent excellent reviews discuss the assessment of surgical risk in the preoperative patient (22,23).

NON-DRUG THERAPIES FOR THE ELDERLY

Sodium restriction may reduce blood pressure in some hypertensives, and the elderly may be no different in this regard. Nevertheless, the older hypertensive may actually consume less sodium than the younger hypertensive. Sodium restriction may potentiate other antihypertensive agents with the possible exception of calcium channel blockers and may also help conserve potassium if on diuretic therapy.

The Working Group on Hypertension in the Elderly has also recommended caloric restriction when appropriate to help lower blood pressure (100).

Although aging is associated with a decline in exercise capacity—which may be due to aging itself, inactivity, or other medical conditions—it may be possible for the elderly to enter into exercise programs (68). Systolic blood pressure reduction of 144 mmHg has been shown to occur in institutionalized men with a mean age of 72 years after an endurance training program. Two other studies have also described significant reduction in resting systolic blood pressure and one of these also found a decline in diastolic blood pressure. Thus, it may be possible for the older hypertensive to benefit from exercise as a non-drug therapy (3,14,81).

Other non-drug treatments of hypertension have less scientific support (39,74). Most studies investigating meditation, biofeedback, and alcohol reduction, for example, have employed younger subjects but, since the effect of placebo therapy has also been shown, as depicted in Table 5, it

Table 5. *Effect of placebo therapy in hypertensives with a mean age of 72 years in the EWPE trial*

Time	Systolic BP[a]	Diastolic BP[a]	n
Baseline	182 ± 16	101 ± 7	424
1 year	172 ± 23	95 ± 12	300
5 years	171 ± 25	95 ± 9	93

Adapted from Amery et al., ref. 2.
[a] Sitting blood pressure ± mean, expressed in mmHg.

is hard to argue too strongly against these adjunctive measures in the older hypertensive. As with younger individuals, the success with long-term non-drug therapies remains to be demonstrated in most instances, so cautious follow-up would be indicated for those so treated. One concern would be that appropriate pharmacotherapy be withheld in the older hypertensive with diastolic hypertension where drug therapy may have the strongest support at the present time. The individual with borderline systolic elevations between 140 and 160 mmHg may be the best candidate for non-drug approaches since much less is known about the benefits or perceived benefits of pharmacotherapy in this group of hypertensives.

PHARMACOTHERAPY OF HYPERTENSION IN THE ELDERLY

Diuretic therapy has been available since 1957 and has formed the basis of the intervention trials and stepped-care. There is little evidence to doubt its efficacy in the older hypertensive based upon the results of the Veterans Administration Cooperative Study, the HDFP study, the EWPE trial, and the Systolic Hypertension in the Elderly Program feasibility trial. Both diastolic and systolic blood pressures may be reduced effectively (1,2,10,33,34,35).

The SHEP trial is currently testing the possible benefits of treating isolated systolic hypertension (as defined by systolic blood pressure of 160 mmHg or greater) with 25 to 50 mg of chlorthalidone daily. This trial is not testing the other possible antihypertensive agents as initial therapy nor is potassium-chloride supplementation nor potassium-retaining pharmacotherapy being investigated.

A feasibility trial has been conducted in which 27,199 men and women over 60 years of age were screened to yield 551 subjects who had isolated systolic hypertension and met other trial criteria (33). Mean systolic blood pressures were 172 ± 11 mmHg and diastolic 75 ± 9 mmHg. It is of interest that 41% lived alone, 11% were current workers, 63% were women, 72% were white, 46% had been treated in the past with antihypertensive medication, 34% had an abnormal funduscopic examination, and 26% took aspirin at least four times weekly.

Chlorthalidone 25 mg daily was initiated in 443 hypertensives and 108 were randomized to placebo. If, after 12 weeks of therapy, systolic blood pressure had not been reduced to less than 160 mmHg or by 20 mmHg (whichever was lower) then the step two regimen of reserpine 0.05 mg twice-daily, metoprolol 50 mg twice-daily, hydralazine 25 mg twice-daily, or matching placebo twice-daily was prescribed in a random fashion. The drugs could be doubled 12 weeks later if needed.

After one year of therapy, 17% of subjects had discontinued the chlorthalidone and 20% had discontinued the placebo therapy. Those who remained in the trial at one year had a remarkable measured compliance of 85%. Significant reductions in blood pressure as compared to placebo were found by intention-to-treat analysis (17 mmHg mean systolic, $p<0.001$). Diastolic hypotension did not appear to be a clinical problem.

After one year of therapy, 56% of the subjects were taking the 25 mg dosage of chlorthalidone and 88% had not required step two medication. Thus, the efficacy of chlor-

thalidone in isolated systolic hypertension in this age group appears established. Side effects appeared no more common in the treated versus placebo groups. Hypokalemia to levels of 3.5 meq/liter occurred in 21% of the diuretic-treated subjects. Serum uric acid was higher in the diuretic group (6.8 versus 5.9 mg/dl, $p<0.001$) but gout occurred in only one subject. Serum cholesterol and creatinine were not significantly greater, and only one subject in the diuretic group developed glucose intolerance that required treatment.

Thus, diuretic therapy appears to be effective and well-tolerated when given to a selected, medically-stable population of elderly patients with systolic hypertension.

Diuretics may initially reduce plasma volume but later appear to reduce total peripheral resistance as their primary mechanism of blood pressure reduction. This effect is maintained even after one year of therapy, even in older subjects (90). Since the older hypertensive may have reduced plasma volume, concerns about volume depletion are not unreasonable but adverse experience in this regard appears to be infrequent. Other issues with diuretic therapy, such as glucose intolerance, gout, and sexual dysfunction, may be less than previously thought in the elderly if the SHEP feasibility trial can be taken at face value. Indapamide has been studied in the elderly and may be associated with little metabolic perturbation (66).

The development of hypokalemia remains a concern in the older patient who may have coronary artery disease and may be more prone to cardiac arrhythmias (60,83). Reversal of diuretic-induced hypokalemia may reduce premature contractions in some but not all hypertensives and also may help reduce diastolic blood pressure by a few millimeters of mercury (30,40,65).

Diuretics also may be useful when the older patient has congestive heart failure or has peripheral edema. In addition, they potentiate all other antihypertensive agents. Other considerations may be cost and the availability of fixed combination preparations which, when appropriate in dose and formulation, reduce the total number of pills the older hypertensive needs to remember to take.

Thiazide or thiazide-like diuretics generally may be taken once-daily but the loop diuretics require twice-daily dosing to be adequate antihypertensive agents. They are not more effective than thiazides for hypertension without renal insufficiency.

Methyldopa has been used as a second step agent in the two trials that have shown improved cardiovascular outcome in patients over age 65 years and has been used extensively as an antihypertensive agent at all ages (1,2,10,34,35,37). In the HDFP trial, overall cessation of this drug was close to 27% whereas, in an analysis of side effects in the older subgroup of HDFP participants aged 60 to 69 years, side effects were severe enough to cause discontinuation in close to 21% of subjects (Table 6). Thus, although this agent may cause orthostatic intolerance, somnolence, dry mouth, and, rarely, hemolytic anemia and abnormal hepatic function, it appears in the HDFP trial not to be less tolerated in the older patient than the younger. Sexual "reactions," for example, occurred only 2% of the time.

Although it is generally felt that this agent

Table 6. *Participants in HDFP with side effects severe enough to cause discontinuation of drug treatment, %*

Drug	Age 60 to 69 years	Age 30 to 69 years
Chlorthalidone	18	21
Spironolactone	17	17
Reserpine	26	29
Methyldopa	21	27
Hydralazine	14	18
Guanethidine	19	27
Other	7	10
Overall	27	33

Adapted from Curb et al., ref. 10.

does not reduce cardiac output, one study has found a reduction in cardiac output in the older hypertensive treated with methyldopa (80). Although these hemodynamic changes have been described, it appears that older hypertensives tolerate methyldopa and the other centrally-acting sympatholytics without exacerbation or precipitation of congestive heart failure. This may be due to the fact that the benefits of blood pressure reduction outweigh any possible negative inotropic effects that may be found. Therapy may be initiated with a dosage as low as 125 mg at bedtime and gradually increased.

The other centrally-acting antihypertensive medications, *clonidine, guanabenz,* and *guanfacine*, may also be useful in treating the older hypertensive. Sedation, dry mouth, and orthostatic intolerance are a concern in some individuals. These agents are usually given in twice-daily doses but some clinicians prefer to give once-daily doses in the evening or at bedtime even though blood pressure control during the latter part of the day may not be achieved. This form of dosing may be more appealing in the hypertensive with side effects to multiple medications, with more severe supine hypertension, or with orthostatic intolerance.

Clonidine is available in a once-weekly application of a transdermal patch which appears to be associated with a lesser side-effect profile than oral clonidine, with the exception of localized skin irritation (67). This form of antihypertensive medication has distinct advantages as far as the ease of administration and may be especially useful when the hypertensive is forgetful, and thus noncompliant, or is visited on a regular basis by family or a visiting nurse. Even if other antihypertensives were omitted most physicians would agree that some medication is better than none, assuming that some blood pressure reduction has occurred.

Reserpine continues to be used in the intervention trials and has a proven track record as far as efficacy and reasonable tolerability. Reserpine's use has been recently reviewed with attention to the elderly (53). Sedation, nasal stuffiness, and exacerbation of peptic symptoms are the major concerns with its use although observations for depression should be made. It is contraindicated in those with a history of previous depression and peptic ulcer disease.

Converting enzyme inhibitors (CEI) have been less enthusiastically forwarded for use in the elderly except when combined with diuretic therapy (70). Recent information suggests that the older and younger hypertensives may have a similar response to this class of antihypertensive (59). CEIs have gained popularity due to their lack of central side effects, usefulness in congestive heart failure, and their tendency not to cause peripheral vascular or orthostatic symptoms. Some elderly hypertensives are very sensitive to the initial dose of the CEI and deserve special caution. Individuals with congestive heart failure, previous diuretic use, and hyponatremia should be monitored carefully and given the smallest possible dose, such as 6.25 mg of captopril or 2.5 mg of enalapril. Caution should be exercised in the hypertensive with renal insufficiency since dosage reductions are necessary and the incidence of adverse reactions to these agents is higher. The elderly hypertensive with severe atherosclerosis, hypertension, and/or renal dysfunction may develop reversible deterioration in renal function when significant renal artery stenosis is present and CEI is added (31,102). Lastly, hyperkalemia may occasionally develop when CEI is added (103). This occurs more often in the presence of mild renal dysfunction, concomitant potassium supplementation, or K-sparing agents. This potassium-retaining property of the CEIs is usually of some benefit, especially when diuretic therapy also is used.

The direct vasodilator *hydralazine* has generally been reserved for use as a third-step agent although some have forwarded its usefulness as a second-step agent in the elderly (100). Reflex increase in heart rate secondary to the vasodilation may be attenuated in the older hypertensive and thus allow its use without beta blocker or sympatholytics that block reflex tachycardia.

Hydralazine is generally well-tolerated in the older hypertensive but headache, gastrointestinal complaints, malaise, and fatigue may occur. Palpitations, chest pain, or myocardial ischemia are uncommon. Hydralazine does not cause orthostatic hypotension. Initial dosage should not exceed 25 mg one- or twice-daily and should be slowly increased to a maximum of probably 200 mg daily. Those with renal insufficiency and blacks are at increased risk of adverse reactions, such as drug-induced lupus syndrome, at higher doses.

Selective alpha blockers reduce peripheral resistance and are associated with less reflex tachycardia than nonselective alpha blockers (51). Tachyphylaxis is not a concern as far as its antihypertensive efficacy but has been found in patients with congestive heart failure. These agents are not associated with exacerbation of asthma, peripheral vascular symptoms, diabetes, or congestive heart failure, and sexual dysfunction is rare. Headache, palpitations, and lassitude may occur but central side effects appear to be fairly rare. Orthostatic hypotension may occur or be exacerbated by these agents and thus they should not be given to the older hypertensive with orthostatic intolerance or demonstrated orthostatic hypotension. The initial dose of both prazosin and terazosin should be no more than 1 milligram at bedtime and diuretic therapy should probably be withheld if possible for a few days to help prevent the rare occurrence of first-dose hypotension. If hypotension occurs, it may last longer if terazosin is used due to terazosin's longer pharmacologic half-life than prazosin. The doses of these drugs should be slowly titrated upwards toward 20 mg, one of the most common errors in usage being a failure to adequately titrate the drug in the absence of side effects.

The *ganglionic blocking agents* guanethidine and guanadrel may induce severe orthostatic hypotension, and for this reason these agents are not appropriate for use in the elderly hypertensive. This may be particularly true in those with baseline isolated systolic hypertension and normal or low-diastolic blood pressure.

The *beta blocking agents* have been extensively used to treat hypertension and have the advantage of being protective in the high-risk acute and postmyocardial infarction, and possibly preventative for initial myocardial infarction, at least as compared to thiazide diuretic (28,85). Beta blockers treat concomitant angina pectoris, certain arrhythmias, tremor, and anxiety, and also have received wide lay-press approval. Previously, older hypertensives had been thought not to respond as well to beta blockade as far as both efficacy in blood pressure reduction and tolerability of side effects are concerned. However, a large multicenter trial, summarized in Table 7, that included a large group of older hypertensives (98) demonstrated that blood pressure reduction was the same to the initial dosage of 25 mg hydrochlorothiazide or 100

Table 7. *Hydrochlorothiazide* versus *Metoprolol in hypertensives aged 60 to 75 years*

	HCTZ 25 mg	Metoprolol 100 mg
Age in years[a]	67.2 ± 4.7	66.4 ± 4.4
Baseline BP[a]	$\frac{188}{108} \pm \frac{18}{7}$	$\frac{186}{108} \pm \frac{18}{6}$
Week 4 BP in mmHg	$\frac{169}{96} \pm \frac{22}{10}$	$\frac{171}{96} \pm \frac{22}{10}$
Percentage of patients with diastolic BP <95 mmHg	47	50
Total drop out rate in percent	5	8

Adapted from Wikstrand, ref. 98.
[a] Mean ± S.D.

mg of metoprolol given once-daily after four weeks of monotherapy in subjects who were aged 60 to 75 years and had moderate hypertension. It is of interest that assessment of well-being scores showed little difference between the thiazide and the beta blocker. Thus, when care is taken to exclude those who have contraindications to beta blockade, beta blocker therapy may be more efficacious and better tolerated in the older hypertensive than previously thought.

Side effects such as fatigue, cool extremities, decreased exercise tolerance, and gastrointestinal complaints may be found. Congestive heart failure, bradycardia, and impaired cardiac conduction, fortunately, are uncommon. Beta blockers should not be given to those elderly hypertensives with congestive heart failure, advanced cardiac conduction disturbances, bradycardia, and asthma.

Agents with significant intrinsic sympathomimetic activity, such as pindolol, may cause less bradycardia and cool extremities than the other beta blockers (48,62). Labetalol combines alpha- and beta-blocking properties and probably causes less reduction in cardiac output than the other beta blockers, but may cause orthostatic hypotension in some patients as well as nasal stuffiness, both of which are usually not seen with the other beta blockers. In addition, this agent may increase the sensitivity to halothane-induced hypotension and a lower dosage of labetalol is indicated when cimetidine is also prescribed (58).

Although much has been made of the central nervous system side effects of the various beta blockers it appears that both the lipophylic and the hydrophylic agents may cause side effects in susceptible individuals, thus reinforcing the need for careful observation with any agent that is chosen.

Metabolic consequences of beta blockade in older hypertensives are probably no different than in younger hypertensives. Selective beta blockers do seem to cause less perturbation of glucose tolerance and, in diabetics who require insulin therapy and a beta blocker, hypoglycemia-induced hypertension and secondary bradycardia is less severe. In addition, recovery from insulin-induced hypoglycemia is more rapid with selective as compared to nonselective beta blockade (43,76,95).

The *calcium channel blockers* have gained rapid acceptance by clinicians caring for older hypertensives because of their efficacy and limited number of contraindications (19,24,26,41,101). They have enjoyed widespread use for the treatment of angina pectoris and therefore their use for hypertension has been an extension of previously developed habits. At the present time three calcium channel blockers are available and there is little evidence that one agent will lower blood pressure more than any other. The differences between the agents rest in their ease of administration and side effect profiles. Nifedipine exhibits little effect on the cardiac conduction system but may cause more peripheral edema, flushing, headache, and occasionally, tachycardia than the other available agents. When given orally and especially after its capsule is severed, the agent may lower blood pressure within 20 to 30 min. This reduction can be quite marked and it may be more appropriate to initiate antihypertensive therapy in the older hypertensive after food ingestion, thereby slowing the absorption of nifedipine and attenuating the onset of blood pressure reduction, as well as lessening any possible vasodilator-related side effects. This agent may be soon available in a slow-release osmotic-pump formulation which should reduce side effects and increase ease of administration as far as dosing frequency is concerned.

Diltiazem and verapamil are similar in that both may have effects on atrio-ventricular conduction and thus are contraindicated in hypertensives with more than first-degree heart block or sick/sinus syndrome. These effects are potentiated by concomitant beta blocker therapy but, using these

agents in otherwise healthy hypertensives, conduction disturbances are rare. It is also rare to develop congestive heart failure with their use in otherwise healthy hypertensives. It is probably true that in most hypertensives the reduction in blood pressure has a more beneficial effect than any possible negative inotropic effect of these calcium channel blockers. The development of pedal edema does not mean that congestive heart failure has developed since this is usually related to the vasodilatory action of these agents. Like nifedipine, diltiazem, at the present time, must be given at least three or four times daily but verapamil is available in a slow-release formulation which allows once- or twice-daily dosing, depending upon the dose required. This clearly is an advantage in the older hypertensive where frequent dosing may be a problem.

The major side effect that limits the usefulness of these two agents in the older hypertensive is the occurrence of abdominal discomfort and constipation. Often constipation is not present but a change in previous bowel habits occurs; a few simple measures may help in this situation. First, before initiation of the calcium channel blocker, adding fiber or preparations such as psyllium to the diet may counteract some of the drug effect. Second, start with the lowest possible dose of the calcium blocker and increase as slowly as the clinical situation allows. Third, other foodstuffs that are known to cause a softening of the stool or increase their frequency may be encouraged.

The addition of calcium channel blockers necessitates a reduction in digoxin dosage and measurement of the serum digoxin level is indicated after their addition (4).

Calcium channel blockers may not be affected by an increased sodium intake but are potentiated by diuretic therapy. They treat coronary symptoms and do not exacerbate asthma, diabetes, peripheral vascular disease and, when given chronically, appear not to cause orthostatic hypotension. They appear not to cause sedation or alter mental function. Thus, these agents, although not perfect, fit in well with older antihypertensive agents as reasonable choices for the elderly hypertensive.

The older hypertensive is more likely to have other medical conditions that may complicate therapy by increasing the total number of individual medications and total number of pills they are required to take intermittently or in a chronic fashion. Both the medical condition itself and the concomitant therapy can conceivably worsen the blood pressure or increase the chance of side effects.

For example, the treatment of arthritis with nonsteroidals may cause sodium retention and interfere with beta blocker, diuretic, or converting enzyme inhibition. Cimetidine, when used for peptide disease, may increase the potency of a given labetalol dose. Initiation of calcium channel blocker increases the digoxin level. Tricyclic antidepressants may interfere with reserpine, the centrally-acting antihypertensives, as well as the ganglionic blockers, and may induce blood pressure reduction and orthostatic hypotension. Levodopa prescribed for Parkinson's disease and sedatives may exacerbate orthostatic hypotension.

In addition, the elderly hypertensive may be unable to open medication containers, may be more forgetful at times, and may require more explicit directions to follow. Compliance-enhancing measures are even more important in these hypertensives and the frequency of office visits may need to be increased. The presence of fixed or limited income may also interfere with obtaining medication in some circumstances and may also affect the nutritional options for the elderly hypertensive. Transportation to and from the health care provider is just one of the social and seemingly "non-medical" issues that may be quite important in achieving improved blood pressure control

in the older hypertensive. Enhanced social support is a desirable goal for improving the health of our older population.

SUMMARY

In summary, the older hypertensive appears to be becoming more common as our population ages. Similarities between aging and hypertension have been demonstrated for some humoral as well as functional characteristics of the endocrine and cardiovascular systems, but it appears that in general hypertension may exacerbate the findings associated with aging.

These changes which result in an elevated blood pressure do increase the cardiovascular risk of the older hypertensive even more than in the younger hypertensive. Evidence has accumulated that supports the notion that established diastolic elevations greater than 90 mm Hg warrant pharmacotherapy, but support for treating isolated systolic hypertension based upon intervention trial data is still wanting. Thus, an individualized approach is indicated for the latter group of hypertensives.

"Quality-of-life" issues are important when treating the older hypertensives since many individuals need to be treated to prevent cardiovascular complications in a few. This is especially important when selecting therapy for isolated systolic hypertension; cautious initiation of therapy, slow titration with attention to detail, and observation for expected and unexpected side effects should help the practitioner deliver the best hypertensive care for this increasingly important segment of the hypertensive population.

ACKNOWLEDGMENT

Supported in part by N.I.H. grant HL 18318.

REFERENCES

1. Amery, A., Birkenhager, W., and Brixko, P., et al. (1985): Mortality and morbidity results from

the European Working Party on High Blood Pressure in the Elderly Trial. *Lancet*, 1:1349–1354.

2. Amery, A., Birkenhager, W., and Brixko, P., et al. (1986): Efficacy of antihypertensive drug treatment according to age, sex, blood pressure, and previous cardiovascular disease in patients over the age of 60. *Lancet*, 2:589–592.

3. Barry, A. J., Daly, J. W., Pruett, E. D. R., Steinmetz, J. R., Page, E. F., Biskhead, N. C., and Rodahl, K. (1966): The effects of physical conditioning on older individuals. I: Working capacity, circulatory-respiratory function and work electrocardiogram. *J. Gerontol.*, 21:182–191.

4. Belz, G. G., Doering, W., Monkes, R., and Matthew, J. (1983): Interaction between digoxin and calcium antagonists and antiarrhythmic drugs. *Clin. Pharmacol. Ther.*, 33:410–417.

5. Carter, A. B. (1970): Hypertensive therapy in stroke survivors. *Lancet*, 1:485–489.

6. Chobanian, A. V. (1988): Arterial wall characteristics in hypertension and aging. In: *Handbook of Hypertension, vol. 11: Hypertension in the Elderly*, edited by A. Amery and J. Staessen. Elsevier Company, Amsterdam (in press).

7. Colandrea, M. A., Friedman, G. D., Nichaman, M. Z., and Lynd, C. D. (1970): Systolic hypertension in the elderly: An epidemiologic assessment. *Circulation*, 41:239–245.

8. Colucci, W. S. (1982): Alpha-adrenergic receptor blockade with prazosin: Consideration of hypertension, heart failure, and potential new applications. *Ann. Int. Med.*, 97:67–77.

9. Conway, J., Whaler, R., and Sannerstadt, R. (1971): Sympathetic nervous activity during exercise in relation to age. *Cardiovasc. Res.*, 5:557–581.

10. Curb, J. D., Borhani, N. O., Blaszkowski, Zimbaldi, N., Fotio, S., and William, W. (1985): Long-term surveillance for adverse effects of antihypertensive drugs. *J. Am. Med. Assoc.*, 253:3263–3268.

11. Curb, D., Borhani, W. O., and Entwisle, G., et al. (1985): Isolated systolic hypertension in 14 communities. *Am. J. Epidemiol.*, 121:362–370.

12. Darmandy, E. M., Offer, J., and Woodhouse, M. A. (1973): The parameters of the aging kidney. *J. Pathol.*, 109:195–203.

13. Davidson, R. A., and Caranasos, G. J. (1987): Should the elderly hypertensive be treated? Evidence from clinical trials. *Arch. Intern. Med.*, 147:1933–1937.

14. deVries, H. A. (1970): Physiological effects of an exercise training regimen upon men aged 52 to 88. *J. Gerontol.*, 25:325–336.

15. Epstein, M., and Hollenberg, N. M. (1976): Age as a determinant of renal sodium conservation in normal man. *J. Lab. Clin. Med.*, 87:411–417.

16. Esler, M. (1981): Age dependence of noradrenaline kinetics in normal subjects. *Clin. Sci.*, 60:217–219.

17. Foster, J. H., Maxwell, M. H., and Franklin, S. S., et al. (1975): Renovascular occlusive disease: Results of operative treatment. *J. Am. Med. Assoc.*, 231:1043–1048.

18. Franklin, S. S., Young, J. D., and Maxwell, M. H., et al. (1975): Operative morbidity and mortality in renovascular disease. *J. Amer. Med. Assoc.*, 231:1148–1153.

19. Frishman, W. H., Weinberg, R., and Peled, H. B. (1984): Calcium-entry blockers for the treatment of severe hypertension and hypertensive crisis. *Am. J. Med.*, 77:35–45.

20. Frohlich, E. D., Grim, C., Labarthe, D. R., Maxwell, M. H., Perloff, D., and Weidman, W. H. (1988): Recommendation for human blood pressure determination by sphygmomanometers: Report of a special task force appointed by the steering committee, American Heart Association. *Hypertension*, 11:210A–222A.

21. Gavras, I., Gavras, H. P., and Chobanian, A. V., et al. (1982): Hypertension and age: Clinical biochemical correlates. *Clin. Exp. Hyp.*, 7:1097–1106.

22. Gerson, M. C., Hurst, J. M., and Hertzberg, V. S. (1985): Cardiac prognosis in noncardiac geriatric surgery. *Ann. Int. Med.*, 103:832–837.

23. Goldman, L. (1983): Cardiac risks and complications of noncardiac surgery. *Ann. Int. Med.*, 98:504–513.

24. Gould, B. A., Hornung, R. S., Mann, S., Balasubramanian, V., and Raftery, E. B. (1982): Slow channel inhibitors, verapamil and nifedipine, in the management of hypertension. *J. Cardiovasc. Pharmacol.*, 4(suppl 3):s369–s373.

25. Gribbin, B., Pickering, T. G., and Sleight, P. (1971): Effect of age and high blood pressure on baroreflex sensitivity in man. *Circ. Res.*, 29:424–431.

26. Halperin, A. K., and Cubeddu, L. X. (1986): The role of calcium channel blockers in the treatment of hypertension. *Am. Heart. J.*, 111:363–382.

27. Havey, R. J., Krumlovsky, F., and del Greco, F., et al. (1985): Screening for renovascular hypertension: Is renal digital-substraction angiography the preferred noninvasive test? *J. Am. Med. Assoc.*, 254:388–393.

28. Hjalmarson, A., Herlitz, J., and Malek, I., et al. (1981): Effect on mortality of metoprolol in acute myocardial infarction: A double-blind randomized trial. *Lancet*, 2:832–837.

29. Hla, K. M., and Feussner, J. R. (1988): Screening for pseudohypertension: A quantitative, non-invasive approach. *Arch. Int. Med.*, 148:673–676.

30. Holland, O. B., Nixon, J. V., and Kuhnert, I. (1981): Diuretic-induced ventricular ectopic activity. *Am. J. Med.*, 70:762–768.

31. Hricik, D. E., Browning, P. J., and Kopelman, R., et al. (1983): Captopril-induced renal insufficiency in patients with bilateral renal-artery stenosis or renal-artery stenosis in a solitary kidney. *N. Engl. J. Med.*, 308:373–376.

32. Hughes, J. H., Dove, H. G., and Gifford, R. W., et al. (1981): Duration of blood pressure elevation in accurately predicting surgical cure of re-

novascular hypertension. *Am. Heart. J.*, 101:408–413.

33. Hulley, S. B., Furberg, C. D., Gurland, B., McDonald, R., Perry, M., Schnaper, H. W., Schoenberger, J. A., Smith, M., and Vogt, T. M. (1985): Systolic Hypertension in the Elderly Program (SHEP): Antihypertensive efficacy of chlorthalidone. *Am. J. Cardiol.*, 56:913–920.

34. Hypertension Detection and Follow-up Program Cooperative Group. (1979): Five-year findings of the Hypertension Detection and Follow-up Program. II: Mortality by race-sex and age. *J. Am. Med. Assoc.*, 242:2572–2577.

35. Hypertension Detection and Follow-up Program Cooperative Group. (1982): Five-year findings of the Hypertension Detection and Follow-up Program. III: Reduction in stroke incidence among persons with high blood pressure. *J. Am. Med. Assoc.*, 247:633–638.

36. Hypertension-Stroke Cooperative Study Group. (1974): Effect of antihypertensive treatment on stroke recurrence. *J. Am. Med. Assoc.*, 229:409–418.

37. Joint National Committee on Detection, Evaluation, and Treatment of High Blood Pressure. (1988): The 1988 Report of the Joint National Committee on Detection, Evaluation, and Treatment of High Blood Pressure (JNC IV). *Arch. Int. Med.*, in press.

38. Kannel, W. B., Wolf, P. A., McGee, D. L., Dawber, T. R., McNamara, P., and Castelli, W. P. (1981): Systolic blood pressure, arterial rigidity, and risk of stroke: The Framingham Study. *J. Am. Med. Assoc.*, 245:1225–1229.

39. Kaplan, N. M. (1985): Non-drug treatment of hypertension. *Ann. Int. Med.*, 102:359–373.

40. Kaplan, N. M., Carnegie, A., Raskin, P., et al. (1985): Potassium supplementation in hypertensive patients with diuretic-induced hypokalemia. *N. Engl. J. Med.*, 312:746–749.

41. Kline, W., Brandt, D., and Vrecko, K. (1983): Role of calcium antagonists in the treatment of essential hypertension. *Circ. Res.*, 52:(suppl I):174–181.

42. Kuramoto, K., Matsushita, S., Kuwajima, I., et al. (1981): Prospective study on the treatment of mild hypertension in the aged. *Jpn. Heart J.*, 22:75–85.

43. Lager, I., Blohme, G., and Smith, U. (1979): Effect of cardioselective and non-selective beta-blockade on the hypoglycaemic response in insulin-dependent diabetics. *Lancet*, 1:458–462.

44. Lakatta, E. G., Gerstenblith, G., and Angell, C. S., et al. (1975): Prolonged contraction duration in aged myocardium. *J. Clin. Invest.*, 55:61–68.

45. Lakatta, E. G., Gerstenblith, G., and Angell, C. S., et al. (1975): Diminished inotropic response of aged myocardium to catecholamines. *Circ. Res.*, 36:262–269.

46. Lake, C. R., Ziegler, M. G., and Coleman, M. D., et al. (1977): Age-adjusted plasma norepinephrine levels are similar in normotensive and hypertensive subjects. *N. Engl. J. Med.*, 296:208–209.

47. Lammy, P. P. (1980): *Prescribing for the Elderly*. PSG Publishing Co., Littleton, Mass.

48. Leclercq, J. F. (1981): Effect of intrinsic sympathetic activity of beta blocker on SA and AV nodes in man. *Eur. J. Cardiol.*, 12:367–375.

49. Levy, D., Anderson, K. M., Savage, D. D., Kannel, W. B., Christiansen, J. C., and Castelli, W. P. (1988): Echocardiographically detected left ventricular hypertrophy: Prevalence and risk factors. The Framingham Heart Study. *Ann. Int. Med.*, 108:7–13.

50. Lipsitz, L. A., Nyquist, R. P., and Wei, J. Y., et al. (1983): Postprandial reduction in blood pressure in the elderly. *N. Engl. J. Med.*, 309:81–89.

51. Lund-Johansen, P. (1975): Hemodynamic changes at rest and during exercise and long-term prazosin therapy for essential hypertension. In: *Prazosin Clinical Symposium Proceedings*. Special report by Postgraduate Medicine, pp. 45–52. Custom Communications (McGraw-Hill Co.), New York.

52. Lund-Johansen, P. (1981): Hemodynamic changes in late hypertension. In: *Hypertension in the young and in the old*, edited by G. Onesti and K. E. Kim, pp. 239–250. Grune and Stratten, New York.

53. Luxenberg, J., and Feigenbaum, L. Z. (1983): The use of reserpine for elderly hypertensive patients. *J. Am. Geriat. Soc.*, 31:556–559.

54. Messerli, F. H., Dreslinski, G. R., Husserl, F. E., Suarez, D. H., and MacPhee, A. A. (1981): Antiadrenergic therapy: Special aspects in hypertension in the elderly. *Hypertension*, 3:II226–II230.

55. Messerli, F. H., Sundgaard-Riise, K., Ventura, H. O., Dunns, F. G., Glade, L. B., and Frohlich, E. D. (1983): Essential hypertension in the elderly: Haemodynamics, intravascular volume, plasma renin activity, and circulating catecholamine levels. *Lancet*, 2:293–296.

56. Messerli, F. H., Ventura, H. O., and Amodeo, C. (1985): Osler's maneuver and pseudohypertension. *N. Engl. J. Med.*, 312:1548–1551.

57. Meyer, J. S., Judd, B. W., Tawakina, T., Rogers, R. L., and Mortel, K. F. (1986): Improved cognition after control of risk factors for multi-infarct dementia. *J. Am. Med. Assoc.*, 256:2203–2209.

58. Michaelson, E., and Frishman, W. H. (1983): Labetalol: An alpha- and beta-adrenoreceptor blocking drug. *Ann. Int. Med.*, 99:553–555.

59. Mulinari, R., Gavras, I., and Gavras, H. P. (1987): Efficacy and tolerability of enalapril monotherapy in mild-to-moderate hypertension in older patients compared to younger patients. *Clin. Ther.*, 9:678–692.

60. Nordrenaug, J. E., and von der Lippe, G. (1983): Hypokalemia and ventricular fibrillation in acute myocardial infarction. *Br. Heart J.*, 50:525–529.

61. O'Callahan, W. G., Fitzgerald, D. J., O'Malley, K., et al. (1983): Accuracy of blood pressure in the elderly. *Br. Med. J.*, 286:1545–1546.

62. Ohlsson, O., and Lindell, S. (1981): The effects

of pindolol and prazosin on hard blood flow in patients with cold extremities and on treatment with beta blockers. *Acta Med. Scand.*, 210:217–219.

63. Olin, J. W., Vidt, D. G., Gifford, R. W., et al. (1985): Renovascular disease in the elderly: An analysis of 50 patients. *J. Am. Col. Cardiol.*, 5:1232–1238.

64. Palmer, B. S., Zeigler, M. G., and Lake, C. R. (1978): Response of norepinephrine and blood pressure to stress increases with age. *J. Gerontol.*, 33:482–487.

65. Papademetriou, V., Fletcher, R., Khatri, M., and Freis, E. D. (1983): Diuretic-induced hypokalemia in uncomplicated systemic hypertension: Effect of plasma potassium correction on cardiac arrhythmias. *Am. J. Cardiol.*, 52:1017–1022.

66. Plante, G. E., and Dessurault, D. L. (1988): Hypertension in elderly patients: A comparative study between indapamide and hydrochlorothiazide. *Am. J. Med.*, 84(suppl 1B):98–103.

67. Popli, S., Daugirdas, J. T., Neubauer, J. A., Hockenberry, B., Hano, J. E., and Ing, T. S. (1986): Transdermal clonidine in mild hypertension: A randomized, double-blind placebo-controlled trial. *Arch. Int. Med.*, 146:2140–2144.

68. Posner, J. D., Gorman, K. M., Klein, H. S., and Woldow, A. (1986): Exercise capacity in the elderly. *Am. J. Cardiol.*, 57:52C–58C.

69. Ram, C. V., Meese, R., and Kaplan, N. M., et al. (1987): Antihypertensive therapy in the elderly: Effects on blood pressure and cerebral blood flow. *Am. J. Med.*, 82(suppl 1A):53–57.

70. Reid, J. L. (1987): Angiotensin converting inhibitors in the elderly. *Br. Med. J.*, 295:943–944.

71. Report by the Management Committee. (1980): The Australian therapeutic trial in mild hypertension. *Lancet*, 1:1261–1267.

72. Report by the Management Committee. (1981): Treatment of mild hypertension in the elderly. *Med. J. Aust.*, 2:398–401.

73. Roccella, E. J. (1985): Hypertension prevalence and the status of awareness, treatment, and control in United States: Final report of the subcommittee on definition and prevalence of the 1984 Joint National Committee. *Hypertension*, 7:457–468.

74. Roccella, E. J. (1986): Non-pharmacological approaches to the control of high blood pressure: Final report of the subcommittee on non-pharmacological therapy of the 1984 Joint National Committee on Detection, Evaluation, and Treatment of High Blood Pressure. *Hypertension*, 8:444–467.

75. Ruff, R. L., Talman, W. T., and Petito, F. (1981): Transient ischemic attacks associated with hypotension in hypertensive patients with carotid artery stenosis. *Stroke*, 12:353–355.

76. Ryan, J. R., LaCorte, W., Jain, A., and McMahon, F. G. (1985): Hypertension in hypoglycemic diabetics treated with beta-adrenergic antagonists. *Hypertension*, 7:443–446.

77. Schoken, D., and Roth, G. (1977): Reduced beta adrenergic receptor concentration in aging man. *Nature*, 267:856–858.

78. Shekelle, R. B., Ostfeld, A. M., and Klawons, H. L., Jr. (1974): Hypertension and the risk of stroke in an elderly population. *Stroke*, 5:71–75.

79. Sos, T. A., Pickering, T. G., and Sniderman, K., et al. (1983): Percutaneous transluminal angioplasty in renovascular hypertension due to atheroma or fibromuscular dysplasia. *N. Engl. J. Med.*, 309:274–279.

80. Sprackling, M. E., Mitchell, J. R. A., Short, A. H., et al. (1981): Blood pressure reduction in the elderly: A randomized controlled trial of methyldopa. *Br. Med. J.*, 283:1151–1153.

81. Stanford, B. A. (1972): Physiologic effects of training upon institutionalized geriatric men. *J. Gerontol.*, 27:451–455.

82. Stein, L., Henry, D. P., and Weinberger, M. H. (1981): Increase in plasma norepinephrine during prazosin therapy for chronic congestive heart failure. *Am. J. Med.*, 70:825–832.

83. Struthors, A. D., Whitesmith, R., and Reid, J. L. (1983): Prior thiazide diuretic treatment increases adrenaline-induced hypokalemia. *Lancet*, 1:1358–1361.

84. Sutton, K. C., Wolfson, S. K., and Kuller, L. H. (1986): Carotid and lower extremity arterial disease in elderly adults with isolated systolic hypertension. *Stroke*, 18:817–822.

85. The Norwegian Multicenter Study Group. (1981): Timolol-induced reduction in mortality and reinfarction in patients surviving acute myocardial infarction. *N. Engl. J. Med.*, 304:801–807.

86. Tifft, C. P. (1983): Renal digital subtraction angiography—A nephrologist's view: A sensitive but imperfect screening procedure for renovascular hypertension. *Cardiovasc. Interven. Radiol.*, 6:231–232.

87. Tifft, C. P. (1988): Are the days of the sphygmomanometer past? *Arch. Int. Med.*, 148:518–519.

88. Topol, E. J., Traill, T. A., and Fortuin, N. J. (1985): Hypertensive hypertrophic cardiomyopathy of the elderly. *N. Engl. J. Med.*, 312:277–283.

89. Traub, Y. M., Shapiro, A. P., Dunjovny, M., et al. (1982): Cerebral blood flow changes with diuretic therapy in elderly subjects with systolic hypertensioon *Clin. Exp. Hypertens.*, [A] 4:1193–1201.

90. Vardan, S., Mookerjec, S., Warner, R., and Smulyan, H. (1983): Systolic hypertension in the elderly: Hemodynamic response to long-term thiazide diuretic therapy and its side effects. *J. Am. Med. Assoc.*, 250:2807–2813.

91. Vardan, S., Mookherjec, S., Warner, R., et al. (1983): Systolic blood hypertension: Direct and indirect blood pressure measurements. *Arch. Int. Med.*, 143:935–938.

92. Vestal, R. E., Wood, A. J., and Shand, D. G. (1979): Reduced beta receptor sensitivity in the elderly. *Clin. Pharmacol. Ther.*, 26:181–186.

93. Veterans Administration Cooperative Study

Group on Antihypertensive Agents. (1972): Effects of treatment on morbidity in hypertension. III. Influence of age, diastolic pressure, and prior cardiovascular disease: further analysis of side effects. *Circulation*, 45:991–1004.

94. Veterans Administration Cooperative Study Group on Antihypertensive Agents. (1974): Effect of antihypertensive treatment on stroke recurrence. *J. Am. Med. Assoc.*, 229:409–418.

95. Waal-Manning, H. J. (1976): Metabolic effects of beta-adrenoreceptor blockers. *Drugs*, 11(suppl 1)):121–126.

96. Wallace, J. D., and Levy, L. L. (1981): Blood pressure after stroke. *J. Am. Med. Assoc.*, 246:2177–2180.

97. Westenend, M., Lenders, J. W. M., and Thein, T. H. (1985): The course of blood pressure after a meal: A difference between young and elderly subjects. *J. Hypertens.*, 3:S417–S419.

98. Wikstrand, J., Westergren, G., Berglund, G., Bracchett, D., Van Couter, A., Feldstein, C. A., Ming, K. S., Kuramoto, K., Landahl, S., Meaney, E., Pedersen, E. B., Rahn, K. H., Shaw, J., Smith, A., and Waal-Manning, H. (1986): Antihypertensive treatment with metoprolol or hydrochlorothiazide in patients aged 60 to 75 years: Report from a double-blind international multi-center study. *J. Am. Med. Assoc.*, 255:1304–1310.

99. Woods, J. W., Pittman, A. W., and Pulliman, C. C., et al. (1976): Renin profiling in hypertension and its use in treatment with propranolol and chlorthalidone. *N. Engl. J. Med.*, 294:1137–1143.

100. Working Group on Hypertension in the Elderly. (1986): Statement on hypertension in the elderly hypertensive patient. *Am. J. Cardiol.*, 52:49D–53D.

101. Yamauchi, K., Furui, H., and Taniguchi, N., et al. (1986): Effects of diltiazem hydrochloride on cardiovascular response, platelet aggregation and coagulating activity during exercise testing in systemic hypertension. *Am. J. Cardiol.*, 57:609–612.

102. Ying, C. Y., Tifft, C. P., and Gavras, H. P., et al. (1984): Renal revascularization in the azotemic hypertensive patient resistant to therapy. *N. Engl. J. Med.*, 311:1070–1075.

103. Zanella, M. T., Mattei, E., and Draibe, S. A., et al. (1985): Inadequate aldosterone response to hyperkalemia during angiotensin converting inhibition in chronic renal failure. *Clin. Pharmacol. Ther.*, 38:613–617.

New Therapeutic Strategies in Hypertension,
edited by Norman M. Kaplan,
Barry M. Brenner, and John H. Laragh.
Raven Press, Ltd., New York © 1989.

Hypertension in Pregnancy

Jay M. Sullivan

Division of Cardiovascular Diseases, The University of Tennessee, Memphis, Tennessee 37232

Hypertension can be induced by pregnancy in previously normotensive women. Alternatively, pregnancy can occur in women with chronic hypertension and is sometimes complicated by superimposed preeclampsia (Fig. 1). The older term "toxemia of pregnancy" refers to a hypertensive disorder associated with pregnancy with two levels of severity, preeclampsia and eclampsia, the etiologies of which remain unknown. Preeclampsia is characterized by edema, proteinuria, and elevated blood pressure appearing after the 24th week of pregnancy. The term eclampsia refers to the development of seizures and coma. Pregnancy-induced hypertension (PIH) can develop with or without preeclampsia or eclampsia. A new classification of the hypertensive disorders of pregnancy has been recommended by a committee of the American College of Obstetricians and Gynecologists. This classification consists of four groups (Table 1).

Elevated blood pressure during pregnancy is a major cause of maternal and perinatal mortality. The incidence of PIH in the United States ranges from 1.6 to 12.6%, averaging about 7%. Chesley (13), using the criteria of an increase of diastolic pressure of 15 mmHg or more and sustained 3 plus proteinuria, found superimposed preeclampsia in only 5.7% of gravidas with chronic hypertension. Recurrences occur in 30% of subsequent pregnancies. A major difficulty in classifying patients lies in making a correct diagnosis on clinical grounds alone. Renal biopsy provides diagnostic certainty, but this procedure carries a high risk of hemorrhage (99). Peripheral vascular resistance and blood pressure fall in early pregnancy, rising toward nonpregnant levels in late pregnancy. Thus, patients with undetected essential or secondary hypertension might present in early pregnancy with blood pressure within normal limits to be misdiagnosed as having PIH when elevated blood pressure is detected later in the course of pregnancy, especially if the blood pressure elevation is accompanied by the mild edema that frequently occurs in otherwise normal pregnancies. In a study of 35 patients with a clinical diagnosis of PIH, characteristic renal pathologic changes were found in only 26% (81). Another study, found the histologic lesions of chronic renal disease in 21% of multigravidas and 43% of primagravidas.

MANAGEMENT

Chamberlain et al. (10), surveyed the practices of 1,093 obstetricians in the management of pregnant women with preexisting hypertension or PIH. Antihypertensive drugs were used frequently, especially methyldopa and diuretics, but those with the least blood pressure elevation were treated with sedatives. PIH was usually treated with bed rest and sedation. The authors noted that although most of the treatments and practices have not been validated by controlled trials, the practices were quite uniform.

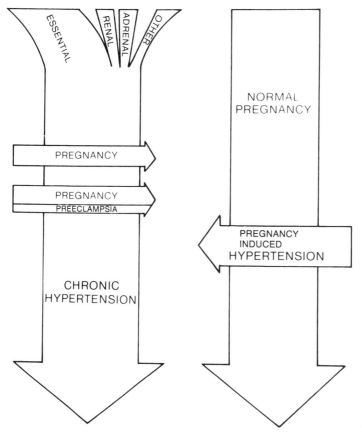

FIG. 1 Interrelationships of natural history of hypertension and pregnancy. (From Sullivan, ref. 106, with permission.)

Activity

Curet and Olsen (17) studied the effect of four hours of daily bed rest in the left lateral decubitus position in 66 patients with chronic hypertension. Therapy with hydralazine was added if diastolic pressure exceeded 110 mmHg. Three perinatal deaths occurred and 38.8% developed superimposed preeclampsia. However, when compared with the outcome of previous preg-

Table 1. *Hypertensive disorders of pregnancy*

1. Pregnancy induced hypertension, without or with preeclampsia or eclampsia
2. Chronic hypertension of whatever cause
3. Chronic hypertension with superimposed preeclampsia
4. Late or "transient" hypertension

nancies, the perinatal mortality rate was lowered from 16.8 to 8.8%. Mathews (71) compared the effects of bed rest and sedation with those of normal activity and nonsedation in the management of 135 patients with nonalbuminuric hypertension in later pregnancy and found no apparent benefit from limitied activity. Little and coworkers (63) compared the effect of systematic relaxation alone or combined with biofeedback in 60 hypertensive pregnancies, finding that the experimental groups had significantly lower blood pressure and fewer hospitalizations than a comparable control group. At present, the weight of evidence suggests that rest is beneficial. However, there are no studies to suggest that increased activity has a beneficial effect. Thus, there appears to be little reason to change the conventional practice of advising periods of rest for hypertensive gravidas.

Plasma Volume in Pregnancy: Therapeutic Implications

Normal pregnancy is accompanied by substantial increases in total body sodium and water. Total body water increases by about 6 to 8 liters; 4 to 6 liters are found in the extracellular compartment (62). Blood volume begins to increase during the first trimester. The rate of increase rises during the second trimester, while during the third trimester the increment is slight, with some finding a modest fall near term (82). An increased plasma and red blood cell volume comprises the increment of blood volume, which has been found to vary from 20 to 100% (82). Plasma volume rises from the 8th week, reaches a peak between the 20th and 32nd week of pregnancy, and remains relatively constant with delivery. The magnitude of the increase appears to be related to the size of the fetus (45). Six to eight weeks after delivery, plasma volume usually returns to nonpregnant levels. Normally, sodium is retained as required by the increase in blood volume and by the size of the conceptus, totaling somewhere between 500 and 900 mEq (38,62). Water is retained at term in a slight excess which varies, from 1 to 2 liters in women without edema, to 5 liters in those with edema. Edema in itself is not a manifestation of underlying pathology, but has been found in 35 to 80% of healthy women with normal pregnancies (91).

The volume receptors of the gravid circulation recognize the volume-expanded state as physiologic. Dietary sodium restriction or sodium-loading result in appropriate changes in plasma-renin activity and aldosterone concentration (121) which are elevated above that found in the nonpregnant state. Diuretic agents or upright posture stimulate aldosterone secretion in normal gravidas (6,19) while exogenous mineralocorticoids cause sodium retention and a fall in aldosterone secretion (122).

Tarazi et al. (109), studied plasma volume in several forms of clinical hypertension and demonstrated that in patients with impaired renal function, blood pressure was directly proportional to plasma volume. In contrast, pressure diuresis determined the volume status of patients with essential hypertension, so that plasma volume was inversely related to diastolic blood pressure in the absence of renal failure. Studies of patients with essential hypertension and pregnancy or with PIH yielded results similar to those of nonpregnant patients with essential hypertension; intravascular volume was diminished.

Although patients with PIH retain sodium and water in excess of that retained in normal pregnancy, several studies have shown that blood volume is contracted in preeclamptic patients (12). Hematocrit and plasma-specific gravity increase in patients with severe preeclampsia. Blekta et al. (5), found that the red blood cell mass of patients who develop PIH does not differ significantly from that of a normal gravida. Plasma volume falls to 30 to 40% of normal in patients with severe preeclampsia (12). Blekta et al. (5), detected a reduction in whole blood volume before preeclampsia was clinically manifest. Lang et al. (57), studied blood rheology in 23 patients with eclampsia and 10 with intrauterine growth retardation and demonstrated significantly increased blood viscosity, along with increased hematocrit and fibrinogen levels.

Arias (1) measured blood volume in 20 patients with chronic hypertension and pregnancy. He found that these patients, as a group, had lower blood volume than normal gravidas, and delivered infants of lower weights. The hypertensive patients who delivered infants of appropriate size for gestational age had a greater degree of volume expansion during pregnancy than those delivered of undersized children or stillbirths. Those patients who did not increase their blood volume by 60 ml/kg or more were likely to deliver growth-retarded children.

Soffronoff and his colleagues (104) measured plasma volume in 51 hypertensive and 35 normotensive gravidas. Although a large range and considerable overlap of values was noted, average volumes in hypertensive gravidas were found to be significantly depressed compared to pregnant women with normal blood pressure. Those hypertensive patients with intravascular volume determinations near those of normotensive patients were found to have a good maternal and fetal outcome. The lowest intravascular volumes were found in pregnancies which were subsequently complicated by severe hypertensive disease and evidence of uteroplacental insufficiency.

Gallery et al. (28), followed the changes in plasma volume which took place during normal and hypertensive pregnancies. In 40 initially normotensive patients who developed hypertension during the third trimester, plasma volume was found to expand normally during the first two trimesters, followed by a significant contraction of plasma volume in the third trimester. The contraction of volume occurred before the development of elevated blood pressure in 29 of the 40 patients. In 30 patients with chronic hypertension and pregnancy, blood pressure was inversely related to plasma volume, while fetal growth was directly related to plasma volume.

Changes in colloid osmotic pressure have been reported in patients with pregnancy-induced hypertension. In a study of 55 pregnancies, Benedetti and Carlson (4) found colloid osmotic pressure to be 22.0 before, and 17.2 mmHg after, delivery in 23 normal subjects while lower values of 17.9 and 13.7 mmHg, respectively, were found in 22 patients with preeclampsia. In contrast, Goodlin et al. (37), found no differences between normal and hypertensive gravidas.

Diet

Sodium manipulation during pregnancy has been studied by several investigators. Robinson (92) studied 1,039 pregnant patients on high-sodium intake, and an equal number on *ad lib* diets, finding fewer complications of pregnancy in the high-salt group. However, the incidence of preeclampsia among primiparas was unchanged by sodium-loading. Zuspan and Bell (126) manipulated dietary sodium in preeclamptic subjects and concluded that the severity of the disease process determined how well sodium was tolerated. Others have found that patients with mild preeclampsia tolerated sodium without difficulty (8,72).

In an uncontrolled study, Foote and Ludbrook (25) examined the effect of a 180 mEq sodium diet on the clinical course of four gravidas with essential hypertension and seven cases of preeclampsia. The patients with preeclampsia did not worsen, however there was not a noticeable improvement in their condition. Three of four patients with essential hypertension responded to a high-salt diet with a fall in blood pressure and a rise in estriol excretion rates, suggesting improved placental perfusion. However, the lack of a suitable control group makes the effect of the added salt difficult to separate from the effects of rest, sedation, and frequent encounters. Individuals vary in their sensitivity to sodium. Patients with essential hypertension are more likely than normotensives to develop an increase in blood pressure when sodium-loaded (108). Therefore, it is unlikely that any study involving a large number of patients will demonstrate a uniformly beneficial or detrimental response to sodium-loading.

Diuretics

Thiazides cause diuresis and saluresis with an initial reduction in extracellular fluid volume, plasma volume, and cardiac output, and an increase in vascular resistance. After two or three months of administration, blood pressure remains reduced in 40% to 50% of hypertensive patients while plasma volume and cardiac output return towards pretreatment levels (125). Thus, the long-term reduction of blood pressure is thought to be due to a fall in peripheral vascular resistance (58) which has been attributed to loss of sodium and water from vascular smooth muscle, thus reducing the degree of encroachment on the cross-sectional areas of the resistance vessels and the responsiveness to pressor agents (112). However, a normalization of the water or sodium content of the arterial walls of animals with experimental hypertension after diuretic treatment has not been observed (113). Tarazi et al. (110), have noted that total body water remains reduced during chronic thiazide therapy. Additionally, plasma-renin activity ordinarily stays elevated during thiazide administration and falls to control levels when thiazides are withdrawn, suggesting that a degree of volume depletion persists during long-term administration.

The use of thiazides during pregnancy has undergone extensive study, and attitudes concerning their use have changed. In early studies Finnerty (24) treated 16 preeclamptic patients with diuretics and noted that blood pressure and proteinuria improved. However, Salerno and his coworkers (97) studied 24 patients with preeclampsia and noted that the disease process appeared to worsen in 11 patients treated with diuretics. MacGillivray (69) studied eight patients with preeclampsia and noted that diuretics did not appear to change the disease process even though the edema improved, suggesting that diuretics treated the signs rather than the cause of the disease.

Finnerty and Bepko (23) later studied approximately 3,000 patients assigned alternatively to groups receiving either prophylactic thiazides or no therapy. A lower incidence of preeclampsia and a lower perinatal mortality rate was noted in the group receiving diuretics. However, Kraus and his colleagues (53) conducted a randomized, controlled study of 195 women who were placed on hydrochlorothiazide and 210 who were placed on placebo. The incidence of superimposed preeclampsia was 6.67% in both groups.

Collins, Yusuf, and Peto (15) have reviewed the results of nine trials of diuretics, involving 7,000 women. While diuretics were found to have a significant effect on blood pressure, there was no significant effect on perinatal mortality. Although the incidence of stillbirth was one-third less in treated patients, the difference was not statistically significant.

Lindheimer and Katz (62) concluded "it remains to be established if the increment in maternal extracellular volume is required for optimal uteroplacental perfusion, but it is noteworthy that in two complications of gravidity, preeclampsia and essential hypertension, intravascular volume is decreased and placental perfusion compromised. Relations between volume status and vascular reactivity need to be clarified. If preeclamptic vasoconstriction is an overcompensation to intravascular volume contraction, sodium salts may well be therapeutic. However, if as in certain experimental models, hypervolemia sensitizes the vascular receptors to the effect of endogenous pressor amines or peptides, excessive salt could be clearly harmful. To date, claims that either salt-loading or its restriction, with or without diuretic therapy, reduces the incidence of preeclampsia are unconvincing when scrutinized critically."

Given the observation that the initiation of diuretic therapy causes a fall in plasma volume, cardiac output, and a rise in vascular resistance, many avoid *adding* thiazide diuretics to the antihypertensive program of pregnant patients, unless needed for the relief of pulmonary edema. Whether it is beneficial or harmful to *continue* diuretic agents as part of the therapeutic program of a patient with chronic hypertension who become pregnant remains to be established. Sibai et al. (101), have demonstrated that chronic thiazide therapy hinders the physiologic expansion of plasma volume that accompanies normal pregnancy. However, in this study of 20 patients, perinatal outcome was not influenced. Until larger studies prove that diuretics do not have an adverse effect on fetal outcome, I believe it to be the safer course to manage essential hypertension without diuretic agents during pregnancy when it is possible to obtain satisfactory control of pressure with other antihypertensive agents.

Plasma Expansion

Another mode of therapy which has been used in attempts to correct the hemoconcentration, contracted intravascular volume, and proteinuria of PIH is the intravenous infusion of noncrystalloid solutions such as dextran and human albumin which has been recommended by several authors. However, published reports include few nonrandomized patients, and did not include suitable control groups receiving concurrent treatment. In a widely cited study, Cloeren et al. (14), studied 20 patients with preeclampsia. Eighteen were found to have central venous pressure, ranging from 0 to -7 cm H_2O, close to those of patients with severe burns or shock. The normal CVP in other patients was attributed to right heart failure. Fifteen patients received treatment with 6% salt-free Macrodex, 10% Rheomacrodex, or 20% low-salt human albumin, in volumes ranging from 100 to 2,500 ml, given over a few hours each day. All patients showed an increase in central venous pressure. The newborn size ranged from the <5 to 95 percentile. IM133-gelatin was used to measure uteroplacental and uterine blood volumes before and after volume expansion in five cases, all showing an increase in uteroplacental blood volume. Diastolic blood pressure fell in eight patients who under-

went continuous monitoring but the magnitude of reduction was not reported. Similar studies have been carried out by Brewer (9) and by MacLean et al. (70), whose results suggested that renal and placental perfusion were improved. Although these studies suggested that preeclamptic patients with a low CVP can receive cautious therapy with plasma expanders without ill effect, the lack of a suitable control group makes it difficult to assess the degree of benefit, if any, received by the patients.

Jouppila et al. (48), have studied the effect of albumin infusion on intervillous blood flow in 13 patients with severe preeclampsia, using intravenous 133 Xe to measure flow. Although serum-albumin concentration and colloid osmotic pressure rose significantly, there was no improvement in intravillous blood flow, leading these investigators to question the value of using infusions of albumin to improve placental circulation in patients with severe preeclampsia.

Goodlin et al. (26), measured plasma volume in 200 patients with various complications of pregnancy to determine if any simple clinical test allowed identification of the hypovolemic patient. They concluded that plasma volume must be measured directly, as no other routine laboratory measurement was predictive. They recommended that expansion of intravascular volume should be a major goal of antenatal care. As pointed out by Redman, (87) this recommendation is based on the assumption that reduced plasma volume causes fetal growth retardation, however, since plasma volume has been shown to be directly related to the size of the conceptus, the reduced plasma volume found in some patients with preeclampsia might be the result, rather than the cause, of a growth-retarded fetus. A randomized, controlled trial is needed to see if expansion of plasma volume has a beneficial effect on the outcome of pregnancy.

Gallery, Mitchell, and Redman (29) infused 500 ml of a volume-expanding solution in 35 patients with PIH and observed a significant fall in blood pressure lasting up to three days. However, the mechanisms of the antihypertensive effect were not clear as the response was not related to the degree of volume expansion nor to the severity of hypertension.

Thus, the pendulum has swung from the liberal use of diuretics during pregnancy to the use of liberal salt diet and plasma expanders. As once was the case with the use of diuretics, large, randomized, controlled studies with monitoring of pulmonary capillary wedge pressure and other hemodynamic variables are now needed to define the place of plasma expanders in the treatment of patients with hypertensive pregnancies. At present, I believe that specific indications such as hypotension should be present before deviating from Pritchard's (83) recommendation that hydration should be limited to crystalloid solution infused at a rate of 60 to 120 ml per hr. It must not be forgotten that arterial blood pressure is the product of total peripheral resistance and cardiac output. If the latter is increased by expansion of blood volume, without reduction of the former, i.e., relieving the vasospasm of PIH, blood pressure will show a further increase. If the increase in pressure is great enough, the patient will be subjected to the acute effects of severe hypertension, cerebral hemorrhage, acute pulmonary edema, and aortic dissection. Additionally, ventricular diastolic relaxation is impaired in chronic hypertension. Therefore, fluid overload leads to pulmonary edema more readily than in those with normal diastolic function (106).

Centrally-Acting Alpha-2 Receptor Agonists

Agents which stimulate central nervous system alpha-2 receptors, thus reducing sympathetic outflow to the periphery, have been used extensively to treat hypertensive patients during pregnancy; the safety of so doing has been established. At present, methyldopa has received the widest investigation in the management of hypertension during pregnancy. Kincaid-Smith et al. (52), treated 32 patients with methyldopa and observed a perinatal loss of 9.3%, which was better than predicted results, and a rate of development of preeclampsia of 38%, which was no better than predicted. Leather et al. (59), treated 22 patients with methyldopa, compared the results with 24 untreated patients. No fetal loss occurred in the 22 patients treated with methyldopa while a fetal loss of 25% was seen in those not treated. Redman et al. (88), conducted a randomized study of 101 patients and 107 controls. The fetal salvage rate was slightly improved, largely because of fewer second trimester abortions. No change was noted in the frequency of superimposed preeclampsia.

Studies of the disposition of methyldopa during pregnancy have shown that methyldopa crosses the placenta and that tissue levels in the fetus are equivalent to those of the mother. Although methyldopa is excreted in breast milk and is absorbed by neonates, the amount does not appear to be high enough to have adverse effects (40,124). Ounsted et al. (77), have reviewed the development during the first four years of life of children born of hypertensive mothers, some of whom were treated with methyldopa. They found that maternal hypertension itself was associated with a slight developmental delay in childhood and that therapy with methyldopa during pregnancy did not worsen the delay and may even have reduced delayed neonatal development.

In a randomized double-blind study of 100 women, Horvath et al. (42), compared clonidine to methyldopa and found no significant differences in blood pressure control or maternal and fetal outcome. Tuimala et al. (114), found clonidine to be effective and well tolerated in the treatment of 82 pregnant patients with either chronic hypertension or PIH. Philippe et al. (78), observed that clonidine did not reduce uteroplacental blood flow during pregnancy.

Sympathetic Blocking Agents

Reserpine, which prevents reuptake of norepinephrine by nerve endings, is not used in pregnancy because it causes severe nasal obstruction in the newborn. Guanethidine and guanadryl, by interfering with impulse transmission by sympathetic ganglia, is seldom used in pregnancy because of the marked postural hypotension commonly associated with the use of these agents.

Beta-adrenergic Receptor Blocking Agents

Propranolol, widely used for the management of essential hypertension, has been used to treat small groups of patients with hypertensive pregnancies. Fetal growth retardation, neonatal bradycardia, and hypoglycemia were described leading to reluctance to use beta blockers during pregnancy on the part of many physicians. Lieberman and colleagues (60) treated nine patients with hypertensive pregnancies and concluded that the probability of fetal neonatal death was increased by propranolol therapy. Pruyn et al. (85), followed ten patients who received propranolol during hypertensive pregnancies, observed evidence of fetal growth retardation, but found no correlation with neonatal hypoglycemia, hyperbilirubinemia, apnea or bradycardia. However, Eliahou et al. (20), treated 25 hypertensive, pregnant patients with propranolol and noted a reduction of predicted fetal wastage. Tcherdakoff et al. (111), studied nine patients and noted good blood pressure control with no increase in fetal mortality. Sotalol (76), and metoprolol (98) have been used to treat small groups of hypertensive patients during pregnancy without notably dangerous side effects. However, a case of neonatal cardiorespiratory depression, hypoglycemia, and growth retardation has

been reported after maternal use of the long-acting compound nadolol (26). Therapy with propranolol or other beta-adrenergic receptor blockers results in a fall in cardiac output and an elevation of peripheral vascular resistance which persist through 10 years of treatment (64). Thus, the hemodynamic effects of beta blockade can be expected to persist throughout pregnancy. Gallery et al. (30,31), randomly allocated 183 hypertensive gravidas to groups treated with either methyldopa or oxprenolol and concluded that although both drugs controlled pressure equally, the outcome of pregnancy, judged by greater fetal growth, was better in the group treated with oxprenolol. There was no evidence of harmful effect on the fetus. Fidler et al. (22), also compared methyldopa to oxprenolol and found no difference in outcome, even though blood pressure was lower in methyldopa-treated patients. Oxprenolol crosses the placenta and is detectable in breast milk (103).

Rubin et al. (94,95), compared atenolol, 100 to 200 mg daily, to placebo in a prospective, randomized double-blind trial which involved 120 women admitted to the hospital because of the development of hypertension during the third trimester of a previously normal pregnancy. Before treatment, blood pressure ranged between 140/90 to 170/110 mmHg. Blood pressure was significantly reduced in patients receiving atenolol, while pressures climbed to levels above 170/110 in one-third of the patients treated with bed rest and placebo. Ten patients in the placebo group, but only three of the atenolol-treated group, developed significant proteinuria. Intrauterine growth retardation, neonatal hypoglycemia, and hyperbilirubinemia occurred equally in the two groups while the symptoms of respiratory distress were seen in only one infant whose mother received placebo. Neonatal bradycardia was more common in infants of atenolol-treated mothers. A follow-up study showed no apparent pediatric complications during the first year of life and the children of atenolol-treated mothers (90). Atenolol is found in breast milk (54). These data indicate that atenolol effectively lowered blood pressure in patients with preeclampsia without worsening maternal or fetal outcome and may reduce the frequency with which protenuria appears and hypertension accelerates.

In a study of 161 women, Hogstedt et al. (41), found that a combination of metoprolol and hydralazine resulted in satisfactory control of mild to moderate hypertension during pregnancy but no improvement in outcome when compared to nonpharmacologic management. Hepatic clearance of metoprolol increases during pregnancy. Metoprolol is found in amniotic fluid and in breast milk (54,61).

Pindolol, a beta blocker with intrinsic sympathomimetic activity, has been reported to lower blood pressure without a reduction in uteroplacental blood flow measured by [113]In scintography (68). Pindolol has little effect on fetal heart rate (46).

Therefore, data exist on both sides of the issue of using beta blockers during pregnancy. The relative risk/benefit ratio of therapy with beta-adrenergic receptor blockers during hypertensive pregnancies remains to be established definitely.

Combined Alpha-Beta Receptor Blocking Agents

Labetalol, a combined alpha and beta blocker, has been demonstrated to lower blood pressure without reducing uteroplacental blood flow measured by the [113]In technique, suggesting that this agent decreases uteroplacental resistance (67,73). Lamming and Symonds (56) treated 19 patients with pregnancy-induced hypertension with either labetalol or methyldopa and observed better blood pressure control and more frequent spontaneous labor in the group treated with labetalol. No adverse fetal effects were noted. Gerard et al., also

reported that labetalol was well-tolerated during pregnancy (34). Nylund et al. (75), reported that labetolol does not lower uteroplacental blood flow. For the treatment of severely elevated blood pressure during pregnancy, labetolol is probably as effective and safe as hydralazine (74). However, experience with the use of labetolol is considerably less. Labetolol is transferred into human breast milk and to amniotic fluid (65).

Alpha-Receptor Blocking Agents

Prazosin, which causes vasodilation by blocking peripheral vascular alpha 1 receptors, has received little study in the management of hypertensive gravidas.

There is no reported use of the long-acting alpha blocker, terazosin, during pregnancy.

Vasodilators

Hydralazine is widely used for the treatment of hypertensive pregnancies, particularly by the intravenous or intramuscular routes when blood pressure is elevated severely. While very effective parenterally, as a long-term oral therapy hydralazine is subject to several, poorly-tolerated side effects. Pregnancy is associated with high cardiac output. Hydralazine, acting as a direct vasodilator and as a reflex, and possibly direct cardiac stimulant, further increases cardiac output while reducing peripheral vascular resistance. Patients note flushing, headache, tachycardia, and palpitations. Hydralazine may induce additional reduction of uteroplacental blood flow. Although Johnson and Clayton (50) found evidence that myometrial [24]Na clearance increased after hydralazine, Gant et al. (32), found evidence that hydralazine causes a reduction in uterine blood flow. Using the [113]In method to measure uteroplacental blood flow, Lunell et al. (66), recently found no reduction after lowering blood pressure in preeclamptic patients with intravenous dihydralazine. Vink et al. (117), treated 33 hypertensive gravidas, whose diastolic blood pressures exceeded 110 mmHg, with dihydralazine, monitoring fetal heart rate for evidence of reduced placental blood flow as arterial pressure was lowered. Fetal heart rate fell in 19 cases, 14 of whom delivered growth-retarded fetuses while only one of 14 whose fetal heart rate did not fall was retarded in growth, suggesting that a reduction in placental blood flow, if it occurs, presents a problem only in certain individuals. Many physicians now limit the use of hydralazine to situations in which severely elevated blood pressure must be controlled quickly for short periods of time before delivery. Jouppila et al. (49), used ^{133}Xe and ultrasonography to study the effect of intravenous dihydralazine on the placental and fetal circulations and found that as blood pressure fell, umbilical vein blood flow increased but there was no change in intervillous blood flow. Kuzniar et al. (55), studied the hemodynamic effect of intravenous hydralazine and found the level of pretreatment vascular resistance tightest in those with preeclampsia, and the predicted response greatest in those with high resistance.

Bott-Kanner et al. (7), examined combination therapy with propranolol and hydralazine in the management of essential hypertension in pregnancy. They found that 13 patients tolerated the regimen without difficulty; blood pressure remained below 140/90 in all cases and none of the patients developed preeclampsia. However, there was one unexplained stillbirth and two cases of hypoglycemia. The combination did not appear to offer an advantage.

Diazoxide is effective in the treatment of many hypertensive emergencies, but has the disadvantage of relaxing the uterine musculature, thus halting labor. It was recommended that this agent must be administered as a rapid intravenous bolus of 300 mg because of prompt binding to plasma proteins. Recent studies show that diazoxide can be given as a minibolus in a dose of 30 mg every 1 to 2 min until blood pressure is controlled. Under these circumstances, the maximum dose required is 150 mg (18). Diazoxide can also be effective as a continuous intravenous infusion in a dose of 15 mg/min (44). Long-term use of diazoxide should be avoided because of sodium retention, hyperglycemia, and hyperuricemia.

Sodium nitroprusside is widely used by internists for the treatment of hypertension or congestive heart failure, but can cause cyanide toxicity in the fetus. This threat has limited the use of this potent agent in the treatment of hypertension during pregnancy. Minoxidil, a potent direct-acting vasodilator, has not been studied in the management of hypertensive pregnancies and must be used with caution.

Angiotensin Converting Enzyme Inhibitors

Several compounds which block various components of the renin-angiotensin system are available or under development, but do not appear to be useful in the management of pregnancy-induced hypertension or hypertension accompaning pregnancy. Sullivan et al. (107), found that intravenous teprotide, an angiotensin converting enzyme inhibitor, had no effect on blood pressure in five patients with PIH until substantial diuresis and reduction of plasma volume was induced by furosemide. Pipkin et al. (79), administered captopril, another converting enzyme inhibitor, to pregnant ewes and rabbits, and observed an increase in perinatal mortality. Francisco and Ferris (27) gave captopril to pregnant rabbits, beginning at the 15th week of gestation. Fetal survival was only 14% in the treated animals, in contrast to 99% in controls, even though blood pressure did not differ between the two groups. In addition, they found that captopril was associated with a fall in uterine vein PGE_2 concentration. When animals are given indomethacin to block uterine synthesis of PGE_2, uterine blood flow fell. In humans, aspirin administered during pregnancy has been associated with high fetal mortality in one study by Turner and Collins (115), but this observation was not confirmed by Shapiro et al. (100). Indeed Wallenberg et al., have reported recently that low-dose aspirin prevents PIH in primigravidas (119).

Plouin and Tchobroutsky (80) reviewed 15 cases of hypertension treated with captopril during pregnancy. While many of the complications appeared to be due to the severity of the mother's disease, two children born to mothers who had also received furosemide, died of neonatal anemia. Rothberg and Lorenz (93) have also reported a case of neonatal renal failure following maternal treatment with captopril.

Given the lack of efficacy in preeclampsia and the potential for fetal harm demonstrated by animal studies, the use of angiotensin converting enzyme inhibitors is considered to be contraindicated during pregnancy.

Calcium Channel Blocking Agents

In the field of cardiovascular therapeutics, an important recent advance has been the introduction of the calcium channel blocking agents. These compounds inhibit the passage of calcium ions into the cell, resulting in a reduction in contractility, vasodilatation, and, since the slow calcium current is required for activity of cardiac conducting tissue, slower transmission of impulses across the A-V node (102). While the first of these agents has been used in Europe since 1962 and many are widely used outside the United States for the treatment of angina pectoris, coronary vasospasm, atrial tachyarrhythmia, and hypertension, only verapamil has received approval for the latter indication in the United States. The three compounds currently available in this country are nifedipine, verapamil, and diltiazem. Nifedipine

is a potent vasodilator, useful in the treatment of vasospastic angina and for the rapid control of severe hypertension. Fluid retention accompanies chronic use of this compound. Verapamil lowers vascular resistance and also reduces myocardial contractility and A-V conduction; thus the agent must be used with caution, or not at all, in patients with heart failure or disorders of cardiac conduction. The properties of diltiazem lie between those of nifedipine and verapamil. Verapamil has been found to lower blood pressure and reverse ventricular hypertrophy in the pregnant SHR (96). Nifedipine has been used successfully to postpone delivery in patients with preterm labor (116). Hypertension, present in 8 of 28 patients, was controlled by nifedipine. Walters and Redman (120) gave oral nifedipine to 21 patients with severe hypertension during pregnancy. The average fall in blood pressure at 20 min was 26/20 mmHg. Headache and flushing were the main side effects. These agents have not been thoroughly investigated relative to the management of essential hypertension during pregnancy, nor of preeclampsia of varying degrees of severity.

Serotonin Receptor Antagonists

Ketanserin has been used to treat 20 postpartum patients with PIH and found to lower blood pressure with minimal side effects (123). However, the effect on fetal outcome has not been studied.

Thus, of the currently available antihypertensive agents, methyldopa has received the widest documented study in the management of pregnant hypertensives, and the children born of mothers so treated have undergone the longest follow-up observation. The weight of presently-available evidence suggests that methyldopa is relatively effective and safe during pregnancy. Until comparable studies demonstrate another antihypertensive agent to be superior, it is reasonable to use methyldopa as the agent of first choice. When methyldopa alone is not effective, hydralazine can be added. The favorable experience with atenolol in a relatively large group of patients with pregnancy-associated hypertension (95) suggest that this agent can be used as an alternative to methyldopa. Evidence is mounting that labetolol and clonidine can also be used safely and effectively during pregnancy.

Precautions in Pregnancy

The potential adverse effects for mother, developing fetus, and newborn are summarized in Table 2.

MANAGEMENT OF PATIENTS WITH PREECLAMPSIA-ECLAMPSIA

The management of patients with preeclampsia-eclampsia or pregnancy-induced hypertension has been the subject of several reviews (21,33,51,83,106). Measures intended to prevent PIH include frequent observation to detect rapid weight gain or rising diastolic pressure. Edema is an early sign, but is not specific because it is common in normal pregnancy. Patients should be instructed to report persistent headache, visual disturbance, or swelling of the face or hands. A beneficial effect from restriction of calories or sodium intake has not been demonstrated convincingly, nor has sodium-loading been of proved benefit. Thiazide diuretics have been used in the past to prevent preeclampsia but a double-blind study has seriously questioned the value of this intervention (53), as has an overview of several studies using diuretics, showing no effect on perinatal mortality (15). Although there is some doubt that preeclampsia can be prevented, progression to eclampsia should be preventable by appropriate therapy. Near term, either induction of labor or cesarean section will achieve such a goal.

When preeclampsia develops earlier in the pregnancy, hospitalization or strict bed rest at home is essential and avoidance of sodium excess appears to be reasonable, although many patients with mild PIH can tolerate salt without difficulty (41). Chesley (11) advocates hospitalization if blood pressure exceeds 140/90, if proteinuria of 1 + or more develops, or if weight repeatedly increases by 3 lb. or more a week. Bed rest, close observation, and sedation are recommended, often resulting in spontaneous diuresis, loss of weight, and a fall in blood pressure. Improvement began within the first 24 hr and blood pressure fell to less than 140/90 by the 5th day in the series of Gilstrap et al. (35). When improvement takes place, the pregnancy can be continued with monitoring for fetal distress or growth retardation by sonogram and/or amniocentesis for the appearance of pulmonary stabilizing phosphorolipids indicating maturity. In the series of Gilstrap et al. (35), worsening of preeclampsia was observed in 6% of patients, necessitating delivery.

Gallery et al. (29), used 500 ml of plasma protein solution to correct intravascular volume contraction in patients with preeclampsia, and reported a fall in blood pressure in most. This report and others have led to the practice of administering large volumes of intravenous fluids to patients with hypertension and pregnancy. However, without adequate hemodynamic monitoring, this practice can lead to pulmonary edema.

Severe preeclampsia is indicated by blood pressure elevation to levels above 160/110, irritability, increasing edema, and proteinuria. Under these circumstances, therapy should be directed towards the prevention of convulsions because they are associated with a major increase in fetal and maternal mortality. Ordinary therapeutic measures include parenteral magnesium sulfate, antihypertensive agents, osmotic diuresis usually with mannitol if oliguria is present, and prompt delivery to prevent progression to eclampsia and fetal death. Magnesium is given primarily to prevent

Table 2. *Antihypertensive therapy during pregnancy: precautions*

Agent	Potential problem
Diuretics	
Furosemide	Maternal: Water and electrolyte depletion
	Newborn: Fetal abnormalities in experimental animals
Thiazides	Maternal: Electrolyte depletion, hypokalemia, gout, hypoglycemia, thrombocytopenia, and hemorrhagic pancreatitis
	Newborn: Thrombocytopenia
Sympathetic Blocking Agents	
Centrally-acting alpha-2 receptor agonists	
Clonidine	Maternal: Drowsiness, dry mouth, rebound hypertension
	Newborn: Inadequate data
Methyldopa	Maternal: Lethargy, fever, hepatitis, positive Coombs test, hemolytic anemia
Agents interfering with impulse transmission	
Guanethidine	Rarely used in pregnancy because of postural hypotension
Reserpine	Maternal: Depression, nasal stuffiness, extrapyramidal signs and increased sensitivities to seizures, peptic ulcer
	Newborn: Increased respiratory tract secretions, nasal congestion, cyanosis, and anorexia
Beta-adrenergic receptor blocking agents	
Atenolol	Maternal: Cardiac failure, bradycardia, bronchospasm, if dose sufficient
	Newborn: Bradycardia
Metoprolol	Maternal: Cardiac failure, bradycardia, bronchospasm
	Newborn: Inadequate data
Propranolol	Maternal: Cardiac failure, bradycardia, bronchospasm
	Newborn: Growth retardation, hypoglycemia, bradycardia, apnea
Combined alpha-beta blocking agents	
Labetolol	Maternal: Cardiac failure, bradycardia, bronchospasm
Alpha-receptor blocking agents	
Prazosin	Maternal: First-dose syncope
	Newborn: Inadequate data
Vasodilators	
Hydralazine	Maternal: Flushing, headache, tachycardia, palpitations, angina pectoris, lupus syndrome
Minoxidil	Maternal: Fluid retention, hirsutism, tachycardia, pericardial effusion
	Newborn: Inadequate data
Sodium Nitroprusside	Maternal: Hypotension
	Newborn: Cyanide toxicity
Angiotensin converting enzyme inhibitors	Maternal: Hypotension, neutropenia, renal failure, proteinuria
	Newborn: Increased perinatal mortality
Calcium-channel blocking agents	Maternal: Prolongation of labor, hypotension heart block, heart failure
	Newborn: Teratogenic or embryocidal in animals at high doses

From Sullivan, ref. 106, with permission.

seizures and, in addition, is a mild vasodilator. Magnesium sulfate, 2 to 4 g of 10 or 23% solution is given intravenously, followed by a continuous infusion of 0.5 to 2.0 g per hr (21). The infusion rate is adjusted to reduce hyperactive deep tendon reflexes to normal levels, without inducing respiratory depression or loss of reflexes, both signs of toxicity. If urine volume falls, magnesium excretion becomes impaired and the rate of infusion must be reduced. Serum magnesium levels provide a helpful guide for therapy, but the length of time required to obtain results from most laboratories limits its usefulness. An intravenous infusion of 4 g given over 4 min results in a plasma concentration of 7 to 9 mEq/l (21). The therapeutic range is considered to lie between 4.8 to 8.4 mEq/l, loss of peripheral reflexes occurs at plasma levels above 10 mEq/l, respiratory muscle depression at levels above 10 mEq/l, and cardiac arrest at levels above 30 mEq/l. An intravenous infusion of 0.5 to 2.0 g per hr after a loading dose should produce levels of 4 to 7 mEq/l. Intramuscular administration offers an alternative route of administration. When given as a bolus injection, magnesium sulfate results in a rise in cardiac index of 15 min duration and a fall in pressure lasting only one hour (16).

Several agents can be used to manage hypertensive emergencies and urgencies during pregnancy (Table 3). Parenteral hydralazine is widely used when additional reduction of blood pressure is necessary. Intravenous doses of 5 to 10 mg, given at 15 min intervals to a diastolic pressure of 90 to 100 mmHg, should be followed by a constant infusion of 5 mg per hr, adjusted to maintain the diastolic pressure between 90 to 100 mmHg. Prolonged infusions will result in compensatory fluid retention beyond that required to correct volume contraction accompaning preeclampsia and may necessitate the use of furosemide, 20 to 40 mg intravenously, to potentiate the antihypertensive effects of hydralazine.

If convulsions develop despite treatment or in the absence of prior therapy, measures should be initiated to prevent additional convulsions, reduce vasospasm, lower blood pressure, and initiate diuresis. The appearance of convulsions is associated with fetal loss in as many as 25% and as high as 25% in maternal mortality. Causes of seizures other than eclampsia should be ruled out. The usual therapeutic measures in obstetrical practice include bed rest in quiet surroundings, with close observation, and parenteral hydralazine and magnesium sulfate. Hydralazine gained popularity with the demonstration that drugs acting upon the autonomic nervous system are relatively ineffective in treating the vasospasm

of patients with acute preeclampsia-eclampsia (3). Recommended anticonvulsive therapy consists of intravenous diazepam, 20 mg.; or amobarbital, 250 mg.; or phenytoin, 0.5–1.0 g, while intravenous furosemide is used to promote diuresis.

If hydralazine does not control blood pressure and delivery is planned within 30 min, intravenous sodium nitroprusside can be used to lower pressure. However, prolonged use can result in fetal cyanide intoxication. Sodium nitroprusside is both an arterial and venous dilator. Thus, this compound can be very effective in improving cardiac failure and pulmonary congestion due to acutely high arterial pressures and the fluid overload which can result from aggressive attempts to correct contraction of plasma volume. Therapy should be monitored with a Swan-Ganz flow-directed pulmonary arterial catheter to allow measurement of left ventricular (pulmonary capillary wedge) filling pressures to guide titration of nitroprusside and furosemide.

Although controversy exists concerning the precise timing of delivery in the patient with eclampsia, there is general agreement that delivery should take place no later than the point when the patient has stabilized under medical therapy. Some authorities advocate delivery as soon as the patient begins to respond to therapy (86).

GOALS OF ANTIHYPERTENSIVE THERAPY

The Joint National Commission on Detection, Evaluation and Management of Hypertension made the following recommendation in its 1984 report (47):

Hypertension during pregnancy may represent the self-limited syndrome of preeclampsia (pregnancy-induced hypertension) or chronic (essential) hypertension. In either situation, treatment of hypertension is beneficial. In women with preeclampsia, antihypertensive therapy has improved fetal survival. There is no clear agreement on the therapy of choice, and each physician must

Table 3. *Management of hypertensive emergencies and urgencies during pregnancy*

Agent	Intramuscular dose	Single dose	Continuous infusion	Onset of action	Maternal adverse effects
Vasodilators					
Diazoxide		50–100 mg bolus	15–30 mg/min over 20–30 min	3–5 min	Nausea, vomiting, hyperglycemia, hyperuricemia, hypotension, flushing, tachycardia, angina
Hydralazine	10–50 mg	10–20 mg	200 mg/L	20–30 min; (IM) 10–12 min (IV)	Tachycardia, palpitations, flushing, headache, vomiting, angina
Sodium nitroprusside			50–100 mg/L	Immediate	Nausea, vomiting, muscle twitching, sweating, thiocyanate intoxication, apprehension
Sympathetic blocking agents					
Labetalol		20–80 mg bolus	2 mg/min	5–10 min	Vomiting, nausea, scalp tingling, burning in throat and groin, pain at injection site, postural hypotension, dizziness
Methyldopa		250–500 mg		2–3 hr	Drowsiness

From Sullivan, ref. 106, with permission.

decide on appropriate therapy for the individual patient. Adverse effects on fetal development must be a concern with any drug during pregnancy. However, there has been no evidence of teratogenicity when antihypertensive drugs have been given throughout pregnancy. Methyldopa has been used extensively in pregnant women, but recent clinical studies indicate that beta-adrenergic blocking drugs are equally effective in controlling blood pressure and improving fetal survival. Because captopril has been demonstrated to increase fetal mortality in pregnant animals, it should probably be avoided during pregnancy.

Attempts to control blood pressure during pregnancy should be mindful of several goals concerned with maternal and fetal welfare (105) (Table 4). Controversy exists about the level to which elevated blood pressure should be lowered in patients with essential hypertension concurrent with pregnancy and in patients with pregnancy-induced hypertension. This dispute will be difficult to resolve until it has been determined whether the human uterine vasculature autoregulates. In the pregnant ewe, uteroplacental blood flow is directly dependent upon arterial pressure, suggesting that this vascular bed does not autoregulate, therefore, lowering blood pressure reduces uteroplacental blood flow in this species (39). In contrast, the uteroplacental blood flow of the pregnant rabbit has been found to remain constant over a range of mean

Table 4. *Goals of antihypertensive therapy during pregnancy*

Maternal
1. Prevention of accelerated hypertension and its complications
2. Prevention of superimposed preeclampsia
3. Prevention of premature atherosclerosis and its complications

Relative to Fetal Well-Being
1. Reduction of fetal wastage
   a. Prevention of prematurity and neonatal death
   b. Prevention of spontaneous abortion and stillbirth
2. Avoidance of drugs with potentially harmful long-term effects

arterial perfusion pressure from 60 to 140 mmHg (118). The relevance of either experiment, which used healthy animals without chronic or pregnancy-induced hypertension, to the problem of human essential hypertension or PIH, remains questionable. Gant and his colleagues (32) have demonstrated that both chronic therapy with thiazide diuretics and acute therapy with either hydralazine or furosemide reduces the metabolic clearance rate of dehydroisoandrosterone sulfate in hypertensive gravidas. If this measurement accurately reflects changes in uteroplacental blood flow under the clinical circumstances in which it was used, it implies that therapy with these particular drugs might be harmful to the fetus while nonetheless protecting the maternal circulatory tree. However, more recent studies, which have used [133]In to measure uteroplacental flow, show that blood pressure can be lowered with agents such as dihydralazine (66) and labetalol (67) without a drop in placental perfusion.

Acting in accord with the concept that diastolic blood pressure of 109 mmHg or less will not damage the maternal vascular tree if sustained for a relatively limited period, Pritchard et al. (84), limited the use of antihypertensive agents to patients whose diastolic pressure exceeded 110 mmHg, in which case intravenous hydralazine was given to prevent the adverse effects of acute severe hypertension. This conservative approach has been applied to 245 consecutive cases with only one maternal death from respiratory arrest in a magnesium sulfate-treated patient.

In a recent review, Naden and Redman (74) concluded that, at present, there is no definite indication for the treatment of mild hypertension during pregnancy but that treatment of moderate hypertension is reasonable, even though the value of such treatment has not been proved. In contrast, as levels of 180/120 mmHg or higher involve a significant risk of cerebral vascular damage, blood pressure should be lowered rapidly to levels no lower than 130/90 mmHg with either parenteral hydralazine or labatolol. Methyldopa, labetolol, or beta blockers were recommended for long-term control of blood pressure during pregnancy.

However, several studies have shown that blood pressure elevation is associated with an adverse outcome of pregnancy. Antihypertensive therapy has not been shown to reduce the subsequent development of preeclampsia, but does appear to reduce fetal wastage and probably prevents the development of short-term complications of hypertension: congestive heart failure, intracerebral hemorrhage, and dissecting aneurysm. Recent studies have also shown that antihypertensive therapy prevents an increase in severity of essential hypertension during pregnancy, although there was often no improvement in fetal outcome (2,43,95). However, clinical studies in this area involve small numbers of patients and are not yet definitive. Continuation of effective antihypertensive therapy during pregnancy plays a part in preventing acceleration of hypertension and the long-term development of premature atherosclerosis. However, this goal could be deferred for a few weeks if antihypertensive therapy were found to have an adverse effect on the outcome of pregnancy. Severely elevated blood pressure, i.e., diastolic levels above 110 mmHg, should not go untreated, as the hypertension might undergo further acceleration and result in intracerebral hemorrhage, the most common cause of death in hypertensive gravidas (89). How little blood pressure elevation requires or benefits from treatment has not been established. Adequately sized, randomized, controlled trials of the effect of various classes of antihypertensive agents on the maternal and fetal complications of pregnancies, stratified by severity of hypertension, are needed to determine whether the reported reduction of uteroplacental blood flow associated with anithypertensive agents is clinically important.

REFERENCES

1. Arias, F. (1975): Expansion of intravascular volume and fetal outcome in patients with chronic hypertension and pregnancy. *Am. J. Obstet. Gynecol.*, 123:610–616.
2. Arias, F., and Zamora, J. (1979): Antihypertensive treatment and pregnancy outcome in patients with mild, chronic hypertension. *Obstet. Gynecol.*, 53:489–494.
3. Assali, N. S. (1954): Hemodynamic effects of hypotensive drugs used in obstetrics. *Obstet. Gynecol. Surv.*, 9:776–794.
4. Benedetti T. J., and Carlson, R. W. (1979): Studies of colloid osmotic pressure in pregnancy-induced hypertension. *Am. J. Obstet. Gynecol.*, 135(3):308–311.
5. Blekta, M., Hlavaty, V., Trnkova, M., Bendl, J., Bendova, L., and Chytil, M. (1970): Volume of whole blood and absolute amount of serum proteins in the early stage of late toxemia of pregnancy. *Am. J. Obstet. Gynecol.*, 106:10–13.
6. Boonshaft, B., O'Connell, J. M. B., Hayes, J. M., and Schreiner, G. E. (1968): Serum renin activity during normal pregnancy: Effect of alterations of posture and sodium intake. *J. Clin. Endocrinol. Metab.*, 28:1641–1644.
7. Bott-Kanner, G., Schweitzer, A., Reisner, S. H., Joel-Cohen, S. J., and Rosenfeld, J. B. (1980): Propranolol and hydralazine in the management of essential hypertension in pregnancy. *Br. J. Obstet. Gynaecol.*, 87:110–114.
8. Bower, D. (1964): The influence of dietary salt intake on preeclampsia. *J. Obstet. Gynaecol. Br. Commonw.*, 71:123–125.
9. Brewer, Th. H. (1963): Administration of human serum albumin in severe acute toxemia of pregnancy. *J. Obstet. Gynaecol. Br. Commonw.*, 70:1001–1004.
10. Chamberlain, G. V. P., Lewis, P. J., Swiet, M. D., and Bulpitt, C. J. (1978): How obstetricians manage hypertension in pregnancy. *Br. Med. J.*, 1:626–629.
11. Chesley, L. C. (1971): Hypertensive disorders in pregnancy, In: *William's Obstetrics*, edited by L. M. Hellman and J. A. Pritchard, p. 685. New York, Appleton-Century-Crofts.
12. Chesley, L. C. (1972): Plasma and red cell volumes during pregnancy. *Am. J. Obstet. Gynecol.*, 112:440–450.
13. Chesley, L. C. (1978): *Hypertensive Disorders in Pregnancy*. New York, Appleton-Century Crofts.
14. Cloeren, S. E., Lippert, T. H., and Hinselmann, M. (1973): Hypovolemia in toxemia of pregnancy: Plasma expander therapy with surveillance of central venous pressure. *Arch. Gynac.*, 215:123–132.
15. Collins, R., Yusuf, S., and Peto, R. (1985): Overview of randomized trials of diuretics in pregnancy. *Br. Med. J.*, 290:17–23.
16. Cotton, D. B., Gonik, B., and Dorman, K. F. (1984): Cardiovascular alterations in severe pregnancy-induced hypertension: Acute effects

of intravenous magnesium sulfate. *Am. J. Obstet. Gynecol.*, 148(2):162–165.

17. Curet, L. B., and Olson, R. W. (1979): Evaluation of a program of bed rest in the treatment of chronic hypertension in pregnancy. *Obstet. Gynecol.*, 53:336–340.

18. Dudley, D. K. (1985): Minibolus diazoxide in the management of severe hypertension in pregnancy. *Am. J. Obstet. Gynecol.*, 151(2):196–200.

19. Ehrlich, E. N., Lugibihl, K., and Taylor, C., et al. (1967): Reciprocal variations in urinary cortisol and aldosterone in response to the sodium-depleting influence of hydrochlorothiazide and ethacrynic acid in humans. *J. Clin. Endocrinol. Metab.*, 27:836–842.

20. Eliahou, H. E., Silverberg, D. S., Reisen, E., Romen, I., Mashiach, S., and Serr, D. M. (1978): Propranolol for the treatment of hypertension in pregnancy. *Br. J. Obstet. Gynaecol.*, 85:431–436.

21. Feinberg, L. E. (1983): Hypertension and Preeclampsia, In: *Medical Care of the Pregnant Patient*, edited by R. S. Abrams and P. Wexler, pp. 161–182. Little Brown & Co., Boston.

22. Fidler, J., Smith, V., Fayers, P., and De Swiet, M. (1983): Randomised controlled comparative study of methyldopa and oxprenolol in treatment of hypertension in pregnancy. *Br. Med. J. (Clin. Res.).*, 286(6382):1927–1930.

23. Finnerty, F. A., Jr., and Bepko, F. J., Jr. (1966): Lowering of the perinatal mortality and the prematurity rate: The value of prophylactic thiazides in juveniles. *JAMA*, 195:429–432.

24. Finnerty, F. A., Jr., Bucklholz, J. H., and Tuckman, J. (1958): Evaluation of chlorothiazide (Diuril) in the toxemia of pregnancy. *JAMA*, 166:141–144.

25. Foote, R. G., and Ludbrook, A. P. R. (1973): The use of liberal salt diet in preeclamptic toxaemia and essential hypertension with pregnancy. *N. Z. Med. J.*, 77:242–245.

26. Fox, R. E., Marx, C., and Stark, A. R. (1985): Neonatal effects of maternal nadaolol therapy. *Am. J. Obstet. Gynecol.*, 152(8):1045–1046.

27. Francisco, L. L., and Ferris, T. F. (1989): The effect of Captopril on uterine PGE synthesis and fetal mortality. *Circ. Res.*, (In press).

28. Gallery, E. D. M., Hunyor, S. N., and Gyory, A. Z. (1979): Plasma volume contraction: A significant factor in both pregnancy-associated hypertension (preeclampsia) and chronic hypertension in pregnancy. *Quart. J. Med.*, 192:593–602.

29. Gallery, E. D., Mitchell, M. D., and Redman, C. W. (1984): Fall in blood pressure in response to volume expansion in pregnancy-associated hypertension (preeclampsia): Why does it occur? *J. Hypertens.*, 2(2):177–182.

30. Gallery, E. D., Ross, M. R., and Gyory, A. Z. (1985): Antihypertensive treatment in pregnancy: Analysis of different responses to oxprenolol and methyldopa. *Br. Med. J. (Clin. Res.).*, 291(6495):563–566.

31. Gallery, E. D., Saunders, D. M., Hunyor, S. N., and Györy, A. Z. (1979): Randomised comparison of methyldopa and oxprenolol for treatment of hypertension in pregnancy. *Br. Med. J.*, 1(6178):1591–1594.

32. Gant, N. F., Madden, J. D., Siiteri, P. K., and MacDonald, P. C. (1976): The metabolic clearance rate of dehydroisoandrosterone sulfate. IV: Acute effects of induced hypertension, and natriuresis in normal and hypertensive pregnancies. *Am. J. Obstet. Gynecol.*, 124:143–148.

33. Gant, N. F., Jr., Worley, R. J. (1980): *Hypertension in Pregnancy: Concepts and Management*, New York, Appleton-Century-Crofts.

34. Gerard, J., Blazquez, G., Lardoux, H., Beausejour, B., Faurie, C., Rousset, D., and Flouvat, B., (1983): Effect of 2 beta-blockers on arterial hypertension during pregnancy: Results of a prospective study on 56 pregnant hypertensive women treated with atenolol and labetalol. *J. Gynecol. Obstet. Biol. Reprod., (Paris).* 12(8):891–900.

35. Gilstrap, L. C., Cunningham, F. G., and Whalle, P. J. (1978): Management of pregnancy-induced hypertension in the nullipapous patient remote from term. *Semin. Perinatol.*, 2:73–81.

36. Goodlin, R. C., Dobry, C. A., Anderson, J. C., Woods, R. E., and Quaife, M. (1983): Clinical signs of normal plasma volume expansion during pregnancy. *Am. J. Obstet. Gynecol.*, 145:1001–1009.

37. Goodlin, R., Kurpershoek, C., and Haesslein, H. (1982): Colloid osmotic pressure changes during hypertensive pregnancy. *Clin. Exp. Hypertens.*, 1:49–56.

38. Gray, M. J., Munro, A. B., and Sims, E. A. H., et al. (1964): Regulation of sodium and total body water metabolism in pregnancy. *Am. J. Obstet. Gynecol.*, 89:760–765.

39. Greiss, F. C., Jr. (1966): Pressure-flow relationship in the gravid uterine vascular bed. *Am. J. Obstet. Gynecol.*, 96:41–47.

40. Hauser, G. J., Almog, S., Tirosh, M., and Spirer, Z. (1985): Effect of alpha-methyldopa excreted in human milk on the breast-fed infant. *Helv. Paediatr. Acta*, 40(1):83–86.

41. Hogstedt, S., Lindberg, B., Peng, D. R., Regardh, C. G., and Rane, A. (1985): Pregnancy-induced increase in metoprolol metabolism. *Clin. Pharmacol Ther.*, 37(6):688–692.

42. Horvath, J. S., Phippard, A., Korda, A., Henderson-Smart, D. J., Child, A., and Tiller, D. J. (1985): Clonidine hydrochloride: A safe and effective antihypertensive agent in pregnancy. *Obstet. Gynecol.*, 66:634–638.

43. Horvath, T. S., Phippard, A., and Smart, D. H., et al. (1982): High risk hypertensive pregnancies: Maternal and fetal outcome. *Clin. Exp. Hypertens.*, 2:21–28.

44. Huysmans, F. T., Thien, T., and Koene, R. A. (1983): Acute treatment of hypertension with slow infusion of diazoxide. *Arch. Intern. Med.*, May;143(5):882–884.

45. Hytten, F. E., and Paintin, D. B. (1963): In-

crease in plasma volume during normal pregnancy. *J. Obstet. Gynaecol. Br. Commw.*, 70:402–407.

46. Ingemarsson, I., Liedholm, H., Montan, S., Westgren, M., and Melander, A. (1984): Fetal heart rate during treatment of maternal hypertension with beta-adrenergic antagonists: A preliminary report. *Acta Obstet. Gynecol. Scand.*, (Suppl) 118:95–97.

47. The Joint National Committee on Detection, Evaluation and Treatment of High Blood Pressure. (1984): The 1984 Report of the Joint National Committee on Detection, Evaluation and Treatment of High Blood Pressure. *Arch. Intern. Med.*, 144:1045–1057.

48. Jouppila, P., Jouppila, R., and Koivula, A. (1983): Albumin infusion does not alter the intervillous blood flow in severe pre-eclampsia. *Acta Obstet. Gynecol. Scand.*, 62:345–348.

49. Jouppila, P., Kirkinen, P., Koivula, A., and Ylikorkala, O. (1985): Effects of dihydralazine infusion on the fetoplacental blood flow and maternal prostanoids. *Obstet. Gynecol.* 65(1):115–118.

50. Johnson, T., and Clayton, C. G. (1957): Diffusion of radioactive sodium in normotensive and preeclamptic pregnancies. *Br. Med. J.*, 1:312–314.

51. Kaplan, N. M. (1986): *Clinical Hypertension, 4th Ed.*, pp. 345–374. Baltimore, Williams and Wilkins Company.

52. Kincaid-Smith, P., Bullen, M., and Mills, J. (1966): Prolonged use of methyldopa in severe hypertension in pregnancy. *Br. Med. J.*, 1:274–276.

53. Kraus, G. W., Marchese, J. R., and Yen, S. S. C. (1966): Prophylactic use of hydrochlorothiazide in pregnancy. *JAMA*, 198:1150–1154.

54. Kulas, J., Lunell, N. O., Rosing, U., Steen, B., and Rane, A. (1984): Atenolol and metoprolol: A comparison of their excretion into human breast milk. *Acta Obstet. Gynecol. Scand.*, (Suppl) 118:65–69.

55. Kuzniar, J., Skret, A., Piela, A., Szmigiel, Z., and Zaczek, T. (1985): Hemodynamic effects of intravenous hydralazine in pregnant women with severe hypertension. *Obstet. Gynecol.*, 66(4):453–458.

56. Lamming, G. D., and Symonds, E. B. (1979): Use of labetalol and methyldopa in pregnancy-induced hypertension. *Br. J. Clin. Pharmacol.*, 8(Suppl 2):217S–222S.

57. Lang, G. D., Lowe, G. D., Walker, J. J., Forbes, C. D., Prentice, C. R. M., and Calder, A. A. (1984): Blood rheology in preeclampsia and intrauterine growth retardation: Effects of blood pressure reduction with labetalol. *Br. J. Obstet. Gynaecol.*, 91:438–443.

58. Lauwers, P., and Conway, J. (1960): Effect of long-term treatment with chlorothiazide on body fluids, serum electrolytes, and exchangeable sodium in hypertensive patients. *J. Lab. Clin. Med.*, 56:401–408.

59. Leather, H. M., Hymphreys, D. M., Baker, P.,

et al. (1968): A controlled trial of hypertensive agents in hypertension in pregnancy. *Lancet*, 2:488–490.

60. Lieberman, B. A., Stirrat, G. M., Cohen, S. L., Beard, R. W., Pinker, G. D., and Belsey, E. (1978): The possible adverse effect of propranolol on the fetus in pregnancies complicated by severe hypertension. *Br. J. Obstet. Gynaecol.*, 85:678–683.

61. Lindeberg, S., Sandstrom, B., Lundborg, P., and Regardh, C. G. (1984): Disposition of the adrenergic blocker metoprolol in the late-pregnant woman, the amniotic fluid, the cord blood and the neonate. *Acta Obstet. Gynecol. Scand.*, (Suppl)118:61–64.

62. Lindheimer, M. D., and Katz, A. L. (1973): Sodium and diuretics in pregnancy. *N. Engl. J. Med.*, 288:891–894.

63. Little, B. C., Hayworth, J., Benson, P., Hall, F., Beard, R. W., Dewhurst, J., and Priest, R. G. (1984): Treatment of hypertension in pregnancy by relaxation and biofeedback. *Lancet*, 1(8382):865–867.

64. Lund-Johansen, P. (1979): Hemodynamic consequences of long-term beta-blocker therapy: A 5-year follow-up study of atenolol. *J. Cardiovasc. Pharmacol.*, 1:487–495.

65. Lunell, N. O., Kulas, J., and Rane, A. (1985): Transfer of labetalol into amniotic fluid and breast milk in lactating women. *Eur. J. Clin. Pharmacol.*, 28(5):597–599.

66. Lunell, N. O., Lewander, R., Nylund, L., Sarby, B., and Thornström, S. (1983): Acute effect of dihydralazine on uteroplacental blood flow in hypertension during pregnancy. *Gynecol. Obstet. Invest.*, 16:274–282.

67. Lunell, N. O., Nylund, L., Lewander, R., and Sarby, B. (1982): Acute effect of an antihypertensive drug, labetalol, on uteroplacental blood flow. *Br. J. Obstet. Gynaecol.*, 89:640–644.

68. Lunell, N. O., Nylund, L., Lewander, R., Sarby, B., and Wager, J. (1984): Uteroplacental blood flow in pregnancy hypertension after the administration of a beta-adrenoceptor blocker, pindolol. *Gynecol. Obstet. Invest.*, 18(5):269–274.

69. MacGillivray, I., Hytten, F. E., Taggart, N., and Buchanan, T. J. (1962): The effect of a sodium diuretic on total exchangeable sodium and total body water in preeclamptic toxaemia. *J. Obstet. Gynaecol. Br. Commonw.*, 69:458–462.

70. Maclean, A. B., Doie, J. R., and Alckin, D. R. (1972): Hypovolemia, pre-eclampsia and diuretics. *Br. J. Obstet. Gynaecol.*, 85:597–601.

71. Mathews, D. D. (1977): A randomized controlled trial of bed rest and sedation or normal activity and non-sedation in the management of non-albuminuric hypertension in late pregnancy. *Br. J. Obstet. Gynaecol.*, 84:108–114.

72. Mengert, W. F., and Tacchi, D. A. (1961): Pregnancy toxemia and sodium chloride. *Am. J. Obstet. Gynaecol.*, 81:601–605.

73. Michael, C. A. (1979): Use of labetalol in the treatment of severe hypertension during preg-

nancy. *Br. J. Clin. Pharmacol.*, 8(Suppl 2):211S–215S.

74. Naden, R. P., and Redman, C. W. (1985): Antihypertension drugs in pregnancy. *Clin. Perinatal.*, 12:521–538.

75. Nylund, L., Lunell, N. O., Lewander, R., Sarby, B.,and Thornstrom, S. (1984): Labetalol for the treatment of hypertension in pregnancy: Pharmacokinetics and effects on the uteroplacental blood flow. *Acta Obstet. Gynecol. Scand.*, (Suppl) 118:71–73.

76. O'Hare, M. F., Russell, C. J., Leahey, W. J., Varma, M. P. S., Murnaghan, G. A., and McDevitt, D. G. (1979): Sotalol in the management of hypertension complicating pregnancy. *Br. J. Clin. Pharmacol.*, 8:390P–391P.

77. Ounsted, M. K., Moar, V. A., Good, F. J., and Redman, C. W. G. (1980): Hypertension during pregnancy with and without specific treatment: The development of the children at the age of four years. *Br. J. Obstet. Gynaecol.*, 87:19–24.

78. Philipp, K., Pateisky, N., Brehm, R., and Skodler, W. (1984): Measurement of uteroplacental circulation in hypertensive therapy with clonidine. *Z. Geburtshilfe Perinatol.*, 188(1):34–36.

79. Pipkin, F. B., Turner, S. R., and Symonds, E. M. (1980): Possible risk with captopril in pregnancy; Some animal data. (Letter), *Lancet*, 1:1256.

80. Plouin, P. F., and Tchobroutsky, C. (1985): Inhibition of angiotensin converting enzyme in human pregnancy. *Presse Med.*, 14(43):2175–2178.

81. Pollack, V. E., and Nettles, J. B. (1960): The kidney in toxemia of pregnancy: A clinical and pathological study based on renal biopsies. *Medicine*, 39:469–526.

82. Pritchard, J. A., (1965): Changes in blood volume during pregnancy and delivery. *Anesthesiology*, 26:393–399.

83. Pritchard, J. A. (1978): Management of severe preeclampsia and eclampsia. *Semin. Perinatal.*, 2:83–97.

84. Pritchard, J. W., Cunningham, F. G., and Pritchard, S. A. (1984): The Parkland Memorial Hospital protocol for treatment of eclampsia: Evaluation of 245 cases. *Am. J. Obstet. Gynecol.*, 148(7):951–963.

85. Pruyn, S. C., Phelan, J. P., and Buchanan, G. C. (1979): Long-term propranolol therapy in pregnancy: Maternal and fetal outcome. *Am. J. Obstet. Gynecol.*, 135:485–489.

86. Reid, D. E. (1972): In: *Principals and Management of Human Reproduction*, edited by D. E. Reid, K. J. Ryan, and K. Benirschke. Saunders, Philadelphia.

87. Redman, C. W. G. (1984): Maternal plasma volume and disorders of pregnancy. *Br. Med. J.*, 288:955–956.

88. Redman, C. W. G., Beilin, L. J., and Bonnar, J., Ounsted, M. K. (1976): Fetal outcome in trial of antihypertensive treatment in pregnancy. *Lancet*, 2:753–756.

89. Report. Department of Health and Social Security. (1979): Report on confidential enquiries into maternal deaths in England and Wales 1973–1975. London, HM50, 21-9.

90. Reynolds, B., Butters, L., Evans, J., Adams, T., and Rubin, P. C. (1984): First year of life after the use of atenolol in pregnancy associated hypertension. *Arch. Dis. Child.*, 59(11):1061–1063.

91. Robertson, E. G. (1971): The natural history of oedema during pregnancy. *J. Obstet. Gynaecol. Br. Commonw.*, 78:520–529.

92. Robinson, M. (1958): Salt in pregnancy. *Lancet*, 1:178–181.

93. Rothberg, A. D., and Lorenz, R. (1984): Can captopril cause fetal and neonatal renal failure? *Pediatr. Pharmacol. (New York)*, 4(3):189–192.

94. Rubin, P. C., Butters, L., Clark, D., Sumner, D., Belfield, A., Pledger, D., Low, R. A., and Reid, J. L. (1984): Obstetric aspects of the use in pregnancy-associated hypertension of the beta-adrenoceptor antagonist atenolol. *Am. J. Obstet. Gynecol.*, 150(4):389–392.

95. Rubin, P. C., Clark, D. M., Sumner, D. J., Low, R. A., Butters, L., Reynolds, B., Steedman, D., and Reid, J. L. (1983): Placebo-controlled trial of atenolol in treatment of pregnancy-associated hypertension. *Lancet*, 1:431–434.

96. Ruskoaho, H. J., and Savolainen, E. R. (1985): Effects of long-term verapamil treatment on blood pressure, cardiac hypertrophy and collagen metabolism in spontaneously hypertensive rats. *Cardiovasc. Res.*, 19(6):355–362.

97. Salerno, L. J., Stone, M. L., and Ditchik, P., (1959): A clinical evaluation of chlorothiazide in prevention and treatment of toxemia of pregnancy. *Obstet. Gynecol.*, 14:188–192.

98. Sandstrom, B. (1978): Antihypertensive treatment with the adrenergic beta-receptor blocker metoprolol during pregnancy. *Gynecol. Invest.*, 9:195–204.

99. Schewitz, L. J., Friedman, I. A., and Pollak, V. E. (1965): Bleeding after renal biopsy in pregnancy. *Obstet. Gynecol.*, 26:295–304.

100. Shapiro, S., Monson, R. R., Kaufman, D. W., Siskind, V., Heihonen, O. P., and Slone, D. (1976): Perinatal mortality and birth weight in relation to aspirin taken during pregnancy. *Lancet*, 1:1375–1376.

101. Sibai, B. M., Grossman, R. A., and Grossman, II. G. (1984): Effects of diuretics on plasma volume in pregnancies with long-term hypertension. *Am. J. Obstet. Gynecol.*, 150(7):831–835.

102. Singh, B. N., Hecht, H. S., Nademane, K., and Chew, Y. C. (1982): Electrophysiological and hemodynamic actions of slow channel blocking compounds. *Progr. Cardiovasc. Dis.*, 25:103–132.

103. Sioufi, A., Hillion, D., Lumbroso, P., Wainer, R., Olivier-Martin, M., Schoeller, J. P., Colussi, D., Leroux, F., and Mangoni, P. (1984): Oxprenolol placental transfer, plasma concentrations in newborns and passage into breast milk. *Br. J. Clin. Pharmacol.*, 18(3):453–456.

104. Soffronoff, E. C., Kaufmann, B. M., and Con-

naughton, J. F. (1977): Intravascular volume determinations and fetal outcome in hypertensive diseases of pregnancy. *Am. J. Obstet. Gynecol.*, 127:4–9.

105. Sullivan, J. M. (1979): Management of essential hypertension during pregnancy. *Clin. Cardiol.*, 2:368–374.

106. Sullivan, J. M. (1986): *Hypertension and Pregnancy*, Yearbook Medical Publishers, Chicago.

107. Sullivan, J. M., Palmer, E. T., Schoeneberger, A. A., Jennings, J. C., Morrison, J. C., and Ratts, T. E. (1978): SQ20,881: Effect on eclamptic-preeclamptic women with postpartum hypertension. *Am. J. Obstet. Gynecol.*, 131:707–715.

108. Sullivan, J. M., and Ratts, T. E. (1988): Sodium-sensitivity in human subjects: Hemodynamic and hormonal correlates. *Hypertension*, 11:717–723.

109. Tarazi, R. C. (1976): Hemodynamic role of extracellular fluid in hypertension. *Circ. Res.*, 38 (Suppl II):II-73–II-83.

110. Tarazi, R. C., Dustan, H. P., and Frohlich, E. D. (1970): Long-term thiazide therapy in essential hypertension: Evidence for persistent alteration in plasma volume and renin activity. *Circulation*, 41:709–717.

111. Tcherdakoff, P. H., Colliard, M., and Berrard, E., et al. (1978): Propranolol in hypertension during pregnancy. *Br. Med. J.*, 2:670.

112. Tobian, L. (1967): Why do thiazide diuretics lower blood pressure in essential hypertension. *Ann. Rev. Pharamcol.*, 7:399–408.

113. Tobian, L., Janecek, J., and Foker, J., et al. (1962): Effect of chlorothiazide on renal juxtaglomerular cells and tissue electrolytes. *Am. J. Physiol.*, 202:905–908.

114. Tuimala, R., Punnonen, R., and Kauppila, E. (1985): Clonidine in the treatment of hypertension during pregnancy. *Ann. Chir. Gynaecol. (Suppl)* 197:47–50.

115. Turner, G., and Collins, E., (1975): Fetal effects or regular salicylate ingestion in pregnancy. *Lancet*, 2:338–339.

116. Ulmsten, U. (1984): Treatment of normotensive and hypertensive patients with preterm labor using oral nifedipine, a calcium antagonist. *Arch. Gynecol.*, 236(2):69–72.

117. Vink, G. J., Moodley, J., and Philpott, R. H. (1980): Effect of dihydralazine on the fetus in the treatment of maternal hypertension. *Obstet. Gynecol.*, 55:519–522.

118. Venuto, R. C., Cox, J. W., Stein, J. H., and Ferris, T. F. (1976): The effect of changes in perfusion pressure on uteroplacental blood flow in the pregnant rabbit. *J. Clin. Invest.*, 57:938–944.

119. Wallenberg, H. C. S., Makovitz, J. W., Dekker, G. A., and Rotmans, P. (1986): Low dose aspirin prevents pregnancy-induced hypertension and pre-eclampsia in angiotensin-sensitive primigravidas. *Lancet*, 1:1–3.

120. Walters, B. N., and Redman, C. W. (1984): Treatment of severe pregnancy-associated hypertension with the calcium antagonist nifedipine. *Br. J. Obstet. Gynaecol.*, 91(4):330–336.

121. Watanabe, M., Meeker, C. L., Gray, M. J., Sims, E. A. H., and Solomon, S. (1963): Secretion of aldosterone in normal pregnancy. *J. Clin. Invest.*, 42:1619–1631.

122. Weinberger, M. H., Kramer, N. J., Grim, C. E., and Petersen, L. P. (1977): The effect of posture and saline loading on plasma renin activity and aldosterone concentration in pregnant, nonpregnant and estrogen treated women, *J. Clin. Endocrinol. Metab.*, 44:69–77.

123. Weiner, C. P., Socol, M. L., and Vaisrub, N. (1984): Control of preeclamptic hypertension by ketanserin, a new serotonin receptor antagonist. *Am. J. Obstet. Gynecol.*, 149(5):496–500.

124. White, W. B., Andreoli, J. W., and Cohn, R. D. (1985): Alpha-methyldopa disposition in mothers with hypertension and in their breast-fed infants. *Clin. Pharmacol. Ther.*, 37(4):387–390.

125. Wilson, I. M., and Freis, E. D. (1959): Relationship between plasma and extracellular fluid volume depletion and the antihypertensive effect of chlorothiazide. *Circulation*, 20:1028–1036.

126. Zuspan, F. P., and Bell, J. D. (1961): Variable salt loading during pregnancy with preeclampsia. *Obstet. Gynecol.*, 18:530–534.

New Therapeutic Strategies in Hypertension,
edited by Norman M. Kaplan,
Barry M. Brenner, and John H. Laragh.
Raven Press, Ltd., New York © 1989.

The Effects of Antihypertensive Therapy on Renal Function

John H. Bauer and Garry P. Reams

Hypertension Section, Division of Nephrology Department of Medicine, University of Missouri, Columbia, Missouri 65212

This chapter will focus on the renal effects of antihypertensive drugs commonly used in the treatment of essential hypertension. Eight generic classes of drugs will be considered:

1. Beta-adrenergic antagonists, including the selective $beta_1$ and nonselective $beta_{1-2}$ adrenergic antagonists, and the $alpha_1$-$beta_{1-2}$-adrenergic antagonists
2. $Alpha_1$-adrenergic antagonists
3. Central $alpha_2$-adrenergic agonists
4. Central and peripheral adrenergic-neuronal blocking agents
5. Peripheral adrenergic-neuronal blocking agents
6. Direct-acting vasodilators
7. Calcium antagonists
8. Angiotensin converting enzyme inhibitors

Each of these classes of antihypertensive drugs will be discussed in terms of their chronic (following oral dosing for weeks or months) effect on glomerular filtration rate (GFR), effective renal plasma flow (ERPF) and/or renal blood flow (RBF), renal vascular resistance (RVR), and salt and water excretion. In this review, an attempt has been made to cite those studies using monotherapy, and employing sensitive indicators for measuring GFR and ERPF. Because many of these studies have employed relatively small samples sizes (<10 patients) and because the interassay coeffi-

cient of variation encountered in exogenous clearance techniques approaches 10%, there is a substantial risk of committing a beta-type statistical error. Because of this possible interpretive error, we have chosen to report not only absolute mean changes, but also the percent changes in GFR, ERPF/RBF, and RVR. From such data, trends become apparent.

Few clinical studies are comparable in their study populations with regard to initial levels of blood pressure or hypertensive end-organ damage; pretreatment mean arterial pressure (MAP), GFR, and ERPF/RBF vary widely both within and between clinical studies reported. Furthermore, few clinical studies employ comparable drug dosages or achieve comparable decreases in MAP. Variable decreases in MAP would be expected to have varying effects on renal hemodynamics. The degree of preexisting arteriolar nephrosclerosis and/or renal vasoconstriction may also influence the effect of therapeutic agents on renal hemodynamics. Thus, it may be inappropriate to characterize one drug versus another drug, within a class, as having a greater or lesser quantitative effect on renal function.

With few exceptions, antihypertensive drugs have not been reported to produce sustained, clinically important, renal function changes in essential hypertensive patients exhibiting a good antihypertensive response. Most of the clearance changes described have not been translated into demonstrable rises in serum urea nitrogen or creatinine, due to the insensitivity of these two serum assays to detect 10 to 20 ml/min/ 1.73 m² clearance changes in patients having normal or near-normal renal function. However, studies assessing renal function responses to antihypertensive drugs have been directed primarily at assessing short-term effects, not long-term effects on the natural progression of the disease.

The natural course of untreated essential hypertension is characterized by slow, but progressive, impairment of renal function (12,39,85,109,110,122,126,139,205). The earliest renal hemodynamic abnormality is a rise in RVR (pre- and postglomerular capillary), followed by a decrease in ERPF/ RBF (37,61,72,73,83,84). Initially, GFR is preserved and the filtration fraction is increased. Subsequently, GFR becomes impaired, resulting from vascular ischemia, but at a rate disproportionately less than ERPF; the high filtration fraction is sustained. Early in essential hypertension, the increase in preglomerular capillary (afferent arteriolar) resistance protects the glomerular capillary bed from the transmission of systemic arterial pressure (53). Although there is an elevated systemic arterial pressure, glomerular capillary pressure (P_{GC}) is normal. Late in essential hypertension, when there has been a substantial reduction in renal mass (i.e., nephrosclerosis), there is a decrease in preglomerular capillary resistance, exposing the glomerular capillary bed to an increase in pressure (53). Experimentally, a sustained rise in P_{GC} is associated with an accelerated rate of glomerular injury, histologically characterized by glomerulosclerosis (3,4,119). Preservation of renal mass appears dependent on maintaining a normal P_{GC}.

The resistance state of the preglomerular and postglomerular (efferent) capillary arterioles may determine if a particular form of antihypertensive therapy will be effective in preventing hemodynamically mediated glomerular injury. If preglomerular capillary resistance declines significantly in response to drug therapy, without a concurrent decrease in postglomerular capillary resistance, the glomerular capillary bed may be exposed to a rise in pressure (although MAP is reduced). If preglomerular capillary resistance is already maximally reduced prior to drug therapy, drug therapy which reduces MAP will also reduce P_{GC}, provided postglomerular capillary resistance is not increased. Experimentally, antihypertensive drugs which reduced both MAP and P_{GC} may have renal protective advantages over drugs which only reduce MAP.

Finally, the therapeutic position of the various classes of antihypertensive drugs in the treatment of essential hypertension should be determined not only by their ability to lower systemic blood pressure, and to preserve or improve ERPF/RBF and GFR, but also by their ability to maintain salt and water homeostasis. There is no simple relationship between the fall in systemic blood pressure and the degree of sodium retention following antihypertensive therapy (104). Renal afferent impulses are probably derived, in part, from baroreceptor-sensed changes in pressure and volume. Increases in sympathetic tone produce renal vasoconstriction. Increased sympathetic nerve activity also stimulates direct proximal tubular sodium reabsorption, probably mediated by alpha-adrenoreceptors. There are several efferent mechanisms that mediate sodium retention: 1) changes in renal hemodynamics, altering physical factors in the proximal tubule (an increase in filtration fraction and RVR will decrease hydrostatic pressure and increase oncotic pressure in the peritubular circulation, enhancing sodium reabsorption); 2) changes in distribution of perfusion between superficial and deep juxtaglomerular (sodium-conserving) nephrons; and 3) active reabsorption of sodium in response to changes in concentration of locally released substances, such as angiotensin II (producing a direct proximal tubular antinatriuretic effect). Furthermore, any decrease in GFR, regardless of etiology, will decrease the filtered load of sodium. Angiotensin II and vasopressin have the potential to increase glomerular mesangial cell contractility, to decrease the glomerular capillary filtering surface area, thus to decrease the ultrafiltration coefficient and GFR. The salt and water effect of any given antihypertensive agent is the net result of these several operative mechanisms. Knowledge of a drug's net pharmacological effect on sodium homeostasis will provide the rationale, and predict the therapeutic efficacy, for using it as a first-step therapy.

THE BETA-ADRENERGIC ANTAGONISTS

The antihypertensive action of beta-adrenergic antagonists depends on the attenuation of sympathetic stimulation through competitive antagonism of catecholamines at beta-adrenoceptors. This competition occurs at postsynaptic beta-adrenoceptors in the heart, beta-adrenoceptors in the brain, and presynaptic beta-adrenoceptors at sympathetic nerve endings in the heart and blood vessels. The net systemic effects are a reduction of heart rate, cardiac output, and MAP. Total peripheral vascular resistance is acutely increased, but may return toward pretreatment levels following prolonged therapy.

The renal effects of the beta-adrenergic antagonists are somewhat controversial. Clearly, catecholamines can modulate renal function in a variety of ways, including alterations in renal hemodynamics, intrarenal perfusion, renin release, and tubular reabsorption of sodium and water. The effects are initiated by the binding of catecholamines to specific receptors. $Beta_1$- and $beta_2$-adrenergic receptor subtypes are distributed differentially within the kidney: $beta_1$ predominate in the juxtaglomerular

granule cells and glomeruli, and $beta_2$ predominate in medullary tubules (78). However, there is little clinical evidence to suggest that the presence of $beta_1$ selectivity in a beta-adrenergic antagonist conveys a specific therapeutic advantage with regard to renal function. To address this issue, both the acute and chronic renal effects of beta-adrenergic antagonists will be reviewed according to the following subclasses:

1. nonselective ($beta_1$ and $beta_2$) adrenergic antagonism (nadolol, propranolol and timolol);
2. nonselective ($beta_1$ and $beta_2$) adrenergic antagonism with intrinsic sympathomimetic activity (pindolol);
3. $beta_1$-selective adrenergic antagonism (atenolol, metoprolol)
4. $beta_1$-selective adrenergic antagonism with intrinsic sympathomimetic activity (acebutolol);
5. nonselective ($beta_1$ and $beta_2$) and $alpha_1$-selective adrenergic antagonism (labetalol).

The Nonselective (Beta$_1$ and Beta$_2$) Adrenergic Antagonists

Renal Effects: Nadolol

Although intravenous nadolol may transiently increase ERPF/RBF (62,81,82), chronic oral nadolol does not appear to be associated with any substantial renal hemodynamic advantage. The initial reports by Britton et al. (27), and Danesh and Brunton (40), demonstrating significant improvement in ERPF (by ^{123}I-Hippuran or ^{125}I-Hippuran), have not been substantiated by other investigators (see Table 1): changes in GFR have ranged from -11 to $+18\%$ and changes in ERPF have ranged from -20 to $+18\%$ (19,26,27,40,41,51,64,132,133,178). RVR is generally unchanged.

Salt and Water Effects: Nadolol

Neither the acute intravenous nor chronic oral administration of nadolol has a

Table 1. *Chronic renal effects of nonselective beta-adrenergic antagonist: Nadolol*

Investigator (year)	N	Mean dose (range)	Duration	Mean arterial pressure			Glomerular filtration rate			Effective renal plasma flow/renal blood flow		
				Control	Nadolol	%	Control	Nadolol	%	Control	Nadolol	%
Britton et al. (1981)												
Normal cardiac output	6	80 mg	2–4 wk	123	105	−15[a]	—	—	—	488 ^{123}I-Hippuran	639	+31[a]
High cardiac output	2	80 mg	2–4 wk	130	113	−13[a]	—	—	—	743 ^{123}I-Hippuran	435	−41[a]
Danesh and Brunton (1981)	7	90 mg (80–160)	4–6 wk	122	103	−19[a]	90 ^{51}Cr-EDTA	90	0	360 ^{125}I-Hippuran	425	+18[a]
O'Connor et al. (1982)	10	96 mg (80–240)	5–7 wk	106	92	−13[a]	113 inulin	118	+4	937 PAH	884	−6
Textor et al. (1982)	15	160 mg (150–240)	4–8 wk	126	113	−10[a]	98 ^{125}I-Iothalamate	87	−11	845 ^{131}I-Hippuran	830	−2
O'Callaghan et al. (1983) Elderly subjects	10	144 mg (80–240)	10 wk	133	113	−15[a]	50 ^{51}Cr-EDTA	53	+6	559 ^{125}I-Hippuran	446	−20[a]
Brater et al. (1984)												
Short-term (blacks)	6	40 mg	1 wk	121	109	−10	82 inulin	89	+9	439 PAH	466	+6
Chronic (blacks)	6	(40–320)	3–11 wk	121	115	−5	82 inulin	97	+18	439 PAH	464	+6
Frohlich et al. (1984)												
1 year	8	88 mg (40–240)	1 yr	115	100	−13[a]	113 creatinine	—	—	647 ^{131}I-Hippuran	649	0
2 year	8	88 mg (40–240)	2 yr	115	100	−13[a]	113 creatinine	—	—	647 ^{131}I-Hippuran	623	−4
Danesh et al. (1984)	7	91 mg (80–160)	4–6 wk	122	103	−16[a]	90 ^{51}Cr-EDTA	91	+1	362 ^{125}I-Hippuran	428	+18[a]
Dupont et al. (1985)	10	80 mg	4 wk	123	106	−14[a]	118 ^{99m}Tc DTPA	111	−6	789 ^{131}I-Hippuran	774	−2
Bauer et al. (1987)	12	103 mg (40–160)	12 wk	116	108	−7[a]	87 inulin	88	+1	357 PAH	331	−6

N, number of subjects; mean dose, mg/day; mean arterial pressure, mmHg; glomerular filtration rate, ml/min (clearance method); effective renal plasma flow, ml/min (clearance method); PAH, para-aminohippurate.
[a] Statistically significant difference.

clinically significant effect on urinary sodium or potassium excretion (19,26,51,133, 178). Plasma volume is unchanged (64,133,178), and body weight (19,51,133, 178) is maintained.

Renal Effects: Propranolol

The chronic oral administration of propranolol in patients with essential hypertension produces modest decreases in GFR (-18 to 0%) and ERPF/RBF (-23 to $+1\%$) (7,9,11,26,41,48,56,57,91,105,114,115,134, 135,137,138,198,203) (see Table 2). RVR is either unchanged or increased. We have reported (11) on the renal response to propranolol therapy in a young group of normotensive subjects; GFR fell 27% and ERPF fell 26%. The renal hemodynamic changes were associated with significant decreases in systemic blood pressure (from 122/70 to 111/65 mmHg) and heart rate (from 60 to 48 beats/min). Following withdrawal of therapy, GFR remained decreased, despite the return of ERPF to normal, suggesting that the sustained decrease in GFR may have been the direct result of ischemic injury secondary to diminished RBF. We have reported (9) subsequently on the renal effects of propranolol therapy in essential hypertensive patients. In this study, propranolol therapy had a modest effect on GFR (-5 to -8%) and ERPF (-5 to -14%). The response of hypertensive patients clearly differed from the response of the normotensive subjects, reflecting the different magnitudes of reductions in heart rate (and presumably cardiac output), systemic blood pressure, and ERPF. Finally, Bakris et al. (7), have demonstrated that propranolol exaggerates the physiologic decrement in GFR and ERPF during orthostasis in normotensive subjects.

Salt and Water Effects: Propranolol

Neither the acute intravenous nor chronic oral administration of propranolol has a significant effect on urinary sodium or potassium excretion (9,26,134,203). Body fluid composition (9,134,161,203) and weight (9,26,134,161,203) are unchanged.

Renal Effects: Timolol

Valvo et al. (185), have reported on the renal response to timolol (10 to 40 mg for 8 weeks) in 14 untreated mild to moderate hypertensive patients: MAP fell 17%, (from 119 to 99 mmHg) and GFR (by 125 I-iothalamate) was unaltered (90 ml/min before and during therapy).

Salt and Water Effects: Timolol

Timolol appears to have no appreciable effect on urinary sodium excretion or body weight (185).

The Nonselective (Beta$_1$ and Beta$_2$) Adrenergic Antagonist with Intrinsic Sympathomimetic Activity

Renal Effects: Pindolol

The chronic oral administration of pindolol has little or no effect on renal function (see Table 3): changes in GFR have varied from -9 to $+2\%$, and changes in ERPF/RBF have varied from -7% to $+28\%$ (24,66,137,187,193,202). Renal vascular resistance is unchanged or decreased. In two studies, intravenous pindolol was administered acutely to patients receiving chronic oral therapy (24,193). In the hypertensive patients with normal kidney function, GFR decreased 15% (from 96 to 82 ml/min/1.73 m^2), and ERPF decreased 9% from (496 to 445/ml/min/1.73 m^2). In the hypertensive patients with mild to moderately impaired GFR (mean inulin clearance 66 ml/min/1.73 m^2), qualitatively similar changes were observed: GFR fell from 69 to 62 ml/min/1.73 m^2, and ERPF fell from 511 to 478 ml/min/ 173 m^2.

Table 2. *Chronic renal effects of non-selective beta-adrenergic antagonist: Propranolol*

Investigator (year)	N	Mean dose (range)	Duration	Mean arterial pressure			Glomerular filtration rate			Effective renal plasma flow/renal blood flow		
				Control	Propranolol	%	Control	Propranolol	%	Control	Propranolol	%
Ibsen and Sederberg-Olsen (1973)												
Short term	12	290 (120–480)	2–3 mo	131	105	−20[a]	100 ^{51}Cr-EDTA	88	−12[a]	—	—	—
Long-term	12	(120–480)	4–5 mo	130	103	−21[a]	100 ^{51}Cr-EDTA	85	−15[a]	—	—	—
Dryer et al. (1975)	11	? (320–540)	2 mo	116	105	−9[a]	120 creatinine ^{51}Cr-EDTA	99	−18[a]	—	—	—
Pedersen (1977)	11	240	3–4 mo	122	109	−13[a]	108 ^{125}I-Iothalamate	104	−4	443 ^{131}I-Hippuran	424	−4
Falch et al. (1978)	10	160	2 wks	139	115	−17[a]	—	—	—	273 ^{131}I-Hippuran	237	−13[a]
O'Connor et al. (1979)	12	170 (80–320)	1 mo	123	92	−31[a]	107 creatinine	91	−15[a]	598 PAH	523	−13[a]
Falch et al. (1979)												
Short-term	13	160	1 mo	138	118	−14	—	—	—	244 ^{131}I-Hippuran	208	−15[a]
Long-term	13		8 mo	138	116	−16[a]	—	—	—	244 ^{131}I-Hippuran	187	−23[a]
Bauer and Brooks (1979)												
Normotensive	8	320	1 mo	87	80	−8[a]	103 inulin	75	−27[a]	418 PAH	308	−26[a]
Wilkinson et al. (1980)	15	221 (75–300)	2 mo	125	110	−12[a]	112 creatinine	92	−18[a]	—	—	—
Lameyer and Hesse (1981)	15	? (210–560)	3 mo	148	113	−24[a]	97 creatinine	96	−1	—	—	—

258

Study	N	Mean dose (range)	Duration	MAP before	MAP after	% change	GFR before	GFR after	% change	ERPF before	ERPF after	% change
Warren and O'Connor (1981)	13	160	1 mo	125	93	-26^a	106 creatinine	94	-11^a	619 PAH	523	-16^a
Pasternack et al. (1982)	14	? (120–240)	2–3 mo	123	107	-13^a	116 51Cr-EDTA	113	-3	691 131I-Hippuran	698	$+1$
Malini et al. (1982)	12	170 (80–320)	3 mo	124	111	-10^a	110 125I-Iothalamate	102	-7	536 131I-Hippuran	434	-19^a
deLeeuw and Birkenthager (1982)	15	240 (120–480)	2 wk	120	95	-21^a	130 creatinine	110	-15	—	—	—
O'Connor and Preston (1982)	15	160 (80–320)	1 mo	113	94	-17^a	104 creatinine	91	-13^a	601 PAH	514	-14^a
Bauer (1983) Short-term	14	149 (80–320)	1–2 mo	112	99	-12^a	85 inulin	81	-5	361	343	-5
Long-term	14	172 (80–320)	5–6 mo	112	97	-13^a	85 inulin	77	-8	361	310	-14
Danesh et al. (1984)	7	206 (160–320)	4–6 wk	124	108	-13^a	97 51Cr-EDTA	86	-11^a	518 121I-Hippuran	412	-20^a
Brater et al. (1984) Short-term (blacks)	6	80	1 wk	114	105	-8	90	78	-13	420 PAH	394	-6
Long-term (blacks)	6	? (80–320)	3–11 wk	114	110	-4	90 inulin	90	0	420 PAH	400	-5
Malini et al. (1984)	12	480	12 wk	123	109	-11^a	109 125I-Iothalamate	101	-7	595 131I-Hippuran	514	-14^a
Bakris et al. (1986) Normotensive—supine	9	160	1 wk	86	83	-3	118 inulin	112	-5	590 PAH	528	-11
Normotensive—upright			20–40 min	93	88	-5	102 inulin	82	-20^a	481 PAH	354	-26^a

N, number of subjects; mean dose, mg/day; mean arterial pressure, mmHg; glomerular filtration rate, ml/min (clearance method); effective renal plasma flow, ml/min (clearance method); PAH, para-aminohippurate.
[a] Statistically significant difference.

259

Table 3. *Clinical renal effect nonselective beta-adrenergic antagonist with intrinsic sympathomimetic activity: Pindolol*

Investigator (year)	N	Mean dose (range)	Duration	Mean arterial pressure			Glomerular filtration rate			Effective renal plasma flow/renal blood flow		
				Control	Pindolol	%	Control	Pindolol	%	Control	Pindolol	%
Wainer et al. (1980)	10	? (10–20)	6 mo	126	111	−12[a]	99 inulin	96	−3	481 PAH	495	+3
Wilcox et al. (1981)	16	29 (10–45)	1–2 mo	121	114	−6[a]	114 51Cr-EDTA	104	−9	411 125I-Hippuran	400	−3
Pasternack et al. (1982)	14	? (10–20)	1.5–2.5 mo	123	106	−14[a]	114 51Cr-EDTA	115	+1	667 131I-Hippuran	713	+7
Boner et al. (1982)	6	? (10–20)	14 wk	123	102	−17[a]	68 inulin	69	+1	398 PAH	511	+28[a]
Gafter et al. (1983)	6	? (5–15)	6–12 mo	118	99	−16[a]	117 inulin	107	−9[a]	539 PAH	500	−7
Van der Meiracker et al. (1986)	10	30 (20–40)	3 wk	116	105	−9[a]	97 125I-Iothalamate	99	+2	996 131I-Hippuran	1031	+3

N, number of subjects; mean dose, mg/day; mean arterial pressure, mmHg; glomerular filtration rate, ml/min (clearance method); effective renal plasma flow, ml/min (clearance method); PAH, para-aminohippurate.
[a] Statistically significant difference.

Salt and Water Effects: Pindolol

Neither the acute intravenous, nor chronic oral administration, of pindolol has a significant effect on urinary sodium or potassium excretion (202). Body fluid composition (117,202) and weight (202) are unchanged.

The Beta₁-Selective Adrenergic Antagonist

Renal Effects: Atenolol

The chronic oral administration of atenolol has no consistent effect on renal function (see Table 4): changes in GFR have varied from -6 to $+6\%$, and changes in ERPF have varied from -16 to $+26\%$ (26,58,133,203). RVR is unchanged.

Salt and Water Effects: Atenolol

Chronic oral therapy usually is not associated with significant effects on urinary sodium or potassium excretion (26). Body fluid composition (47,58,203) and weight (192,203) are unchanged.

Renal Effects: Metoprolol

The chronic oral administration of metoprolol appears to have little or no effect on renal function (see Table 5): GFR changes have varied from -2 to $+2\%$, and ERPF changes have varied from -2 to 0% (102,145,170,172). RVR is unchanged.

Salt and Water Effects: Metoprolol

Chronic oral therapy is not associated with significant effects on urinary sodium or potassium excretion (172). Body fluid composition (145,172) and weight (172) are unchanged.

The Beta₁-Selective Adrenergic Antagonist with Intrinsic Sympathomimetic Activity

Renal Effects: Acebutolol

There are two reports in the literature (22,46) on the chronic (1 to 3 months) renal

effects of acebutolol (800 to 1,000 mg/min): a modest decrease in MAP was associated with no change in creatinine clearance, but a 16% decrease in RBF (by ^{131}I-hippuran) (from 641 to 538 ml/min).

Salt and Water Effects: Acebutolol

Chronic oral therapy is not associated with significant effects on urinary sodium or potassium excretion (22). Body fluid composition and weight are unchanged (46).

The Nonselective (B₁ and B₂) and Alpha₁ and Selective Adrenergic Antagonist

Renal Effects: Labetalol

The chronic oral administration of labetalol has no consistent effect on renal function (see Table 6): GFR changes have varied from -18% to $+9\%$, and ERPF changes have varied from -26 to $+14\%$ (94,103, 115,144,186,197,210). Renal vascular resistance is unchanged.

Salt and Water Effects: Labetalol

Chronic oral therapy is not associated with significant changes in urinary sodium or potassium excretion (94,199). However, chronic oral therapy may be associated with increases in plasma volume (89,144,199), total blood volume (199), extracellular fluid volume (144), and/or body weight (27,52) changes which are reversible on discontinuation of labetalol monotherapy (199).

Summary: Beta-adrenergic Antagonists

In general, beta-adrenergic antagonists have little or no clinical effect on GFR, ERPF/RBF, RVR, urinary sodium or potassium excretion, body fluid composition, or body weight. There are no consistent, long-term data that suggest that beta₁-selectivity, with or without partial agonist activity, or combined alpha-beta-adrenergic

Table 4. *Chronic renal effects beta$_1$-selective adrenergic antagonist: Atenolol*

Investigator (year)	N	Mean dose (range)	Duration	Mean arterial pressure			Glomerular filtration rate			Effective renal plasma flow/renal blood flow		
				Control	Atenolol	%	Control	Atenolol	%	Control	Atenolol	%
Falch et al. (1979)												
Short-term	13	100	2 mo	130	112	−14[a]	—	—	—	243 ^{131}I-Hippuran	213	−12
Long-term			4 mo	130	114	−12[a]	—	—	—	243 ^{131}I-Hippuran	205	−16
Waal-Manning and Bolli (1980)	10	100	2 mo	120	107	−11[a]	79 ^{51}Cr-EDTA	74	−6	444 ^{125}I-Hippuran	431	−3
Wilkinson et al. (1980)	15	221 (75–300)	2 mo	125	108	−14[a]	112 creatinine	106	−5	—	—	—
Dreslinski et al. (1982)	10	100	1 mo	109	99	−9[a]	107 creatinine	102	−5	461 ^{131}I-Hippuran	498	+8
O'Callaghan et al. (1983) Elderly subjects	10	? (100–200)	3 mo	130	108	−17[a]	56 ^{51}Cr-EDTA	58	+4	513 ^{131}I-Hippuran	646	+26[a]
Brater et al. (1984)												
Short-term (blacks)	6	50	1 wk	121	115	−5	78 inulin	75	−4	391 PAH	380	−3
Long-term (blacks)	6	100	11 wk	121	120	0	78 inulin	83	+6	391 PAH	448	+15

N, number of subjects; mean dose, mg/day; mean arterial pressure, mmHg; glomerular filtration rate, ml/min (clearance method); effective renal plasma flow, ml/min (clearance method); PAH, para-aminohippurate.
[a] Statistically significant difference.

Table 5. *Chronic renal effects beta$_1$-selective adrenergic antagonist: Metoprolol*

Investigator (year)	N	Mean dose (range)	Duration	Mean arterial pressure			Glomerular filtration rate			Effective renal plasma flow/renal blood flow		
				Control	Metoprolol	%	Control	Metoprolol	%	Control	Metoprolol	%
Rasmussen and Rasmussen (1979)	7	230 (100–400)	5 mo	127	107	−16[a]	90 ^{51}Cr-EDTA	92	+2	—	—	—
Lameyer and Hesse (1981)	10	? (150–300)	3 mo	148	115	−22[a]	97 creatinine	98	+1	—	—	—
Standgaard et al. (1982)												
Short-term	14	? (100–200)	1–6 wk	132	111	−16[a]	95 ^{51}Cr-EDTA	93	−2	523 ^{131}I-Hippuran	511	−2
Long-term	9	? (100–200)	3–6 mo	134	107	−20[a]	97 ^{51}Cr-EDTA	95	−2	554 ^{131}I-Hippuran	545	−2
Sugino et al. (1984)	9	? (100–300)	5–7 wk	116	100	−14[a]	124 inulin	122	−2	504 PAH	504	0

N, number of subjects; mean dose, mg/day; mean arterial pressure, mmHg; glomerular filtration rate, ml/min (clearance method); effective renal plasma flow, ml/min (clearance method); PAH, para-aminohippurate.
[a] Statistically significant difference.

Table 6. *Chronic renal effects nonselective beta-adrenergic and alpha$_1$-adrenergic antagonist: Labetalol*

Investigator (year)	N	Mean dose (range)	Duration	Mean arterial pressure			Glomerular filtration rate			Effective renal plasma flow/renal blood flow		
				Control	Labetalol	%	Control	Labetalol	%	Control	Labetalol	%
Keusch et al. (1980)	18	1,460 (300–2000)	6 wk	131	117	−11[a]	100 ^{51}Cr-EDTA	82	−18[a]	498 PAH	370	−26[a]
Larsen and Pedersen (1980)	6	1,700 (1200–2400)	? mo	119	106	−11[a]	123 ^{125}I-Iothalamate	114	−7	450 ^{131}I-Hippuran	476	+6
Zech et al. (1980)	45	? (400–1800)	2–4 mo	157	127	−19[a]	64 creatinine	65	+2	—	—	—
Rasmussen and Nielsen (1981)	11	875 (300–1200)	1–4 mo	?	?	?	97	97	0	—	—	—
Valvo et al. (1981)	10	690 (500–1000)	6 mo	135	107	−21[a]	103 ^{51}Cr-EDTA	106	+3	—	—	—
Malini et al. (1982)	12	240 (200–600)	3 mo	126	109	−13[a]	111 ^{125}I-Iothalamate	121	+9	510 ^{131}I-Hippuran	582	+14[a]
Wallin (1985)	17	870 (400–2400)	2 wk	127	111	−13[a]	80 inulin	77	−4	401 PAH	382	−5

N, number of subjects; mean dose, mg/day; mean arterial pressure, mmHg; glomerular filtration rate, ml/min (clearance method); effective renal plasma flow, ml/min (clearance method); PAH, para-aminohippurate.
[a] Statistically significant difference.

antagonism, confer unique renal pharmacological effects, compared to nonselective (beta$_1$-beta$_2$) adrenergic antagonism. The intrarenal hemodynamic effects of beta-adrenergic antagonists are unknown. They generally do not lower RVR, hence they are unlikely to adversely affect glomerular capillary pressure. To the degree that they inhibit renin release, they may reduce the intrarenal generation of angiotensin II, preferentially reducing postglomerular capillary resistance. Most, if not all, of the beta-adrenergic antagonists preserve renal function during long-term use.

The most severe alterations in renal function have been described only in patients receiving propranolol therapy. Among the patients receiving propranolol therapy, the most severe alterations have been described in normotensive subjects (11). These subjects experienced the greater reduction in their MAP (to 80 mmHg), compared to the hypertensive patients (MAP range from 92 to 118 mmHg). If one plots the relationship between the percent change in ERPF as a function of the absolute MAP obtained following therapy in those chronic propranolol studies in which MAP was decreased to ≤110 mmHg, there is a significant relationship (r = 0.902, p < 0.001) between the percent reduction in ERPF and the absolute reduction in MAP (17). As MAP falls below the renal autoregulatory threshold (80 to 100 mmHg), ERPF falls.

In addition to the systemic effect (reduced cardiac output, reduced renal perfusion, impaired renal autoregulation), several intrarenal mechanisms have been proposed to account for the reported decreases in renal function observed following beta-adrenergic antagonist therapy: blockade of beta receptors (presumably beta$_1$ receptors), increased (unopposed) activity of the alpha-adrenoceptor system, inhibition of renal vasodilatory hormones (prostaglandins, kallikrein-kinin system), dopaminergic activation, and/or direct nephrotoxicity. There is virtually no evidence of direct nephrotoxicity.

Although there has been considerable conjecture on the mechanisms for the "variable effect of different beta-adrenergic antagonist on renal hemodynamics" (54,55), we believe this is unwarranted. Long-term results in hypertensive patients are inconsistent for most of the beta-adrenergic antagonists. Only propranolol has been thoroughly studied. There are no double blind, comparative studies reported between propranolol and the beta-adrenergic antagonists. Few studies, using a beta-adrenergic antagonist as monotherapy, achieved absolute MAP responses ≤100 mmHg: 2 of 10 with nadolol, 7 of 17 with propranolol, 1 of 1 with timolol, 1 of 6 with pindolol, 1 of 6 with atenolol, 1 of 4 with metoprolol, 1 of 2 with acebutolol, and 0 of 7 with labetalol. Since the response in the majority of drug intervention studies did not threaten renal autoregulation, it is not surprising that renal function was preserved.

Finally, the chronic oral administration of beta-adrenergic antagonists (with the exception of labetalol) usually have no effect on sodium, potassium, or free water excretion. Body fluid composition and body weight are unchanged. As such, this class of drugs may be prescribed as monotherapy for the treatment of hypertensive disease, without concern for the development of drug tolerance.

ALPHA$_1$-ADRENERGIC ANTAGONISTS

Alpha$_1$-adrenoceptor antagonists induce dilation of both resistance (arterial) and capacitance (venous) vessels by selectively inhibiting postjunctional alpha$_1$-adrenoceptors. The net effect is a decrease in peripheral vascular resistance. Reflex tachycardia and the attendant increase in cardiac output does not predictably occur. This is due to their low affinity for prejunctional alpha$_2$-adrenoceptors, which modulate the local control of norepinephrine from sympathetic nerve terminals by a negative feedback mechanism. There are currently two alpha$_1$-

adrenergic antagonists in clinical use: prazosin hydrochloride and terazosin hydrochloride.

Renal Effects: Prazosin

The long-term (1–6 months) administration of prazosin monotherapy (1–20 mg) has no consistent effect on renal function (see Table 7): GFR changes have varied from −8 to +1% and ERPF changes have varied from −2 to +8% (15,98,112,142). RVR is decreased.

Salt and Water Effects: Prazosin

Chronic (6 months) prazosin therapy has no effect on sodium or potassium excretion, urine flow rate, urine osmolality, or free water clearance (8,15,159). However, chronic prazosin therapy (15,90,112,159) may be associated with significant increases in plasma volume, extracellular fluid volume (15,90,112), interstitial fluid volume (15), total body water (15), and/or body weight (8).

Renal Effects: Terazosin

The short-term (8 weeks) administration of terazosin monotherapy (2 to 20 mg) has no significant effect on creatinine clearance (22a,59) (see Table 7).

Salt and Water Effects: Terazosin

The short-term (4 to 8 weeks) administration of terazosin has no significant effect on urinary sodium or potassium excretion, plasma volume, blood volume, exchangeable sodium, or body weight (59). However, results of multicenter studies suggest that terazosin monotherapy may be associated with an increase in body weight, and a 10% incidence of peripheral edema (42,43).

Summary: Alpha$_1$-adrenergic Antagonists

In general, alpha$_1$-adrenergic antagonists have little or no clinical effect on GFR or ERPF/RBF. RVR is reduced, probably mediated by reducing preglomerular capillary resistance via inhibition of alpha$_1$-mediated, noradrenergic-dependent, vasoconstriction. The intrarenal hemodynamic effects of alpha$_1$-adrenergic antagonists are unknown. However, if they selectively decrease preglomerular capillary resistance, they may increase glomerular capillary pressure, unless postglomerular capillary resistance is reduced concurrently.

The fractional sodium excretion is reduced, and the extracellular fluid compartment expanded. The mechanism(s) responsible for fluid retention accompanying the long-term administration of alpha$_1$-adrenergic antagonists is (are) unknown, but may be mediated by increased (unopposed) activity of renal alpha$_2$-adrenoceptors. Salt and water retention, which accompanies the administration of prazosin and terazosin, may limit their antihypertensive effectiveness as monotherapy.

Central Alpha$_2$-Adrenergic Agonists

Central alpha$_2$-adrenoceptor agonists have a direct effect on specific pre- and postsynaptic alpha$_2$-adrenoceptors in the central nervous system vasomotor center (nucleus of the tractus solitarious) located in the dorsal portion of medulla oblongata. Stimulation of these receptors diminishes sympathetic outflow and increases parasympathetic outflow to the heart via the vagus nerve. The net effect is a decrease in peripheral vascular resistance and a slowing of the heart rate; cardiac output is either unchanged or mildly decreased. There are currently 4 central alpha$_2$-adrenergic agonists in clinical use: Methyldopa (L-alpha-methyl-3, 4-dihydroxyphenylalanine), Clonidine hydrochloride, Guanabenz acetate, and Guanfacine monohydrochloride.

Table 7. *Chronic renal effects alpha$_1$-adrenergic antagonist: Prazosin and terazosin*

Investigator (year)	N	Mean dose (range)	Duration	Mean arterial pressure			Glomerular filtration rate			Effective renal plasma flow/ renal blood flow		
				Control	Alpha$_1$-antagonist	%	Control	Alpha$_1$-antagonist	%	Control	Alpha$_1$-antagonist	%
Prazosin monotherapy												
Koshy et al. (1977)	6	? (4–20)	8 wk	?	?	?	144 inulin	145	+1	621 PAH	606	−2
Preston et al. (1979)	10	7 (3–15)	4 wk	119	102	−14[a]	114 creatinine	105	−8	593 PAH	637	+7
McNair et al. (1980)	12	? (1.5–20)	2–6 mo	129	123	−5	95 ^{51}Cr-EDTA	93	−2	—	—	—
Bauer et al. (1984)	14	6 (2–20)	3–6 wk	108	99	−8[a]	85 inulin	85	0	371 PAH	399	+8
Terazosin monotherapy												
Ferrier et al. (1986)	9	12 (5–20)	8 wk	121	113	−7[a]	95 creatinine	89	−6	—	—	—
Beretta-Piccoli et al. (1986)	17	13 (2–20)	8 wk	120	112	−6[a]	102 creatinine	98	−4	—	—	—

N, number of subjects; mean dose, mg/day; mean arterial pressure, mmHg; glomerular filtration rate, ml/min (clearance method); effective renal plasma flow, ml/min (clearance method); PAH, para-aminohippurate.
[a] Statistically significant difference.

Renal Effects: Methyldopa

The short-term (6–29 days) oral administration of methyldopa (0.5–2.0 g/day) has no consistent effect on renal function (see Table 8): GFR changes have varied from −14 to +28%, ERPF changes have varied from −4 to +31% (28,75,121,163,200), whereas RVR is decreased.

Salt and Water Effects: Methyldopa

Grabie et al. (75), found that both the acute and short-term (1 week) administration of 1.0 g methyldopa to 10 hypertensive patients was associated with decreases in the fractional sodium excretion and urine flow rate, but no change in urine osmolality or free water clearance. Short-term administration was associated with a 0.6 kg weight gain and a positive sodium balance of 318 mEq. Retention of salt and water, with weight gain and edema formation, appears unrelated to the degree of blood pressure reduction (21,45,167). It is most likely to occur in patients with severe degrees of hypertension and in patients with severe renal insufficiency. However, at least two clinical trials report that methyldopa, given as monotherapy for a period of six months, had no significant effect on body weight (88,194).

Renal Effects: Clonidine

The short-term (1 to 3 months) administration of clonidine (0.2 to 1.2 mg) has no consistent effect on renal function (see Table 8): changes in GFR have varied from −1 to +6%, changes in ERPF/RBF have varied from −8 to +16% (38,123,180), whereas RVR is reduced.

Salt and Water Effects: Clonidine

Although clonidine acutely decreases sodium excretion (136,151), its chronic administration has no consistent effect on sodium excretion (20,23,38,206). At least four clinical trials report that clonidine, given as monotherapy for periods of 3 months or longer, had no significant effect on body weight (34,128,180,196,206).

Renal Effects: Guanabenz

The long-term (7 days to 24 weeks) administration of guanabenz (8 to 64 mg) has no consistent effect on renal function (see Table 8): changes in GFR have varied from −18 to +9%, and changes in ERPF have varied from −17 to +17% (10,68,125). Although RVR is reduced during short-term therapy, the reduction may not be sustained during long-term therapy (10).

Salt and Water Effects: Guanabenz

Bosanac et al. (25), have reported that guanabenz acutely decreases the fractional excretion of sodium, urine flow rate, and free water clearance. In contrast, Gehr et al. (68), have reported that guanabenz acutely increases both fractional sodium excretion and free water clearance. However, neither change was sustained following one week of monotherapy. We have reported that guanabenz has no effect on fractional sodium or potassium excretion at either 3 to 6 weeks, or 5 to 6 months of drug therapy (10). However, guanabenz increased urine flow rate 30 to 36%, decreased urine osmolality 38 to 43%, and increased free water clearance 50 to 52%, respectively, at 3 to 6 weeks and at 5 to 6 months of drug therapy. Guanabenz has no long-term effect on body fluid composition or body weight (10,80,195).

Renal Effects: Guanfacine

The long-term (24–42 months) administration of guanfacine, 2–15 mg/day, to 10 patients with essential hypertension, has been reported to produce a 23% increase in GFR (by ^{51}Cr-EDTA), (from 81 to 100 ml/min) (154).

Table 8. *Chronic renal effects of central alpha₁-adrenergic agonists: Methyldopa, clonidine, guanabenz*

Investigator (year)	N	Mean dose (range)	Duration	Mean arterial pressure			Glomerular filtration rate			Effective renal plasma flow/renal blood flow		
				Control	Alpha₂-agonist	%	Control	Alpha₂-agonist	%	Control	Alpha₂-agonist	%
Methyldopa monotherapy												
Weil et al. (1963)	9	? (500–2000)	10 days	150	113	−25[a]	71 creatinine	91	+28	362 PAH	450	+24
Sannerstedt et al. (1963)	11	? (500–2000)	6–19 days	134	120	−10[a]	108 inulin	101	−6	520 PAH	546	+5
Mohammed et al. (1968)	8	? (1000–2750)	7–13 days	162	121	−25[a]	71 inulin	76	+7	302 PAH	350	+31
Broadwell et al. (1972)	7	?	9 days	?	?	−?	86 inulin	75	−13	390 PAH	432	+11
Grabie et al. (1980)	8	1500	7 days	128	108	−16[a]	114 creatinine/ ³H-inulin	98	−14	344 PAH	329	−4
Clonidine monotherapy												
Cohen et al. (1979)	13	0.4 (0.2–0.6)	1 mo	105	84	−20[a]	109 creatinine	111	+2	631 PAH	613	−3
Thananopavarn et al. (1982)	16	0.6	3 mo	126	107	−15[a]	106 ⁹⁹ᵐTc DTPA	105	−1	711 ¹³¹I-Hippuran	653	−8
Morgan (1983)	8	0.6 (0.3–1.2)	? wk	127	112	−12[a]	95 ¹²⁵I-Iothalamate	101	+6[a]	380 ¹³¹I-Hippuran	440	+16[a]
Guanabenz monotherapy												
Bauer (1983)	17	20 (8–64)	24 wk	113	100	−12[a]	84 inulin	69	−18[a]	369 PAH	306	−17
Mosley et al. (1984)	14	16 (8–32)	5–7 wk	112	100	−11[a]	92 creatinine	100	+9	469 ¹³¹I-Hippuran	551	+17
Gehr et al. (1986)	8	16	7 days	103	98	−5	118 inulin	115	−3	534 PAH	605	+13

N, number of subjects; mean dose, mg/day; mean arterial pressure, mmHg; glomerular filtration rate, ml/min (clearance method); effective renal plasma flow, ml/min (clearance method); PAH, para-aminohippurate.
[a] Statistically significant difference.

Salt and Water Effects: Guanfacine

The acute intravenous administration of guanfacine is associated with a marked decrease in urinary flow, sodium and potassium excretion, secondary to the marked decrease in perfusion and filtration (154). These effects are less pronounced after acute oral administration (154). However, prolonged therapy (8 weeks) has no effect on plasma volume, total blood volume (92), or body weight (60).

Summary: Central Alpha$_2$-Adrenergic Agonists

In general, central alpha$_2$-adrenergic agonists have little or no sustained clinical effect on GFR or ERPF/RBF. RVR is reduced, probably mediated by reducing preglomerular capillary resistance, via reduced levels of circulating catecholamines (hence, reduced renal alpha-adrenoceptor stimulation). The intrarenal hemodynamic effects of central alpha$_2$-adrenergic agonists are unknown. However, if they selectively decrease preglomerular capillary resistance, they may increase glomerular capillary pressure. Such would have the potential to produce hemodynamic injury, unless postglomerular capillary resistance was concurrently reduced.

Fractional sodium and potassium excretion are unchanged following chronic therapy; initial sodium retention, when it occurs, is probably related to the observed initial acute reduction in GFR (hence, filtered load of sodium). Body fluid composition and weight are not altered. Clinical trials for all of these drugs suggest that some patients can be treated effectively with monotherapy for long periods without clinically apparent weight gain or edema formation. Guanabenz may produce a water diuresis via inhibition of vasopressin; increased alpha$_2$-adrenergic stimulation has been shown to inhibit vasopressin activity by a central depression of vasopressin release, and by altered tubular responsiveness to vasopressin (10,71).

CENTRAL AND PERIPHERAL ADRENERGIC-NEURONAL BLOCKING AGENT: RESERPINE

Reserpine acts both within the central nervous system and in the peripheral sympathetic nervous system. It effectively depletes stores of norepinephrine and 5-hydroxytryptamine by competitively inhibiting the uptake of dopamine by storage granules and by preventing the incorporation of norepinephrine into protective chromaffin granules. The net effect is a decrease in peripheral vascular resistance, heart rate, and cardiac output.

Renal Effects: Reserpine

Moyer et al. (127), have measured GFR (by inulin) and ERPF (by PAH) in eight hypertensive patients in the supine position, following the oral administration of 3 to 6 mg reserpine/day for 3 months. A 24 mmHg decrease in MAP (from 152 to 128 mmHg) was associated with a 6% decrease GFR (from 109 to 102 ml/min), a 2% increase in ERPF (from 585 to 596 ml/min), and a 13% decrease in RVR. Reusch (152) performed similar studies in 8 hypertensive patients, and found similar results.

Salt and Water Effects: Reserpine

Moyer et al. (127), have reported that reserpine has no effect on the renal excretion of water or electrolytes, either after intravenous or oral administration for 3 months. These observations were confirmed by Kogsgaard (99); furthermore, he was unable to demonstrate any significant effect of reserpine (2 to 4.5 mg/day for 6 days) on plasma volume, extracellular fluid volume, total body water, or body weight. Melick and McGregor (118) studied 18 hypertensive patients treated with reserpine, rauwiloid, or raudixin, for a period of 28 to 119 days; although the patients had an average weight gain of 2.2 kg, the investigators were unable to demonstrate a significant change in the extracellular fluid space. They suggested that the weight gain was, in part, due to an increase in appetite associated with reserpine therapy. However, fluid retention, with the appearance of edema formation, may occur (140,157).

Summary: Reserpine

Reserpine has little or no clinical effect on GFR or ERPF/RBF. RVR is reduced, probably mediated by reduced sympathetic stimulation of renal alpha-adrenoceptors. The intrarenal hemodynamic effects of reserpine are unknown. Reserpine, used in combination with a diuretic and direct acting vasodilator, has no effect on postglomerular capillary resistance vessels; glomerular capillary pressure remains elevated despite drug-induced falls in systemic blood pressure, and hemodynamic injury is accelerated (4). Fractional sodium and potassium excretion are unchanged and body fluid composition and weight are generally not altered, permitting the effective monotherapeutic use of this drug.

PERIPHERAL ADRENERGIC-NEURONAL BLOCKING AGENTS

Peripheral adrenergic-neuronal blocking agents act by interfering with the release of norepinephrine at the adrenergic postganglionic nerve terminal, without having a significant effect on the central nervous system. Acutely, there is a substantial reduction in cardiac output, caused partly by diminished venous return (due to venodilation), and partly by the blockade of sympathetic beta-adrenergic effects on the heart, whereas peripheral vascular resistance is unchanged. However, following long-term therapy, peripheral vascular resistance is decreased, along with modest decreases in heart rate and cardiac output. There are currently two peripheral adrenergic-neuronal blocking agents in clinical use: guanethidine sulfate, and guanadrel sulfate.

Renal Effects: Guanethidine

Smith (166) has measured creatinine clearance in seven hypertensive patients at 3-month intervals, treated for one year with guanethidine. Pretreatment mean creatinine clearance was 92 ml/min, at 6 months it was 56 ml/min, and at 12 months it was 59 ml/min, representing a 39% decrease in GFR.

Salt and Water Effects: Guanethidine

Richardson and Wyso (153), have reported that guanethidine acutely decreases the fractional sodium excretion, urine flow rate, and free water clearance. Fluid retention, with edema formation, occurs following both short-term and long-term therapy (44,131,153,156,157,165,166,191,201). Increases in plasma volume, total blood volume, exchangeable sodium, and body weight have been reported from as early as 1 week to as long as 12 months, following 15 to 75 mg/day guanethidine therapy (44, 131,153,156,157,165,166,191,201).

Renal Effect: Guanadrel

Cangiano and Bloomfield (35) have measured GFR (by ^{125}I Iothalamate) and ERPF (by ^{131}I-hippuran) in six hypertensive patients treated from 7 to 60 days with guanadrel (25–400 mg daily). A decrease of 28-mmHg in the supine MAP (from 142 to 124 mmHg) was associated with a 9% decrease in the GFR (from 116 to 105 ml/min), a 12% decrease in ERPF (from 386 to 336 ml/min), and a 5% decrease in RVR. In the erect position, MAP fell further (from 149 to 106 mmHg), and was associated with further declines in renal function: GFR fell 29% (from 96 to 68 ml/min), and ERPF fell 40% (from

321 to 191 ml/min). However, RVR increased 120%.

Salt and Water Effects: Guanadrel

Studies on the effects of guanadrel on the renal handling of sodium and water have not been reported in hypertensive man.

Summary: Peripheral Adrenergic Neuronal Blocking Agent

Guanadrel and guanethidine decrease GFR and ERPF/RBF following acute, short-term, and long-term therapy. Reduction in renal function is probably secondary to the drug's peripheral sympatholytic action. The antihypertensive response is characterized by a reduction in cardiac output; reduced renal perfusion pressure leads to reduced GFR and ERPF/RBF. The impaired peripheral adrenergic transmission, and the resulting blockade of the baroreceptor reflex, magnifies these responses when the patient is in the upright position. RVR is reduced secondary to the peripheral sympatholytic action. The intrarenal hemodynamic effects of the peripheral adrenergic neuronal blocking agents are unknown. Long-term data with guanethidine suggest that these drugs may be injurious to the kidney.

The filtered load and fractional excretion of sodium is decreased (secondary to reduced GFR and renal perfusion pressure), leading to fluid retention and weight gain. Tolerance will develop during monotherapy, unless a diuretic is added to control the antinatriuretic effect of these drugs.

DIRECT-ACTING VASODILATORS

Direct-acting vasodilators may have an effect on both arterial resistance and venous capacitance; however, both of the currently available oral drugs, hydralazine and minoxidil, are highly selective for the resistance vessels. Their mechanism of vascular relaxation, and reasons for selectivity, are unknown. The net effect is a decrease in peripheral vascular resistance, associated with a compensatory increase in heart rate and cardiac output. The latter is related, in part, from withdrawal of parasympathetic tone.

Chronic Renal Effects: Hydralazine

Vanderkolk et al. (188), have measured GFR (by inulin) and ERPF (by PAH) in seven hypertensive patients, before and after 11 to 15 weeks of continuous treatment with hydralazine. Hydralazine (75 to 150 mg), given as a single oral dose before the beginning of the chronic treatment period, had no significant effect on GFR, but increased ERPF 36% (from 385 to 523 ml/min), and decreased RVR 40%. The same oral dose, given at the end of the chronic treatment period, had no significant effect on any of the parameters studied, suggesting that tolerance to the renal effects of hydralazine occurred during prolonged oral therapy.

Salt and Water Effects: Hydralazine

Hydralazine acutely decreases sodium and water excretion in hypertensive patients (93). Fluid retention and edema formation may occur with chronic therapy (32,97).

Renal Effects: Minoxidil

The long-term addition of minoxidil to essential hypertensive patients, receiving concurrent diuretic and beta-adrenergic blocker therapies, has a variable effect on GFR and ERPF. Gilmore et al. (69) have reported that minoxidil, given as monotherapy for one week, produced a 9% increase in GFR (by inulin) (from 99 to 108 ml/min), and no change in ERPF (by PAH) (387 ml/min prior to, versus 393 ml/min following, drug); when minoxidil was added to a beta-adrenergic blocker, there was no change in either parameter. Gottlieb et al. (74), have made similar observations. However, Bryan et al. (31), observed that the addition of minoxidil to a diuretic and a beta-adrenergic blocker for 4 to 6 weeks, compared to placebo, was associated with a 14% decrease in creatinine clearance (from 116 to 100 ml/min), and a 13% decrease in ERPF (by PAH) (from 420 to 367 ml/min). Greminger et al. (76), have reported a 10% decrease in creatinine clearance from 93 to 84 ml min during 12 months of minoxidil therapy. We have observed (unpublished data) that triple drug therapy, employing a diuretic, beta-adrenergic blocker, and minoxidil, administered for 12 weeks to 15 essential hypertensive patients, was associated with a 15% decrease in GFR (by inulin) (from 91 to 77 ml/min/1.73 m^2), a 17% decrease in ERPF (from 291 to 241 ml/min/1.73 m^2), and a 9% decrease in RVR. It has been suggested that renal function may deteriorate more rapidly in patients with essential hypertension treated with minoxidil, having base-line serum creatinines greater than 1.5 mg/dl, compared to patients having base-line serum creatinines less than 1.5 mg/dl (33).

Salt and Water Effects

Short-term and long-term administration of minoxidil causes progressive sodium retention, and an increase in body weight appropriate to the degree of sodium retention (31,33,69,74,76,77). Plasma volume and total blood volume are increased (31). The degree of sodium and water retention correlates with the dose administered, the duration of therapy, and the patient's degree of renal impairment (33). Rigid salt restriction, coupled with the use of potent diuretics, is required to maintain body weight close to pretreatment levels.

Summary: Direct Acting Vasodilator

Hydralazine and minoxidil have a similar antihypertensive mechanisms of action;

however, minoxidil has a substantially greater hypotensive effect. The two direct acting vasodilators have qualitatively similar short-term renal effects: GFR and ERPF are probably preserved in patients with normal renal function. RVR is decreased, related to relaxation of the resistance vessels. Long-term renal effects are more controversial, especially in patients with impaired renal function. Experimentally, hydralazine (and presumably minoxidil) used in combination with a diuretic and reserpine does not decrease postglomerular capillary resistance (4). Stimulation of the renin-angiotensin system would be expected to increase postglomerular capillary resistance. Although systemic blood pressure is reduced, glomerular capillary pressure is increased. Each has the potential to precipitate and/or accelerate hemodynamic glomerular injury.

Hydralazine and minoxidil therapy are both accompanied by retention of sodium and water, and expansion of plasma and extracellular fluid volumes. This is particularly evident when the hypotensive effect is severe, or when renal insufficiency is pronounced. Tolerance develops rapidly without concurrent diuretic therapy. Retention of sodium and water is not related to reductions in GFR or ERPF; it has been suggested that vasodilation increases sodium reabsorption in the proximal convoluted tubule of the nephron (211).

CALCIUM ANTAGONISTS

A large number of calcium entry blocking drugs are currently undergoing clinical investigation. They are a chemically heterogenous group of drugs, sharing a common antihypertensive mechanism of action: interference with entry of calcium into smooth muscle cells of resistance arterioles through potential-sensitive channels. Systemic vascular resistance is reduced; heart rate and cardiac output are maintained or increased. There are three calcium antag-

onists currently available: the benzothiazepine derivative, diltiazem hydrochloride;
the dihydropyridine derivative, nifedipine;
and the diphenylalkylamine derivative, verapamil hydrochloride.

Renal Effects: Diltiazem

Studies in patients with primary or secondary renal disease (with or without hypertension) have suggested that chronic
oral diltiazem therapy (doses ranging from
30 to 120 mg/day, from one week to three
months) tended to increase GFR and ERPF,
the latter demonstrating the greatest and
most consistent change (124,158,182,183).
We have reported (174) that diltiazem mon-
otheray in essential hypertensive patients
had no overall effect on GFR or ERPF (see
Table 9); calculated filtration fraction was
unchanged, compared to control, and RVR
was decreased 22%. However, in eight patients with initially impaired GFR (≤80 ml/
min/1.73 m^2), there were marked increases
in GFR (48%) and ERPF (39%), whereas
RVR was decreased (22%). Six of these
eight patients, maintained on diltiazem
monotherapy for a period of 24 weeks, have
demonstrated sustained improvement in
renal function (175).

Salt and Water Effects: Diltiazem

The intravenous administration of diltiazem to patients with essential hypertension (0.5 mg/kg bolus dose), and patients
with primary or secondary renal disease
(with or without hypertension) (10 to 40 mg
over 10 min to 2 hr), has been reported to
increase both urinary flow rate and/or urinary sodium excretion (65,149,183). Diltiazem had no consistent effect on urinary
potassium excretion. However, the chronic
oral administration of diltiazem, in doses up
to 480 mg/day, has not been associated with
generalized fluid retention, as evidenced by
changes in body fluid composition or weight
gain (65,149,175).

Renal Effects: Nifedipine

Bruun et al. (29), have reported that nifedipine, prescribed for 12 weeks (mean
dose 51 mg/day), had no effect on GFR (see
Table 9). However, we have reported (148)
that nifedipine, prescribed for 4 weeks
(mean dose 58 mg/day), increased GFR
13%, and ERPF 20% (see Table 9). Calculated filtration fraction was unchanged,
compared to control, and RVR was decreased 25%. The observed renal responses
were independent of the patient's initial
level of GFR, and were independent of the
patient's level of blood pressure control.
Urinary albumin excretion rate was unchanged.

Salt and Water Effects: Nifedipine

The acute intravenous administration of
nifedipine (1 mg) to patients with essential
or renal hypertension has been reported to
increase urinary flow rate and sodium clearance (96,207). Similar results have been reported following the acute oral or sublingual
administration of nifedipine (10 to 20 mg)
(100,106,184). There is no significant effect
on potassium excretion. Chronic studies,
however, do not suggest sustained diuretic
or natriuretic effects; chronic nifedipine
therapy (in doses ranging to 120 mg/day)
does not significantly alter urinary electrolyte excretion, plasma volume, or body
weight (29,116,148).

Renal Effects: Verapamil

The chronic oral administration of verapamil, prescribed in doses ranging from 240
to 480 mg/day, from one to 12 weeks, has
no adverse effect on GFR or ERPF
(101,160,169) (see Table 9). Calculated filtration fraction is unchanged, compared to
control, and RVR is decreased.

Salt and Water Effects: Verapamil

Neither acute oral administration of verapamil (160 mg) nor chronic oral therapy

Table 9. *Chronic renal effects of calcium antagonist: Diltiazem, nifedipine, verapamil*

Investigator (year)	N	Mean dose (range)	Duration	Mean arterial pressure			Glomerular filtration rate			Effective renal plasma flow/renal blood flow		
				Control	Ca^{++} antagonist	%	Control	Ca^{++} antagonist	%	Control	Ca^{++} antagonist	%
Diltiazem monotherapy												
Sunderrajan et al. (1986)	18	360 (240–480)	8 wk	121	108	−11[a]	91 inulin	91	0	336 PAH	362	+8
Nifedipine monotherapy												
Bruun et al. (1986)	18	51 (40–80)	12 wk	126	113	−10[a]	78 ^{51}Cr-EDTA	77	−1	—	—	—
Reams et al. (1988)	26	58 30–120	4 wk	120	106	−12[a]	90 inulin/ ^{99m}Tc DTPA	102	+13[a]	358 PAH	428	+20[a]
Verapamil monotherapy												
Sorensen et al. (1985)	11	? (240–360)	6 wk	118	109	−8[a]	108 ^{125}I-Iothalamate	112	+4	428 ^{131}I-Hippuran	434	+1
Kubo et al. (1986)	9	347 (240–480)	1 wk	133	103	−23[a]	95 inulin	103	+8	752 PAH	775	+3
Schmieder et al. (1987)	10	372 (240–480)	12 wk	114	98	−14[a]	100 creatinine	106	+6	749 ^{131}I-Hippuran	829	+11

N, number of subjects; mean dose, mg/day; mean arterial pressure, mmHg; glomerular filtration rate, ml/min (clearance method); effective renal plasma flow, ml/min (clearance method); PAH, para-aminohippurate.
[a] Statistically significant difference.

(doses ranging to 480 mg/day for up to six weeks), has been reported to have a significant effect on urinary flow rate, free water clearance, or sodium and potassium excretion, in either normotensive subjects or hypertensive patients (101,106,107,160,169). Blood volume and body weight are unchanged (101,107,160,169).

Summary: Calcium Antagonist

Calcium antagonist have been demonstrated to maintain or improve ERPF and GFR (in the presence of a marked reduction in MAP), and to decrease RVR. These renal findings may be independent of the drug effects on systemic blood pressure (148). There are at least two potential mechanisms for the observed increases in GFR and/or ERPF: 1) reversal of angiotensin II-induced vasoconstriction (mesangium and/or efferent arteriolar tone), and 2) reversal of norepinephrine-induced vasoconstriction (afferent arteriolar tone). The effect of calcium entry blockers to prevent an increase in cytosol-ionized calcium would be expected to decrease the sensitivity of the renal vasculature and the mesangium to both angiotensin II and norepinephrine. Indeed, several investigators have demonstrated that diltiazem, nifedipine, and/or verapamil attenuate the intrarenal effects of exogenously administered angiotensin II and norepinephrine (16). Diltiazem and verapamil may also differentially effect alpha-adrenergic receptors; both drugs have been reported to preferentially antagonize postsynatpic (voltage activated calcium channel) alpha$_2$-adrenergic receptors (16). Selective interference with the vasoconstrictor action of norepinephrine on the afferent arteriole (suggesting a greater density of alpha$_2$-adrenergic receptors), while leaving intact its action on the efferent arteriole (suggesting a greater density of alpha$_1$-adrenergic receptors) would be expected to increase GFR. Our observations of hypertensive patients (when GFR is increased, filtration fraction is unchanged) suggest a differential

attenuating effect of norepinephrine on the afferent (preglomerular) capillary bed, but we do not exclude the possibility of a concurrent reversal of a direct angiotensin II effect on the glomerulus (mesangium) or postglomerular capillary bed. Reversal of angiotensin II-mediated efferent arteriolar vasoconstriction might be expected to disproportionately enhance ERPF, decreasing the filtration fraction. However, calcium antagonists do not alter the filtration fraction, either acutely or chronically. Experimentally, the acute infusion of calcium antagonists has been reported to reduce glomerular capillary pressure (2). These findings suggest that calcium antagonists dilate both pre- and postglomerular capillary resistance beds. If calcium antagonists do reduce both pre- and postglomerular capillary resistances (i.e., maintain normal glomerular capillary pressure), they may provide long-term renal protection.

All of the calcium antagonists induce an acute natriuresis and diuresis. The effect appears to be independent of any vascular action of the drugs, and most likely is due to a direct effect on both proximal segments and/or segments more distally located than the loop of Henle (155,208,209). However, none of the calcium antagonists have been demonstrated to sustain clinically important effects on salt and water excretion. This conclusion is supported by the absence of an observed effect on serum electrolytes, body fluid composition, or body weight. However, anecdotal case reports do attest to the potential for these drugs to produce localized, peripheral edema. The frequency or mechanism for this potential side effect is unclear.

ANGIOTENSIN CONVERTING ENZYME INHIBITORS

Angiotensin converting enzyme (ACE) inhibitors lower blood pressure by decreasing total peripheral vascular resistance; there is usually little change in cardiac output, heart rate, or pulmonary wedge pressure. The mechanism(s) responsible for the lowering of vascular resistance include: 1) inhibition of circulating levels of angiotensin II and aldosterone, 2) inhibition of tissue levels of angiotensin II (vascular endothelium, brain, kidney), 3) potentiation of the vasodepressor kallikrein-kinin system, 4) sympathoinhibitory effects via inhibition norepinephrine release, inhibition postjunctional pressor responses to angiotensin II and/or norepinephrine, and/or interference with sympathetic reflexes, and 5) alteration in prostanoid metabolism (direct and/or indirect via an increase in tissue bradykinin). It has also been suggested that ACE inhibition may inhibit vasopressin secretion. Declines in both aldosterone and vasopressin secretion would be expected to enhance the renal excretion of sodium and water, respectively. There are currently three ACE inhibitors in clinical use: captopril, enalapril, and lisinopril.

Renal Effects: Captopril

Although the administration of captopril (37.5 to 75 mg/day) to essential hypertensive patients for 5 to 10 days has been reported to increase creatinine clearance 14% (from 87 to 99 ml/min), and ERPF 14% (by PAH) (from 478 to 543 ml/min) (162), the long-term administration of captopril, given as monotherapy or in combination with a diuretic, is not associated with significant changes in GFR or ERPF (5,49,95,141,143, 181,190) (see Table 10). Calculated filtration fraction is either unchanged or decreased, compared to control, and RVR is decreased. In general, investigators have not reported significant changes in 24-hour urinary protein excretion. However, proteinuria (over 1 g/day), sometimes sufficient to produce nephrotic syndrome, has been reported to occur in 1.2% of patients (63). In patients without a history of renal disease who received doses of ≤150 mg/dl, the incidence may be as low as 0.2%. In patients with evidence of renal disease, at doses >150 mg/dl, the incidence may approach

3.5%. Findings of membranous nephropathy, with epimembranous electron-dense deposits on renal biopsy, suggest the possibility of an immune-complex glomerulopathy, perhaps related to the sulfhydryl structure of captopril (36,87,108,113,171, 176,179). In these patients, proteinuria may subside despite continued drug therapy, and is reversible on discontinuation of therapy.

Salt and Water Effects: Captopril

The short-term administration of captopril produces sodium loss and potassium retention (1,6,30,67,86,120). These changes are most marked in patients with normal and high-plasma-renin activity (6). Potassium retention is associated with mild increases in the serum potassium concentration (6,67). During chronic therapy, plasma volume, extracellular fluid volume, and body weight are unchanged (1,30,143,173, 177,181,190).

Renal Effects: Enalapril

The long-term administration of enalapril, given as monotherapy, is not associated with significant changes in GFR, although ERPF may be mildly increased (130,146,164) (see Table 10). Calculated filtration fraction is unchanged, compared to control, and RVR is decreased. In a single study, reporting the long-term effects of enalapril-hydrochlorothiazide combination therapy, GFR was observed to increase 16%, and ERPF to increase 19%, compared to control values (146) (see Table 10). In patients with essential hypertension and impaired renal function (GFR ≤ 80 ml/min/ 1.73 m^2), we have observed (18) marked improvement in renal function with either enalapril monotherapy or enalapril-hydrochlorothiazide combination therapy, sustained for up to three years: GFR increased from 60 to 80 ml/min/1.73 m^2 and ERPF increased from 256 to 376 ml/min/ 1.73 m^2. Such changes suggest that strict blood pressure control with enalapril, or en-

Table 10. *Chronic renal effects of angiotensin converting enzyme inhibitors: Captopril, enalapril, lisinopril*

Investigator (year)	N	Mean dose (range)	Duration	Mean arterial pressure			Glomerular filtration rat			Effective renal plasma flow/renal blood flow		
				Control	ACEI	%	Control	ACEI	%	Control	ACEI	%
Captopril monotherapy												
Pessina et al. (1981)	10	300 (150–500)	7 wk	123	114	−7[a]	122 ^125I-Iothalamate	88	−28[a]	534 ^131I-Hippuran	471	−12
Kiowski et al. (1982)	8	325 (150–450)	4 wk	132	116	−12[a]	140 ^125I-Iothalamate	142	+1	490	521	+6
Duchin and Willard (1984)	12	163 (150–300)	4–6 wk	114	100	−12[a]	112 inulin	117	+4	604 PAH	701	+16
Rasmussen et al. (1986)	14	? (75–150)	8 wk	124	114	−8[a]	83 ^51Cr-EDTA	83	0	—	—	—
Ando et al. (1986)	12	37.5 (75–150)	2 wk	118	104	−12[a]	—	—	—	419 ^131I-Hippuran	480	+15
Captopril and diuretic combination therapy												
Duchin and Willard (1984)	8	300	6 wk	128	99	−23[a]	115 inulin	113	−2	559 PAH	650	+16
Ventura et al. (1985)	12	? (50–150)	12 wk	111	96	−14[a]	102 creatinine	111	+9	733	764	+4
Thomsen et al. (1986)	10	? (75–150)	6 wk	124	101	−19[a]	94 ^125I-Iothalamate	86	−9	387 ^131I-Hippuran	382	−1
Enalapril monotherapy												
Navis et al. (1983)	11	15 (10–40)	12 wk	119	106	−11[a]	102 ^125I-Iothalamate	103	+1	413 ^131I-Hippuran	445	+8[a]
Simon et al. (1983)	21	40	12 wk	110	101	−8[a]	103 creatinine	110	+7[a]	690 ^131I-Hippuran	774	+12[a]
Reams and Bauer (1986)	9	18 (10–40)	96 wk	119	94	−21[a]	98 inulin	98	0	397 PAH	421	+6
Enalapril and diuretic combination therapy												
Reams and Bauer (1986)	20	21 (10–40)	96 wk	121	92	−24[a]	82 inulin	95	+16[a]	330 PAH	394	+19[a]
Lisinopril monotherapy												
Giorgi et al. (1986)	12	40 (20–80)	24 wk	129	109	−16[a]	—	—	—	537 ^131I-Hippuran	495	−8
Reams and Bauer (1988)	19	48 (20–80)	12 wk	115	101	−12[a]	92 inulin	88	−4	324 PAH	321	−1

N, number of subjects; mean dose, mg/day; mean arterial pressure, mmHg; glomerular filtration rate, ml/min (clearance method); effective renal plasma flow, ml/min (clearance method); PAH, para-aminohippurate.
[a] Statistically significant difference.

alapril-hydrochlorothiazide therapy, may reverse and/or attenuate the development and/or progression of hypertensive nephrosclerosis. Finally, at least two investigators have reported that enalapril therapy is associated with a significant decrease in 24-hr urinary protein excretion (14,146,164).

Salt and Water Effects: Enalapril

Short-term administration of enalapril tends to produce sodium loss and potassium retention (111,129). Sufficient potassium retention may mildly increase the serum potassium concentration (13,14). Long-term administration of enalapril (20 to 40 mg) has no significant effect on fractional sodium or potassium excretion, although serum potassium levels may remain mildly elevated (13,14,18,111,129,130,146,164). Enalapril therapy has been reported to decrease urine osmolality and to increase free water clearance, both indices of urinary diluting ability (14). These changes are sustained during both short- and long-term therapy (146). The increased free water clearance could be mediated by either suppression of vasopressing release or inhibition of its hydroosmotic effect on the renal colleting duct. Red cell mass, plasma volume, interstitial, extracellular and intracellular fluid volumes, total body water, and body weight are unchanged (13,14,50).

Renal Effects: Lisinopril

The long-term administration of lisinopril, given as monotherapy, is not associated with significant changes in GFR or ERPF, regardless of the initial level of GFR (70,147) (see Table 10). With prolonged therapy (52 weeks), the calculated filtration fraction and RVR are decreased, compared to control (147). Twenty-four hr urinary protein excretion is unchanged (147).

Salt and Water Effects: Lisinopril

Lisinopril has been reported to produce an acute diuresis, which is not sustained beyond eight days of continuous therapy (79). Potassium retention may occur, as evidenced by a mild increase in the serum potassium concentration (189). Body weight is unchanged (70,147).

Summary: Angiotensin Converting Enzyme Inhibitors

Angiotensin converting enzyme inhibitors have been demonstrated to produce a variety of renal responses related to interruption of the integrity of the intrarenal renin-angiotensin system. Experimentally, ACE inhibition has been demonstrated to decrease glomerular capillary pressure via their ability to lower both systemic blood pressure and postglomerular capillary pressure (3,4,119). Hemodynamic-mediated glomerular injury is prevented. In essential hypertension, ACE inhibitor therapy has been demonstrated to maintain or improve ERPF and GFR (in the presence of marked reductions in MAP), to reduce RVR, and to decrease the transglomerular passage of albumin.

Most intriguing is the report suggesting that ACE inhibition may be protective of the essential hypertensive kidney. (18) Sustained improvement in renal perfusion and glomerular filtration are not generally observed with other classes of antihypertensive drugs (with the possible exception of calcium antagonists). Sodium restriction and/or diuretic therapy appears to amplify this effect. Hollenberg and co-workers (163,204) have reported that 40 to 50% of patients with essential hypertension fail to increase their ERPF, or fail to enhance their renal vascular responsiveness, to angiotensin II when shifted from a low- to a high-sodium intake. Such patients have been termed "nonmodulators". In these patients, ACE inhibition restores ERPF to normal (150). The clinical importance and drug specificity of these observations with enalapril remain to be determined, but suggest that ACE inhibitor therapy may reverse the pathophysiology of essential hypertensive renal disease by attenuating the effects of renal (tissue) angiotensin II.

Finally, ACE inhibitors have been demonstrated to reset sodium and water homeostasis (via an initial natriuresis and sustained water diuresis), and to spare potassium loss. Acute pharmacologic interruption of the renin-angiotensin-system probably leads to the natriuresis through local, intrarenal (angiotensin II-mediated) mechanisms, since the response occurs too quickly to be attributed to a decrease in plasma-aldosterone concentration. However, long-term effects on salt and water excretion are less clear. Absence of changes in plasma volume, extracellular fluid volume, and body weight suggest that salt and water homeostasis is restored, perhaps related to attenuated humoral responses of angiotensin II and/or aldosterone. The acute antikaluretic effect of ACE inhibitors does correlate with acute changes in aldosterone metabolism (serum concentration and/or urinary excretion). Since clinically significant potassium retention may occur, especially in the presence of renal disease, the concurrent administration of potassium supplements, potassium sparing diuretics, and/or drugs impairing potassium excretion should be avoided.

REFERENCES

1. Aldigier, J. C. Plonn, P. F., Guyene, T. T., Thibonnier, M., Corvol, P., and Menard, J. (1982): Comparison of the humoral and renal effects of captopril in severe essential and renovascular hypertension. *Am. J. Cardiol.*, 49:1447–1452.

2. Anderson, S., Clarey, L. E., Riley, S. L., and Troy, J. L. (1988): Acute infusion of calcium channel blockers reduces glomerular capillary pressure in rats with reduced renal mass. *Kidney Internat.*, 33:371. (abstr.)

3. Anderson, S., Meyer, T. W., Rennke, H. G., and Brenner, B. M. (1985): Control of glomerular hypertension limits glomerular injury in rats with reduced renal mass. *J. Clin. Invest.*, 76:612–619.

4. Anderson, S., Rennke, H. G., and Brenner, B. M. (1986): Therapeutic advantage of converting enzyme inhibitors in arresting progressive renal disease associated wtih systemic hypertension in the rat. *J. Clin. Invest.*, 77:1993–2000.

5. Ando, K., Kujita, T., Ito, Y., Noda, H., and Yamashita, K. (1986): The role of renal hemodynamics in the antihypertensive effect of captopril. *Am. Heart J.* 111:347–352.

6. Atlas, S. A., Case, D. B., Sealey, J. E., Laragh, J. H., McKinstry, D. N. (1979): Interruption of the renin-angiotensin system in hypertensive patients by captopril induces sustained reduction in aldosterone secretion, potassium retention and natriuresis. *Hypertension*, 1:274–280.

7. Bakris, G. L., Wilson, D. M., Burnett, Jr., J. C. (1986): The renal, forearm and hormonal responses to standing in the presence and absence of propranolol. *Circulation*, 74:1061–1065.

8. Barbieri, C., Ferrari, C., Caldara, R., Rampini, P., Crossignarri, R. M., and Bergonzi, M. (1981). Effects of chronic prazosin treatment on the renin-angiotensin-aldosterone system in man. *J. Clin. Pharmacol.*, 21:418–423.

9. Bauer, J. H. (1983): Effects of propranolol therapy on renal function and body fluid composition. *Arch. Intern. Med.*, 143:927–931.

10. Bauer, J. H. (1983): Effects of guanabenz therapy on renal function and body fluid composition. *Arch. Intern. Med.*, 143:1163–1170.

11. Bauer, J. H., and Brooks, C. S. (1979): The long-term effect of propranolol therapy on renal function. *Am. J. Med.*, 66:405–410.

12. Bauer, J. H., Brooks, C. S., and Burch, R. N. (1982): Renal function and hemodynamic studies in low and normal renin essential hypertension. *Arch. Intern. Med.*, 142:1317–1323.

13. Bauer, J. H., and Gaddy, P. (1985): Effects of enalapril alone and in combination with hydrochlorothiazide, on renin-angiotensin-aldosterone, renal function, salt and water excretion and body fluid composition. *Am. J. Kidney Dis.*, 6:222–232.

14. Bauer, J. H., and Jones, L. B. (1984): Comparative studies: Enalapril versus hydrochlorothiazide as first-step therapy for the treatment of primary hypertension. *Am. J. Kidney Dis.*, 4:55–62.

15. Bauer, J. H., Jones, L. B., and Gaddy, P. (1984): Effects of prazosin therapy on blood pressure, renal function and body fluid composition. *Arch. Intern. Med.*, 144:1196–1200.

16. Bauer, J. II., and Reams, G. (1987): Short- and long-term effects of calcium entry blockers on the kidney. *Am. J. Cardiol.*, 59:66A–71A.

17. Bauer, J. H., and Reams, G. P. (1987): Beta-adrenergic antagonists and the kidney. In: *Pharmacotherapy of Renal Disease and Hypertension*, edited by W. M. Bennett and D. A. McCarron. *Contemporary Issues in Nephrology, Vol. 17*, pp. 223–254. Churchill Livingstone, New York.

18. Bauer, J. H., Reams, G. P., and Lal, S. M. (1987): Renal protective effect of strict blood pressure control with enalapril therapy. *Arch. Intern. Med.*, 147:1397–1400.

19. Bauer, J. H., Reams, G. P., and Lau, A. L.

(1987): A comparison of betaxolol and nadolol on renal function in essential hypertension. *Am. J. Kid. Dis.*, 10:109–112.

20. Baum, V. P. (1966): Experimentelle untersuchungen zur Nierenhamodynamik und zum Verhalten der elecktrolyte nach einmaliger Verabreichung von 2-(2,6-dichlorphenylamino)-2-imidazolin-hydrochlorid. *Arzneimittelforsch*, 16:1162–1165.

21. Bayliss, R. I. S., and Harvey-Smith, E. A. (1962): Methyldopa in the treatment of hypertension. *Lancet*, i:763–768.

22. Begg, E., Munn, S., and Bailey, R. R. (1979): Acebutolol in the treatment of patients with hypertension and renal functional impairment. *N. Z. Med. J.*, 89:293–295.

22a. Beretta-Piccoli, C., Ferrier, C., Weidmann, P. (1986): α_1-Adrenergic blockade and cardiovascular pressor responses in essential hypertension. *Hypertension* 8:407–414, 1986.

23. Bock, K. D., Heimsoth, V., Merguet, P., and Schoenermark, J. (1966): Klinische und klinishexperimentelle untersuchungen mit einer neuen blutdrucksenkinden substanz: Dichlorophenylamino-imidazolin. *Dutsch. Med. Wochenschr.*, 91:1761–1770.

24. Boner, G., Wainer, E., and Rosenfeld, J. B. (1982): Effects of pindolol on renal functions II: Effects of intravenous and prolonged oral dosing. *Clin. Pharmacol. Ther.*, 32:423–427.

25. Bosanac, P., Dubb, J., Walker, B., Goldberg, M., and Agus, Z. S. (1976): Renal effect of guanabenz: A new antihypertensive. *J. Clin. Pharmacol.*, 16:631–636.

26. Brater, D. C., Anderson, S., Kaplan, N. M., and Rain, C. V. S. (1984): Beta-adrenergic blockade alone does not decrease renal perfusion in black hypertensives. *J. Hypertens.*, 2:43–48.

27. Britton, K. E., Gruenewald, S. M., and Nimmon, C. C. (1981): Nadolol and renal hemodynamics. In: *International Experience with Nadolol a Long-acting β-blocking Agent*. Royal Society of Medicine International Congress and Symposium Series No. 37, pp. 77–85. Academic Press, Inc. (London) Ltd. and the Royal Society of Medicine, London.

28. Broadwall, E. K., Myhre, E., Stenback, O., and Hansen, T. (1972): The effect of methyldopa on renal function in patients with renal insufficiency. *Acta Med. Scand.*, 191:339–341.

29. Bruun, N. E., Ibsen, H., Nielsen, F., Nielsen, M. D., Moelbak, A. G., and Hartling, O. J. (1986): Lack of effect of nifedipine on counterregulatory mechanisms in essential hypertension. *Hypertension*, 8:655–661.

30. Brunner, H. R., Gavras, H., Waeber, B., Kershaw, G. R., Turini, G. A., Vukovich, R. A., McKinstry, R. A., and Gavras, I. (1979): Angiotensin converting enzyme inhibitor in long-term treatment of hypertensive patients. *Ann. Intern. Med.*, 90:19–23.

31. Bryan, P. K., Hoobler, S. W., Rosenzweig, J., Weller, J. M., and Purdy, J. M. (1977): Effect of minoxidil on blood pressure and hemodynam-

ics in severe hypertension. *Am. J. Cardiol.*, 39:796–801.

32. Byyny, R. L., Nies, A. S., LoVerde, M. E., and Mitchell, W. D. (1987): A double-blind, randomized, controlled trial comparing pinacidil to hydralazine in essential hypertension. *Clin. Pharmacol. Ther.*, 42:50–57.

33. Campese, V. M. (1981): Minoxidil: A review of its pharmacological properties and therapeutic use. *Drugs*, 22:257–278.

34. Campese, V. M., Romoff, M., Telfer, N., Weidmann, P., and Massry, S. G. (1981): Role of sympathetic nerve stimulation and body sodium-volume state in the antihypertensive action of clonidine in essential hypertension. *Kidney Int.*, 18:351–357.

35. Cangiano, J. L., and Bloomfield, D. K. (1969): Hemodynamic effects of a new antihypertensive agent, guanadrel sulfate. *Curr. Ther. Res.*, 11:736–744.

36. Case, D. B., Atlas, S. A., Mouradian, J. A., Frishman, R. A., Sherman, R. L., and Laragh, J. H. (1980): Proteinuria during long-term captopril therapy. *JAMA*, 244:346–349.

37. Chasis, H., and Redish, J. (1941): Effective renal blood flow in the separate kidneys of subjects with essential hypertension. *J. Clin. Invest.*, 20:655–661.

38. Cohen, I. M., O'Connor, D. T., Preston, R. A., and Stone, R. A. (1979): Reduced renovascular resistance by clonidine. *Clin. Pharmacol. Ther.*, 26:572–577.

39. Corcoran, A. C., Taylor, R. D., and Page, I. H. (1948): Functional patterns in renal disease. *Ann. Intern. Med.*, 28:560–582.

40. Danesh, B. J. Z., and Brunton, J. (1981): Nadolol and renal hemodynamics. In: *International Experience with Nadolol a Long-acting β-Blocking Agent*. Royal Society of Medicine International Congress and Symposium Series No. 37, pp. 87–95. Academic Press, Inc. (London) Ltd. and the Royal Society of Medicine, London.

41. Danesh, B. J. Z., Brunton, J., and Sumner, D. J. (1984): Comparison between short-term renal hemodynamic effects of propranolol and nadolol in essential hypertension: A crossover study. *Clin. Sci.*, 67:243–248.

42. Dauer, A. D. (1986): Terazosin: An effective once-daily monotherapy for the treatment of hypertension. *Am. J. Med.*, 80(Suppl 5B):29–34.

43. Deger, G. (1986): Comparison of the safety and efficacy of once-daily terazosin versus twice-daily prazosin for the treatment of mild to moderate hypertension. *Am. J. Med.*, 80(Suppl 5B):62–67.

44. Dollery, C. T., Emslie-Smith, D., and Milne, M. D. (1960): Clinical and pharmacological studies with guanethidine in the treatment of hypertension. *Lancet*, ii:381–387.

45. Dollery, C. T., and Harington, M. (1962): Methyldopa in hypertension: Clinical and pharmacological studies. *Lancet*, i:760–763.

46. Dreslinski, G. R., Aristimuno, G. G., Messerli, F. H., Suarez, D. H., and Frohlich, E. D. (1979):

Effects of beta blockade with acebutolol on hypertension, hemodynamics and fluid volume. *Clin. Pharmacol. Ther.*, 26:562–565.

47. Dreskinski, G. R., Messerli, F. H., Dunn, F. G., Svarey, D. H., Reisin, E., and Frohlich, E. D. (1982): Hemodynamics, biochemical and reflexive changes produced by atenolol. *Circulation*, 65:1365–1368.

48. Dryer, J. I. M., Kloppenberg, P. W. C., Festen, J., van't Laar, A., and Benraad, T. J. (1975): Intra-patient comparison of treatment with chlorthalidone, spironolactone and propranolol in normoreninemic essential hypertension. *Am. J. Cardiol.*, 36:716–721.

49. Duchin, K. L., and Willard, D. A. (1984): The effect of captopril on renal hemodynamics in hypertensive patients. *J. Clin. Pharmacol.*, 24:351–359.

50. Dunn, F. G., Oigman, W., Ventura, H. O., Messerli, F. H., Kobrin, I., and Frohlich, E. D. (1984): Enalapril improves systemic and renal hemodynamics and allows regression of left ventricular mass in essential hypertension. *Am. J. Cardiol.*, 53:105–108.

51. Dupont, A. G., Vanderniepen, P., Bossuyt, A. M., Jonckheer, M. H., and Six, R. O. (1985): Nadolol in essential hypertension: Effect on ambulatory blood pressure, reanl hemodynamics and cardiac function. *Br. J. Clin. Pharmacol.* 20:93–99.

52. Dux, S., Grosskopf, I., Boner, G., and Rosenfeld, J. B. (1986): Labetalol in the treatment of essential hypertension: a single blind dose ranging study. *J. Clin. Pharmacol.*, 26:346–350.

53. Dworkin, L. D., and Feiner, H. D. (1986): Glomerular injury in uninephrectomized spontaneously hypertensive rats: A consequence of glomerular capillary hypertension. *J. Clin. Invest.*, 77:797–809.

54. Epstein, M., and Oster, J. F. (1985): Beta blockers and renal function: A reappraisal. *J. Clin. Hypertens.*, 1:85–99.

55. Epstein, M., Oster, J. R., and Hollenberg, N. K. (1985): β-blockers and the kidney: Implications for renal functions and renin release. *Physiologist*, 28:53–63.

56. Falch, D. K., Odegaard, A. E., and Norman, N. (1978): Renal plasma flow and cardiac output during hydralazine and propranolol treatment in essential hypertension. *Scand. J. Clin. Invest.*, 38:143–146.

57. Falch, D. K., Odegaard, A. E., and Norman, N. (1979): Decreased renal plasma flow during propranolol treatment in esssential hypertension. *Acta Med. Scand.*, 205:91–95.

58. Falch, D. K., Paulsen, A. Q., Odegaard, A. E., and Norman, N. (1979): Central and renal circulation, electrolytes, body weight, plasma aldosterone and renin during atenolol treatment in essential hypertension. *Curr. Ther. Res.*, 26:813–820.

59. Ferrier, C., Beretta-Piccoli, C., Weidmann, P., and Mordasini, R. (1986): Alpha₁-adrenergic blockade and lipoprotein metabolism in essential hypertension. *Clin. Pharmacol. Ther.*, 40:525–530.

60. Fillingim, J. M., Blackshear, J. L., Strauss, A., and Strauss, M. (1986): Guanfacine as monotherapy for systemic hypertension. *Am. J. Cardiol.*, 57:50E–54E.

61. Foa, P. P., Woods, W. W., Peet, M. M., and Foa, N. (1941): Effective renal blood flow, glomerular filtration rate and tubular excretory mass in arterial hypertension. *Arch. Intern. Med.*, 69:822–835.

62. Foley, J., Penner, B., and Fung, H. (1981): Short-term renal hemodynamic effects of nadolol and metoprolol in normotensive and hypertensive subjects. *Clin. Pharmacol. Ther.*, 29:245. (abstr.)

63. Frohlich, E. D., Cooper, R. A., and Lewis, E. J. (1984): Review of the overall experience of captopril in hypertension. *Arch. Intern. Med.*, 144:1441–1444.

64. Frohlich, E. D., Messerli, F. H., Deslinski, G. R., and Kobrin, I. (1984): Long-term renal hemodynamic effects of nadolol in patients with essential hypertension. *Am. Heart J.* 108:1141–1143.

65. Funyu, T., Nigawara, K., Ohno, K., Hamada, W., and Yagihashi, Y. (1974): Effects of benzothiazepine derivative (CRD-401) on blood pressure, excretion of electrolytes and plasma renin activity. *Jpn. J. Nephr.*, 16:529–536.

66. Gafter, U., Holtzman, E., Rosenthal, T., Stern, N., Zevin, D., and Levi, J. (1983): Effect of pindolol on renal function in hypertensive patients. *Isr. J. Med. Sci.*, 19:563–565.

67. Gavras, H., Brunner, H. R., Turini, G. A., Kershaw, G. R., Tifft, C. P., Cuttelad, S., Gavras, I., Vukovich, R. A., and McKinstry, D. N. (1978): Antihypertensive effect of the oral angiotensin converting enzyme inhibitor SQ 14225 in man. *N. Eng. J. Med.*, 298:991–995.

68. Gehr, M., MacCarthy, E. P., and Goldberg, M. (1986): Guanabenz: A centrally acting natriuretic antihypertensive drug. *Kidney Internat.*, 29:1203–1208.

69. Gilmore, E., Weil, J., and Chidsey, C. (1970): Treatment of essential hypertension with a new vasodilator in combination with beta-adrenergic blockade. *N. Eng. J. Med.*, 282:521–527.

70. Giorgi, D. M. A., Giorgi, M. C. P., de Almcida Burdmann, E., Silva, H. B., and Marcondes, M. (1986): Effects of MK-521 (Lisinopril) on the renal plasma flow and renin-angiotensin-aldosterone system in patients with essential hypertension. *J. Hypertens.*, 4(Suppl 5):S420–S422.

71. Goldberg, M., and Gehr, M. (1985): Effects of alpha-2 agonists on renal function in hypertensive humans. *J. Cardiovas. Pharmacol.*, 7(Suppl 8):S34–S37.

72. Goldring, W., Chasis, H., Ranges, H. A., and Smith, H. W. (1941): Effective renal blood flow in subjects with essential hypertension. *J. Clin. Invest.*, 20:637–653.

73. Gomez, D. M. (1951): Evaluation of renal resistance, with special reference to changes in es-

senntial hypertension. *J. Clin. Invest.*, 30:1143–1155.

74. Gottleib, T. B., Katz, F. H., and Chidsey, C. A. (1972): Combined therapy with vasodilator drugs and beta-adrenergic blockade in hypertension. *Circulation*, 45:571–582.

75. Grabie, M., Nussbaum, P., Goldfarb, S., Walker, B. R., Goldberg, M., and Agus, Z. S. (1980): Effects of methyldopa on renal hemodynamics and tubular function. *Clin. Pharmacol. Ther.*, 27:522–527.

76. Greminger, P., Foerster, E., Vetter, H., Baumgart, P., and Vetter, W. (1986): Minoxidil and captopril in severe hypertension. *Klin. Wochenschr.*, 64:327–332.

77. Grim, C. E., Luft, F. C., Grim, C. M., Klotman, P. E., Van Huysse, J. W., Weinberger, M. H. (1979): Rapid blood pressure control with minoxidil. *Arch. Intern. Med.*, 139:529–533.

78. Healy, D. P., Munzel, P. A., and Insel, P. A. (1985): Localization of B_1 and B_2-adrenergic receptors in rat kidney by autoradiography. *Circ. Res.*, 57:278–284.

79. Hodsman, G. P., Zabludowski, J. R., Zoccali, C., Fraser, R., Morton, J. J., Murray, G. D., and Robertson, J. I. S. (1984): Enalapril (MK421) and its lysine analogue (MK521): A comparison of acute and chronic effects on blood pressure, renin-angiotensin system and sodium excretion in normal man. *Br. J. Clin. Pharmac.*, 17:233–241.

80. Holland, O. B., Fairchild, C., and Gomez-Sanchez, C. E. (1981): Effect of guanabenz and hydrochlorothiazide on blood pressure and plasma renin activity. *J. Clin. Pharmacol.*, 21:133–139.

81. Hollenberg, N. K. (1982): Introduction: B-adrenergic blocking agents—the treatment of hypertension and the kidney. In: *The Hemodynamics of Nadolol*, edited by N. K. Hollenberg. Second International Symposium. Royal Society of Medicine International Congress and Symposium Series No. 51, pp. 1–8. Academic Press, Inc. (London) Ltd. and the Royal Society of Medicine, London.

82. Hollenberg, N. K., Adams, D. F., McKinstry, D. N., Williams, G. H., Borucki, L. J., and Sullivan, J. M. (1979): B-adrenoceptor-blocking agents and the kidney: Effect of nadalol and propranolol on the renal circulation. *Br. J. Clin. Pharmac.* 7(Suppl 2):219s–225s.

83. Hollenberg, N. K., Adams, D. F., Solomon, H., Chenity, W. R., Burger, B. M., Abrams, H. L., and Merrill, J. P. (1975): Renal vascular tone in essential and secondary hypertension. *Medicine*, 54:29–44.

84. Hollenberg, N. K. Borucki, L. J., and Adams, D. F. (1978): The renal vasculature in early essential hypertension: Evidence for a pathogenetic role. *Medicine*, 57:167–178.

85. Hollenberg, N. K., Epstein, M., Basch, R. I., and Merrill, J. P. (1969): "No Man's Land" of the renal vasculature. *Am. J. Med.*, 47:845–854.

86. Hollenberg, N. K., Megas, L. G., Williams, G. H., Katz, J., Garnic, J. D., and Harrington, D.

P. (1981): Sodium intake and renal responses to captopril in normal man and in essential hypertension. *Kidney Int.*, 20:240–245.

87. Hoorntje, S. J., Donker, A. J. M., Prins, E. J. L., and Weening, J. J. (1980): Membranous glomerulopathy in a patient on captopril. *Acta Med. Scand.*, 208:325–329.

88. Horwitz, D., Pettinger, W. A., Orvis, H., Thomas, R. E., and Sjoersdma, A. (1967): Effects of methyldopa in fifty hypertensive patients. *Clin. Pharmacol. Ther.*, 8:224–234.

89. Hunyor, S. N., Bauer, G. E., Ross, M., and Larkin, H. (1980): Labetalol and propranolol in mild hypertensives: Comparison of blood pressure and plasma volume effects. *Aust. N. Z. J. Med.*, 10:162–166.

90. Ibsen, H., Rasmussen, K., Aerenlund Jensen, H., and Leth, A. (1978): Changes in plasma volume and extracellular fluid volume after addition of prazosin to propranolol treatment in patients with hypertension. *Scand. J. Clin. Lab. Invest.*, 38:425–429.

91. Ibsen, H., and Sederberg-Olsen, P. (1973): Changes in glomerular filtration rate during long-term treatment with propranolol in patients with arterial hypertension. *Clin. Sci.*, 44:129–134.

92. Jain, A. K., Hiremath, A., Michael, R., Ryan, J. R., and McMahon, F. G. (1985): Clonidine and guanfacine in hypertension. *Clin. Pharmacol. Ther.*, 37:271–276.

93. Judson, W. E., Hollander, W., and Wilkins, R. W. (1956): The effect on intravenous apresoline on cardiovascular and renal function in patients with and without congestive heart failure. *Circulation*, 13:664–674.

94. Keusch, G., Weidmann, P., Ziegler, W. H., de Chatel, R., and Reubi, F. C. (1980): Effects of chronic alpha and beta adrenoceptor blockade with labetolol on plasma catecholamines and renal function in hypertension. *Klin. Wochenschr.*, 58:25–29.

95. Kiowski, W., Van Brummelen, P., Hulthen, L., Amann, F. W., Buhler, F. R. (1981): Antihypertensive and renal effects of captopril in relation to renin activity and bradykinin-induced vasodilation. *Clin. Pharmacol. Ther.*, 31:677–684.

96. Klutsch, V. K., Schmidt, P., Grosswendt, J. (1972): Der einfluss von BAY a 1040 auf die Nierenfunktion des hypertonikers. *Arzneim Forsch.*, 22:377–380.

97. Koch-Weser, J. (1974): Vasodilator drugs in the treatment of hypertension. *Arch. Intern. Med.*, 133:1017–1027.

98. Koshy, M. C., Mickley, D., Bourgoignie, J., and Blaufox, M. D. (1977): Physiological evaluation of a new antihypertensive agent: Prazosin HCl. *Circulation*, 55:533–537.

99. Krogsgaard, A. R. (1957): The effect of reserpine on the electrolyte and fluid balance in man. *Acta Med. Scand.*, 159:127–132.

100. Krusell, L. R., Christensen, C. K., and Pedersen, O. L. (1987): Acute natriuretic effect of nifedipine in hypertensive patients and normoten-

sive controls: A proximal tubular effect? *Eur. J. Clin. Pharmacol.*, 32:121–126.

101. Kubo, S. H., Cody, R. J., Covit, A. B., Feldschuh, J., and Laragh, J. H. (1986): The effects of verapamil on renal blood flow, renal function and neurohormonal profiles in patients with moderate to severe hypertension. *J. Clin. Hypertens.*, 3:38s–46s.

102. Lameyer, L. D. F., and Hesse, C. J. (1981): Metoprolol in high renin hypertension. *Ann. Clin. Res.*, 13(Suppl 30):16–22.

103. Larsen, J. S., and Pedersen, E. B. (1980): Comparison of the effects of propranolol and labetalol on renal hemodynamics at rest and during exercise in essential hypertension. *Eur. J. Clin. Pharmacol.*, 18:135–139.

104. Ledingham, J. G. G. (1981): Implications of antihypertensive therapy on sodium balance and sodium and water retention. *Br. J. Clin. Pharmac.*, 12:15s–21s.

105. de Leeuw, P. W., and Birkenhager, W. A. (1982): Renal response to propranolol treatment in hypertensive humans. *Hypertension*, 4:125–131.

106. Leonetti, G., Cuspidi, C., Sampieri, L., Terzoli, L., and Zanchetti, A. (1982): Comparison of cardiovascular, renal, and humoral effects of acute administration of two calcium channel blockers in normotensive and hypertensive subjects. *J. Cardiovas. Pharmacol.*, 4(Suppl 3):S319–S324.

107. Leonetti, G., Sala, C., Bianchini, C., Terzoli, L., and Zanchetti, A. (1980): Antihypertensive and renal effects of orally administered verapamil. *Eur. J. Clin. Pharmacol.*, 18:375–382.

108. Lewis, E. J., (1982): Proteinuria and abnormalities of the renal glomerulus in patients with hypertension. *Clin. Exp. Pharmacol. and Physiol.*, (Suppl 7):105–115.

109. Lindeman, R. D., Tobin, J. D., and Shock, N. W. (1984): Association between blood pressure and the rate of decline in renal function with age. *Kidney Internat.*, 26:861–868.

110. Ljungman, S., Aurell, M., Hartford, M., Wikstrand, J., Wilhelmsen, L., Berglund, G. (1980): Blood pressure and renal function. *Acta Med. Scand.*, 208:17–25.

111. McNabb, W. R., Noomohamed, F. H., Brooks, B. A., Till, A. E., and Lant, A. F. (1985): Effects of repeated doses of enalapril on renal function in man. *Br. J. Clin. Pharmacol.*, 19:353–361.

112. McNair, A., Rasmussen, S., Nielsen, P. E., Rasmussen, K. (1980): The antihypertensive effect of prazosin on mild to moderate hypertension, changes in plasma volume, extracellular volume and glomerular filtration rate. *Acta Med. Scand.*, 207:413–416.

113. Madeddu, P., Ena, P., Dessi-Fulgheri, P., Glorioso, N., Cerimele, D., and Rappelli, A. (1986): Captopril-induced proteinuria in hypertensive psoriatic patients. *Nephron*, 44:358–360.

114. Malini, P. L., Strocchi, E., and Ambrosioni, E. (1984): Comparison of the effects of prizidilol and propranolol on renal hemodynamics at rest and during exercise. *Br. J. Clin. Pharmac.*, 17:251–255.

115. Malini, P. L., Strocchi, E., Negroni, S., Ambrosioni, E., and Magnani, B. (1982): Renal hemodynamics after chronic treatment with labetalol and propranolol. *Br. J. Clin. Pharmac.*, 13:S123–S126.

116. Marone, C., Luisoli, S., Bomio, F., Beretta-Piccoli, C., Bianchetti, M. G., and Weidmann, P. (1985): Body sodium-blood volume state, aldosterone and cardiovascular responsiveness after calcium entry blockade with nifedipine. *Kidney Internat.*, 28:658–665.

117. Matsunaga, M., Hara, A., Ogino, K., Motohara, S., Saito, M., Yamamoto, J., and Pak, C. H. (1977): The effects of beta-adrenergic blocking agents on the blood pressure, plasma renin activity and hemodynamics of hypertensive patients. *Jpn. Heart J.*, 18:24–30.

118. Melick, R., and McGregor, M. (1957): Reserpine and extracellular-fluid volume. *N Eng. J. Med.*, 256:1000–1002.

119. Meyer, T. W., Anderson, S., Rennke, H. G., and Brenner, B. M. (1987): Reversing glomerular hypertension stabilizes established glomerular injury. *Kidney Internat.*, 31:752–759.

120. Mimran, A., Brunner, H. R., Turini, G. A., Waeber, B., and Brunner, D. (1979): Effect of captopril on renal vascular tone in patients with essential hypertension. *Clin. Sci.*, 57:421S–423S.

121. Mohammed, S., Hanenson, I. B., Magenheim, H. G., and Gaffney, T. E. (1968): The effects of alpha-methyldopa on renal function in hypertensive patients. *Am. Heart J.*, 76:21–27.

122. Morduchowicz, G., Boner, G., Ben-Bassat, M., and Rosenfeld, J. B. (1986): Proteinuria in benign nephrosclerosis. *Arch. Intern. Med.*, 146:1513–1516.

123. Morgan, T. (1983): The use of centrally acting antihypertensive drugs in patients with renal disease. *Chest*, 83(Suppl):383–386.

124. Mori, K., Hiromoto, N., Shiraishi, J., Fukushige, M., and Nihira, H. (1973): Clinical experience with CRD-401, a benzthiazepine derivative, for hypertension associated with various renal diseases. *Acta Urol. Jpn.*, 19:175–179.

125. Mosley, C., O'Connor, D. T., Taylor, A., Slutsky, R. A., and Cervenka, J. (1984): Comparative effects of antihypertensive therapy with guanabenz and propranolol on renal vascular resistance and left ventricular mass. *J. Cardiovas. Pharmacol.*, 6:S757–S761.

126. Moyer, J. H., Heider, C., Pevey, K., and Ford, R. V. (1958): The effect of treatment on the vascular deterioration associated with hypertension, with particular emphasis on renal function. *Am. J. Med.*, 24:177–192.

127. Moyer, J. H., Hughes, W., and Huggins, R. (1954): The cardiovascular and renal hemodynamic response to the administration of reserpine. *Am. J. Med. Sci.*, 227:640–648.

128. Mroczek, W. J., Davidov, M., and Finnerty, F. A. (1972): Prolonged treatment with clonidine:

Comparative antihypertensive effects alone and with a diuretic agent. *Am. J. Cardiol.*, 30:536–541.

129. Navis, G., de Jong, P. E., Donker, A. J. M., van der Hem, G. K., and de Zeeuw, D. (1985): Effects of enalaprilic acid on sodium excretion and renal hemodynamics in essential hypertension. *J. Clin. Hypertens.*, 1:228–238.

130. Navis, G. J., de Jong, P. E., Donker, A. J. M., and de Zeeuw, D. (1983): Effects of enalapril on blood pressure and renal hemodynamics in essential hypertension. *Proc. Eur. Dial. Transplant Assoc.*, 20:577–581.

131. Novack, P. (1961): The effect of guanethidine on renal, cerebral, and cardiac hemodynamics. In: *Hypertension-Recent Advances*, edited by A. N. Brest and J. H. Moyer, pp. 444–448. Lea and Febiger, Philadelphia.

132. O'Callaghan, W. G., Laher, M. S., McGarry, K., O'Brien, E., and O'Malley, K. (1983): Antihypertensive and renal hemodynamic effects of atenolol and nadolol in elderly hypertensive patients. *Br. J. Clin. Pharmac.*, 6:417–421.

133. O'Connor, D. T., Barge, A. P., and Duchin, K. L. (1982): Preserved renal perfusion during treatment of essential hypertension with the beta blocker Nadolol. *J. Clin. Pharmacol.*, 22:187–195.

134. O'Connor, D. T., Preston, R. A. (1982): Urinary kallikrein activity, renal hemodynamics and electrolyte handling during chronic beta blockade with propranolol in hypertension. *Hypertension*, 4:742–749.

135. O'Connor, D. T., Preston, R. A., and Sasso, E. H. (1979): Renal perfusion changes during treatment of essential hypertension: Prazosin versus propranolol. *J. Cardiovas. Pharmacol.*, 1(Suppl 1):S38–S42.

136. Onesti, G., Schwartz, A. B., Kim, K. E., Swartz, C., and Brest, A. N. (1974): Pharmacodynamic effects of new antihypertensive drug, catapres (ST-155). *Circulation*, 39:671–676.

137. Pasternack, A., Porsti, P., and Poyhonen, L. (1982): Effect of pindolol and propranolol on renal function of patients with hypertension. *Br. J. Clin. Pharmac.*, 13:S241–S244.

138. Pedersen, E. B. (1977): Effect of sodium loading and exercise on renal hemodynamics and urinary sodium excretion in young patients with essential hypertension before and during propranolol treatment. *Acta Med. Scand.*, 201:365–373.

139. Pedersen, E. B., and Kornerup, H. J. (1976): Renal hemodynamics and plasma renin in patients with essential hypertension. *Clin. Sci. and Mol. Med.*, 50:409–414.

140. Perera, G. A. (1955): Edema and congestive failure related to administration of Rauwolfia serpentina. *J. Am. Med. Assoc.*, 159:439.

141. Pessina, A. C., Gatta, A., Semplicini, A., Rossi, G. P., Casiglia, E., Milani, L., Amodio, P., Merkel, C., Pagnan, A., and DalPalu, C. (1981): Hypotensive and renal effects of captopril. *Eur. J. Clin. Invest.*, 11:409–413.

142. Preston, R. A., O'Connor, D. J., Stone, R. A. (1979): Prazosin and renal hemodynamics: Arteriolar vasodilation during therapy of essential hypertension in man. *J. Cardiovas. Pharmacol.*, 1:277–286.

143. Rasmussen, S., Leth, A., Ibsen, H., Nielsen, M. D., Nielsen, F., and Giese, J. (1986): Converting enzyme inhibition in mild and moderate essential hypertension II. *Acta Med. Scand.*, 219:29–36.

144. Rasmussen, S., and Nielsen, P. E. (1981): Blood pressure, body fluid volumes and glomerular filtration rate during treatment with labetalol in essential hypertension. *Br. J. Clin. Pharmac.*, 12:349–353.

145. Rasmussen, S., and Rasmussen, K. (1979): Influence of metoprolol, alone and in combination with a thiazide diuretic, on blood pressure, plasma volume, extracellular volume and glomerular filtration rate in essential hypertension. *Europ. J. Clin. Pharmacol.*, 15:305–310.

146. Reams, G. P., and Bauer, J. H. (1986): Long-term effects of enalapril monotherapy and enalapril/hydrochlorothiazide combination therapy on blood pressure, renal function and body fluid composition. *J. Clin. Hypertens.*, 2:55–63.

147. Reams, G. P., and Bauer, J. H. (1988): Effect of lisinopril monotherapy on renal hemodynamics. *Am. J. Kidney Dis.*, 11:499–507.

148. Reams, G. P., Hamory, A., Lau, A., and Bauer, J. H. (1988): Effect of nifedipine on renal functions in patients with essential hypertension. *Hypertension*, 11:452–456.

149. Reams, G. P., Lau, A., Messina, C., Villarreal, D., and Bauer, J. H. (1987): Efficacy, electrocardiographic and renal effects of intravenous diltiazem for essential hypertension. *Am. J. Cardiol.*, 60:78I–84I.

150. Redgrave, J., Robinowe, S., Hollenberg, N. K., and Williams, G. H. (1985): Correction of abnormal renal blood flow response to angiotensin II by converting enzyme inhibition in essential hypertension. *J. Clin. Invest.*, 75:1285–1290.

151. Reubi, F. C., Vorburger, C., and Butikofer, E. (1974): A comparison of the short-term and long-term hemodynamic effects of antihypertensive drug therapy.In: *Catapres in Hypertension*, edited by M. E. Conolly, pp. 113–125. Butterworths, London.

152. Reusch, C. S. (1962): The cardiorenal hemodynamic effects of antihypertensive therapy with reserpine. *Am. Heart J.*, 64:643–649.

153. Richardson, D. W., and Wyso, E. M. (1960): Human pharmacology of guanethidine. *Ann. NY Acad. Sci.*, 88:944–955.

154. Roeckel, A., and Heidland, A. (1980): Acute and chronic renal effects of guanfacine in essential and renal hypertension. *Br. J. Clin. Pharmac.*, 10:141s–149s.

155. Romero, J. C., Raij, L., Granger, J. P. Ruilope, L. M., and Rodicio, J. L. (1987): Multiple effects of calcium entry blockers on renal function in hypertension. *Hypertension*, 10:140–151.

156. Ronnov-Jessen, V. (1963): Blood volume during

treatment of hypertension with guanethidine. *Acta Med. Scand.*, 174:307–310.

157. Safar, M. E., Weiss, Y. A., Corvol, P. L., Menard, J. E., London, G. M., and Millez, P. L. (1975): Antihypertensive adrenergic blocking agents: Effects on sodium balance, the renin-angiotensin system, and hemodynamics. *Clin. Sci. Mol. Med.*, 48:593–595.

158. Sakurai, T., Kurita, T., Nagano, S., and Sonoda, T. (1972): Antihypertensive vasodilating and sodium diuretic actions of D-cis-isomer of benzothiazepine derivative (CRD-401). *Acta Urol. Jap.*, 18:695–707.

159. Scharf, S. C., Lee, H. B., Wexler, J. P., Blaufox, M. D. (1984): Cardiovascular consequences of primary antihypertensive therapy with prazosin hydrochloride. *Am. J. Cardiol.*, 53:32A–36A.

160. Schmieder, R. E., Messerli, F. H., Garavaglia, G. E., and Nunez, B. D. (1987): Cardiovascular effects of verapamil in patients with essential hypertension. *Circulation*, 75:1030–1036.

161. Sederberg-Olsen, P., and Ibsen, H. (1972): Plasma volume and extracellular fluid volume during long-term treatment with propranolol in essential hypertension. *Clin. Sci.*, 43:165–170.

162. Shionoiri, H., Yasuda, G., Takagi, N., Oda, H., Young, S. C., Miyajima, E., Umemura, S., Gotoh, E., Sesoko, S., Uneda, S., and Kaneko, Y. (1987): Renal hemodynamics and comparative effects of captopril in patients with benign or malignant essential hypertension or chronic renal failure. *Clin. Exp. Theor. Prac.*, A9:543–549.

163. Shoback, D. M., Williams, G. H., Moore, T. J., Dluhy, R. G., Podolsky, S., and Hollenberg, N. K. (1983): Defect in the sodium-modulated tissue responsiveness to angiotensin II in essential hypertension. *J. Clin. Invest.*, 72:2115–2124.

164. Simon, G., Morioka, S., Snyder, D. K., and Cohn, J. N. (1983): Increased renal plasma flow in long-term enalapril treatment of hypertension. *Clin. Pharmacol. Ther.*, 34:459–465.

165. Smith, A. J. (1965): Clinical features of fluid retention complicating treatment with guanethidine. *Circulation*, 31:485–489.

166. Smith, A. J. (1965): Fluid retention produced by guanethidine. *Circulation*, 31:490–496.

167. Smith, W. M., Bachman, B., Galante, J. G., Nanowell, E. G., Johnson, W. P., Koch, C. E. Jr., Korfmacher, S. D., Thurm, R. H., and Bromer, L. (1966): Co-operative clinical trial of alpha-methyldopa. *Ann. Intern. Med.*, 65:657–671.

168. Sonnerstedt, R., Bojs, G., Varnauskas, E., and Werko, L. (1963): Alpha-methyldopa in arterial hypertension: Clinical, renal and hemodynamic studies. *Acta Med. Scand.*, 174:53–67.

169. Sorensen, S. S., Thomsen, O. O., Danielsen, H., and Pedersen, E. B. (1985): Effect of verapamil on renal plasma flow, glomerular filtration rate and plasma angiotensin II, aldosterone and arginine vasopressin in essential hypertension. *Eur. J. Clin. Pharmacol.*, 29:257–261.

170. Strandgaard, S., Ehmgreen, J., Christensen, T. E., Laursen, S. W. (1982): Effect of short-term and long-term treatment with metoprolol on renal blood flow and glomerular filtration rate in hypertensive patients with a normal kidney function. *Dan. Med. Bull.*, 29:287–289.

171. Sturgill, B. C., and Shearlock, K. T. (1983): Membranous glomerulopathy and nephrotic syndrome after captopril theray. *JAMA*, 250:2343–2345.

172. Sugino, G., Barg, A. P., and O'Connor, D. T. (1984): Renal perfusion is preserved during cardioselective B-blockade with metoprolol in hypertension. *Am. J. Kidney Dis.*, 3:357–361.

173. Sullivan, J. M., Ginsburg, B. A., and Ratts, T. E. (1979): Hemodynamic and antihypertensive effects of captopril, an orally active angiotensin converting enzyme inhibitor. *Hypertension*, 1:397–401.

174. Sunderrajan, S., Reams, G., and Bauer, J. H. (1986): Renal effects of diltiazem in primary hypertension. *Hypertension*, 8:238–242.

175. Sunderrajan, S., Reams, G., and Bauer, J. H. (1987): Long-term renal effects of diltiazem in essential hypertension. *Am. Heart J.*, 114:383–388.

176. Sunderrajan, S., Luger, A., and Bauer, J. H. (1983): Captopril-induced membranous glomerulopathy. *South. Med. J.*, 76:1294–1297.

177. Tarazi, R. C., Bravo, E. L., Fuoad, F. M., Omvik, P., and Cody, R. J. (1980): Hemodynamic and volume changes associated with captopril. *Hypertension*, 2:576–585.

178. Textor, S. C., Fouad, F. M., Bravo, E. L., Tarazi, R. C., Vidt, D. G., and Gifford, R. W. (1982): Redistribution of cardiac output to the kidneys during oral nadolol administration. *N. Eng. J. Med.*, 307:601–605.

179. Textor, S. C., Gephardt, G. N., Bravo, E. L., Tarazi, R. C., Fouad, F. M., Tubbs, R., and McMahon, J. T. (1983): Membranous glomerulopathy associated with captopril therapy. *Am. J. Med.*, 74:705–712.

180. Thananopavarn, C., Golub, M. S., Eggena, P., Barrett, J. D., and Sambhi, M. P. (1982): Clonidine, a centrally acting sympathetic inhibitor, as monotherapy for mild to moderate hypertension. *Am. J. Cardiol.*, 49:153–158.

181. Thomsen, O. O., Danielsen, H., Sorensen, S. S., and Pedersen, E. B. (1986): Effect of captopril on renal hemodynamics and the renin-angiotensin-aldosterone and osmoregulatory systems in essential hypertension. *Eur. J. Clin. Pharmacol.*, 30:1–6.

182. Tojo, S., Shishido, H., and Yamamoto, S. (1972): Effects of CRD-401 on blood pressure and renal function. *Jpn. J. Clin. Exp. Med.*, 49:1958–1966.

183. Tsuchiya, N., Watanabe, K., Ajiro, H., and Tojo, S. (1975): Action of diltiazem hydrochloride (CRD-401) on diseased kidney. *Jpn. J. Clin. Exp. Med.*, 52:611–621.

184. Tsunoda, K., Abe, K., Omata, K., Kudo, K., Sato, M., Kohzuki, M., Tanno, M., Seino, M., Yasujima, M., and Yoshinaga, K. (1986): Hy-

potensive and natriuretic effects of nifedipine in essential hypertension. *J. Clin. Hypertens.*, 3:263–270.

185. Valvo, E., Gammaro, L., Tessitore, N., Fabris, A., Ortalda, V., Bedogna, V., and Maschio, G. (1984): Effects of timolol on blood pressure, systemic hemodynamics, plasma renin activity and glomerular filtration rate in patients with essential hypertension. *Int. J. Clin. Pharmacol. Ther. and Toxicol.*, 22:156–161.

186. Valvo, E., Previato, G., Tessitore, N., Oldrizzi, L., Gammaro, L., Corgnati, A., and Maschio, G. (1981): Effects of the long-term administration of labetalol on blood pressure, hemodynamics and renal function in essential and renal hypertension. *Curr. Ther. Res.*, 29:634–643.

187. Van den Meiracker, A. H., Man in 't Veld, A. J., Ritsema van Eck, H. J., Schalekamp, M. A. D. H. (1986): Systemic and renal vasodilation after beta adrenoceptor blockade with pindolol: A hemodynamic study on the onset and maintenance of its antihypertensive effect. *Am. Heart J.*, 112:368–374.

188. Vanderkolk, K., Dontas, A. S., and Hoobler, S. W. (1954): Renal and hypotensive effects of acute and chronic oral treatment with 1-hydrazinophthalazine in hypertension. *Am. Heart J.*, 48:95–101.

189. Van Schaik, B. A. M., Geyskes, G. G., and Boer, P. (1987): Lisinopril in hypertensive patients with and without renal failure. *Eur. J. Clin. Pharmacol.*, 32:11–16.

190. Ventura, H. O., Frohlich, E. D., Messerli, F. H., Kobrin, I., and Kardon, M. B. (1985): Cardiovascular effects and regional blood flow distribution associated with angiotensin converting enzyme inhibitor (captopril) in essential hypertension. *Am. J. Cardiol.*, 55:1023–1026.

191. Villarreal, H., Exaire, J. E., Rubio, V., and Davila, H. (1964): Effect of guanethidine and bretylium tosylate on systemic and renal hemodynamics in essential hypertension. *Am. J. Cardiol.*, 14:633–640.

192. Waal-Manning, H. J., and Bolli, P. (1980): Atenolol versus placebo in mild hypertension: Renal, metabolic and stress antipressor effects. *Br. J. Clin. Pharmacol.*, 9:533–560.

193. Wainer, E., Boner, G., and Rosenfeld, J. B. (1980): Effects of pindolol on renal function. *Clin. Pharmacol. Ther.*, 28:575–580.

194. Walker, B. R., Deitch, M. W., Schneider, B. E., and Hare, L. E. (1967): Comparative antihypertensive effects of guanabenz and methyldopa. *Clin. Ther.*, 4:275–284.

195. Walker, B. R., Deitch, M. W., Schneider, B. E., Hare, L. E., and Gold, G. A. (1981): Long-term therapy of hypertension with guanabenz. *Clin. Ther.*, 4:217–228.

196. Walker, B. R., Hare, L. E., and Deitch, M. W. (1982): Comparative antihypertensive effects of guanabenz and clonidine. *J. Int. Med. Res.*, 10:6–14.

197. Wallin, J. D. (1985): Adrenoceptors and renal functions. *J. Clin. Hypertens.*, 1:171–178.

198. Warren, S. E., O'Connor, D. T., Cohen, I. M., and Mitas, J. A. (1981): Renal hemodynamic changes during long-term antihypertensive therapy. *Clin. Pharmacol. Ther.*, 29:310–317.

199. Weidmann, P., DeChatel, R., Ziegler, W. H., Flammer, J., and Reubi, F. (1978): Alpha and beta adrenergic blockade with orally administered labetalol in hypertension. *Am. J. Cardiol.*, 41:570–576.

200. Weil, M. H., Barbour, B. H., and Chesne, R. B. (1963): Alpha-methyldopa for the treatment of hypertension. *Circulation*, 28:165–174.

201. Weil, J. V., and Chidsey, C. A. (1968): Plasma volume expansion resulting from interference with adrenergic function in normal man. *Circulation*, 37:54–61.

202. Wilcox, C. S., Lewis, P. S., Peart, W. S., Sever, P. S., Osikowska, B. A., Suddle, S. A. J., Bluhm, M. M., Veall, N., and Lancaster, R. (1981): Renal function, body fluid volumes, renin, aldosterone and noradrenaline during treatment of hypertension with pindolol. *J. Cardiovas. Pharmacol.*, 3:598–611.

203. Wilkinson, R., Stevens, I. M., Pickering, M., and Robson, V. (1980): A study of the effects of atenolol and propranolol on renal function in patients with essential hypertension. *Br. J. Clin. Pharmac.*, 10:51–59.

204. Williams, G. H., Tuck, M. L., Sullivan, J. M., Dluhy, R. G., and Hollenberg, N. K. (1982): Parallel adrenal and renal abnormalities in young patients with essential hypertension. *Am. J. Med.*, 72:907–914.

205. Yamada, T., Ishihara, M., Ichikawa, K., and Hiramatsu, K. (1980): Proteinuria and renal function during antihypertensive treatment for essential hypertension. *J. Am. Geriat. Soc.*, 28:114–117.

206. Yeh, B. K., Nantel, A., and Goldberg, L. I. (1977): Antihypertensive effect of clonidine. *Arch. Intern. Med.*, 127:233–237.

207. Yokoyama, S., and Kaburagi, T. (1983): Clinical effects on intravenous nifedipine on renal function. *J. Cardiovas. Pharmacol.*, 5:67–71.

208. Zanchetti, A., and Leonetti, G. (1985): Natriuretic effect of calcium antagonists. *J. Cardiovas. Pharmacol.*, 7(Suppl 4):S33–S37.

209. Zanchetti, A., Stella, A., and Golin, R. (1985): Adrenergic sodium handling and the natriuretic action of calcium antagonists. *J. Cardiovas. Pharmacol.*, 7(Suppl 6):S194–S198.

210. Zech, P., Pozet, N., Sassard, J., and Vincent, M. (1980): Le labetalol, bloqueur des recepteurs alpha et beta-adrenergiques. *Nouv. Presse. Med.*, 9:1087–1090.

211. Zins, G. R. (1974): Alterations in renal function during vasodilator therapy. In: *Recent Advances in Renal Physiology and Pharmacology*, edited by L. G. Wesson and G. M. Fanelli, pp. 165–186. University Park Press, Baltimore.

New Therapeutic Strategies in Hypertension,
edited by Norman M. Kaplan,
Barry M. Brenner, and John H. Laragh.
Raven Press, Ltd., New York © 1989.

Hypertension with Diabetes

Sharon Anderson and Barry M. Brenner

Renal Division and Department of Medicine, Brigham and Women's Hospital, and The Harvard Center for The Study of Kidney Diseases, Harvard Medical School, Boston, Massachusetts 02115

Systemic hypertension is a serious adverse consequence of diabetes mellitus, contributing appreciably to cardiovascular morbidity and mortality (65,66) by acceleration of diabetic micro- and macrovascular complications. Both hypertension and the diabetic state contribute to vascular injury. Elevated arterial pressure enhances shear stress on endothelial cells, as well as increased transcapillary pressure gradients. Nonenzymatic protein glycosylation, induced by hyperglycemia, contributes as well (17), as glycosylation of hemoglobin impairs oxygen delivery to vascular tissues, while glycosylation of low-density lipoprotein enhances atherogenicity. Glycosylation of collagen stimulates binding of low-density lipoprotein, and nonenzymatic glycosylation of capillary basement membranes may contribute to thickening and increased permeability (17). Thus, hypertension and metabolic abnormalities together render the hypertensive diabetic patient at high risk for vascular complications.

That systemic hypertension is a complication of the diabetic state, rather than a late consequence of diabetic glomerulopathy, has been established by observations that hypertension precedes both proteinuria and renal insufficiency (40,99). Type I diabetics exhibit statistical elevations in blood pressure, albeit still within the normal range, when the urinary albumin excretion rate (AER) is still within normal limits (40,93). During the stage of incipient nephropathy, when microalbuminuria is present, but prior to the development of persistent proteinuria, blood pressures are clearly higher than those in normal subjects (40,53,85,93,135). The incidence of hypertension prior to development of renal disease is even higher in Type II diabetes (108). A multicenter study in the United Kingdom found the prevalence of hypertension to be as high as 40% in males and 53% in females with newly-diagnosed Type II diabetes (121). Once overt diabetic glomerulopathy is present, with urinary protein excretion greater than 500 mg/day and impaired renal function, systemic hypertension is found in the majority of diabetic patients (53,106,108,127), and severity of hypertension correlates inversely with level of renal function (108).

The prevalence of hypertension in Type I and Type II diabetic patients, as found in a representative study by Hasslacher and colleagues (54), is depicted in Fig. 1. Prevalence of hypertension (defined as blood pressure >160/95 mmHg) increases with diabetes duration in both Type I (Fig. 1A) and Type II (Fig. 1B) diabetics, and accelerates when proteinuria is present (54,108). Of note, surprisingly few studies have directly addressed the relationship between blood pressure and degree of metabolic control (43). While blood pressures may tend to be higher during periods of poor control (50), glycemic control and levels of blood pressure generally do not correlate well (65).

289

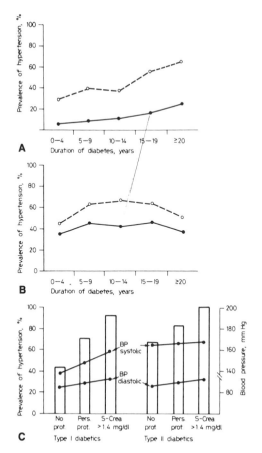

FIG. 1. Prevalence of hypertension in (**A**) Type I (n = 82) and (**B**) Type II (n = 168) diabetics with (○) and without (●) proteinuria. (**C**) Longitudinal measurements of blood pressure and hypertension in 52 Type I and 63 Type II diabetic patients who developed proteinuria. (From Ritz et al., ref. 108, with permission.)

PATHOGENESIS OF HYPERTENSION IN DIABETES

Multiple hormonal and vascular abnormalities play a role in the pathogenesis of hypertension in diabetes (33,59,108). Expansion of plasma volume, stimulated by hyperglycemia and enhanced proximal tubule sodium reabsorption brought about by both glycosuria (70) and insulin action (31), may contribute to volume-dependent hypertension in the early stages of diabetes. Exchangeable body sodium is increased

prior to the development of hypertension (129). Once hypertension is present, blood pressure is positively correlated to exchangeable sodium (41,42). Later in the course, declining renal function stimulates further plasma volume expansion, and the volume-dependent form of hypertension common to all forms of end-stage renal disease.

In general, the renin-angiotensin-aldosterone system is depressed in diabetes (8,24,41), but vascular reactivity to angiotensin II may be increased (129). Moreover, diabetic patients exhibit elevated levels of plasma-angiotensin I converting enzyme (76), which may contribute to increases in angiotensin II even when plasma-renin concentration is not markedly elevated. Increasing circulating angiotensin II levels have been correlated with hypertension (13), and elevations of both circulating angiotensin II levels (13) and plasma-inactive-renin levels (79) may be markers of risk for microvascular complications. Similarly, while plasma-catecholamine levels are usually normal or suppressed (41,129), vascular reactivity to catecholamines is enhanced (130). Taken together, these findings suggest that sodium retention and abnormalities in vascular reactivity act in concert to predispose diabetic patients to systemic hypertension (129).

Exogenous insulin therapy may also play a role in the hypertension of diabetes. Insulin directly stimulates sodium reabsorption in the distal nephron (31), an effect which may result in extracellular fluid volume expansion, increased cardiac output, enhanced pressor responsiveness to angiotensin II and norepinephrine, and thus to hypertension (123). In addition, insulin administration may induce an increase in plasma-norepinephrine levels, leading to venous constriction, a rise in capillary pressure, and a reduction in plasma volume, thereby stimulating the sympathetic nervous system (22,51). Counteracting this potential hypertensive effect, however, insulin appears to exert a direct vasodilatory effect in skeletal muscle in the dog (75), although such an action has yet to be confirmed in humans (22). Less well substantiated potential contributory actions of insulin include enhancing pressor responsiveness (19), and stimulation of renin secretion during hypoglycemic episodes (55).

Studies in diabetic rats suggest that vascular responsiveness to the vasopressor hormones angiotensin II, norepinephrine, and vasopressin is depressed early in the course of diabetes, but later returns toward normal (69,104). The role of these vasopressor substances in hypertension was further evaluated using blocking agents. The angiotensin I converting enzyme inhibitor (CEI) captopril reduced blood pressure throughout the 12-week course of the study, whereas administration of a specific V_1 vasopressin inhibitor was without effect, and blockade of the sympathetic nervous system with propranolol and phentolamine reduced blood pressure only after 12 weeks of diabetes. These authors concluded that the hypertension in experimental diabetes is caused mainly by exacerbation of the renin-angiotensin system early in the course, but that later the main factor may be overactivity of the sympathetic nervous system (69,104).

Abnormalities in red blood cell sodium-lithium countertransport have recently been implicated in the pathogenesis of hypertension in diabetes. Countertransport activity is abnormal in patients with essential hypertension (18), and maximal velocity rates are higher in patients with diabetic glomerulopathy than in patients with uncomplicated diabetes or with nondiabetic renal disease (82). Conceivably, enhanced transport rates may reflect increased activity of the renal tubule brush border sodium-hydrogen exchanger (128), contributing to the enhanced sodium retention in diabetic patients. Both parental hypertension and abnormal countertransport activity appear to predispose to risk of diabetic nephropathy

in patients with Type I diabetes (71,82,122). Taken together, these observations suggest that the association between sodium-lithium countertransport activity, diabetic nephropathy, and arterial blood pressure may be at least partially genetically determined in Type I diabetes. Transport rates do not appear elevated in hypertensive Type II diabetic patients (118).

Both decreased distensibility of the vascular bed (38) and later in the course of diabetes, fixed vascular lesions, may contribute to hypertension. In addition, it has been suggested that the abnormal hemorrheology of diabetes, and in particular decreased red blood cell deformability (81), may contribute to hypertension in this disease, possibly by stimulation of the renin-angiotensin system.

EFFECTS OF SYSTEMIC HYPERTENSION ON PROGRESSION OF DIABETIC MICROANGIOPATHY

Once present, hypertension accelerates the rate at which diabetic complications worsen. Elevation of blood pressure shortens the time interval between onset of diabetes and occurrence of both renal failure and retinopathy (53,68). Cardiovascular death of diabetic patients on hemodialysis correlates with predialysis blood pressure status (109). The incidence of retinopathy is increased in diabetic patients with hypertension (68), but definitive data regarding the potential beneficial effect of blood pressure reduction on diabetic retinopathy is lacking (15). Of the microvascular complications of diabetes, glomerulopathy has been the most extensively studied. After 5 years of diabetes, 95% of hypertensive, but only 35% of normotensive diabetics with proteinuria, have progressed to renal failure (Fig. 2) (108). Conversely, those patients who are spared from these microvascular complications exhibit comparatively low blood pressures even after decades of diabetes (16).

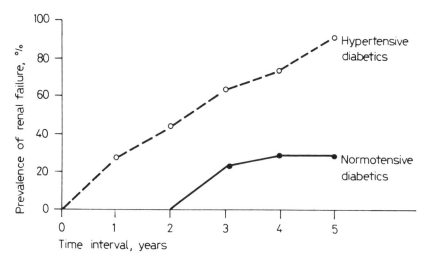

FIG. 2. Onset of renal failure (serum creatinine >1.4 mg/dl) in 48 proteinuric Type I diabetic patients with or without hypertension. (From Ritz et al., ref. 108, with permission.)

The most convincing evidence for the role of systemic hypertension in the acceleration of diabetic nephropathy comes from studies, primarily in Scandinavia, demonstrating that blood pressure control slows the progression of diabetic renal disease (Table 1). In these studies, rates of decline in glomerular filtration rate (GFR) and increase in urinary albumin excretion rate (AER) most often have been compared in individual patients before and after blood pressure is lowered by antihypertensive therapy. In 1976, Mogensen (89) reported that reduction of systemic arterial pressure from 162/103 to 144/95 with antihypertensive therapy significantly slowed rates of decline in GFR and increase in AER in 6 patients with heavy proteinuria and normal, but deteriorating, renal function. Subsequent studies (Table 1) have confirmed this observation in patients with persistent proteinuria but fairly normal renal function (57,90,98), and extended the beneficial effect of blood pressure control to those patients with overt diabetic nephropathy (14,116), as well as to those with incipient nephropathy (AER >15 μg/min but less than clinical proteinuria, 0.5 g/day) (21,84,137). Indeed, administration of the

CEI enalapril reduces blood pressure, filtration fraction, and AER in normotensive diabetic patients with normal values for AER (102).

HYPERTENSION AND EXPERIMENTAL DIABETIC GLOMERULOPATHY

Animal models offer the opportunity to study the role of hypertension in the initiation and pathogenesis of diabetic glomerulopathy. A clinically relevant model of conventionally-treated diabetes mellitus accrues from the administration of insulin in doses sufficient to maintain stable moderate hyperglycemia. In analogy witih many patients with early Type I diabetes (91,92), these rats are normotensive, but exhibit elevated values for the GFR as compared to normal rats (61,138,139). Single nephron hyperfiltration results from reductions in intrarenal vascular resistances, which allow elevation of the glomerular capillary plasma flow rate, Q_A. The decrease in afferent arteriolar resistance is proportionately greater than that in efferent resistance, and therefore mean glomerular capillary hydraulic pressure ($\bar{P}_{GC}$) is also elevated. Although glomerular capillary pressures can-

Table 1. *Effects of antihypertensive therapy on renal function*

Ref.	No. of patients	Duration	Drug	SBP (mmHg) Pre	SBP (mmHg) Post	AER Pre	AER Post	AER Δ Pre	AER Δ Post	GFR (ml/min/1.73 m²) Pre	GFR (ml/min/1.73 m²) Post	GFR Δ (ml/min/mo) Pre	GFR Δ (ml/min/mo) Post
						Incipient nephropathy							
21	6	5.4 yr	Metoprolol	135 ± 9 / 93 ± 9	125 ± 5* / 83 ± 6	131 ± 5 µg/min	56 ± 4*,[a] µg/min	+18 ± 17%	−17 ± 15%	149 ± 6	144 ± 11	—	—
84	10	6 mo	Enalapril	137 ± 7 / 82 ± 8	124 ± 13*,† / 72 ± 9	124 (27–380) µg/min	37*,† (21–382) µg/min	+6 mg/mo	−8 mg/mo*,†	130 ± 23	141 ± 24*	—	—
						Overt nephropathy (Normal GFR)							
98	11	6 yr	Metoprolol Hydralazine Furosemide[b]	143 ± 10 / 96 ± 7	129 ± 7* / 84 ± 7	1038 ± 514 µg/min	504 ± 322* µg/min	—	—	80 ± 17	60 (24–81)	−0.89 ± 0.33	−0.22 ± 0.17*,[c]
90	6	6 yr	Metoprolol Hydralazine Furosemide[d]	162 ± 14 / 103 ± 9	144 ± 11* / 95 ± 8	3.9 ± 3.4 g/day		+107%/yr	+5%/yr	86		−1.23 ± 0.8	−0.49 ± 0.5*
57	16	12 wk	Captopril	147 ± 11 / 94 ± 6	135 ± 13*,† / 86 ± 7	1460 ± 844 µg/min	1010 ± 746*,† µg/min	—	—	99 ± 19	93 ± 25*	—	—
						Overt nephropathy (Reduced GFR)							
14	14	2 yr	Captopril[e]	163 ± 13 / 97 ± 6	155 ± 14* / 94 ± 6	2.9 ± 2.0 g/day	2.8 ± 1.9 g/day	—	—	—	—	−10.3 ± 7.8	−5.5 ± 3.9*,[f]
116	10	8 wk	Captopril[g]	151 ± 10 / 83 ± 5	146 ± 7 / 80 ± 5	10.6 ± 2.2 g/day	6.1 ± 1.4* g/day	—	—	SCr 4.7 ± 0.7 mg/dl	5.0 ± 0.7 mg/dl	—	—

Values are means ± S.D.

SBP, systemic blood pressure; AER, urinary albumin excretion rate; GFR, glomerular filtration rate.

* $p < 0.05$ versus Pre; † $p < 0.05$ versus placebo.

[a] geometric mean × / ÷ tolerance factor.

[b] 10/11 patients; 1 received prazosin, spironolactone and furosemide.

[c] decline in GFR was 0.10 ± 0.13 ml/min/mo. during years 3 to 6.

[d] all on propranolol, then metoprolol; 4 on hydralazine, 1 switched to prazosin; 3 on furosemide.

[e] additional drugs: furosemide (13), thiazide (1), metoprolol (2).

[f] ml/min/yr; during second year, decline in GFR averaged only −2.4 ml/min/yr.

[g] captopril added to previous antihypertensive regimens.

not be measured in humans, the observed increases in renal-plasma flow account for only about 50 to 60% of the increase in GFR (23,91). Findings of an increased filtration fraction have been taken to suggest that intraglomerular pressure may be elevated (88), suggesting that the hemodynamic pattern in moderately hyperglycemic rats is analogous to that in human diabetics.

After a period of months, diabetic rats develop familiar morphologic changes, including renal hypertrophy (112), enlargement of glomerular size (86,105), glomerular basement-membrane thickening (105), mesangial matrix thickening (86), and hyaline deposition and glomerular sclerosis (86,138,139). Since experimental diabetes in the rat usually is not accompanied by overt systemic hypertension (61,114,138, 139), these renal hemodynamic and morphologic abnormalities occur despite the absence of systemic hypertension. While hypertension may accelerate both clinical (53,89,99) and experimental glomerulopathy (see below), it is not a prerequisite for experimental (138,139) or, in fact, clinical diabetic nephropathy (33,127).

Experimental studies indicate that the adverse effects of systemic hypertension on progression of renal disease may depend upon the intraglomerular hemodynamic consequences (3). Afferent arteriolar resistance determines the fraction of systemic arterial pressure which is transmitted to the glomerular capillary network. In some models, such as the spontaneously hypertensive rat, relative afferent arteriolar vasoconstriction prevents glomerular capillary hypertension, and the kidney is relatively protected from the development of glomerular sclerosis (7,39). In other models, however, including experimental diabetes, relative afferent-arteriolar vasodilation allows the development of glomerular-capillary hypertension, which in turn is associated with progressive proteinuria and glomerular sclerosis (3,4,60,138,139).

Systemic hypertension appears to contribute to diabetic glomerulopathy by aggravation of the abnormal glomerular-microcirculatory hemodynamics (4,60). With the institution of two-kidney Goldblatt hypertension, a striking intensification of glomerular lesions is observed in the unclipped kidney of diabetic rats, while the clipped kidney is substantially protected from glomerular injury (87). Though renal hemodynamics were not studied, unilateral renal artery clipping intensifies glomerular hypertension in the contralateral kidney which is intact (111); it seems likely that enhanced glomerular capillary hypertension produced this acceleration of diabetic renal injury.

Experimental diabetic glomerulopathy is also accelerated when diabetes is induced in the spontaneously hypertensive rat (SHR): glomerular injury in hypertensive diabetic rats is greater than that in rats with hypertension alone (9,27,103) (Table 2). Albuminuria and mesangial expansion were enhanced in each of these studies, though correlated more with diabetes than with hypertension per se (27). Micropuncture studies have reported conflicting results in this model. In one study, elevation of $\bar{P}_{GC}$ was noted in diabetic hypertensive rats, though not in rats with diabetes or hypertension alone (9), while others did not document glomerular hypertension in diabetic SHRs with either moderate or severe hyperglycemia (96). In the latter study, however, evidence of glomerular injury was found only in the deep glomeruli (96), which are presumed to exhibit higher glomerular capillary pressures and flows than are the superficial glomeruli accessible to micropuncture.

EFFECTS OF ANTIHYPERTENSIVE THERAPY IN EXPERIMENTAL DIABETIC GLOMERULOPATHY

Studies in the diabetic rat have also elucidated the mechanisms by which antihypertensive therapy slows the progression of diabetic glomerulopathy (Table 2). In the

Table 2. Effects of superimposed hypertension and of antihypertensive therapy in experimental diabetes

Reference	Group	Duration (months)	SBP mmHg	$\bar{P}_{GC}$ mmHg	AER mg/d	Mesangial expansion	Other morphology
87	C	4	127 ± 4	—	—	~0.2	
	DM		135 ± 4	—	—	~0.6[a]	
	DM/GH		234 ± 6[a,b]	—	—	~1.8[b]	
103	SHR	6	181 ± 2	—	28 ± 1	↑1/12	
	SHR/DM		168 ± 2[a]	—	74 ± 17[a]	↑4/9	
	SHR/DM/TRX		140 ± 2[a,b]	—	23 ± 2[a]	normal	
9	WKY	6	109 ± 2	43 ± 1	normal	15 ± 3	
	WKY/DM		114 ± 1	48 ± 1[a]	normal	27 ± 1[a]	
	SHR		159 ± 4[c]	44 ± 1	normal	22 ± 2[a]	
	SHR/DM		168 ± 3[c]	53 ± 1[a,c]	normal	26 ± 2[a]	
	SHR/DM/TRX		112 ± 3[a,b]	47 ± 1[b]	normal	16 ± 2[b]	
27	WKY	8	136 ± 5	—	—	↑ by DM but not by SBP	GBM thickening ↑ by both DM and SBP
	WKY/DM		128 ± 4	—	3		
	SHR		224 ± 7[a]	—	20[c]		
	SHR/DM		194 ± 7[c]	—	70[a,c]	↑SBP	
	SHR/DM/CEI		~145[b]	—	8[b]		
138	C	14	119 ± 3[d]	53 ± 1	25 ± 6	—	Glomerular sclerosis ↑ only in untreated DM rats
	DM		117 ± 4	63 ± 2[a]	111 ± 22[a]	—	
	DM/CEI		98 ± 2[a,b]	50 ± 1[b]	18 ± 3[b]	—	
64	C	3	117 ± 3		8 ± 0.2	—	
	DM		133 ± 3[a]		71 ± 18[a]	—	
	DM/CEI		108 ± 3[b]		36 ± 3[b]	—	
	DM/CCB		114 ± 2[b]		58 ± 10	—	
45	C	9	117 ± 3		12 ± 3	—	
	DM		130 ± 3		45 ± 10[a]	—	
	DM/H		106 ± 5[a,b]		41 ± 9[a,b]	—	
	DM/CEI		114 ± 3[a,b]		2 ± 1[b]	—	
6	C	16	126 ± 4		14 ± 3	—	
	DM		147 ± 4		57 ± 9[a]	—	
	DM/TRX		114 ± 4[b]		42 ± 13[a,b]	—	
	DM/CEI		124 ± 5[b]		3 ± 0.4[b]	—	

Values are means ± S.E.M.

SBP, systolic blood pressure; $\bar{P}_{GC}$, glomerular capillary pressure; AER, urinary albumin excretion rate; C, nondiabetic control; DM, diabetic; GH, Goldblatt hypertension; SHR, spontaneously hypertensive rat; TRX, triple therapy; WKY, Wistar-Kyoto rat; CEI, converting enzyme inhibitor; CCB, calcium channel blocker; H, hydralazine.

[a] $p < 0.05$ versus nondiabetic control.
[b] $p < 0.05$ versus untreated diabetes.
[c] $p < 0.05$ versus comparable WKY.
[d] mean arterial pressure under anesthesia.

normotensive, moderately hyperglycemic Munich-Wistar rat, the CEI enalapril was administered in a dose which modestly lowered systemic arterial pressure by about 15 mmHg (138) (Fig. 3A). Despite this modest effect, and the absence of any changes in glycemic control (Fig. 3A), CEI therapy selectively controlled glomerular capillary hypertension, without affecting the supranormal single nephron GFR (SNGFR) and Q_A (Fig. 3B). Control of glomerular hypertension was associated with limitation of AER (Fig. 3C) and glomerular injury to levels seen in nondiabetic control rats. Thus, these findings confirm the earlier results with dietary protein restriction (139) that amelioration of hemodynamic abnormalities affords protection even in the absence of any changes in metabolic control. Although glomerular hemodynamics were not studied, CEI therapy also has been shown to limit albuminuria, mesangial expansion, and glomerular basement-membrane thickening in the diabetic SHR (27), as well as to reduce blood pressure, filtration fraction (possibly reflecting $\overline{P}_{GC}$), and proteinuria in uninephrectomized diabetic rats (64).

In relatively short-term studies, administration of reserpine, hydralazine and hydrochlorothiazide ("triple therapy") lowers blood pressure (9,103) and $\overline{P}_{GC}$ (9), and limits mesangial expansion (9,103) and proteinuria (103) in the diabetic SHR. In contrast, however, hydralazine alone affords no protection against development of diabetic glomerulopathy, despite reduction of blood pressure to levels comparable to those achieved with CEI (45). Studies in nondiabetic models of progressive renal disease have indicated that effective antihypertensive control with triple therapy prevents glomerular hypertension and injury in some models (35,95) but limits neither in others (5,36). In the moderately hyperglycemic diabetic rat, a recent preliminary report suggests that while reduction of blood pressure with triple therapy slows the development of albuminuria in this model, the

effect is only to delay the development of injury, whereas comparable blood pressure control with CEI appears to prevent the development of diabetic glomerulopathy (6). In the uninephrectomized diabetic rat, excellent control of systemic blood pressure with verapamil resulted in no reduction in filtration fraction or proteinuria (64). Taken together, these studies suggest that reduction in blood pressure *per se* may afford protection in the presence of severe hypertension, but that a substantial beneficial effect on slowing the progression of diabetic glomerulopathy may be most successfully achieved when antihypertensive therapy results in control of glomerular capillary hypertension.

ANTIHYPERTENSIVE THERAPY AND THE PROGRESSION OF CLINICAL DIABETIC GLOMERULOPATHY

Numerous clinical studies have established that control of systemic hypertension slows the development of diabetic glomerulopathy. This beneficial effect is found virtually irrespective of the specific pharmacologic agents used. As is demonstrated in Table 1, successful antihypertensive therapy is associated with stabilization of both albumin excretion and GFR. These beneficial effects have been documented in patients with incipient nephropathy, as well as in patients with overt diabetic glomerulopathy. However, the experimental studies in diabetic rats, as well as in other models of progressive glomerulopathy, suggest that all antihypertensive agents may not prove equally efficacious in slowing glomerular injury.

In patients with nondiabetic renal disease, several recent studies suggest that CEI therapy may be superior to conventional combination regimens in reducing proteinuria and in preventing renal functional deterioration (56,83,110). Long-term, prospective clinical studies of this issue are currently lacking in diabetic as well as in

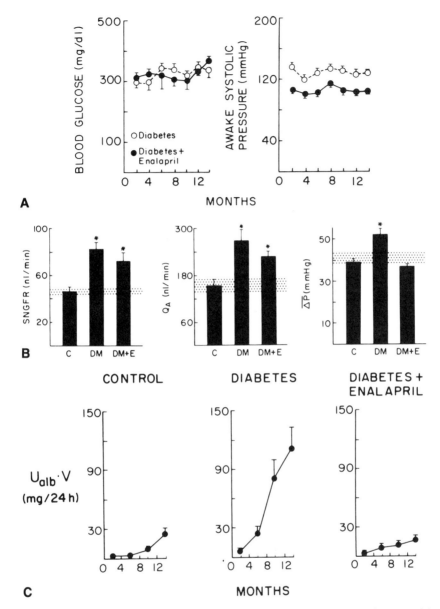

FIG. 3. Effects of enalapril (E) therapy on development of glomerulopathy in rats with diabetes mellitus (DM). Values are means ± SEM; horizontal bands depict normal ranges. **(A)** Values for blood glucose were comparable in DM rats and DM rats treated with enalapril, whereas values for awake systolic blood pressure were slightly lower in enalapril-treated rats. **(B)** Glomerular hemodynamics in nondiabetic control (C), DM, and DM + E rats. Values for the single nephron glomerular filtration rate (SNGFR) and glomerular capillary plasma flow rate (Q_A) were comparably elevated in DM and DM + E rats. Enalapril selectively normalized values for $\overline{\Delta P}$, the glomerular transcapillary hydraulic pressure gradient. **(C)** Serial values for 24-hr urinary albumin excretion ($U_{alb} \cdot V$). Aging control rats showed a slight increase over time. Development of albuminuria was markedly accelerated by diabetes, but maintained at levels comparable to those seen in nondiabetic rats in diabetic rats treated with enalapril. (From Zatz et al., ref. 138, with permission.)

nondiabetic renal disease. However, several recent observations suggest that interventions such as dietary protein restriction and CEI therapy, which reduce $\overline{P}_{GC}$ in the rat, also may have comparable glomerular hemodynamic effects in patients.

That the beneficial effects of CEI are not entirely due to reduction in systemic pressure is suggested by a recent study of enalapril therapy in normotensive diabetic patients with persistent microalbuminuria. After six months on this regimen, which reduced mean arterial pressure from 98 to 90 mmHg, GFR increased slightly and AER fell (84), whereas placebo therapy ameliorated neither. In patients with severe diabetic nephropathy, a substantial decrease in proteinuria was noted after an 8-week course of therapy with the CEI captopril. In this study, captopril was added to the existing antihypertensive regimen in doses which did not further reduce systemic blood pressure (116). In each of these studies, absence of a marked reduction in systemic arterial pressure strongly suggests that the reduction in proteinuria resulted from a decrease in $\overline{P}_{GC}$, most likely due to inhibition of angiotensin II formation and subsequent relaxation of efferent (postglomerular) arteriolar tone.

Finally, despite the evidence of a correlation between increased exchangeable sodium in diabetes, and some evidence for a beneficial effect of dietary sodium restriction (97), an intriguing recent observation suggests that diuretic therapy may in fact accelerate the decline in renal function in diabetic patients (126).

In addition to pharmacologic therapy of systemic and glomerular hypertension, dietary interventions may protect the kidney as well. Dietary protein restriction, which has no effect on blood pressure in experimental diabetes, reduces glomerular capillary pressure (139), and slows the development of glomerulopathy (134,139) in diabetic rats. This nutritional therapy has been reported to slow the decline of GFR in diabetic patients over one year (37,140), and in these patients, blood pressure tended to fall as well. Together with observations that dietary protein restriction reduces albuminuria in diabetic patients (26,37,140), these observations suggest that this intervention may reduce $\overline{P}_{GC}$ in patients as well.

TREATMENT OF HYPERTENSION IN DIABETES

Given the magnitude of microvascular and cardiovascular complications of diabetes, aggressive treatment of hypertension is mandatory. In diabetic patients, just as in patients with essential hypertension, a reasonable first step is to implement dietary and lifestyle changes which affect blood pressure. Such general measures include weight loss, reduction of sodium intake, cessation of cigarette smoking, regular exercise, and discontinuance of medications known to raise blood pressure. In the diabetic patient, obesity decreases sensitivity of peripheral tissues to insulin and contributes to hypertension. Adherence to the high-carbohydrate, low-fat American Diabetes Association diet is generally recommended. In diabetic patients, a diet with low-sodium, low-fat, and high-fiber content has been demonstrated to exert a significant antihypertensive effect (97), and represents a reasonable initial approach. However, the majority of hypertensive diabetic patients will eventually require pharmacologic therapy. In addition to concerns over the intrarenal hemodynamic consequences of pharmacologic therapy, and thus to protection from microvascular complications, attention must be paid to the potential side effects of various therapeutic agents which may limit their use in this population (25,58,63,100,107,113,115). Detailed discussions of each class of available antihypertensive agents are found elsewhere in this volume; the following will address those issues of particular concern in diabetic patients.

DIURETICS

Thiazide diuretics, in widespread general use for essential hypertension, exhibit several metabolic side effects which limit their utility in diabetic patients, including impaired glucose tolerance (47,94,115) and elevation of serum triglyceride and cholesterol levels, and particularly of low-density and very low-density lipoprotein cholesterol fractions (48,131,133). In addition, the incidence of impotence and orthostatic hypotension may be higher in diabetics on thiazide diuretics (25,33,77). Loop diuretics such as furosemide are less diabetogenic than thiazides, although they may cause hypokalemia.

BETA-ADRENERGIC RECEPTOR ANTAGONISTS

Beta-adrenergic receptor antagonists may also prove problematic in diabetic patients, particularly in Type II diabetics, although it should be noted that the important metabolic side effects are associated with beta$_2$-adrenergic receptors and may be lessened with a more selective beta-blocker. Beta$_2$-blockade may prolong hypoglycemic episodes by impairment of peripheral glycogenolysis in muscle and lipolysis in adipose tissue, thereby reducing substrates for gluconeogenesis and ketogenesis (25,63,125). Moreover, beta$_2$-blockade may impair glucagon secretion (125). Administration of propranolol delays the recovery of blood glucose level after hypoglycemia, an effect not seen with the more cardioselective agents metoprolol, atenolol, or acebutolol (29,72). However, some investigators (29), but not others (101), report potentiation of the hypoglycemic effects of insulin with acebutolol, a cardioselective agent with membrane-stabilizing properties which may inhibit glucose release from the liver in response to hypoglycemia. Of note, clinical experience has not always confirmed this risk in diabetic patients (11,49).

In one study of 150 patients treated with beta-blockers for 8 months, the frequency of hypoglycemic episodes was no higher than in diabetic patients not receiving the drugs, despite the fact that 86% of these patients were taking nonselective beta-blockers (11). Nevertheless, cardioselective agents may be preferable in this patient population.

Nonselective beta-blockade poses the theoretical risk of lessening patient perception of hypoglycemic symptoms, though long-term studies suggest that this is an infrequent adverse effect (11). In addition, the hemodynamic response to hypoglycemia may be altered, since the normal response to hypoglycemia includes increased catecholamine stimulation of beta$_2$-adrenergic receptors, causing vasodilatation and reduction in blood pressure. When nonselective beta-blockers are used, however, the increase in catecholamines leads to unopposed alpha-adrenergic stimulation, causing vasoconstriction and elevation of blood pressure (78), that might precipitate unacceptable levels of hypertension. Again, this complication may be avoided by using a cardioselective beta-blocker (33,63,125).

These agents may also impact on glycemic control, since they may impair the normal insulin release which results from stimulation of beta-adrenergic receptors, as well as allow unopposed stimulation of pancreatic alpha-adrenergic receptors which inhibit insulin release. Studies of the effects of beta-blockade on acute (20) and chronic (136) glycemic control have tended to support the notion that blood glucose levels are higher following the usual stimuli in the presence of these agents, although this effect may be lessened by the use of cardioselective beta-blockers (124) and may also be obviated by adjustment of the insulin regimen.

In addition to interfering with glucose homeostasis, beta-blockers may contribute to cardiovascular risk by increasing serum triglycerides and decreasing high-density lipoprotein fractions (133). Most studies have found increases in serum triglycerides, and all beta-blockers except pindolol (which possesses intrinsic sympathomimetic activity) decrease high-density lipoproteins (133). However, cardioselective beta-blockers also have less effect on lipid levels than do nonselective agents. Labetolol, a combined alpha- and beta-adrenergic blocker, may be less likely to adversely affect serum lipid levels (44,80).

Another potential risk is aggravation of hyperkalemia, through suppression of renin release, particularly when the juxtaglomerular apparatus is already compromised by renal disease or neuropathy. Finally, nonselective beta-blockade in diabetic patients may aggravate peripheral microvascular disease, a complication which is less frequent with selective beta-blockers (63,125).

ALPHA-ADRENERGIC ANTAGONISTS

As noted above, these agents may have important effects on glycemic control, since alpha-adrenergic stimulation inhibits pancreatic insulin release. Administration of the selective $alpha_1$-adrenergic blocker prazosin for one week has been reported to improve glucose tolerance in patients with chemical diabetes (10), perhaps reflecting some degree of $alpha_2$-antagonism. Of note, several studies with prazosin have demonstrated decreases in total cholesterol and triglyceride levels, and increases in high density lipoprotein levels (67,74,129). The major adverse effects of this class of drugs are orthostatic hypotension (63) and sexual dysfunction (77), which may be troublesome in diabetic patients with even minor neuropathy.

SYMPATHOLYTIC AGENTS

The $alpha_2$-adrenergic agonists (clonidine, methyldopa, guanabenz) are sometimes used in treatment of diabetic patients. Administration of clonidine has been re-

ported to increase the glycemic response to intravenous glucose, but to have no significant effect on long-term glycemic control (52). Methyldopa does not affect glucose metabolism, but reports of effects on cholesterol metabolism are conflicting. Some investigators have documented reduction in high-density lipoproteins (2,73), while another study found an overall reduction in low-density lipoproteins (34). Clonidine and guanabenz have been reported to reduce total cholesterol levels when given alone, but not when given with a diuretic (67). However, the inhibitory action of these agents on sympathetic responses may contribute substantially to orthostatic hypotension and to sexual dysfunction in the diabetic patient.

PERIPHERAL VASODILATORS

Administration of potent peripheral vasodilators such as hydralazine and minoxidil may prove disadvantageous in diabetic patients, as aggravation of sodium retention and stimulation of the sympathetic nervous system with induction of tachycardia may contribute to volume-related hypertension as well as risk of cardiovascular incidents. These side effects may be lessened by concurrent administration of loop diuretics and cardioselective beta-blockers. These agents do not appear to offer significant metabolic side effects nor to aggravate orthostatic hypotension or sexual problems (63,77).

CALCIUM CHANNEL BLOCKERS

Calcium channel blockers, which are receiving increased use in the hypertensive population in general, also tend not to cause the troublesome metabolic side effects which characterize thiazide diuretics (120). Of some theoretical concern, however, is that calcium influx is an essential step in insulin release, and calcium channel blockers have been shown to inhibit insulin release *in vitro* in the isolated perfused rat pancreas (115). However, this effect has not been well documented in the intact animal or, for that matter, in patients. Clinical studies have found somewhat conflicting results, with aggravation of hyperglycemia noted in some (1,30) but not in most studies (12,46,119,120).

CONVERTING ENZYME INHIBITORS

While angiotensin I converting enzyme inhibitors may offer a special benefit to the diabetic kidney, certain aspects of these agents must be watched in the diabetic patient. On the one hand, their metabolic profile is optimal, in that they do not appear to impair glucose tolerance nor to raise cholesterol levels. Administration of the CEI captopril with a thiazide diuretic has been reported to block the rise in total cholesterol seen with the diuretic alone (132). Nor do diabetic patients per se fall into the high-risk category (collagen vascular disease with renal insufficiency) for development of neutropenia. However, it should be remembered that their aldosterone-suppressing actions may promote hyperkalemia, a special concern in a population with an increased risk of hyporeninemic hypoaldosteronism (30). This risk may be enhanced when CEI are administered with potassium-sparing diuretics or potassium supplements (117), while concomitant use of a loop diuretic may counteract the hyperkalemic effect of CEI.

In addition, the presence of known renovascular disease (bilateral renal artery stenosis or stenosis of a single renal artery) may be a relative contraindication to use of these drugs, which have been shown to precipitate renal failure in such patients (28,62), presumably by reducing efferent arteriolar tone in a situation where glomerular filtration is critically dependent upon maintenance of efferent arteriolar resistance.

SUMMARY AND IMPLICATIONS

Recent advances in the treatment of hyperglycemia and hypertension have not yet begun to have a substantial impact on the incidence of end-stage renal disease in patients with diabetes mellitus. Nonetheless, enhanced understanding of the risk factors for development of diabetic complications, together with improved hypoglycemic technology, recognition of optimal dietary therapies, and an expanded antihypertensive pharmacopeia, generate optimism that the diabetic state need not lead to devastating microvascular complications. These newer strategies will require validation with long-term, prospective, controlled studies. In addition, several important questions will need to be addressed in future studies. First, how can we identify those patients at risk for diabetic complications who are perhaps candidates for earlier and more aggressive intervention? The recent demonstration that patients who develop diabetic renal disease are more likely to have a parent with essential hypertension (71,122) suggests a genetic susceptibility, and reported abnormalities in red blood cell sodium-lithium countertransport (71,82) offer a promising avenue of investigation of this question. Second, at what point should preventive measures be instituted? While it may be imprudent to wait until renal function is severely compromised, universal application of these interventions at the time diabetes is diagnosed will prove inappropriate, unnecessary, and possibly perilous for those patients not destined to suffer serious complications of the disease. Although short-term studies of CEI therapy in normotensive diabetic patients show promise, currently available data does not justify the widespread use of antihypertensive therapy in normotensive patients. Finally, the suggestion from the animal studies that antihypertensive agents such as CEI which reduce glomerular capillary pressure afford superior protection to other antihypertensive regimens requires careful comparison studies in diabetic patients. These caveats notwithstanding, further investigation into the mechanisms of hemodynamic injury may reveal nutritional and pharmacologic strategies that will provide successful, and readily achievable, means for conferring protection against the debilitating complications of diabetes mellitus.

REFERENCES

1. Abadie, E., and Passa, P. H. (1984): Diabetogenic effects of nifedipine. *Br. Med. J.*, 289:437–438.
2. Ames, R. P., and Hill, P. (1982): Antihypertensive therapy and the risk of coronary heart disease. *J. Cardiovasc. Pharmacol.*, 4 (Suppl. 2):S206–S212.
3. Anderson, S., and Brenner, B. M. (1987): Role of intraglomerular hypertension in the initiation and progression of renal disease. In: *Perspectives in Hypertension. Vol. I. The Kidney in Hypertension*, edited by Kaplan, N., Brenner, B. M., and Laragh, J. H., pp. 67–76. Raven Press, New York.
4. Anderson, S., and Brenner, B. M. (1988): The hemodynamic basis of glomerulopathy in diabetes mellitus. In: *Perspectives in Hypertension. Vol. II. Endocrine Mechanisms in Hypertension*, edited by Kaplan, N., Brenner, B. M., and Laragh, J. H. pp. 91–104. Raven Press, New York.
5. Anderson, S., Rennke, H. G., and Brenner, B. M. (1986): Therapeutic advantage of converting enzyme inhibitors in arresting progressive renal disease associated with systemic hypertension in the rat. *J. Clin. Invest.*, 77:1993–2000.
6. Anderson, S., Rennke, H. G., Garcia, D. L., and Brenner, B. M. (1989): Short and long term effects of antihypertensive therapy in the diabetic rat. *Kidney Int.* (in press).
7. Arendshorst, W. J., and Beierwaltes, W. H. (1979): Renal and nephron hemodynamics in spontaneously hypertensive rats. *Am. J. Physiol.*, 236:F246–F251.
8. Ballermann, B. J., Skorecki, K. L., and Brenner, B. M. (1984): Reduced glomerular angiotensin II receptor density in early untreated diabetes mellitus in the rat. *Am. J. Physiol.*, 247:F110–F116.
9. Bank, N., Klose, R., Aynedjian, H. S., Nguyen, D., and Sablay, L. B. (1987): Evidence against increased glomerular pressure initiating diabetic nephropathy. *Kidney Int.*, 31:898–905.
10. Barbieri, C., Ferrari, C., Borzio, M., Piepoli, V., and Caldara, R. (1980): Metabolic effects of chronic prazosin treatment. *Horm. Metab. Res.*, 12:331–334.
11. Barnett, A. H., Leslie, D., and Watkins, P. J. (1980): Can insulin-treated diabetics be given beta-adrenergic-blocking drugs? *Br. Med. J.*, 280:976–978.
12. Bhatnagar, S. K., Amin, M. A. A., and Al-Yusuf, A. R. (1984): Diabetogenic effects of nifedipine. *Br. Med. J.*, 289:19.

13. Bjorck, S., Delin, K., Herlitz, H., Larson, O., and Aurell, M. (1984): Renin secretion in advanced diabetic nephropathy. *Scand. J. Urol. Nephrol.*, 79:S53–S57.
14. Bjorck, S., Nyberg, G., Mulec, H., Granerus, G., Herlitz, H., and Aurell, M. (1986): Beneficial effects of angiotensin converting enzyme inhibition on renal function in patients with diabetic nephropathy. *Br. Med. J.*, 293:471–474.
15. Bock, K. D. (1984): Regression of retinal vascular changes by antihypertensive therapy. *Hypertension*, 6 (Suppl. III):III-58–III-162.
16. Borch-Johnsen, K., Nissen, R. N., and Nerup, J. (1985): Blood pressure after 40 years of insulin-dependent diabetes. *Diabetic Nephrop.*, 4:11–12.
17. Brownlee, M., Vlassara, H., and Cerami, A. (1984): Nonenzymatic glycosylation and the pathogenesis of diabetic complications. *Ann. Intern. Med.*, 101:527–537.
18. Canessa, M., Adragna, N., Solomon, H. S., Connolly, T. M., and Tosteson, D. C. (1980): Increased sodium-lithium countertransport in red cells of patients with essential hypertension. *N. Engl. J. Med.*, 302:772–776.
19. Cavaliere, T. A., Taylor, D. G., Kerwin, L. J., and Antonaccio, M. J. (1980): Cardiovascular effect of alloxan diabetes in normotensive and spontaneously hypertensive rats. *Pharmacology*, 20:211–223.
20. Cerasi, E., Luft, R., and Efendic, S. (1972): Effect of adrenergic-blocking agents on insulin response to glucose infusion in man. *Acta Endocrinol. (Scand.)*, 69:335–346.
21. Christensen, C. K., and Mogensen, C. E. (1985): Effect of antihypertensive treatment on progression of incipient diabetic nephropathy. *Hypertension*, 7(Suppl. II):II-109–II-113.
22. Christensen, N. J. (1983): Acute effects of insulin on cardiovascular function and noradrenaline uptake and release. *Diabetologia*, 25:377–381.
23. Christiansen, J. S., Gammelgard, J., Frandsen, M., et al. (1981): Increased kidney size, glomerular filtration rate, and renal plasma flow in short term insulin-dependent diabetics. *Diabetologia*, 20:451–456.
24. Christlieb, A. R. (1974): Renin, angiotensin and norepinephrine in alloxan diabetes. *Diabetes*, 23:962–970.
25. Christlieb, A. R. (1982): Treating hypertension in the patient with diabetes mellitus. *Med. Clin. N. Am.*, 66:1373–1388.
26. Cohen, D. L., Dodds, R., and Viberti, G. C. (1987): Effect of protein restricted diet in insulin-dependent diabetics at risk of nephropathy. *Br. Med. J.*, 294:795–798.
27. Cooper, M. E., Allen, T. J., Macmillan, P., Bach, L., Jerums, G., and Doyle, A. E. (1988): Genetic hypertension accelerates nephropathy in the streptozotocin diabetic rat. *Am. J. Hypertension*, 1:5–10.
28. Curtis, J. J., Luke, R. G., Whelchel, J. D., Diethelm, A. G., Jones, P., and Dustan, H. P.

(1983): Inhibition of angiotensin-converting enzyme in renal-transplant recipients with hypertension. *N. Engl. J. Med.*, 308:377–381.

29. Deacon, S. P., Karunanayake, A., and Barnett, D. (1977): Acebutolol, atenolol, and propranolol and metabolic responses to acute hypoglycaemia in diabetics. *Br. Med. J.*, 274:1255–1257.

30. DeFronzo, R. A. (1980): Hyperkalemia and hyporeninemic hypoaldosteronism. *Kidney Int.*, 17:118–134.

31. DeFronzo, R. A. (1981): The effect of insulin on renal sodium metabolism: A review with clinical implications. *Diabetologia*, 21:165–171.

32. Donnelly, J., and Harrower, A. D. M. (1980): Effect of nifedipine on glucose tolerance and insulin secretion in diabetic and non-diabetic patients. *Curr. Med. Res. Opin.*, 6:690–693.

33. Drury, P. L. (1983): Diabetes and arterial hypertension. *Diabetologia*, 24:1–9.

34. Dujovne, C. A., DeCoursey, S., and Krehbiel, C., et al. (1984): Serum lipids in normo- and hyperlipidemics after methyldopa and propranolol. *Clin. Pharmacol. Ther.*, 36:157–162.

35. Dworkin, L. D., Grosser, M., Feiner, H., Ullian, M., Randazzo, J., and Parker, M. (1989): Renal vascular effects of antihypertensive therapy in the uninephrectomized SHR. *Kidney Int.*, 35:790–798.

36. Dworkin, L. D., Feiner, H. D., and Randazzo, J. (1987): Glomerular hypertension and injury in desoxyorticosterone-salt rats on antihypertensive therapy. *Kidney Int.*, 31:718–724.

37. Evanoff, G. V., Thompson, C. S., Brown, J., and Weinman, E. J. (1987): The effect of dietary protein restriction on the progression of diabetic nephropathy: A 12-month follow-up. *Arch. Intern. Med.*, 147:492–495.

38. Faris, I., Agerskov, K., Henriksen, O., Lassen, N. A., and Parving, H. H. (1982): Decreased distensibility of a passive vascular bed in diabetes mellitus: An indicator of microangiopathy. *Diabetologia*, 23:411–414.

39. Feld, L. G., Van Liew, J. B., Brentjens, J. R., and Boyland, J. W. (1981): Renal lesions and proteinuria in the spontaneously hypertensive rat made normotensive by treatment. *Kidney Int.*, 20:606–614.

40. Feldt-Rasmussen, B., Borch-Johnsen, K., and Mathiesen, E. R. (1985): Hypertension in diabetes as related to nephropathy: Early blood pressure changes. *Hypertension*, 7 (Suppl. II):II-18–II-20.

41. Feldt-Rasmussen, B., Mathiesen, E. R., Deckert, T., Giese, J., Christensen, N. J., Bent-Hansen, L., and Nielsen, M. D. (1987): Central role for sodium in the pathogenesis of blood pressure changes independent of angiotensin, aldosterone and catecholamines in Type I (insulin-dependent) diabetes mellitus. *Diabetologia*, 30:610–617.

42. Feriss, J. B., O'Hare, J. A., Cole, M., Kingston, S. M., Twomey, B. M., and O'Sullivan, D. J. (1986): Blood pressure in diabetic patients: Relationships with exchangeable sodium and renin activity. *Diabetic Nephrop.*, 5:27–30.

43. Ferriss, J. B., O'Hare, J. A., Kelleher, C. C. M., Sullivan, P. A., Cole, M. M., Ross, H. F., and O'Sullivan, D. J. (1985): Diabetic control and the renin-angiotensin system, catecholamines, and blood pressure. *Hypertension*, 7 (Suppl. II):II-58–II-63.

44. Frishman, W., Michelson, E., Johnson, B., et al. (1983): Multiclinic comparison of labetalol to metoprolol in treatment of mild-to-moderate systemic hypertension. *Am. J. Med.*, 75(4A):54–67.

45. Fujihara, C. K., Gianella-Neto, D., Cavaleiro, A. M. S., Wajchenberg, B. L., Marcondes, M., and Zatz, R. (1987): Lowering of arterial pressure with hydralazine therapy does not prevent albuminuria in experimental diabetes rats. *Hypertension*, 9:539 (abstr.).

46. Giugliano, D., Torella, R., Cacciapuoti, F., Gentile, S., Verza, M., and Varricchio, M. (1980): Impairment of insulin secretion in man by nifedipine. *Eur. J. Clin. Pharmacol.*, 18:395–398.

47. Goldner, M. G., Zarowitz, H., and Akgun, S. (1960): Hyperglycemia and glycosuria due to thiazide derivatives administered in diabetes mellitus. *N. Engl. J. Med.*, 262:403–405.

48. Grimm, R. H., Jr., Leon, A. S., Hunninghake, D. B., et al. (1981): Effects of thiazide diuretics on plasma lipids and lipoproteins in mildly hypertensive patients: A double-blind controlled trial. *Ann. Intern. Med.*, 94:7–11.

49. Groop, L., and Totterman, K. J. (1982): Propranolol does not inhibit sulfonyl-urea-stimulated insulin secretion in patients with non-insulin-dependent diabetes mellitus. *Acta Endocrinol. (Copenh.)*, 100:410–415.

50. Gundersen, H. J. G. (1974): Peripheral blood flow and metabolic control in juvenile diabetes. *Diabetologia*, 10:225–231.

51. Gundersen, H. J. G., and Christensen, N. J. (1977): Intravenous insulin causing loss of intravascular water and albumin and increased adrenergic nervous activity in diabetics. *Diabetes*, 26:551–557.

52. Guthrie, G. P., Miller, R. E., Kotchen, T. A., and Koening, S. H. (1983): Clonidine in patients with diabetes and mild hypertension. *Clin. Pharmacol. Ther.*, 34:713–717.

53. Hasslacher, C., Ritz, E., Terpstra, J., Gallasch, G., Kunowski, G., and Rall, C. (1985): Natural history of nephropathy in Type I diabetes: Relationship to metabolic control and blood pressure. *Hypertension*, 7 (Suppl. II):II-74–II-78.

54. Hasslacher, C., Stech, W., and Ritz, E. (1985): Blood pressure and metabolic control as risk factors for nephropathy in Type I (insulin-dependent) diabetes. *Diabetologia*, 28:6–11.

55. Hedeland, H., Dymling, J. F., and Hokfelt, B. (1972): The effect of insulin-induced hypoglycemia on plasma renin activity and urinary catecholamines before and following clonidine in man. *Acta Endocrinol. (Copenh.)*, 71:321–330.

56. Heeg, J. E., de Jong, P. E., van der Hem, G. K., and de Zeeuw, D. (1987): Reduction of proteinuria by angiotensin converting enzyme inhibition. *Kidney Int.*, 32:78–83.

57. Hommel, E., Parving, H. H., Mathiesen, E., Edsberg, B., Nielsen, M. D., and Giese, J. (1986): Effect of captopril on kidney function in insulin-dependent diabetic patients with nephropathy. *Br. Med. J.*, 293:467–470.

58. Horan, M. J., and Page, L. B., eds. (1988): Drug side effects, drug-drug interactions, drug resistance, and patient compliance in the management of hypertension. *Hypertension*, 11 (Suppl. 2).

59. Hostetter, T. H. (1986): Diabetic Nephropathy. In: *The Kidney*. 3rd ed., edited by Brenner, B. M. and Rector, F. C., Jr., pp. 1377–1402. W. B. Saunders Co., Philadelphia.

60. Hostetter, T. H., Rennke, H. G., and Brenner, B. M. (1982): The case for intrarenal hypertension in the initiation and progression of diabetic and other glomerulopathies. *Am. J. Med.*, 72:375–380.

61. Hostetter, T. H., Troy, J. L., and Brenner, B. M. (1981): Glomerular hemodynamics in experimental diabetes mellitus. *Kidney Int.*, 19:410–415.

62. Hricik, D. E., Browning, P. J., Kopelman, R., Goorno, W. E., Madias, N. E., and Dzau, V. J. (1983): Captopril-induced functional renal insufficiency in patients with bilateral renal-artery stenoses or renal-artery stenosis in a solitary kidney. *N. Engl. J. Med.*, 308:373–376.

63. Husserl, F. E., and Messerli, F. H. (1981): Adverse effects of antihypertensive drugs. *Drugs*, 22:88–210.

64. Jackson, B., Debrevi, L., Whitty, M., and Johnston, C. I. (1986): Progression of renal disease: Effects of different classes of antihypertensive therapy. *J. Hypertension*, 4 (Suppl. 5):S269–S271.

65. Janka, H. U., and Dirschedl, P. (1985): Systolic blood pressure as a predictor for cardiovascular disease in diabetes: A 5-year longitudinal study. *Hypertension*, 7 (Suppl. II):II-90–II-94.

66. Kannel, W. B. (1976): Diabetes and cardiovascular disease: The Framingham Study. 18-year follow-up. *Cardiol. Digest*, 11:11–15.

67. Kirkendall, W. M., Hammond, J. J., Thomas, J. C., et al. (1978): Prazosin and clonidine for moderately severe hypertension. *J. Am. Med. Assoc.*, 240:2553–2556.

68. Knowler, W. C., Bennett, P. H., and Ballantin, E. J. (1980): Increased incidence of retinopathy in diabetics with high blood pressure. *N. Engl. J. Med.*, 203:645–650.

69. Kohlmann, D., Jr., Bossolan, D., Zanella, M. T., Ramos, O. L., and Ribeiro, A. B. (1987): Hypertension in experimental diabetes mellitus: Role for major vasopressor systems. (abstr.). *Hypertension*, 9:531.

70. Kokko, J. P. (1973): Proximal tubule potential difference: Dependence of glucose, HCO_3, and amino acids. *J. Clin. Invest.*, 52:1362–1367.

71. Krolewski, A. S., Canessa, M., Warram, J. H., et al. (1988): Predisposition to hypertension and susceptibility to renal disease in insulin-dependent diabetes mellitus. *N. Engl. J. Med.*, 318:140–145.

72. Lager, I., Bhohme, G., and Smith, U. (1979): Effect of cardioselective and non-selective β-blockade on the hypoglycaemic response in insulin-dependent diabetics. *Lancet*, 1:458–462.

73. Leon, A. S., Agre, J., Grimm, R., et al. (1982): Plasma lipid changes with aldomet and propranolol during treatment of hypertension. *Circ.*, 2:37. (abstr.)

74. Leren, P., Gelgeland, A., Holme, I., et al. (1980): Effect of propranolol and prazosin on blood lipids: The Oslo study. *Lancet*, 2:4–6.

75. Liang, C. S., Doherty, J. U., Faillace, R., et al. (1982): Insulin infusion in conscious dogs: Effects on systemic and coronary hemodynamics, regional blood flows, and plasma catecholamines. *J. Clin. Invest.*, 69:1321–1336.

76. Lieberman, J., and Sastre, A. (1980): Serum angiotensin-converting enzyme: Elevation in diabetes mellitus. *Ann. Intern. Med.*, 93:825–826.

77. Lipson, L. G. (1984): Treatment of hypertension in diabetic men: Problems with sexual dysfunction. *Am. J. Cardiol.*, 53:46A–50A.

78. Lloyd-Mostyn, R. M., and Oram S. (1975): Modification by propranolol of cardiovascular effects of induced hypoglycaemia. *Lancet*, 1:1213–1215.

79. Luetscher, J. A., Kraemer, F. B., Wilson, D. M., Schwartz, H. C., and Bryer-Ash, M. (1985): Increased plasma inactive renin in diabetes mellitus: A marker of microvascular complications. *N. Engl. J. Med.*, 312:1412–1417.

80. McGonigle, R. J. S., Williams, L., Murphy, M. J., et al. (1981): Labetalol and lipids. *Lancet*, 1:163.

81. McMillan, D. E. (1983): The effect of diabetes on blood flow properties. *Diabetes*, 32 (Suppl. 2):56–63.

82. Mangili, R., Bending, J. J., Scott, G., Li, L. K., Gupta, A., and Viberti, G. C. (1988): Increased sodium-lithium countertransport activity in red cells of patients with insulin-dependent diabetes and nephropathy. *N. Engl. J. Med.*, 318:146–150.

83. Mann, J., and Ritz, E. (1987): Preservation of kidney function by use of converting enzyme inhibitors for control of hypertension. *Lancet*, 2:622.

84. Marre, M., Chatellier, G., Leblanc, H., Guyenne, T., Menard, J., and Passa, P. (1988): Prevention of diabetic nephropathy with enalapril in normotensive diabetics with microalbuminuria. *Br. Med. J.*, 297: 1092–1095.

85. Mathiesen, E. R., Oxenboll, D., Johansen, K., Svendsen, P. A., and Deckert, T. (1984): Incipient nephropathy in type I insulin-dependent diabetes. *Diabetologia*, 26:406–410.

86. Mauer, S. M., Michael, A. F., Fish, A. J., and Brown, D. M. (1972): Spontaneous immuno-

globulin and complement deposition in glomeruli of diabetic rats. *Lab. Invest.*, 27:488–494.

87. Mauer, S. M., Steffes, M. W., Azar, S., Sandberg, S. K., and Brown, D. M. (1978): The effects of Goldblatt hypertension on development of the glomerular lesions of diabetes mellitus in the rat. *Diabetes*, 27:738–744.

88. Mogensen, C. E. (1976): Renal function changes in diabetes. *Diabetes*, 25:872–879.

89. Mogensen, C. E. (1976): Progression of nephropathy in long-term diabetes with proteinuria and effect of initial antihypertensive treatment. *Scand. J. Clin. Lab. Invest.*, 36:383–388.

90. Mogensen, C. E. (1982): Long-term antihypertensive treatment inhibiting progression of diabetic nephropathy. *Br. Med. J.*, 285:685–688.

91. Mogensen, C. E., and Andersen, M. J. F. (1975): Increased kidney size and glomerular filtration rate in untreated juvenile diabetes: Normalization by insulin treatment. *Diabetologia*, 11:221–224.

92. Mogensen, C. E., and Christensen, C. K. (1984): Predicting diabetic nephropathy in insulin-dependent patients. *N. Engl. J. Med.*, 311:89–93.

93. Mogensen, C. E., and Christensen, C. K. (1985): Blood pressure changes and renal function in incipient and overt diabetic nephropathy. *Hypertension*, 7 (Suppl. II):II-64–II-73.

94. Murphy, M. B., Lewis, P. J., Kohner, E., Schumer, B., and Dollery, C. T. (1982): Glucose intolerance in hypertensive patients treated with diuretics: A fourteen-year follow-up. *Lancet*, 2:1293–1295.

95. Neugarten, J., Feiner, H. D., Schacht, R. G., Liu, D. T., and Baldwin, D. S. (1985): Nephrotoxic serum nephritis with hypertension: Amelioration by antihypertensive therapy. *Kidney Int.*, 28:135–139.

96. O'Donnell, M. P., Kasiske, B. L., Daniels, F. X., and Keane, W. F. (1986): Glomerular haemodynamic function in long-term diabetic rats with systemic hypertension. *J. Hypertens.*, 4 (Suppl. 5):S248–S250.

97. Pacy, P. J., Dodson, P. M., Kubicki, A. J., Fletcher, R. F., and Taylor, K. G. (1984): Comparison of the hypotensive and metabolic effects of bendrofluazide therapy and high fibre, low fat, low sodium diet in diabetic subjects with mild hypertension. *J. Hypertens.*, 2:215–220.

98. Parving, H. H., Andersen, A. R., Smidt, U. M., Hommel, E., Mathiesen, E. R., and Svendsen, P. A. (1987): Effect of antihypertensive treatment on kidney function in diabetic nephropathy. *Br. Med. J.*, 294:1443–1447.

99. Parving, H. H., Andersen, A. R., Smidt, U. M., Oxenboll, B., Edsberg, B., Christiansen, J. S. (1983): Diabetic nephropathy and arterial hypertension. *Diabetologia*, 24:10–12.

100. Passa, P. (1980): Le traitement de l'hypertension arterielle chez les diabetiques. *Diabete Metab.*, 6:287–298.

101. Passa, P., Bouvier, P., Assan, R., and Canivet, J. (1978): Effects of acebutolol (cardio-selective beta blocker) on insulin-induced hypoglycaemia in diabetic patients. *Diabetologia*, 13:424.

102. Pedersen, M. M., Schmitz, A., Bjerregaard Pedersen, E., Danielsen, H., and Christiansen, J. S. (1988): Acute and long-term renal effects of angiotensin converting enzyme inhibition in normotensive, normoalbuminemic insulin-dependent diabetic patients. *Diabetic Medicine*, 5:562–565.

103. Rabkin, R., Petersen, J., Kitaji, J., Marck, B., Murphy, W., and Muirhead, E. E. (1984): Effect of antihypertensive therapy on the kidney in spontaneously hypertensive rats with diabetes. *Kidney Int.*, 25:205. (abstr.).

104. Ramos, O. L. (1988): Diabetes mellitus and hypertension. *Hypertension*, 11 (Suppl. I):I-14–I-18.

105. Rasch, R. (1981): Studies on the prevention of glomerulopathy in diabetic rats. *Acta Endocrinol.*, (Suppl. 242):43–44.

106. Reubi, F. C., Franz, K. A., and Horber, F. (1985): Hypertension as related to renal function in diabetes mellitus. *Hypertension*, 7 (Suppl. II):II-21–II-28.

107. Ritz, E., and Hasslacher, Ch. (1984): Genesis and treatment of hypertension in diabetes mellitus. *Diab. Nephropathy*, 3:2–8.

108. Ritz, E., Hasslacher, C., Tschope, W., Koch, M., and Mann, J. F. E. (1987): Hypertension in diabetes mellitus. *Contr. Nephrol.*, 54:77–85.

109. Ritz, E., Strumpf, C., Katz, F., Wing, A. J., and Quellhorst, E. (1985): Hypertension and cardiovascular risk factors in hemodialyzed diabetic patients. *Hypertension*, 7 (Suppl. II):II-118–II-124.

110. Ruilope, L. M., Miranda, B., Morales, J. M., Rodicio, J. L., Romero, J. C., and Raij, L. (1989): Converting enzyme inhibition in chronic renal failure. *Am. J. Kidney Dis.*, 13:120–126.

111. Schweitzer, G., and Gertz, K. H. (1979): Changes of hemodynamics and ultrafiltration in renal hypertension of rats. *Kidney Int.*, 15:134–143.

112. Seyer-Hansen, K., Hansen, J., and Gundersen, H. S. G. (1980): Renal hypertrophy in experimental diabetes: A morphometric study. *Diabetologia*, 18:501–505.

113. Skillman, T. G. (1986): Pitfalls of antihypertensive drugs in diabetes. In: *New Concepts in Diabetes Management*, edited by Siperstein, M. D., pp. 3–14. Vol. 6. HP Publishing Co., New York.

114. Steffes, M. W., Brown, D. M., and Mauer, S. M. (1978): Diabetic glomerulopathy following unilateral nephrectomy in the rat. *Diabetes*, 27:35–41.

115. Struthers, A. D., Murphy, M. B., and Dollery, C. T. (1985): Glucose tolerance during antihypertensive therapy in patients with diabetes mellitus. *Hypertension*, 7 (Suppl. II):II-95–II-101.

116. Taguma, Y., Kitamoto, Y., Futaki, G., Ueda, H., Monma, H., Ishikazi, M., Takahashi, H., Sekino, H., and Sasaki, Y. (1985): Effect of cap-

topril on heavy proteinuria in azotemic diabetics. *N. Engl. J. Med.*, 313:1617–1620.

117. Textor, S. C., Bravo, E. L., Fouad, F. M., and Tarazi, R. C. (1982): Hyperkalemia in azotemic patients during angiotensin-converting enzyme inhibition and aldosterone reduction with captopril. *Am. J. Med.*, 73:719–725.

118. Trevisan, M., Vaccaro, O., Laurenzi, M., de Chiara, F., di Muro, M., Iacone, R., and Franzese, A. (1988): Hypertension, non-insulin-dependent diabetes, and intracellular sodium metabolism. *Hypertension*, 11:264–268.

119. Trost, B. N., and Weidmann, P. (1984): Effects of nitrendipine and other calcium antagonists on glucose metabolism in man. *J. Cardiovasc. Pharmacol.*, 6:S986–S995.

120. Trost, B. N., Weidmann, P., and Beretta-Piccoli, C. (1985): Antihypertensive therapy in diabetic patients. *Hypertension*, 7 (Suppl. II):II-102–II-108.

121. United Kingdom Prospective Diabetes Study. (1985): III. Prevalence of hypertension and hypotensive therapy in patients with newly diagnosed diabetes: A multicenter study. *Hypertension*, 7 (Suppl. II):II-8–II-13.

122. Viberti, G. C., Keen, H., and Wiseman, M. J. (1987): Raised arterial pressure in parents of proteinuric insulin dependent diabetics. *Br. Med. J.*, 295:515–517.

123. Vierhapper, H. (1985): Effect of exogenous insulin on blood pressure regulation in healthy and diabetic subjects. *Hypertension*, 7 (Suppl. II):II-49–II-53.

124. Waal-Manning, H. J. (1976): Metabolic effects of β-adrenoreceptor blockers. *Drugs*, 11 (Suppl. 1):121–126.

125. Waal-Manning, H. J. (1979): Can beta blockers be used in diabetic patients? *Drugs*, 17:157–160.

126. Walker, W. G., Hermann, J., and Yin, D. P. (1987): Hypertension and diuretic Rx as risk factor for diabetic nephropathy. *Proc. Xth Int. Congr. Nephrol.*, 37. (abstr.)

127. Watkins, P. J., Blainey, J. D., Brewer, D. B., Fitzgerald, M. G., Malins, J. M., O'Sullivan, D. J., and Pinto, J. A. (1972): The natural history of diabetic renal disease. *Quarterly J. Med. New Series*, XLI, 164:437–456.

128. Weber, A. B. (1986): Red-cell lithium-sodium countertransport and renal lithium clearance in hypertension. *N. Engl. J. Med.*, 314:198–201.

129. Weidmann, P. (1980): Recent pathogenic aspects in essential hypertension and hypertension

associated with diabetes mellitus. *Klin. Wschr.*, 58:1071–1089.

130. Weidmann, P., Betetta-Piccoli, C., and Trost, B. N. (1985): Pressor factors and responsiveness in hypertension accompanying diabetes mellitus. *Hypertension*, 7 (Suppl. II):II-33–II-42.

131. Weidmann, P., Gerber, A., and Mordasini, R. (1983): Effects of antihypertensive therapy on serum lipoproteins. *Hypertension*, 5 (Suppl. III):III-120–III-131.

132. Weinberger, M. H. (1982): Comparison of captopril and hydrochlorothiazide alone and in combination in mild to moderate essential hypertension. *Brit. J. Clin. Pharmacol.*, 14:127S–131S.

133. Weinberger, M. H. (1985): Antihypertensive therapy and lipids: Evidence, mechanisms, and implications. *Arch. Intern. Med.*, 145:1102–1105.

134. Wen, S.-F., Huang, T.-P., and Moorthy, A. V. (1985): Effects of low protein diet on experimental diabetic nephropathy in the rat. *J. Lab. Clin. Med.*, 106:589–597.

135. Wiseman, M. J., Viberti, G. C., Mackintosh, D., Jarrett, R. J., and Keen, H. (1984): Glycaemia, arterial pressure and microalbuminuria in type I insulin-dependent diabetes mellitus. *Diabetologia*, 26:401–405.

136. Wright, A. D., Barber, S. G., Kenall, M. J., and Poole, P. H. (1979): Beta-adrenreceptor-blocking drugs and blood sugar control in diabetes mellitus. *Br. Med. J.*, 278:159–161.

137. Zanella, M. T., Salgado, B. J. L., Kohlman, O., Jr., and Ribeiro, A. B. (1987): Converting enzyme inhibition: A therapeutical option for diabetic hypertensive patients. *Hypertension*, 9:543. (abstr.)

138. Zatz, R., Dunn, B. R., Meyer, T. W., Anderson, S., Rennke, H. G., and Brenner, B. M. (1986): Prevention of diabetic glomerulopathy by pharmacological amelioration of glomerullar capillary hypertension. *J. Clin. Invest.*, 77:1925–1930.

139. Zatz, R., Meyer, T. W., Rennke, H. G., and Brenner, B. M. (1985): Predominance of hemodynamic rather than metabolic factors in the pathogenesis of diabetic glomerulopathy. *Proc. Nat. Acad. Sci. (USA)*, 82:5963–5967.

140. Zeller, K. R., Jacobson, H., and Raskin, P. (1987): The effect of dietary protein modification on renal function in diabetic nephropathy: Preliminary report of an ongoing study. *Kidney Int.*, 31:225A (abstr).

Subject Index

A

A–64,662, 126
Acebutolol, 72–74
  black patient, 74
  comparative studies, 73
  diabetes, 299
  dose interval studies, 73
  elderly patient, 74
  lipids, 74, 92
  lipoprotein, 92
  pharmacologic properties, 72, 92
  renal effects, 261
  salt effects, 261
  trials vs. placebo, 72–73
  vs. atenolol, 73–74
  vs. hydrochlorothiazide, 73
  vs. mefruside, 74
  vs. nitrendipine, 74
  vs. propranolol, 73
  water effects, 261
Acute inflammatory disease
  alpha blocker, 62
  prazosin, 62
Adenosine receptor agonist, 1341–135
Aging, 115. *See also* Elderly patient
  arterial wall, 213
  drug withdrawal, 174
  hypertension characteristics, 213–215
Alcohol, 10
  stroke, 10
Aldosterone, 101–102
Alpha–1-adrenergic blocker
  low-renin hypertension, 163
  renal effects, 265–270
Alpha–2 receptor agonist, pregnancy, 237–238
Alpha-adrenergic antagonist, diabetes, 300
Alpha-adrenergic receptor, clonidine, 34
Alpha blocker, 51–63
  acute inflammatory disease, 62
  asthma, 61
  central hemodynamics, 51
  co-existing diseases, 59–62
  congestive heart failure, 59–60
  diabetes, 61–62
  dosages, 57–58
  dose effect relationship, 58
  drug interactions, 62–63
  efficacy, 57–58
  elderly patient, 59, 222–223
  kidney failure, 61
  lipid, 53–57

  lipoprotein, 53–57
  peripheral hemodynamics, 53
  plasma renin activity level, 165
  pregnancy, 59
  renal failure, 60
  response determinants, 58
  response predictors, 58
  selective action, 165
  side effects, 57
Alpha receptor, subtypes, 51
Alpha-receptor blocking agent, pregnancy, 239
Amiloride, 19, 27–28
Angiotensin, 144–146
Angiotensin converting enzyme inhibitor, 97–107, 127
  beta blocker, 84
  blood pressure, 99
  calcium channel blocker, 103
  cardiac output, 99
  cardiovascular disorder, 205
  central nervous system, 102
  cerebrovascular disease, 105
  clinical use, 102–103
  co-therapy, 102–103
  congestive heart failure, 105, 203, 205
  coronary heart disease, 105
  development, 97–98
  diabetes, 105
  diuretics, 102–103
  dosage, 106
  heart rate, 99
  hemodynamic effects, 99–100
  hypertensive emergency, 183
  mechanisms of action, 101–102
  metabolic effects, 106
  monotherapy, 102
  peripheral nervous system, 102
  peripheral vascular disease, 105
  pharmacokinetics, 98–99
  pregnancy, 105, 240–241
  pulmonary disease, 105
  quality of life, 107
  regional blood flow, 99–100
  renal effects, 276–280
  renal failure, 104
  renin-angiotensin system, 100–101
  renovascular hypertension, 102–104
  side effects, 106–107
  treatment initiation, 106
Angiotensin I, 144

Angiotensin I converting enzyme inhibitor, 128
    diabetes, 301
Angiotensin II, 97, 101, 144
    diabetes, 290
Angiotensin II receptor antagonist, 127–129
Aortic aneurysm, threatened rupture, 190
Aortic dissection
    beta blocker, 204–205
    central sympatholytics, 203, 204
Apamin, 131
Appointment keeping, 2
Arrhythmia, 203
Arterial baroreflex, calcium blocker, 117
Arterial wall, aging vs. hypertension, 213
Aspartic proteinase family, 125
Asthma, alpha blocker, 61
Atenolol, 74–77
    elderly patient, 76
    hypertensive emergency, 183
    lipids, 76–77, 92
    lipoprotein, 92
    pharmacologic properties, 72, 92
    pregnancy, 238–239
    renal effects, 261, 262
    salt effects, 261
    severe hypertension, 184
    side effects, 76
    urgent hypertension, 187, 188
    vs. alpha-blocking agents, 75–76
    vs. angiotensin-converting enzyme inhibitor, 75
    vs. captopril, 75
    vs. doxazosin, 75–76
    vs. lisinopril, 75
    vs. nifedipine, 75
    vs. verapamil, 75
    water effects, 261
Atopic airways disease, prazosin, 61
Atrial natriuretic factor, 200
Atrial natriuretic peptide
    blood pressure, 145
    electrolyte homeostasis, 145
    mechanism of action, 131
    modulators, 129–130
    properties, 129
Australian National Blood Pressure Study, 215
Autoregulation, 191–192

B
Balloon angioplasty, 159
Baroreceptor abnormality, 200
Baroreflex mechanism, clonidine, 35
Behavior modification, 2
Bendroflumethiazide, 19
Benzthiazide, 19
Beta blocker, 71–93
    angiotensin converting enzyme inhibitor, 84

    aortic dissection, 204–205
    calcium-entry blocker, 84
    cardiovascular disorder, 204–205
    clinical effects, 42
    clinical range, 42
    combination therapy, 84
    coronary artery disease, 204–205
    diabetes, 299–300
    elderly patient, 84, 223–224
    high-renin hypertension, 162–163
    lipids, 84–85
    low-renin hypertension, 163
    pharmacodynamic properties, 72
    plasma renin activity level, 165
    prazosin, 62
    pregnancy, 238
    proposed mechanisms, 71, 72
    renal effects, 255–265
    selective action, 165
    trial evaluation, 71–72
    vs. alpha-blocking agents, 84
    vs. thiazides, 19–20
Betaloc, 83–84
    vs. diuretics, 83–84
Bevantolol, 77
    diuretics, 77
    pharmacodynamic properties, 72
    vs. atenolol, 77
Bisoprolol, 78
    dose-finding studies, 78
    lipids, 78, 92
    lipoprotein, 92
    pharmacodynamic properties, 72
    pharmacologic properties, 92
    vs. atenolol, 78
Black patient
    acebutolol, 74
    diltiazem, 120
    diuretics, 20
    drug withdrawal, 174–175
    nicardipine, 120
    nifedipine, 120
    nitrendipine, 120
    sectral, 74
    thiazides, 20
    verapamil, 120
Blocadren, 91
    bendrofluazide, 91
    combination therapy, 91
    diuretics, 91
    vs. hydrochlorothiazide, 91
Blood pressure
    angiotensin converting enzyme inhibitor, 99
    atrial natriuretic peptide, 145
    renin-angiotensin-aldosterone system, 145
BM 14190, 80
    vs. metroprolol, 80

Bopindolol, 78–79
  dose-finding studies, 79
  lipids, 79, 92
  lipoprotein, 92
  pharmacologic properties, 92
Bradycardia, 203
Bradykinin, 102
BRL 34,915, 130, 132
BTS–49465, 135, 136
Bucindolol, 79–80
  chronic effects, 79
  pharmacodynamic properties, 72
  vs. hydrochlorothiazide, 79–80
  vs. oxprenolol, 80
Bumetanide, 19, 27
BW A575C, 127, 128

C
Caffeine, 10
Calcium
  high-renin hypertension, 153–156
  hypotensive action, 9
  low-renin hypertension, 153–156
  supplementation, 8–9
  vasoconstriction, 153–156
Calcium antagonist, 115–121
  angiotensin converting enzyme inhibitor, 103
  beta blocker, 84
  cardiovascular disorder, 205–206
  coronary artery disease, 203, 205–206
  diabetes, 300–301
  elderly patient, 224–225
  hypertensive emergency, 193–195
  peripheral vascular disease, 203, 205–206
  plasma renin activity level, 165
  pregnancy, 241
  selective action, 165
  urgent hypertension, 183–187
Calcium blocker
  arterial baroreflex, 117
  elderly patient, 115–121
    cardiovascular counter-regulation, 118
  low-renin hypertension
  mode of action, 117–118
  pathophysiological antihypertensive
    response rationale, 115–117
  prognosticators, 115
  renal effects, 273–276
Capillary arteriole, 254
Captopril
  diabetes, 301
  elderly patient, 222
  high-renin hypertension, 162
  pharmacokinetics, 98–99
  pregnancy, 240–241
  renal effects, 277, 278
  salt effects, 277

  urgent hypertension, 187, 188
  water effects, 277
Captopril test, 159–161
  evaluation, 161
  plasma-renin response, 160, 161
  procedures, 161
Cardiac hypertrophy, angiotensin converting
    enzyme inhibitor, 104
Cardiac output, angiotensin converting
    enzyme inhibitor, 99
Cardiovascular complications, 1, 2
  decreased risk, 2
Cardiovascular disorder
  angiotensin converting enzyme inhibitor, 205
  antihypertensive therapy, 203–207
  beta-blocker, 204–205
  calcium antagonist, 205–206
  central sympatholytics, 204
  diuretics, 203–204, 207
  hypertension, 199–207
  vasodilator agent, 205
Carteolol, pharmacodynamic properties, 72
Carvedilol, 80
  pharmacodynamic properties, 72
  vs. metroprolol, 80
Catecholamine
  guanabenz, 37
  reserpine, 40
Celiprolol, 80–81
  lipids, 92
  lipoprotein, 92
  pharmacologic properties, 92
  vs. placebo, 80–81
  vs. propranolol, 81
Central nervous system, angiotensin
    converting enzyme inhibitor, 102
Central sympatholytics
  aortic dissection, 203, 204
  cardiovascular disorder, 204
Centrally acting antihypertensive agent, 33–46
  alternative delivery systems, 43–44
  clinical effects, 41–43, 42
  clinical range, 42
  diuretics, 41–42
  elderly patient, 44–45
  indications, 33
  left ventricular hypertrophy, 45–46
  pharmacology, 33
  side effects, 33
Cerebral autoregulation, 191
Cerebrovascular disease, angiotensin
    converting enzyme inhibitor, 105
cGMP, 135–136
CGP 38560, 126
Chicago Stroke Study, 215
Chlorothiazide, 17, 19
Chlorthalidone, 19
  elderly patient, 45, 220

Cholesterol
    diuretics, 24–26
    thiazides, 24–26
Circulation
    adrenergic regulation, 116
    angiotensinergic regulation, 116
Clonidine, 34–36
    alpha-adrenergic receptor, 34
    alternative delivery systems, 43–44
    atrial emptying index, 46
    baroreflex mechanism, 35
    diabetes, 300
    drawbacks, 166
    elderly patient, 45, 221
    hemodynamic effects, 36
    hypertensive emergency, 196
    left ventricular hypertrophy, 46
    maximum dose, 41
    prazosin, 42–43
    pregnancy, 237–238
    presynaptic receptor, 34
    propranolol, 42, 43
    range, 41
    renal effects, 268, 269
    renin-angiotensin-aldosterone system, 35
    salt effects, 268
    side effects, 34, 36
    skin reaction, 44
    starting dose, 41
    transdermal, 43–44
        advantages, 44
        clinical range, 44
        efficacy, 44
    urgent hypertension, 187
    water effects, 268
Compensated hypertrophy, 189–190
Compound 9, 135–136
Concor, 78
    dose-finding studies, 78
    lipids, 78
    vs. atenolol, 78
Conduction abnormality, 203
Congenital heart disease, 3
Congestive heart failure, 189–190, 202
    alpha blocker, 59–60
    angiotensin converting enzyme inhibitor,
        203, 205
    diastolic dysfunction, 190
    diuretics, 203–204
    high-renin hypertension, 152–153
    low-renin hypertension, 152–153
    myocardial dilation, 190
    prazosin, 59–60
    systolic dysfunction, 190
    vasodilator agent, 203, 205
Converting enzyme inhibitor, 148–149
    elderly patient, 222
    high-renin hypertension, 162

    low-renin hypertension, 163
    medium-renin hypertension, 164
    plasma renin activity level, 165
    selective action, 165
Corgard, 85
    combination therapy, 85
    diuretics, 85
    vs. placebo, 85
    vs. prazosin, 85
Coronary artery disease, 201–202
    beta blocker, 204–205
    calcium antagonist, 203, 205–206
Coronary autoregulation, myocardial ischemia,
        191–192
Coronary heart disease
    angiotensin converting enzyme inhibitor, 105
    diuretics, 17
    exercise, 11
    thiazides, 17
Cortical collecting duct, 28
Cromakalim, 130, 132
Cushing's syndrome, 161

D
Diabetes
    acebutolol, 299
    alpha-adrenergic antagonist, 300
    alpha blocker, 61–62
    angiotensin converting enzyme inhibitor, 105
    angiotensin I converting enzyme inhibitor,
        301
    angiotensin II, 290
    beta blocker, 62, 299–300
    calcium channel blocker, 300–301
    captopril, 301
    clonidine, 300
    diuretics, 299
    guanabenz, 300
    hyperkalemia, 300
    hypertension, 289–302
        diabetic glomerulopathy, 292–298
        diabetic microangiopathy, 291–292
        insulin therapy, 290
        pathogenesis, 290–291
        prevalence, 289–290
        renal failure, 291–292, 293
        treatment, 298
        Type I, 289
        Type II, 289
    labetolol, 300
    methyldopa, 300
    pindolol, 300
    prazosin, 61–62, 300
    propranolol, 62
    renin-angiotensin-aldosterone system, 290
    sympatholytic agent, 300
    thiazides, 62
    vasodilator, 300

Diaminopyridine, 131
Diastolic pressure
    90 to 105 mmHg, 1
        nonpharmacologic therapy, 5
    above 105 mmHg, 1
    low, complications, 3
    risk, 141–142
Diazoxide, 194
    hypertensive emergency, 193, 194
    pregnancy, 240
Digital subtraction angiography, 160
Dihydralazine, 194
    hypertensive emergency, 193, 194
Dilevalol, 81
    lipids, 92
    lipoprotein, 92
    pharmacodynamic properties, 72
    pharmacologic properties, 92
    vs. placebo, 81
Diltiazem
    black patient, 120
    elderly patient, 120, 224
    low-renin patient, 120
    pregnancy, 241
    renal effects, 274, 275
    salt effects, 274
    urgent hypertension, 183–184
    water effects, 274
Diuretics, 17–29
    angiotensin converting enzyme inhibitor,
        102–103
    benefits, 17–18
    bevantolol, 77
    black patient, 20
    blocadren, 91
    cardiovascular disorder, 203–204, 207
    centrally acting antihypertensive agent, 41–
        42
    cholesterol, 24–26
    clinical effects, 42
    clinical range, 42
    congestive heart failure, 203–204
    corgard, 85
    coronary heart disease, 17
    diabetes, 299
    diuretic-induced metabolic disturbances, 17
    efficacy, 17, 19–20
    elderly patient, 20, 118, 219–220
    extracelular fluid volume, 18
    glucose intolerance, 23–24
    hypercholesterolemia, 24–26
    hyperuricemia, 23
    hypokalemia, 21
    hypomagnesemia, 23
    inderal, 88
    inderide, 88
    indications, 28–29
    iset, 86

labetalol, 81–82
    lipids, 24–26
    low-dose therapy, 17
    low-renin hypertension, 163
    magnesium, 23
    mechanism of action, 18–20
    metabolic effects, 20–21, 26
    nadolol, 85
    normodyne, 81–82
    oxprenolol, 86
    pindolol, 87
    plasma renin activity level, 165
    potassium, 20–23
    pregnancy, 234–236
    propranolol, 88
    ranestol, 77
    selective action, 165
    side effects, 20–26, 26
    timolide, 91
    timolol, 91
    trandate, 81–82
    trasicor, 86
    triglyceride, 24–26
    ventrical premature beat, 21
    visken, 87
Dopamine receptor agonist, 132–134
    subtypes, 132
Doxazosin
    dosages, 57–58
    dose effect relationship, 58
    efficacy, 57
    elderly patient, 59
    hemodynamic effects, 52
    lipid, 53, 54
    renal function, 55
    response determinants, 58
    response predictors, 58
    side effects, 57
    total peripheral resistance, 51
Drowsiness, 33
    methyldopa, 40
Drug withdrawal, 171–179
    age, 174
    antihypertensive therapy duration, 175
    black patient, 174–175
    cardioprotective effect loss, 178
    clinical characteristics, 175
    demographic factors, 174–175
    economic advantages, 178–179
    follow-up, 173, 174
    hazards, 177–178
    loss to follow-up, 177
    medical advantages, 178
    natural history hypothesis, 177
    normotension mechanism, 176–177
        baroreceptor resetting, 176
        structural regression, 176–177
    nutritional interventions, 175–176

Drug withdrawal (*contd.*)
    percentage successful, 173
    pretreatment blood pressure level, 175
    race, 174–175
    rationale, 171
    sodium, 175
    studies, 171–173
    withdrawal syndrome, 177–178
Dry mouth, 33
DU 29,373, 133, 134

E
Edema, 242
Elderly patient, 211–225. *See also* Aging
    acebutolol, 74
    alpha blocker, 59, 222–223
    atenolol, 76
    beta blocker, 84, 223–224
    calcium blocker, 115–121
        cardiovascular counter-regulation, 118
    calcium channel blocker, 224–225
    captopril, 222
    cardiovascular hemodynamics, 214
    centrally acting antihypertensive agent, 44–
        45
    chlorthalidone, 45, 220
    clonidine, 45, 221
    converting enzyme inhibitor, 222
    diltiazem, 120, 224
    diuretics, 20, 118, 219–220
    doxazosin, 59
    enalapril, 222
    evaluation, 218–219
    ganglionic blocking agent, 223
    guanabenz, 45, 221
    guanadrel, 223
    guanethidine, 223
    guanfacine, 221
    humoral findings, 214
    hydralazine, 222
    hydrochlorothiazide, 223
    hypertension characteristics, 213–215
    hypertension definition, 211–212
    hypertension prevalence, 212–213
    hypertension risks, 215
    hypokalemia, 220
    inderal, 90
    inderide, 90
    labetalol, 223
    methyldopa, 40, 45, 221
    metoprolol, 223
    nicardipine, 120
    nifedipine, 120, 224
    nitrendipine, 120
    non-drug therapies, 219
    pharmacotherapy, 219–225
    pindolol, 223
    placebo therapy, 219
    prazosin, 59, 222
    propranolol, 90
    reserpine, 221–222
    sectral, 74
    side effects, 221
    tenormin, 76
    terazosin, 59, 222
    thiazides, 20, 221
    treatment benefits, 215, 218
    treatment contraindications, 218
    treatment indications, 218
    verapamil, 120, 224
Electrolyte homeostasis
    atrial natriuretic peptide, 145
    renin-angiotensin-aldosterone system, 145
Enalapril
    elderly patient, 222
    high-renin hypertension, 162
    pharmacokinetics, 98–99
    renal effects, 277–279
    salt effects, 279
    water effects, 279
Endothelium-derived relaxing factor, 135
ES-305, 126
Esmolol
    hypertensive emergency, 195
    pharmacodynamic properties, 72
Essential hypertension
    high-renin hypertension, 152
    low-renin hypertension, 152
Ethacrynic acid, 19, 27
Ethanol, 10
    stroke, 10
European Working Party on High Blood
        Pressure in the Elderly, 215–217
Exercise, 10–11
    coronary heart disease, 11
    hyperinsulinemia, 10
    insulin, 6, 10
    isometric, 11
    isotonic, 10
    weight loss, 6, 11
Extracellular fluid volume
    diuretics, 18
    thiazides, 18

F
Fat, 9–10
Fenoldopam, 132–134
Fish oil, 9–10
Flosequinan, 135, 136
Fluoxetine, 7
Framingham Heart Study, 215
Furosemide, 19, 27, 194
    hypertensive emergency, 194, 195

G

Ganglionic blocking agent, elderly patient, 223
Glucose intolerance
    diuretics, 23–24
    thiazides, 23–24
Goldblatt hypertension
    high-renin hypertension, 149–151
    low-renin hypertension, 148–151
Guanabenz, 36–37
    catecholamine, 37
    competitive binding studies, 36
    diabetes, 300
    drawbacks, 166
    elderly patient, 45, 221
    hemodynamic effects, 36
    left ventricular hypertrophy, 46
    maximum dose, 41
    mechanism of action, 36
    metabolic effects, 37
    range, 41
    renal effects, 268, 269
    renal function, 37
    salt effects, 268
    side effects, 36
    starting dose, 41
    water effects, 268
Guanadrel
    elderly patient, 223
    renal effects, 271–272
    salt effects, 272
    water effects, 272
Guanethidine
    drawbacks, 166
    elderly patient, 223
    renal effects, 271
    salt effects, 271
    water effects, 271
Guanfacine, 37–38
    elderly patient, 221
    hemodynamic effects, 36
    maximum dose, 41
    range, 41
    renal effects, 268
    salt effects, 270
    side effects, 36
    starting dose, 41
    water effects, 270

H

H–142, 126
Heart
    diastolic abnormality, 200
    systolic abnormality, 200
Heart Attack Primary Prevention in
    Hypertension, 23–24
Heart rate, angiotensin converting enzyme
    inhibitor, 99

High-fiber diet, 9
High-renin hypertension, 145–153
    beta blocker, 162–163
    calcium, 153–156
    captopril, 162
    clinical examples, 147
    congestive heart failure, 152–153
    converting enzyme inhibitor, 162
    drug therapy, 162–163
    enalapril, 162
    essential hypertension, 152
    Goldblatt hypertension, 149–151
    malignant hypertension, 151–152
    MK–422, 154
    nephrotic syndrome, 153
    pathophysiology differences, 147
    renovascular hypertension, 151–152
    saralasin, 148
    sodium, 154–156
    treatments, 147
    vascular sequelae, 147
Hydralazine, 194
    chronic renal effects, 272
    drawbacks, 166
    elderly patient, 222
    hypertensive emergency, 193, 194
    pregnancy, 239, 239–240
    salt effects, 272
    water effects, 272
Hydrochlorothiazide, 19
    elderly patient, 223
Hypercalcuria, 9
Hypercholesterolemia
    diuretics, 24–26
    thiazides, 24–26
Hyperinsulinemia, 6
    exercise, 10
Hyperkalemia, diabetes, 300
Hypertension. *See also* Specific type
    cardiovascular characteristics, 199–201
    cardiovascular disorder, 199–207
    clinical heterogeneity, 141–142
    diabetes, 289–302
        diabetic glomerulopathy, 292–298
        diabetic microangiopathy, 291–292
        insulin therapy, 290
        pathogenesis, 290–291
        prevalence, 289–290
        renal failure, 291–292, 293
        treatment, 298
        Type I, 289
        Type II, 289
    diagnosis, 1–2
    emergency. *See* Hypertensive emergency
    endocrinologic heterogeneity, 142–143
    etiology, alcohol, 10
    female patient, 1
    high-renin. *See* High-renin hypertension

Hypertension (*contd.*)
    identifying curable forms, 158–161
    low-renin. *See* Low-renin hypertension
    pharmacologic heterogeneity, 142
    prevention, weight loss, 7
    renal function, natural course, 254
    severe. *See* Severe hypertension
    therapy
        drop-out, 2
        goals, 2, 3
        renal function effects, 253–280
        strategies, 2–3
    treatment
        goals, 158
        strategy, 157–166
    urgent. *See* Urgent hypertension
Hypertension Detection and Follow-Up
        Program, 175–176, 215
Hypertensive emergency, 187–190
    angiotensin enzyme inhibitor, 183
    atenolol, 183
    calcium antagonist, 193–195
    clonidine, 196
    diazoxide, 193, 194
    dihydralazine, 193, 194
    esmolol, 195
    furosemide, 194, 195
    hydralazine, 193, 194
    intravenous agents, 192–196
    ketanserin, 196
    labetalol, 183, 192–193, 194
    nifedipine, 183
    nitrate, 193
    nitroprusside, 193, 194
    pregnancy, 244, 245
        hydralazine, 244
        sodium nitroprusside, 244
    propranolol, 195
    reserpine, 195–196
    sodium nitroprusside, 193, 194
    urapidil, 196
    verapamil, 193–195
Hypertensive encephalopathy, 187–189
Hyperuricemia
    diuretics, 23
    thiazides, 23
Hypokalemia
    diuretics, 21
    elderly patient, 220
    thiazides, 20–21
        mechanism, 21
    treatment, 22–23
    ventricular arrhythymia, 21–22
Hypomagnesemia
    diuretics, 23
    thiazides, 23
Hypotension, drug-induced, 191

I
Imidazole derivative, 129
Indapamide, 19, 26–27
    lipids, 27
    mechanisms, 26–27
    side effects, 27
Inderal, 89–90
    combination therapy, 89
    diuretics, 88
    elderly patient, 90
    lipids, 90
    quality of life, 89–90
    vs. angiotensin-converting enzyme
        inhibitors, 88–90
    vs. atenolol, 88
    vs. calcium-entry blockers, 89
    vs. diltiazem, 89
    vs. metoprolol, 88
    vs. nifedepine, 89
    vs. oxprenolol, 88
    vs. prazosin, 89
    vs. verapamil, 89
Inderide, 89–90
    combination therapy, 89
    diuretics, 88
    elderly patient, 90
    lipids, 90
    quality of life, 89–90
    vs. angiotensin-converting enzyme
        inhibitors, 88–90
    vs. atenolol, 88
    vs. calcium-entry blockers, 89
    vs. diltiazem, 89
    vs. metoprolol, 88
    vs. nifedepine, 89
    vs. oxprenolol, 88
    vs. prazosin, 89
    vs. verapamil, 89
Inflammatory disease, acute, 62
Insulin
    exercise, 6, 10
    weight reduction, 6
Intravenous load reduction, 190
Intrinsic sympathomimetic activity, 71
Iset, 86
    combination therapy, 86
    diuretics, 86
    lipids, 86
    vs. calcium-entry blockers, 86
    vs. nitrendipine, 86
Isradipine, 131

K
Ketanserin, 131–132, 133
    hypertensive emergency, 196
Kidney, 143–144
    failure, alpha blocker, 61

L
Labetalol, 81–83, 194
  diabetes, 300
  diuretics, 81–82
  dose-ranging studies, 81
  elderly patient, 82, 223
  hypertensive emergency, 183, 192–193, 194
  lipids, 83, 92
  lipoprotein, 92
  pharmacodynamic properties, 72
  pharmacologic properties, 92
  renal effects, 261, 264
  salt effects, 261
  severe hypertension, 184
  side effects, 83
  urgent hypertension, 187, 188
  vs. atenolol, 82
  vs. hydrochlorothiazide, 82
  vs. nifedipine, 82
  vs. prazosin, 82
  water effects, 261
Left ventricular hypertrophy
  centrally acting antihypertensive agent, 45–46
  clonidine, 46
  guanabenz, 46
  methyldopa, 45–46
Left ventricular systolic function, abnormal, 10
Lipids, 206
  acebutolol, 74, 92
  alpha blocker, 53–57
  atenolol, 76–77, 92
  beta blocker, 84–85
  bisoprolol, 78, 92
  bopindolol, 79, 92
  celiprolol, 92
  concor, 78
  dilevalol, 92
  diuretics, 24–26
  doxazosin, 53, 54
  indapamide, 27
  inderal, 90
  inderide, 90
  iset, 86
  labetalol, 83, 92
  metaprolol, 92
  normodyne, 83
  oxprenolol, 86, 92
  pindolol, 87–88, 92
  propranolol, 90, 92
  sandonorm, 79
  sectral, 74
  tenormin, 76–77
  terazosin, 53, 54
  thiazides, 24–26
  trandate, 83
  trasicor, 86

  visken, 87–88
Lipoprotein
  acebutolol, 92
  alpha blocker, 53–57
  atenolol, 92
  bisoprolol, 92
  bopindolol, 92
  celiprolol, 92
  dilevalol, 92
  labetalol, 92
  metoprolol, 92
  oxprenolol, 92
  pindolol, 92
  propranolol, 92
Lisinopril, 84
  pharmacokinetics, 99
  renal effects, 278, 279
  salt effects, 279
  water effects, 279
Loop diuretics, 27
  indications, 27
Lopressor, 83–84
  vs. diuretics, 83–84
Low-renin hypertension, 146–153
  alpha–1-adrenergic blocker, 163
  beta blocker, 163
  calcium, 153–156
  calcium blocker
  clinical examples, 147
  congestive heart failure, 152–153
  converting enzyme inhibitor, 163
  diuretics, 163
  drug therapy, 163–164
  essential hypertension, 152
  Goldblatt hypertension, 148–151
  malignant hypertension, 151–152
  MK–422, 154
  nephrotic syndrome, 153
  pathophysiology differences, 147
  renovascular hypertension, 151–152
  saralasin, 148
  sodium, 148–149, 154–156
  treatments, 147
  vascular sequelae, 147
Low-renin patient
  diltiazem, 120
  nicardipine, 120
  nifedipine, 120
  nitrendipine, 120
  verapamil, 120

M
Magnesium
  diuretics, 9, 23
  supplementation, 9–10
  thiazides, 9, 23

Malignant hypertension
  high-renin hypertension, 151–152
  low-renin hypertension, 151–152
Medical Research Council study, 88, 172–173
Medium-renin hypertension
  converting enzyme inhibitor, 164
  drug therapy, 164–166
    empiric process, 164, 165
Membrane-stabilizing activity, 71
Mentation, methyldopa, 40
Methylclothiazide, 19
Methyldopa, 38–40
  diabetes, 300
  drawbacks, 166
  drowsiness, 40
  elderly patient, 40, 45, 221
  hemodynamic effects, 36
  left ventricular hypertrophy, 45–46
  maximum dose, 41
  mentation, 40
  norepinephrine, 39
  periperhal action, 39
  positive direct Coomb's test, 40
  pregnancy, 237, 241–242
  range, 41
  renal effects, 268, 269
  salt effects, 268
  side effects, 36
  as single-agent therapy, 39–40
  starting dose, 41
  water effects, 268
Metolazone, 19
Metoprolol, 83–84, 84
  elderly patient, 223
  lipids, 92
  lipoprotein, 92
  pharmacodynamic properties, 72
  pharmacologic properties, 92
  pregnancy, 239
  renal effects, 261, 263
  salt effects, 261
  vs. diuretics, 83–84
  water effects, 261
Minoxidil, 130
  drawbacks, 166
  renal effccts, 272–273
  salt effects, 273
  water effects, 273
MK–422
  high-renin hypertension, 154
  low-renin hypertension, 154
Monoclonal antirenin antibody, 125–126
Multiple Risk Factor Intervention Trial, 17
Myocardial dilation, congestive heart failure,
    190
Myocardial infarction, 57
  antihypertensive therapy, 207
Myocardial ischemia, coronary autoregulation,
    191–192

N
Nadolol, 85
  combination therapy, 85
  diuretics, 85
  pharmacodynamic properties, 72
  renal effects, 255, 256
  salt effects, 255–257
  vs. placebo, 85
  vs. prazosin, 85
  water effects, 255–257
National Health and Nutrition Examination
    Survey, 212
Nephrotic syndrome
  high-renin hypertension, 153
  low-renin hypertension, 153
Nicardipine
  black patient, 120
  elderly patient, 120
  low-renin patient, 120
Nifedipine
  black patient, 120
  elderly patient, 120, 224
  hypertensive emergency, 183
  low-renin patient, 120
  prazosin, 62
  pregnancy, 241
  renal effects, 274, 275
  salt effects, 274
  severe hypertension, 184
  urgent hypertension, 184–186, 188
    combined therapy, 186
    resistance, 186
  water effects, 274
Nitrate, hypertensive emergency, 193
Nitrendipine
  black patient, 120
  elderly patient, 120
  low-renin patient, 120
Nitroprusside, 194
  hypertensive emergency, 193, 194
  pregnancy, 240
Nonpharmacologic therapy, 5–12
  rationale, 5
    controlled trials, 5
Norcpinephrine
  methyldopa, 39
  reserpine, 40
Normodyne, 81–83
  combination studies, 82
  diuretics, 81–82
  dose-ranging studies, 81
  elderly patient, 82–83
  lipids, 83
  side effects, 83
  vs. atenolol, 82
  vs. hydrochlorothiazide, 82
  vs. nifedipine, 82
  vs. prazosin, 82
Nutrition, pregnancy, 234

O

Obesity, 206
  distribution, 6
  upper body, 6, 7
Omega–3 fatty acid, 9–10
Oxprenolol, 86
  combination therapy, 86
  diuretics, 86
  lipids, 86, 92
  lipoprotein, 92
  pharmacodynamic properties, 72
  pharmacologic properties, 92
  vs. calcium-entry blockers, 86
  vs. nitrendipine, 86

P

Parathyroid hormone, 9
Patient education, 2
PD 117,519, 134, 135
Penbutolol, pharmacodynamic properties, 72
Pepstatin, 125, 126
Peripheral blood-renin assay, 159
Peripheral nervous system, angiotensin
      converting enzyme inhibitor, 102
Peripheral vascular disease
  angiotensin converting enzyme inhibitor, 105
  calcium antagonist, 203, 205–206
  vasodilator agent, 203, 205
Phenoxybenzamine, 51
Phentolamine, 51
Pheochromocytoma, 51, 161
Pinacidil, 130, 132
Pindolol, 87–88
  combination therapy, 87
  diabetes, 300
  diuretics, 87
  elderly patient, 223
  lipids, 87–88, 92
  lipoprotein, 92
  pharmacologic properties, 72, 92
  pregnancy, 239
  renal effects, 257, 260
  salt effects, 261
  vs. alpha-blocking agents, 87
  vs. calcium-entry blockers, 87
  vs. nifedipine, 87
  water effects, 261
Plasma expansion, pregnancy, 236–237
Plasma-renin value, 159
Plasma volume, pregnancy, 233–234
Polyclonal antirenin antibody, 125–126
Polythiazide, 19
Potassium
  sodium, 8
  supplementation, 8
  thiazides, 20–23
  ventricular ectopy, 22

Potassium efflux stimulator, 130–131
Potassium-sparing diuretics, 27–28
  hyperkalemia, 28
  side effects, 28
Prazosin, 51
  acute inflammatory disease, 62
  atopic airways disease, 61
  beta blocker, 62
  clonidine, 42–43
  congestive heart failure, 59–60
  diabetes, 61–62, 300
  dosages, 57–58
  dose effect relationship, 58
  drug interactions, 62–63
  efficacy, 57
  elderly patient, 59, 222
  hemodynamic effects, 52
  nifedipine, 62
  pregnancy, 59, 239
  renal effects, 266, 267
  renal failure, 60
  renal function, 55
  renin-angiotensin system, 58
  response determinants, 58
  response predictors, 58
  salt effects, 266
  side effects, 57
  total peripheral resistance, 51
  urgent hypertension, 187
  verapamil, 62
  water effects, 266
Preeclampsia
  intravascular volume contraction, 242
  prevention, 242
  severe, 242–244
  treatment, 242
Preeclampsia-eclampsia, 242–244
Pregnancy, 231–247
  activity, 232–233
  alpha–2 receptor agonist, 237–238
  alpha blocker, 59
  alpha-receptor blocking agent, 239
  angiotensin converting enzyme inhibitor,
      105, 240–241
  antihypertensive therapy goals, 244–247
  antihypertensive therapy precautions, 243
  atenolol, 238–239
  beta blocker, 238
  calcium blocking agent, 241
  captopril, 240–241
  classification, 231, 232
  clonidine, 237–238
  diazoxide, 240
  diltiazem, 241
  diuretics, 234–236
  hydralazine, 239, 239–240
  hypertensive emergency, 244, 245
    hydralazine, 244
    sodium nitroprusside, 244

Pregnancy (*contd.*)
  management, 231–241
  methyldopa, 237, 241–242
  metoprolol, 239
  nifedipine, 241
  nitroprusside, 240
  nutrition, 234
  pindolol, 239
  plasma expansion, 236–237
  plasma volume, 233–234
  prazosin, 59, 239
  propranolol, 238, 240
  reserpine, 238
  serotonin receptor antagonist, 241–242
  sodium, 234
  sodium nitroprusside, 240
  sympathetic blocking agent, 238
  teprotide, 240
  urgent hypertension, 244, 245
    hydralazine, 244
    sodium nitroprusside, 244
  vasodilator, 239–240
  verapamil, 241
Presynaptic receptor, clonidine, 34
Primary aldosteronism, diagnosis, 161
Propranolol, 88–90
  atrial emptying index, 46
  clonidine, 42, 43
  combination therapy, 89
  diabetes, 62
  diuretics, 88
  elderly patient, 90
  hypertensive emergency, 195
  lipids, 90, 92
  lipoprotein, 92
  pharmacologic properties, 72, 92
  pregnancy, 238, 240
  quality of life, 89–90
  renal effects, 257, 258–259
  salt effects, 257
  vs. angiotensin-converting enzyme
    inhibitors, 88–90
  vs. atenolol, 88
  vs. calcium-entry blockers, 89
  vs. diltiazem, 89
  vs. metoprolol, 88
  vs. nifedepine, 89
  vs. oxprenolol, 88
  vs. prazosin, 89
  vs. verapamil, 89
  water effects, 257
Prostaglandin, 102
Pulmonary circulation, abnormalities, 201
Pulmonary disease, angiotensin converting
    enzyme inhibitor, 105
Pulmonary edema, acute, 190

Q
Quinethazone, 19
Quinpirole, 132–134

R
R28935, 133, 134
Race, drug withdrawal, 174–175
Ranestol, 77
  diuretics, 77
  vs. atenolol, 77
Reinforcement, 2
Relaxation, 11–12
Renal artery stenosis, 159
  bilateral, 161
Renal autoregulation, renal failure, 191
Renal disease, chronic bilateral, 161
Renal failure, 190
  alpha blocker, 60
  angiotensin converting enzyme inhibitor, 104
  apparent, 190
  prazosin, 60
  renal autoregulation, 191
  true acute deterioration, 190
Renal function
  doxazosin, 55
  hypertension, natural course, 254
  prazosin, 55
Renal vein renin study, 160
Renin, 125, 144
  aspartic acid residues, 125
Renin-angiotensin-aldosterone system
  blood pressure, 145
  clonidine, 35
  diabetes, 290
  electrolyte homeostasis, 145
Renin-angiotensin system, 97
  angiotensin converting enzyme inhibitor,
    100–101
  components, 98
  new antihypertensive drugs, 125–129
  prazosin, 58
Renin inhibitor, 125–127
Renin profile, 161–162
Renin-sodium profile, 159, 161–162
Renin system, 143–145
Renovascular disease, 159–161
Renovascular hypertension
  angiotensin converting enzyme inhibitor,
    102–104
  high-renin hypertension, 151–152
  low-renin hypertension, 151–152
Reserpine
  catecholamine, 40
  drawbacks, 166
  elderly patient, 221–222
  hemodynamic effects, 36

Pregnancy (*contd.*)
  hypertensive emergency, 195–196
  maximum dose, 41
  mechanism, 40–41
  norepinephrine, 40
  pregnancy, 238
  range, 41
  renal effects, 270
  salt effects, 270–271
  serotonin, 40
  side effects, 36
  starting dose, 41
  water effects, 270–271
RIP, 126
Risk, 141–142

S
S 2395, 90–91
  dosage studies, 91
  vs. acebutolol, 91
Sandonorm, 78–79
  dose-finding studies, 79
  lipids, 79
Saralasin, 127, 129
  high-renin hypertension, 148
  low-renin hypertension, 148
SC 32,796, 134, 135
SC 46542, 130
SCRIP, 126
Sectral, 72–74
  black patient, 74
  dose interval studies, 73
  elderly patient, 74
  lipids, 74
  trials vs. placebo, 72–73
  vs. atenolol, 73–74
  vs. hydrochlorothiazide, 73
  vs. mefruside, 74
  vs. nitrendipine, 74
  vs. propranolol, 73
Selectol, 80–81
  vs. placebo, 80–81
  vs. propranolol, 80–81
Serotonergic receptor agonist, 131–132
Serotonergic receptor antagonist, 131–132
Serotonin, reserpine, 40
Serotonin receptor antagonist, pregnancy, 241–242
Severe hypertension, 183–197
  atenolol, 184
  clinical features, 184
  diagnosis, 183
  labetalol, 184
  nifedipine, 184
  significance, 183–184
  urgency vs. emergency, 184

Sex differences, 1–2
SKF 82526, 132–134
Skin reaction, clonidine, 44
Smoking, 12
Sodium
  arterial wall overload, 19
  drug withdrawal, 175
  high-renin hypertension, 154–156
  low-renin hypertension, 148–149, 154–156
  moderate reduction, 8
  potassium, 8
  pregnancy, 234
  vasoconstriction, 153–156
Sodium nitroprusside
  hypertensive emergency, 193, 194
  pregnancy, 240
Sotalol, pharmacodynamic properties, 72
Spironolactone, 19, 27–28
SQ 27,786, 127, 128
SQ 28,853, 127, 128
SQ 29,072, 130
SR 42,128, 126
Statine, 126
Stroke
  alcohol, 10
  ethanol, 10
  incidence, 216
  threatened, 189
Sympathetic blocking agent, pregnancy, 238
Sympathetic nervous system, 33
  vasoconstriction, 158
Sympatholytic agent, diabetes, 300
Systemic vascular resistance, 199
Systemic vasculature, 200–201
Systolic Hypertension in the Elderly Program, 212–213
Systolic pressure, rise during exercise, 10–11

T
Tenormin, 74–77
  elderly patient, 76
  lipids, 76–77
  side effects, 76
  vs. alpha-blocking agents, 75–76
  vs. captopril, 75
  vs. doxazosin, 75–76
  vs. lisinopril, 75
  vs. nifedipine, 75
  vs. verapamil, 75
Teprotide, pregnancy, 240
Terazosin
  dosages, 57–58
  efficacy, 57
  elderly patient, 59, 222
  lipid, 53, 54
  renal effects, 266, 267

Reserpine (contd.)
  salt effects, 266
  side effects, 57
  water effects, 266
Tertatolol, 90–91
  dosage studies, 91
  pharmacodynamic properties, 72
  vs. acebutolol, 91
Tetraethylaminonium, 131
Thiazide, efficacy, 17, 19–20
Thiazides, 17
  benefits, 17–18
  black patient, 20
  cholesterol, 24–26
  coronary heart disease, 17
  diabetes, 62
  diuretic-induced metabolic disturbances, 17
  efficacy, 17
  elderly patient, 20, 221
  extracelular fluid volume, 18
  glucose intolerance, 23–24
  hypercholesterolemia, 24–26
  hyperuricemia, 23
  hypokalemia, 20–21
    mechanism, 21
  hypomagnesemia, 23
  indications, 28–29
  lipids, 24–26
  magnesium, 23
  magnesium deficiency, 9
  mechanism of action, 18–20
  metabolic effects, 20–21, 26
  potassium, 20–23
  side effects, 20–26, 26
  triglyceride, 24–26
  vs. beta-blockers, 19–20
Thyroid disease, 161
Timolide, 91
  bendrofluazide, 91
  combination therapy, 91
  diuretics, 91
  vs. hydrochlorothiazide, 91
Timolol, 91
  bendrofluazide, 91
  chronic renal effects, 257
  combination therapy, 91
  diuretics, 91
  pharmacodynamic properties, 72
  salt effects, 257
  vs. hydrochlorothiazide, 91
  water effects, 257
Total peripheral resistance
  doxazosin, 51
  prazosin, 51
Trandate, 81–83
  diuretics, 81–82
  dose-ranging studies, 81
  elderly patient, 82–83

lipids, 83
  side effects, 83
  vs. atenolol, 82
  vs. hydrochlorothiazide, 82
  vs. nifedipine, 82
  vs. prazosin, 82
Trasicor, 86
  combination therapy, 86
  diuretics, 86
  lipids, 86
  vs. calcium-entry blockers, 86
  vs. nitrendipine, 86
Triamterene, 19, 27–28
Trichlormethiazide, 19
Triglyceride
  diuretics, 24–26
  thiazides, 24–26

U
U71.038, 126
Urapidil, 133, 134
  hypertensive emergency, 196
Urgent hypertension, 184–187
  atenolol, 187, 188
  calcium antagonist, 183–187
  captopril, 187, 188
  clonidine, 187
  diltiazem, 183–184
  follow-up therapy, 187
  labetalol, 187, 188
  nifedipine, 184–186, 188
    combined therapy, 186
    resistance, 186
  prazosin, 187
  pregnancy, 244, 245
    hydralazine, 244
    sodium nitroprusside, 244
  verapamil, 183

V
Valvular heart disease, 203
Vascular disease, 202
Vasoconstriction, 157–158
  angiotensin II, 158
  calcium, 153–156
  low-plasma-renin value, 158
  mechanisms, 158
  sodium, 153–156
  sympathetic nervous system, 158
Vasodilator
  diabetes, 300
  pregnancy, 239–240
  renal effects, 272–273
Vasodilator agent
  cardiovascular disorder, 205
  congestive heart failure, 203, 205

Vegetarian diet, 9
Ventrical premature beat, diuretics, 21
Ventricular arrhythmia, 203
  hypokalemia, 21–22
Ventricular ectopy, potassium, 22
Verapamil, 115, 194
  black patient, 120
  elderly patient, 120, 224
  hypertensive emergency, 193–195
  low-renin patient, 120
  prazosin, 62
  pregnancy, 241
  renal effects, 274, 275
  salt effects, 274–276
  urgent hypertension, 183
  water effects, 274–276
Veterans Administration study, 172
Visken, 87–88
  combination therapy, 87

diuretics, 87
lipids, 87–88
vs. alpha-blocking agents, 87
vs. calcium-entry blockers, 87
vs. nifedipine, 87
Volume overload, 206

W
Weight loss, 6–8
  exercise, 11
  fluoxetine, 7
  metabolic rate, 7
Weight reduction
  diet type, 6
  exercise, 6
  insulin, 6
  very low-calorie diet, 6–7

DATE DUE
DATE DE RETOUR

FEB 1 , 1990		
MAR 3 1990		
DEC 1 7 1992		
NOV 2 1 1995		
OCT 2 1997		
Nov 1st 1997		
Nov 12th		

NLR 178